AOTRAUMA

Stephen L Kates | Olivier Borens

Principles of Orthopedic Infection Management

Principles of Orthopedic Infection Management Stephen L Kates, Olivier Borens

AOTRAUMA

Stephen L Kates | Olivier Borens

Principles of Orthopedic Infection Management

Includes 6 videos and over 800 images and illustrations

Library of Congress Cataloging-in-Publication Data is available from the publisher.

Hazards

Great care has been taken to maintain the accuracy of the information contained in this publication. However, the publisher, and/or the distributor, and/or the editors, and/or the authors cannot be held responsible for errors or any consequences arising from the use of the information contained in this publication. Contributions published under the name of individual authors are statements and opinions solely of said authors and not of the publisher, and/or the distributor, and/or the AO Group.

The products, procedures, and therapies described in this work are hazardous and are therefore only to be applied by certified and trained medical professionals in environments specially designed for such procedures. No suggested test or procedure should be carried out unless, in the user's professional judgment, its risk is justified. Whoever applies products, procedures, and therapies shown or described in this work will do this at their own risk. Because of rapid advances in the medical sciences, AO recommends that independent verification of diagnosis, therapies, drugs, dosages, and operation methods should be made before any action is taken.

Although all advertising material which may be inserted into the work is expected to conform to ethical (medical) standards, inclusion in this publication does not constitute a guarantee or endorsement by the publisher regarding quality or value of such product or of the claims made of it by its manufacturer.

Legal restrictions

Distribution by Georg Thieme Verlag, Rüdigerstrasse 14, 70469 Stuttgart, Germany, and Thieme New York, 333 Seventh Avenue, New York, NY 10001, USA

ISBN: 978-3-13-241075-6
e-ISBN: 978-3-13-241076-3

1 2 3 4 5 6

Foreword

When the AO Foundation was founded in Switzerland in 1958, a revolution began in the management of fractures. Similarly, hip joint replacement was a major breakthrough in the treatment of osteoarthritis. Unfortunately, orthopedic implant-associated infection then became a serious problem compromising functional results. Hans Willenegger, one of the five founders of AO, therefore dedicated a significant part of his career to studying the management of complications following internal bone fixation. He and others rapidly realized that implant material as well as the bone sequesters increased susceptibility to infection and promoted microbial persistence on nonvital surfaces.

Initially, the therapeutic approach was mainly surgical. It has been recognized that not only the degree of severity of the trauma, but also the type of bone fixation influence the pattern of bone necrosis in a typical way. The pillars of surgical treatment were then defined as:

- Debridement of necrotic bone and soft tissue
- Removal of implant material
- Osteoplastic measures such as autogenous bone grafting

In case of failure, infected nonunions became an important subject. Unfortunately, even adding systemic antibiotics or antiseptics failed to result in reliable healing of posttraumatic osteomyelitis. Success rates remained low, the number of required surgical interventions high, and late recurrence was rather frequent.

A few dedicated microbiologists and infectious disease specialists demonstrated that microorganisms persist as biofilm on implants, and withstand not only host defences but also most antimicrobial agents. It was observed that the efficacy of an antibiotic in implant-associated infection required activity on nongrowing bacteria. Furthermore, it could be shown that even such antibiotics act only on young biofilms. Based on these observations, treatment algorithms were developed for the management of implant-associated osteomyelitis and periprosthetic joint infection.

Over the last two decades, it has been realized that the treatment success of orthopedic implant-associated infection has been heavily dependent on correct management. Thus, a dedicated team of orthopedic surgeons, infectious disease specialists, microbiologists, plastic surgeons, and pathologists are now required for optimal treatment results. It is an important message from this book to train such specialized teams to improve the success rate of orthopedic implant-associated infection treatment.

This book gives an overview of the important field of orthopedic infection. The first section deals with the basic principles of such infections. These principles facilitate the understanding of pathogenesis, diagnosis, and management of infections of the musculoskeletal system. It became clear that therapeutic success can only be considered after 1–2 years, therefore, patients must be followed up for at least this period of time to rapidly diagnose and treat any possible recurrences, and to evaluate the treatment results of a cohort. The second section of the book deals with the different types of infections and offers specific advice on how to manage a variety of situations. In the third section, typical case examples allow the reader to see how the knowledge explained in the preceding chapters works in practice. These case examples help the reader to get an impression of the reasoning of the specialists in managing such infections.

A collaboration nearly as long as their professional lives links the authors of this Foreword in the treatment of musculoskeletal infections. We have realized that by doing so, the mutual promotion of knowledge in the field continues to grow. We are convinced that further progress can only be achieved by the constant acquisition of new fields of knowledge. It is up to you to devote yourself to this task.

Peter E. Ochsner, MD
Orthopedic surgeon

Werner Zimmerli, MD
Infectious diseases specialist

Foreword

The authors are to be congratulated – this book is a must for anyone treating the musculoskeletal system, and especially so for surgeons. There are many complications in medicine, as in life, but for a surgeon, infection is the most dreaded and especially so when it is iatrogenic, ie, we are responsible! This treatise is remarkable as it is so comprehensive, covering the basics, the science, organisms, how they colonize, multiply, biofilm, and even the host response. This is followed by techniques and algorithms for diagnosis, treatment principles, and antibiotics, and how these are applied to surgical situations including acute and chronic infections, postfracture/nonunion, and other orthopedic implant surgeries involving arthroplasty, the spine, sports injuries, open fractures, and wounds. Finally, there is a long list of case examples of common infectious scenarios involving the musculoskeletal system.

This book is an unbelievable resource for any surgeon, not only to treat and manage musculoskeletal infections, but better still to understand why and hopefully prevent such from happening in the future.

David L Helfet, MD
Professor of Orthopaedic Surgery
Weill Medical College of Cornell University
Director, Orthopaedic Trauma Service
Hospital for Special Surgery/New York Presbyterian Hospital

Preface

When serving as chairs and faculty of various AOTrauma courses on infection over the years, we have had the opportunity to get to know each other and to share our knowledge and thoughts about the things that affect our daily practice. During one snowy afternoon in December, we realized that despite our shared concern over the impact of infection on our patients and their families, there was very little literature and indeed no orthopedic text book that covered the sorts of things we felt were important. Few books really dealt with the problem adequately, and many were written specifically for and by infection specialists. No book really combined the daily practical needs of both the surgeon and the infection specialist.

It was our great pleasure then to be able to liaise with medical colleagues and education experts to propose the development of this text at a time when infection had come to light as a critical and highly overlooked factor in orthopedic treatment. We especially wanted to ensure there was a focus on a team approach to treating infection, involving microbiologists, orthopedic surgeons, and infection specialists. Our main goal for the book was to provide a basic knowledge for all of these professionals on how to approach the problem, and equally importantly, on how to prevent it.

We are extremely pleased that we were able to involve opinion leaders from a wide range of fields and specialties to join us and contribute to the book. We were especially motivated to ensure that the book offered the reader a practical approach to infection treatment, with many real patient cases on how the authors treated their own orthopedic infection challenges.

Interest in the topic of infection is increasing dramatically, and we note the AO has greatly increased the number of courses and other educational activities covering this topic in recent years. We are extremely proud to be at the forefront of this new focus, and to be able to genuinely recommend this book to our colleagues and counterparts involved in researching, analyzing, or treating orthopedic infection.

Stephen L Kates
Olivier Borens

Acknowledgments

Production and publication of the Principles of Orthopedic Infection Management would not have been possible without the dedication and support of an extensive list of contributors. From AO surgeons donating their time within the various education committees and working groups, to our many colleagues that volunteered case notes and images, to staff within our own medical practices, and to the teams at AOTrauma and AO Education Institute, we thank you for assisting us to develop this worthwhile publication.

While there are many people to thank, we would especially like to mention these individuals:

- Kodi Kojima and the other members of the AOTrauma Education Commission, for recognizing the educational opportunity and for providing the resources in approving the development of this publication
- Urs Rüetschi, Robin Greene, and Michael Cunningham from the AO Education Institute, for their guidance and expertise, and for enabling extensive resources and staff to prepare this publication to its fullest capacity
- The authors, our colleagues from around the world, who donated many hours to provide chapters, cases, and images, and also to those not even involved specifically with this work, but who otherwise share in the spirit of fraternity when it comes to education and training
- David Helfet, Peter Ochsner, and Werner Zimmerli for writing the Forewords to this book
- Carl Lau, Manager Publishing and Amber Parkinson, Project Manager for their professional support
- Jecca Reichmuth, Tamara Aepli, and Rolf Joray (Nougat design) for their illustration work
- Tom Wirth from Nougat design and Roman Kellenberger, the graphic designers, responsible for the overall layout of this book and for taking in the many rounds of editorial corrections
- Mike Laws and Thomas Lopathka for their expertise and assistance in producing the videos
- And lastly, to our own families for their support and encouragement throughout this project.

Stephen L Kates
Olivier Borens

Contributors

Editors

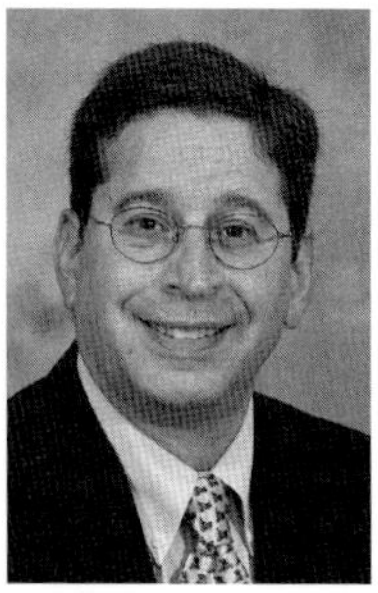

Stephen L Kates, MD
Professor and Chair of Orthopaedic Surgery
Virginia Commonwealth University
Richmond, VA 23284
USA

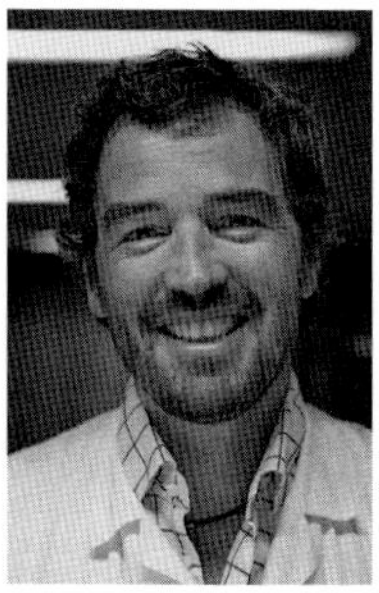

Olivier Borens, MD
Professor and Médecin chef
Unité de Traumatologie
Unité de Chirurgie Septique
Service d'Orthopédie et de Traumatologie
Bureau BH10-230
Rue du Bugnon 46
1011 Lausanne
Switzerland

Authors

Volker Alt, Dr med, Dr biol hom
Professor
Department of Trauma, Hand
and Reconstructive Surgery
University Hospital Giessen-Marburg
Campus Giessen
Rudolf-Buchheim-Str. 7
35385 Giessen
Germany

Mathieu Assal, PD Dr med
Clinique La Colline
Avenue de Beau-Séjour 6
1206 Genève
Switzerland

Jorge Daniel Barla, MD
Orthopedics
Hospital Italiano de Buenos Aires
Potosi 4247
C1181ACH Buenos Aires
Argentina

Caleb Behrend, MD
Rothman Institute
999 Route 73 N, Suite 3RD
Marlton, NJ 08053
USA

Karen Bentley, MS
Director
Electron Microscope Shared Research Laboratory
Pathology and Laboratory Medicine
University of Rochester Medical Center
575 Elmwood Avenue
Rochester, NY 14642
USA

Olivier Borens, MD
Professor and Médecin chef
Unité de Traumatologie
Unité de Chirurgie Septique
Service d'Orthopédie et de Traumatologie
Bureau BH10-230
Rue du Bugnon 46
1011 Lausanne
Switzerland

Antonia F Chen, MD, MBA
Assistant Professor
Sidney Kimmel Medical College
Associate Director of Research
Rothman Institute
Thomas Jefferson University Hospital
Philadelphia, PA 19107
USA

Anna Conen, MD, MSc
Deputy Head Physician
Division of Infectious Diseases and Hospital Hygiene
Kantonsspital Aarau
Tellstrasse
5001 Aarau
Switzerland

Stéphane Corvec, PharmD, PhD, HDR
Associate Professor, MCU-PH
Clinical Microbiologist
Nantes University Hospital
Bacteriology and Hygiene Department
Biology Institute
9 Quai Moncousu
44093 Nantes, Cedex 01
France

Xavier Crevoisier, PD Dr med
Médecin chef
Site Hôpital Orthopédique
Service d'Orthopédie et de Traumatologie
Avenue Pierre Decker 4
1011 Lausanne
Switzerland

John L Daiss, PhD
Research Associate Professor
Center for Musculoskeletal Research
University of Rochester Medical Center
601 Elmwood Ave, Box 665
Rochester, NY 14642
USA

Craig J Della Valle, MD
Professor of Orthopaedic Surgery
Chief, Division of Adult Reconstructive Surgery
Rush University Medical Center
1611 West Harrison Street, Suite 300
Chicago, IL 60612
USA

Lorenzo Drago, PhD
Chief of Clinical Chemistry and Microbiology Lab
IRCCS Istituto Ortopedico Galeazzi
Via R. Galeazzi 4
20161 Milano
Italy

Christopher J Drinkwater, MD, FRACS
Chief, Adult Reconstruction Division
Director, Evarts Joint Center
Associate Professor of Orthopaedics
University of Rochester Medical Center
601 Elmwood Avenue
Rochester, NY 14642
USA

Lisca Drittenbass, Dr med
Centre de Chirurgie du Pied et de la Cheville
Clinique La Colline
Avenue de Beau-Séjour 6
1206 Genève
Switzerland

George SM Dyer, MD, FACS
Assistant Professor, Orthopaedic Surgery
Harvard Medical School
Program Director, Harvard Combined Orthopaedic Residency
Orthopaedic Upper Extremity Surgeon
Brigham and Women's Hospital
75 Francis St
Boston, MA 02115
USA

AJ Electricwala, MS, DNB(Orth)
Assistant Professor
Sancheti Hospital
16 Shivajinagar
Pune 411005
Maharashtra State
India

John C Elfar, MD, FACS
Director, Hand and Upper Extremity Fellowship
Director, Center for Orthopaedic Population Studies
Department of Orthopaedics
Division of Sports Medicine
University of Rochester Medical Center
601 Elmwood Ave
Rochester, NY 14642
USA

Alain Farron, MD
Professor
Chef de Service
Service d'Orthopédie et de Traumatologie
Bureau HO/06/1644
Avenue Pierre Decker 4
1011 Lausanne
Switzerland

A Samuel Flemister Jr, MD
School of Medicine and Dentistry
University of Rochester Medical Center
601 Elmwood Ave, Box 665
Rochester, NY 14642
USA

Arthur Grzesiak, Dr méd
Médecin-hospitalier
Service d'Orthopédie et Traumatologie
Chasseral 20
2300 Chaux-de-Fonds
Switzerland

Peter J Haar, MD, PhD
Director of Medical Student Education for Radiology
Assistant Professor of Radiology
Virginia Commonwealth University Medical Center
1250 East Marshall Street
Richmond, VA 23219
USA

Sven Hungerer, PD Dr med
Head of Department for Reconstructive Joint Surgery
BG Trauma Center Murnau
Professor-Küntscherstr. 8
82418 Murnau
Germany

Peter JL Jebson, MD
Instructor, Grand Rapids Medical Education Partners
Associate Professor
Michigan State College of Medicine
Chief, Department of Orthopedics
Spectrum Health Medical Group
Chief, Orthopedic Health Clinical Service Line
Spectrum Health System
Grand Rapids, MI
USA

Christian Kammerlander, PD MD
Vice Director
Department for General, Trauma and Reconstructive Surgery
Ludwig Maximilian University Munich
Campus Grosshadern
Marchioninistrasse 15
81377 Munich
Germany

Stephen L Kates, MD
Professor and Chair of Orthopaedic Surgery
Virginia Commonwealth University
Richmond, VA 23284
USA

Anjan P Kaushik, MD
Attending Physician, Orthopaedic Surgery
Hancock Orthopedics
Hancock Regional Hospital
1 Memorial Square
Greenfield, IN 46140
USA

James F Kellam, MD, FRCS(C), FACS, FRCSI(Hon)
UTHealth, The University of Texas
McGovern Medical School
Department of Orthopaedic Surgery
6431 Fannin St
Houston, TX 77030
USA

Johan Lammens, MD, PhD
Professor
Orthopaedic Department
UZ Leuven
Weligerveld 1
3212 Pellenberg
Belgium

Tak-Wing Lau, MBBS, FRCS(Ed) (Orth), FHKAM (Orth), FHKCOS
Associate Consultant
Division of Orthopaedic Trauma
Queen Mary Hospital
102 Pokfulam Rd
Pokfulam
Hong Kong

Martin A McNally, MD, FRCS(Ed), FRCS (Orth)
The Bone Infection Unit
Nuffield Orthopaedic Centre
Oxford University Hospitals
Windmill Road
Oxford OX3 7HE
UK

Paul W Millhouse, MD, MBA
Research Fellow
Thomas Jefferson University
1015 Walnut St, Suite 509
Philadelphia, PA 19107
USA

Mario Morgenstern, Dr med
Department of Traumatology
University Hospital Basel
Spitalstrasse 21
4031 Basel
Switzerland

T Fintan Moriarty, PhD
Research Scientist
AO Research Institute Davos
Clavadelerstrasse 8
7270 Davos
Switzerland

Kohei Nishitani, MD PhD
Staff Physician
Department of Orthopaedic Surgery
Graduate School of Medicine
Kyoto University
54 Shogoin Kawaharacho
Sakyo-ku Kyoto 606-8507
Japan

Peter E Ochsner, Dr med
Professor
Emeritus Extraordinarius in Orthopaedics
University of Basel
Rüttigasse 7
4402 Frenkendorf
Switzerland

Chang-Wug Oh, MD
Professor
Department of Orthopedic Surgery
Kyungpook National University Hospital
50,2-ga, Samdok
Chunggu
Daegu 700-721
Korea

Jong-Keon Oh, MD
Director
Department of Orthopedic Surgery
Korea University Guro Hospital
#148, Gurodong-ro, Guro-gu
Seoul 08308
Korea

Kailash Patil, MBBS, DOrth, DNB(Orth), MNAMS
Assistant Professor
Department of Joint Replacement and Sports Injury
Sancheti Institute for Orthopedics
and Rehabilitation
16 Shivajinagar
Pune 411005
Maharashtra State
India

Javad Parvizi, MD, FRCS
Director of Clinical Research
Rothman Institute
Thomas Jefferson University Hospital
Sheridan Building, Suite 1000
125 S 9th Street
Philadelphia, PA 19107
USA

María Eugenia Portillo, PhD
Department of Microbiology
Complejo Hospitalario de Navarra
C/Irunlarrea
31008 Pamplona, Navarra
Spain

Virginia Post, PhD
Postdoctoral Research Fellow
AO Research Institute Davos
Clavadelerstrasse 8
7270 Davos
Switzerland

R Geoff Richards, MSc, PhD, FBSE
Director
AO Research Institute Davos
Clavadelerstrasse 8
7270 Davos
Switzerland

David C Ring, MD, PhD
Associate Dean for Comprehensive Care
Professor of Surgery
The University of Texas at Austin
Dell Medical School
1400 Barbara Jordan Avenue
Suite 1.114
Austin, TX 78723
USA

Carlo L Romanò, MD
Director
Centro di Chirurgia Ricostruttiva e delle Infezioni Osteo-articolari
IRCCS Istituto Ortopedico Galeazzi
Via R. Galeazzi 4
20161 Milano
Italy

Yoav Rosenthal, MD
Department of Orthopaedic Surgery
Rabin Medical Center
Petah Tikva 49100
Israel

Luciano Rossi, MD
Italian Hospital from Buenos Aires
Department of Trauma
Peron 4190
C1199ABB Buenos Aires
Argentina

Parag Sancheti, MS(Orth), DNB(Orth), MCh, FRCS(Ed)
Professor and Chairman
Sancheti Institute for Orthopaedics
and Rehabilitation
16 Shivajinagar
Pune 411005
Maharashtra State
India

Edward M Schwarz, PhD
Professor of Orthopaedics
Director, Center for Musculoskeletal Research
University of Rochester Medical Center
601 Elmwood Avenue
Rochester, NY 14642
USA

Parham Sendi, MD
Lecturer in Infectious Diseases
Department of Infectious Diseases
Bern University Hospital
University of Bern
3010 Bern
Switzerland

Ashok Shyam, MBBS, MS(Orth)
Consultant Orthopaedic Surgeon and Research Head
Sancheti Institute for Orthopaedics
and Rehabilitation
16 Shivajinagar
Pune 411005
Maharashtra State
India

Theddy Slongo, MD
Department of Paediatric Surgery, Paediatric Trauma
and Orthopaedics
University Children's Hospital
Freiburgstr. 7
3010 Bern
Switzerland

Christoph Sommer, Dr med
Chefarzt Unfallchirurgie
Departement Chirurgie
Kantonsspital Graubünden
Loëstrasse 170
7000 Chur
Switzerland

Andrej Trampuz, MD
Professor
Center for Septic Surgery
Charité - University Medicine Berlin
Campus Virchow-Klinikum
Mittelallee 4
13353 Berlin
Germany

Alexander R Vaccaro, MD, PhD
Rothman Institute
925 Chestnut Street
Philadelphia, PA 19107
USA

Steven Velkes, MBChB
Head of Orthopedic Surgery
Rabin Medical Center
Petah Tikva 49100
Israel

Josephina A Vossen, MD, PhD
Assistant Professor
MCV Hospitals and Physicians
VCU Health System
1250 E Marshall St
Richmond, VA 23298
USA

Zhao Xie, MD, PhD
Professor and Vice Director
Department of Orthopaedic Surgery
Southwest Hospital
Third Military Medical University
#30 Gaotanyan St
400038 Chongqing
China

Erlangga Yusuf, MSc, MD, PhD
Department of Medical Microbiology
and Infection Control
University Hospital Brussels (UZ Brussel)
Laarbeeklaan 101
1090 Jette
Belgium

Charalampos G Zalavras, MD, PhD
Professor of Orthopaedic Surgery
Keck School of Medicine
University of Southern California
LAC and USC Medical Center
1200 North State Street
Los Angeles, CA 90033
USA

Michael J Zegg, MD
Department for Trauma Surgery
University Hospital Innsbruck
Anichstrasse 35
6020 Innsbruck
Austria

Werner Zimmerli, MD
Professor in Internal Medicine
and Infectious Diseases
Interdisciplinary Unit for Orthopaedic Infections
Kantonsspital Baselland
Rheinstrasse 26
4410 Liestal
Switzerland

Matthias A Zumstein, PD Dr med
Section Head
Shoulder, Elbow and Sports Medicine
Department of Orthopaedics and Traumatology
University of Bern, Inselspital
3010 Bern
Switzerland

Front matter

Section 1
Principles

Section 2
Special situations

Section 3
Cases

Section 1

Principles

Section 1
Principles

1 Implant-associated biofilm

Kohei Nishitani, Karen de Mesy Bentley, John L Daiss

1 Basics

The steady increase in the use of total joint replacement (TJR) as the treatment for arthritis and other severe joint pathologies attests to its enormous success in improving the mobility and quality of life for millions of patients around the world [1]. While they are rare, implant-associated infections remain TJR's most feared, devastating, and costly consequences [2–14]. In addition to the struggles of patients compelled to undergo extensive antibiotic therapy, revision surgery, and, in some cases, the tragedy of arthrodesis or amputation, the financial costs of implant-associated orthopedic infections are a multi-billion dollar burden for health care providers worldwide [2].

Many species of bacteria can cause implant-associated orthopedic infections, but the staphylococci predominate, particularly the human commensals *Staphylococcus aureus* and *Staphylococcus epidermidis*. Some of the major challenges with implant-associated orthopedic infections are that they are hard to diagnose, persist against antibiotic therapy, and are prone to recurrence. These traits are largely attributable to the "lifestyle" that pathogens adopt in the presence of an orthopedic implant. We are accustomed to thinking that bacteria naturally grow in suspension cultures like those typically used in laboratories, but most, if not all, species of bacteria thrive in a genetically programmed, alternative lifestyle known as biofilm.

This chapter will cover some of the main features of biofilms including how they are made, how they interact with the host immune response, and how they complicate detection and therapy. The authors will describe additional lifestyles of bacteria that may be alternatives or complements to biofilms, and will briefly enumerate strategies for overcoming biofilm infections. Even though orthopedic infections are caused by many species of bacteria and some biofilms are polymicrobial, the focus will be on the most challenging pathogens in orthopedic implants, *S aureus* and *S epidermidis*.

In surgical specimens, biofilms are not always easy to identify. In **Fig 1-1**, images are presented of *S aureus* biofilm on the cement of an infected femoral component. It appears as a shiny, reddish area that turns black when treated with osmium tetroxide (**Fig 1-1b**). Scanning electron micrographs of this and other implant-associated biofilms reveal some of the features depicted in **Fig 1-1c–f**, including single and clustered cocci often in association with conspicuous fibrin filaments.

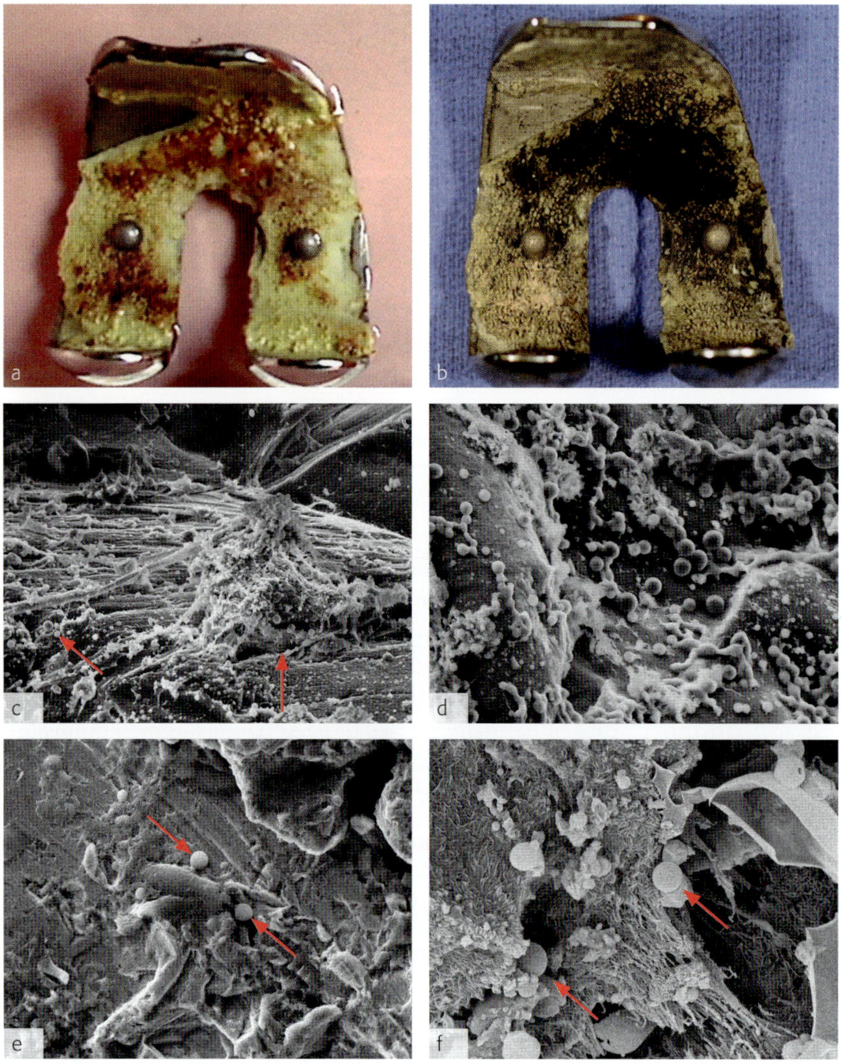

Fig 1-1a–f Biofilms observed on orthopedic hardware explanted from humans.
This example features an infected femoral component removed from a patient and fixed in 2.5% glutaraldehyde/4.0% paraformaldehyde for imaging by scanning electron microscopy. Scanning electron microscopy micrographs of biofilm from this implant and others (**c–f**):

- **a** Pale yellow cement on implant's inverse side displaying red-brown biofilm.
- **b** Same implant after 1.0% osmium tetroxide staining (now black) showing the extent of the patient's biofilm covering the cement of the implant.
- **c** From the implant in **b**, fibrin cables supporting the colonization of *Staphylococcus aureus* indicated by red arrows (x 3,000).
- **d** Colonies of *S aureus* covering the cement surface of the implant in **b** (x 5,000).
- **e** Cocci (arrows) on the surface from an infected tibial implant (x 3,000).
- **f** Higher magnification from an infected patellar implant displaying fibrin which serves as a scaffold for *S aureus* cocci (arrows) within biofilm (x 10,000).

2 Definition of a biofilm

Our understanding that bacteria grow in biofilms is surprisingly new [15, 16]. In fact, the term biofilm was first used in 1981 [17], and it was not until the early 1980s that the first publications demonstrated the adhesion and growth of bacteria on multiple types of medical devices including sutures [18, 19], pacemakers [20, 21], indwelling catheters [22], and orthopedic implants [23]. We now recognize that bacterial biofilms are responsible for at least 65% of bacterial infections in humans including recurrent lung infections and diabetic wounds [24]. In addition, we now understand that bacterial biofilms are the predominant lifestyle of bacteria in their natural aquatic or soil environments [24].

Based on his years of pioneering observations, William Costerton, PhD, provided a compact definition of a biofilm: "A structured community of bacterial cells enclosed in a self-produced polymeric matrix adherent to an inert or living surface" [25]. Biofilm formation is a coordinated activity among many bacterial cells, sometimes even among multiple bacterial species. As previously noted, essentially all bacteria can form biofilms, and many biofilms consist of multiple bacterial species. Founder biofilm-forming species sometimes create the necessary conditions for the recruitment of additional species so that biofilms can develop into complex communities. Even within a single species biofilm, bacteria in discrete zones, such as at the bottom or the top of the biofilm, will make characteristic adaptations giving rise to a structured community sometimes equated with differentiation within the tissues of higher organisms (**Fig 1.2**) [26].

The self-produced matrix, generically referred to as extracellular polymeric substance (EPS), is composed of hydrophilic, sparingly soluble biopolymers that can be produced and secreted in abundance creating an environment where bacteria can survive in the face of environmental stresses like nutrient limitation, water flow, or dehydration. The EPS is often referred to as a slime layer because of its combination of adhesive and cohesive properties. Many EPS are produced by polymerizing available sugars such as the α1,3-linked glucose polymer synthesized from extracellular sucrose in familiar dental biofilms made by *Streptococcus mutans*. In *S aureus* and *S epidermidis* the most prominent biofilm EPS is polymerized-N-acetylglucosamine (PNAG), although the relative abundance of this widely used polymer varies substantially from strain to strain.

The need for an inanimate foreign body in biofilm formation is discussed in detail in part 4 of this chapter. It has been widely understood that foreign bodies provide a nidus for the establishment of biofilm infections dramatically reducing the bacterial load required for infection. Biofilms can also form on soft tissue in the form of microcolonies, but the most difficult to eradicate biofilms clinically are implant-associated.

Compared to the relatively unbridled planktonic growth of bacteria in rich media typical of laboratory experiments, biofilms are a survival mode that is relatively costly in terms of cell divisions but provide huge advantages in terms of ability to survive hostile assaults resulting from environmental shifts or host responses. Moreover, the adaptations necessary for biofilm formation are coordinated by an elaborate genetic program that includes shifts in cellular metabolism and cooperation among bacterial cells.

3 What is biofilm?

Biofilms are often perceived as static fortresses where bacteria find shelter like people gathering in a castle to seek refuge from invaders. Biofilms are indeed fortresses providing shelter from both immunological and medical interventions such as neutrophils and antibiotics. But this concept is far too limited. Biofilms are also dynamic communities that undergo their own lifecycle of attachment, accumulation/maturation, and dispersal. In addition, they are incubators for at least two subsets of bacteria that adopt distinctive lifestyles; each contributes to the persistence of orthopedic infections.

In vitro studies of biofilm formation have revealed a cooperative, multistep process typically described as attachment, maturation, and dispersal [27–31]. Sensing some environmental stressor such as the innate immune response, individual bacterial cells begin to synthesize high intracellular levels of cyclic di-AMP, which shifts gene expression towards products that contribute to biofilm formation [32, 33]. Among the activated genes are those encoding microbial surface components recognizing adhesive matrix molecules (MSCRAMMs), which function as adhesions, cell wall-associated, and secreted molecules that mediate attachment to host proteins likely to be abundant at a wound site such as collagen, fibrin, vitronectin, and fibronectin [34]. In vitro this is approximated by precoating plastic surfaces with human plasma [35].

Following MSCRAMM-mediated attachment, the adherent staphylococci divide and begin the synthesis of PNAG, by the activation of the *ica* operon that encodes a series of

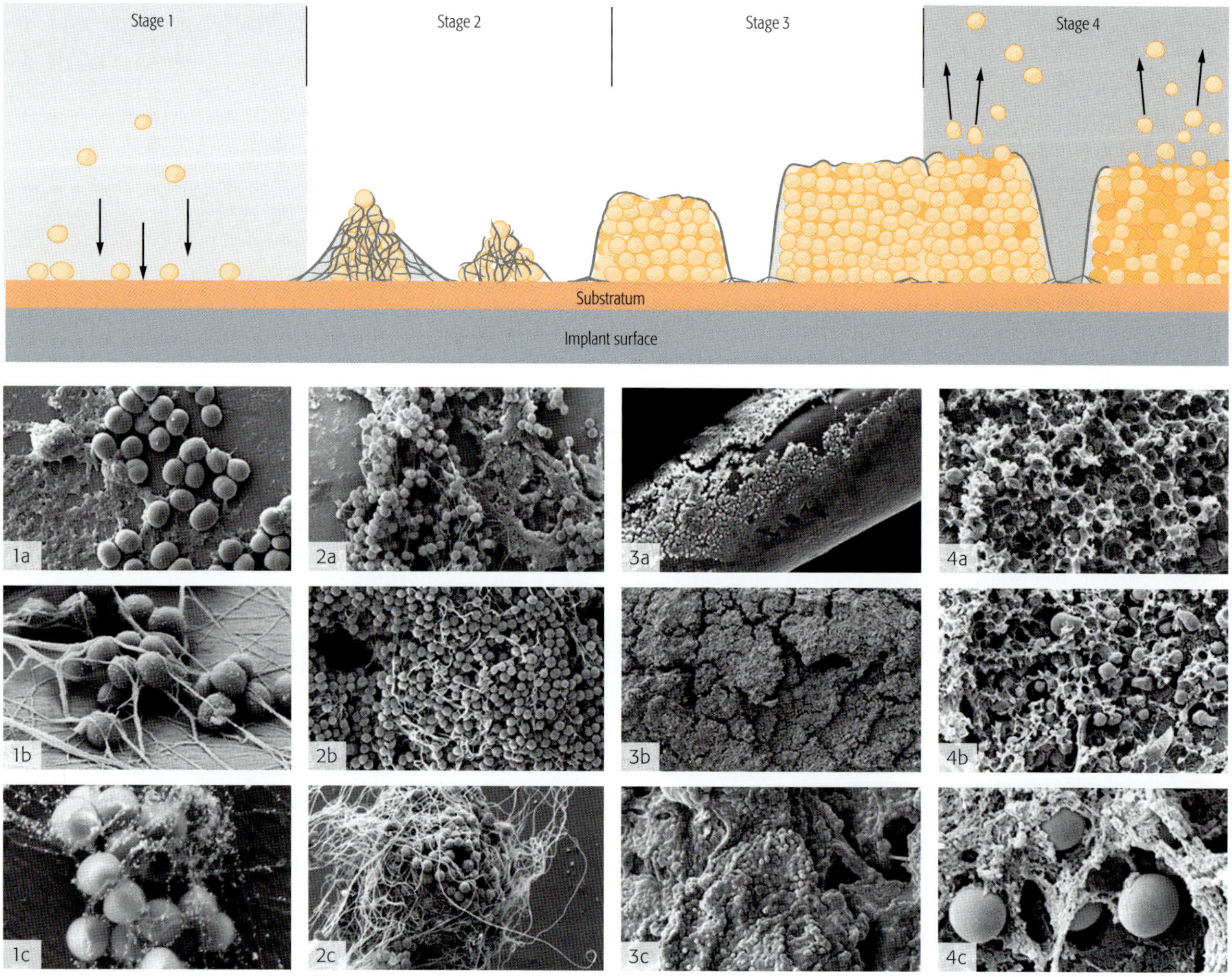

Fig 1-2 Stages of biofilm development: models and corresponding scanning electron microscopy images. Biofilm development is typically described as proceeding in three or four steps: attachment, accumulation/maturation, and dispersal. These stages are depicted diagrammatically above the corresponding scanning electron microscopy images of the various biofilm stages taken from in vitro and in vivo experimental models.

1a Example of in vitro attachment of *Staphylococcus aureus* cocci incubated in a flow chamber system where bacteria are circulated over a surface of a stainless steel wire (x 10,000).

1b In vitro: *S aureus* cocci using fibrin to secure attachment to the wire's surface (x 20,000).

1c In vitro: *S aureus* cocci (similar to (**1b**) labeled with antifibrin antibodies using immunogold labeling and scanning electron microscopy imaging. Note the bright white dots (30 nm gold particles) on filaments confirming the identity of fibrin (x 30,000).

2a–c In vitro series of scanning electron microscopy images of *S aureus* forming larger clusters of cocci entwined with fibrin filaments facilitating a stronger attachment to the wire's metal surface (x 5,000).

3a Mature biofilm uniformly coating a round pin which was removed from a mouse tibia infected for 14 days by the methicillin-sensitive *S aureus* strain UAMS-1 (x 200).

3b Example of the thicker biofilm formed by *S aureus* UAMS-1 Δ*agr* on a transtibial metal implant 14 days postinfection (x 150). *Staphylococcus aureus* cocci with deletion of the *agr* gene cannot disperse so they accumulate producing a thicker biofilm.

3c Higher magnification scanning electron microscopy image of (**3b**) showing the build-up of *S aureus* biofilm lacking the *agr* gene. (Note: *S aureus* UAMS-1 Δ*agr* was the gift from the laboratory of Dr Paul Dunman at the University of Rochester Medical Center, Department of Microbiology and Immunology.)

4a Example of *S aureus* UAMS-1 leaving behind empty lacunae suggesting full biofilm maturation and dispersal of the bacteria (x 5,000).

4b Example of nondispersal by *S aureus* UAMS-1 Δ*agr* cocci which remain within matrix components and have fewer well-defined lacunae (x 5,000).

4c Example of lacunae with four *S aureus* UAMS-1 cocci embedded in matrix components in a biofilm present on a transtibial implant after 14 days of infection (x 30,000).

enzymes and membrane proteins that polymerize, transport, and partially deacetylate the growing polymer chains that can reach lengths of thousands of saccharide units. To promote PNAG synthesis, the bacteria reduce functions associated with cell division such as protein and DNA synthesis, increase arginase, and urease mobilize the required nitrogen [36, 37]. In vitro, many strains of *S aureus* and *S epidermidis* produce primarily PNAG for their EPS. Some secrete proteins primarily associated with biofilms. For example, *S aureus* biofilms in cattle are characterized by the abundance of biofilm-associated protein, polymerized N-acetylglucosamine, and *S epidermidis* implant-associated biofilms have high levels of accumulation-associated protein. Some *S aureus* biofilms display high levels of SasG [38–40]. Others secrete extracellular DNA and proteins in a process that resembles apoptosis in eukaryotic cells [41, 42]. The resulting matrix limits access to the immune system's elements, specifically neutrophils and macrophages, and may contribute to the enhanced antibiotic resistance observed in biofilms [27, 28, 30, 37].

Many investigators have observed modulation of biofilm formation in vitro by the presence or absence of endogenous nucleases, proteases, or glycosidases [43–46]. The precise roles of these enzymes are not yet clear, but their roles are not strictly degradative. For example, the accumulation-associated protein expressed in *S epidermidis* must be proteolytically cleaved to contribute to biofilm formation [47]. There are reports that secreted proteases are used essentially as weapons, as competing species battle for contested sites [48–50]. These observations have raised the hope that biofilms can be readily treated with EPS-degrading enzymes. To date, therapeutic treatment with degradative enzymes has not progressed and the notion may be simplistic when one considers how dynamic biofilms are [51].

As the biofilm matures, the bacteria continue to divide, and local resources become limiting; two additional strategies for survival are initiated. Some of the bacteria undergo mutations that dramatically reduce their metabolic requirements [52, 53] or they shift into a dormant, antibiotic-resistant, persistent state [54, 55]. Others, in response to quorum sensing, mediated by the accumulation of secreted autoinducing peptides, activate the master controller gene, accessory gene regulator (*agr*), which governs the expression of a group of secreted virulence factors including α-hemolysin (Hla) and the phenol-soluble modulins [30, 37, 56–58]. Activation of *agr* has become associated with the initiation of disassembly of the biofilm and dispersal of bacterial cells to expand the biofilm or populate new surfaces [29, 30, 56, 57]. These stages are shown schematically in **Fig 1-2**, together with scanning electron microscopy images depicting comparable stages observed from in vitro and in vivo biofilms.

Biofilms in vivo are woefully undercharacterized [59, 60]. As an initial effort, the authors are working to describe the natural history of biofilms that form on a flat metal wire in our mouse model of implant-associated *S aureus* osteomyelitis [61]. In this model, an *S aureus* contaminated, flat stainless steel wire is inserted into the tibia of a mouse and left in place for days to weeks. Then it is removed and examined by scanning electron microscopy. The authors' initial objectives have been to:

- Measure the growth of the biofilm across the implant surface
- Identify the structural features that develop as the biofilm matures using scanning electron microscopy as the primary readout

The main features of the in vitro model described above may apply in vivo, but there are many additional factors to consider such as foreign bodies, the innate immune response, high levels of plasma proteins, and limited availability of essential nutrients such as iron Fe++ [62].

On day 1, the pin is covered with neutrophils and few bacteria are observed even though we know that bacteria are proliferating in the vicinity of the pin (**Fig 1-3a**). Possibly there are soft-tissue reservoirs of *S aureus* that attach to the pin surface after day 1 or clumps of fibrin-agglutinated *S aureus* that manage to establish a nascent biofilm [63–65] while fending off neutrophils, or perhaps phagocytized *S aureus* escape from phagocytes [66–68] to populate the pin surface. In any case, the presence of abundant neutrophils in the mouse tibia makes it unlikely that the simple adhesion step described in in vitro models will apply in vivo.

By day 4, the pin surface is dotted with clusters of *S aureus* always in association with fibers that are 0.02–0.1 µm in diameter (**Fig 1-3b**), presumably fibrin resulting from the action of coagulase or vWbp (see part 4 of this chapter). That host-derived structures are components of the in vivo biofilms, and possibly essential ones, has not been anticipated in the in vitro models. Similarly, it appears that 7–10 µm cells, presumably neutrophils, become incorporated into the biofilm. By day 7 (**Fig 1-3c**), clusters of *S aureus* are visible with a prominent coating of an uncharacterized matrix, possibly the PNAG of the in vitro models. Finally, on day 14 (**Fig 1-3d**), regions with a film comprised of a fibrous, finely woven mesh are evident and dimpled with depressions of lacunae exactly the size of *S aureus* giving the appearance that the bacteria had resided in the mesh and then emigrated, perhaps the result of the activation of *agr*, and the expression of dispersal-related proteins like the phenol-soluble modulins [28, 30, 56, 57]. After 28 days, *S aureus* are seldom observed by scanning electron microscopy on the pins and colony-forming units are rarely recovered following vigorous extraction of the pin. However, *S aureus* RNA can be extracted and identified by RNA sequencing, suggesting the presence of persister cells [54, 55].

There are many open questions. Even though the removed implants rarely have bacterial colony-forming units after day 28, the tibiae remain culture positive. If the implant is not the only reservoir for the infecting pathogen, where do the bacteria reside? Can the previously populated pin be repopulated or is the depopulated surface irreversibly fouled? Do the *S aureus* populations of the implant cycle through multiple forms possibly with some of the other forms described in part 5 of this chapter?

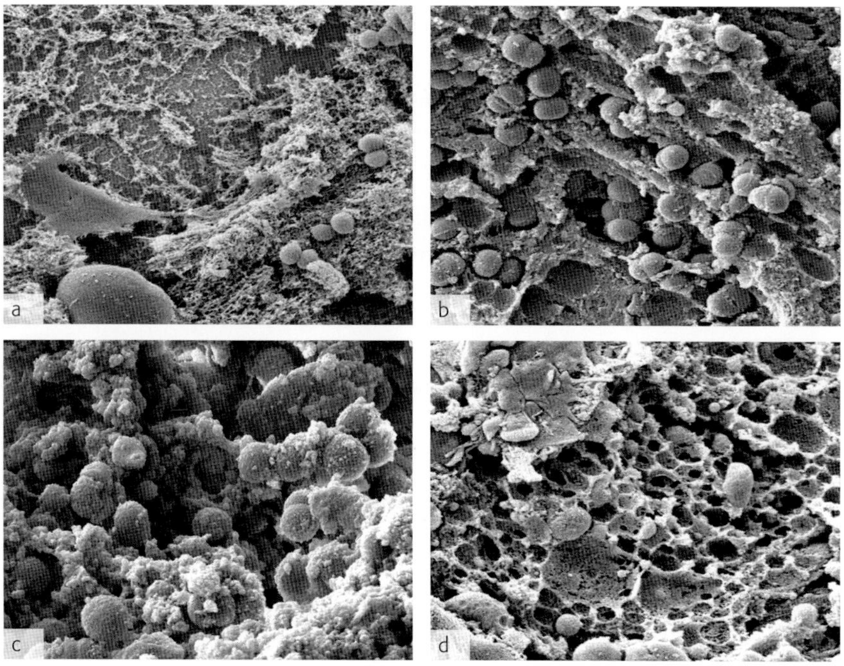

Fig 1-3a–d Stages of biofilm development observed in the mouse transtibial implant model. Shown are the scanning electron microscopy images of the time course of biofilm maturation in the C57BL/6 mouse infected with methicillin-sensitive *Staphylococcus aureus* (SH1000) [75]. *Staphylococcus aureus*-inoculated stainless steel implants were surgically placed in mouse tibiae, implants were harvested at the indicated time point, then implants were observed by scanning electron microscopy.

- **a** At day 1, fuzzy structures which are presumably from host fibrin were observed on the wire surface, and *S aureus* existed as single or small clusters. Note that host immune cells are found elsewhere on the implant.
- **b** At day 4, *S aureus* were evident as larger clusters surrounded by honeycomb matrix.
- **c** At day 7, *S aureus* cocci are embedded in biofilm matrix or extracellular polymeric substance.
- **d** At day 14, few cells are observed on the surface, but many shallow bacterium-sized depressions are observed. The authors named these depressions "empty lacunae" and believe they represent sites from which cocci dispersed. After day 14, *S aureus* biofilm shows almost no morphological change, indicating that the maturation of the *S aureus* biofilm is complete in 14 days or less.

4 Interaction between biofilm and implant

Many kinds of foreign bodies are placed into patients. These include devices intended to last decades such as total joint replacements and heart valves, as well as temporary devices like intravenous and indwelling urinary tract catheters. Among surgeons, it is generally recognized that foreign bodies significantly increase the risk of infection. Especially in severely ill or immunocompromised patients, foreign bodies are responsible for 60–70% of hospital-acquired infections [69]. Surgeons have been aware of this since the early 20th century because of the association of abscesses with surgical stitches. In the 1950s, the risk of foreign bodies was dramatically demonstrated by artificial infection using human volunteers [70]. This sensational study showed that only 100 cocci with a silk suture could cause a suppurative infection, whereas 100,000 cocci were required in the absence of the foreign body. In cases involving sutures, staples, and indwelling catheters, it is easy to remove the foreign body if infection is suspected; however, diagnosis and corrective intervention are far more complicated in deep-seated implants.

There are several routes for bacteria to cause an implant-associated infection. One common route is the direct local spread from exposure at the time of surgery. These infections are frequently evident within 30 days of surgery. Many other implant-associated infections are secondary to infections of other tissues that are spread due to proximity, such as infections in the feet of the patients with vascular insufficiency, or by bacteremia such as hematogenous osteomyelitis, which is more a common cause of acute osteomyelitis in prepubertal children and in vertebral osteomyelitis of the elderly [71–73].

As described in part 3 of this chapter, the initial step of the implant-associated infection is bacterial adhesion to host proteins adsorbed on the implant surface using their MSCRAMMs. Once bacteria have attached to the implant surface, they can increase the cell number by both cell division and accretion of planktonic cells. In fact, the implant surface serves as both a secure anchorage site that facilitates increase in biomass, and it enables the attached bacteria to have access to other host factors that may be valuable in biofilm development. For example, *S aureus* can polymerize fibrinogen into potentially protective fibrin through the action of coagulase and von Willebrand factor-binding protein. Bacteria use these host materials to build up the biofilm matrix together with bacterial own EPS, on the implant surface. Thus, the implant provides two important things to bacteria: stable anchorage and access to materials. An example is presented in **Fig 1-3a** where cocci are attached to fibrous material, presumably fibrin. Biofilm formation is often regarded as the defining feature of the chronic stage of infection providing the pathogen with protection from host immunity and antibiotics. However, in human infections, it is not clear exactly where to draw the line between acute and chronic phases of infection. It probably differs among bacterial strains, initial bacterial inoculum, and efficiency of the host immune response. Clinically, patients whose infection resolves in fewer than 3 weeks may be candidates for implant retention [74]. However, in the authors' murine model, *S aureus* biofilm is initiated almost immediately after infection, and matures within as few as 7–14 days [75]. If biofilm building follows the same time course in humans, a robust biofilm would be expected in as little as 2 weeks, thereby necessitating implant removal.

Following the principle that prevention of infection is more effective than treating it, many investigators have attempted to identify attributes that will make orthopedic implants resistant to infection. Stainless steel and titanium alloys are the most common metal materials for orthopedic implants. Many believe that the higher cost of titanium is offset by it superior resistance to infection. Consequently, the differences between stainless steel and titanium implants have been the subjects of considerable inquiry. Regarding attachment, the initial step for biofilm formation, the relative merits between these materials are still controversial. Ha et al found more *S epidermidis* attachment to titanium alloy (Ti-6-4) than to stainless steel (316SS), however, reported the opposite for *Mycobacterium tuberculosis* [76], and Gracia et al and Koseki et al reported no difference between titanium and stainless steel using *S epidermidis* [77, 78]. In the present authors' studies, no differences have been observed in adhesion of *S aureus* in the presence of human plasma on stainless steel or titanium K-wires using a flow-chamber model [79]. While the metal composition of the implant may not provide a demonstrable advantage in preventing bacterial adhesion, multiple reports [80, 81] and a systematic review [82] conclude that roughness of the implant surface is a critical factor. Initial adhesion of *S aureus* to a model implant was less in electropolished pure titanium or titanium alloy (Ti-6Al-7Nb) than to relatively rough commercial titanium or titanium alloy (Ti-6Al-7Nb) [80].

Even though the superiority of titanium may not be evident from initial attachment experiments, its superior resistance to infection has been consistently observed in vivo. For example, in rabbit studies using dynamic compression plates, the 35% infection rate reported for titanium alloy was less than half the 75% infection rate of otherwise identical steel plates [83]; similar observations were made for intramedullary nails where the infection rate was 82% for stainless steel and 59% for titanium [84]. In a recent review article, Harris et al suggest that the discrepancies between in vitro and in vivo experiments lie in the fact that soft tissue adheres firmly to titanium implant surfaces, while steel implants are known to elicit the formation of a fibrous capsule, enclosing a liquid-filled void [85]. Although these studies show the difference of infection rates or bacterial burden on implants, direct evidence of mature bacterial biofilm is not clearly described and further studies are warranted to better understand the difference in biofilm formation in different materials.

In human studies, two reports conclude that titanium is more resistant to bacterial infection than stainless steel. In a randomized controlled trial of external fixation devices for distal radial fracture, Pieske et al report a higher rate of removal resulting from severe pin-track infection, and of pin loosening in the stainless steel group than in the titanium alloy group (5% versus 0%, 10% versus 5%, respectively) [86]. In a separate nonrandomized controlled trial study of transfixation of toe deformities, Clauss et al reported that titanium alloy wires displayed superior outcomes in terms of recurrence of deformity and patients' pain (39% versus 13%, 48% versus 22%, respectively). Furthermore, in their biofilm analyses, titanium alloy wires resulted in higher resistance against bacteria than stainless steel wires ($P < .05$) [87]. These two clinical trials both involved percutaneous fixation; the superiority of titanium in closed implant fixation has not yet been conclusively demonstrated in humans. Though titanium implants increase the surgical costs, in the subcutaneous fixation for high risk of infection cases, such as open fracture, toe fixation, or in compromised patients, usage of titanium implants may be beneficial for patients.

Extensive research has been undertaken to prevent biofilm formation by treating the implant surface. Efforts to prevent the initial bacterial attachment to the implant have included polishing the metal surface [88], coating it with TiO2 [89, 90], and adding surfactants [91]. Staphylococci have their own proteins that promote aggregation or modify host proteins such as fibrinogen or fibronectin to promote initial adhesion and subsequent biofilm formation. Attempts to counter the attachment of bacterial aggregates have included coating implants with human serum albumin [92], polyethylene glycol (PEG) [80], hydroxyapatite [93], and chitosan [94] have shown some benefit in vitro. Coating implants with silver, a known antimicrobial, decreases the attachment of bacteria [95, 96], as does coating with iodine [97]. Antibiotic-laden metallic implants have been studied since the 1950s and have shown some promise, however, they are not available commercially at present.

Although an implant surface or a bony sequestrum is a favorable site for bacterial biofilm formation, living bone surface is not. One attribute of the living bone surface is the presence of communities of numerous osteoblasts and osteoclasts on the endosteum, and periosteal cells and fibroblasts on periosteum. Several investigators have attempted to promote the selective growth of host-cell populations on the implant surface. Coating the surface with specific titanium [98], or poly-L-lysine-grafted-polyethylene glycol (PLLg-PEG) facilitated the adhesion of host cells to the implant surface and inhibited the attachment of bacteria [85, 98]. Though these cells do not directly combat bacteria, increasing these host cells on the implant surface leads to early soft-tissue coverage and/or bone mineralization on the implant surface and results in less biofilm formation.

5 Pathogenesis of implant-associated infections

The primary and earliest host response to bacteria is an acute inflammatory reaction, led by the rapid recruitment of neutrophils into the infection site. Neutrophils are the first line of host defense against bacteria and patients who have genetic or acquired neutrophil insufficiencies are prone to developing frequent and life-threatening infections [99]. On the surface of an infected implant, neutrophils are observed in the very early stages of the infection (**Fig 1-3a**). Activation of complement proteins opsonizes bacteria facilitating their ingestion by phagocytes including the infiltrating neutrophils and resident macrophages. Cytokines, such as interleukin-1 (IL-1), IL-6, and tumor necrosis factor (TNF) are released and act as chemotactic factors and activators of phagocytic cells. These initial responders of the host defense against bacteria are elements of innate immunity which use ancient mechanisms evolutionarily conserved from insects [100]. In innate immunity, all immunocompetent cells recognize "foreign and dangerous" structures characteristic of bacteria via toll-like receptors (TLRs) [101]. By using a variety of TLRs, neutrophils recognize bacterial lipopolysaccharides, peptidoglycans, bacterial DNA, and other pathogen-associated molecular patterns: for example, TLR9 binds bacterial DNA and TLR4 recognizes lipopolysaccharides [102].

In the acute inflammatory phase, increases will be observed in several serological tests, notably white blood-cell count, C-reactive protein, erythrocyte sedimentation rate, and procalcitonin. Locally, the four classic signs of inflammation: pain, heat, redness, and swelling, are usually observed due to the local vasodilation and chemotaxis of inflammatory cells, primarily neutrophils. In many cases, orthopedic implant infections can cause osteomyelitis. In bone, osteoblasts also express TLRs 2, 4, and 9, and respond to bacterial structures to produce antimicrobial peptides, chemokines and inflammatory cytokines, and receptor activator of nuclear factor kappa-B ligand (RANKL) [103, 104]. By the influence of RANKL and other proinflammatory cytokines, osteoclast precursors mature into osteoclasts. Osteoclasts also secrete cytokines and chemokines, which induce chemotaxis of additional precursors and promote osteoclastogenesis [105, 106]. By these amplifying cascades, osteoclasts participate in paracrine and autocrine regulation of massive bone resorption in osteomyelitis. Bacterial toxins themselves also have a strong stimulatory effect on osteoclasts by directly affecting osteoclast generation, survival, and activation; and by indirectly promoting the production of RANKL and other osteoclastogenic factors [107, 108]. Moreover, biofilm can directly regulate various host cells to induce RANKL and cause bone resorption [109]. This bone resorption causes the loosening of the implant, which is often observed as a radiolucent line in plain x-rays or computed tomographic images, and implant loosening is another cause of the pain in the infected patient. In classic osteomyelitis, the local osteolysis is followed by the formation of the involucrum, which is a ring of new reactive bone surrounding the infection site and fragments of dead bone called sequestra. In implant-associated infection cases, though it is not as typical as classic sequestrum and involucrum, bone resorption and reactive bone formation are observed. Although necrotic bone is formed as early as 10 days postinfection, plain x rays are unable to detect sequestrum or sclerotic bone for many weeks [110].

Chronic infections can last years or even decades and are frequently resistant to medical or surgical intervention. The chronic stage generally produces more infection-related bone damage and requires more aggressive intervention. Extensive antibiotic therapy in combination with irrigation and debridement is sometimes sufficient for the elimination of many infecting microorganisms. However, once *S aureus* has been confirmed by culture, the standard of care for TJR patients is two-stage exchange arthroplasty which features removal of the primary implant and debridement followed by weeks or months of antibiotic therapy [9, 74]. Remarkably, 30% of patients never achieve the criteria for reimplantation. While reimplantation is attempted in about 70% of infected patients, as many as 10–20% become reinfected. Thus, the combined failure rate for *S aureus*-infected TJR approaches 50%.

Some reinfections result from different microorganisms, but most recurrent infections are with the same strain as the initial infection [111]. What is the physical basis for this remarkable persistence? Multiple citations attest that these *S aureus* infections can persist for over 60 years [112, 113]. In addition to biofilms, we are becoming aware of still other "lifestyles" of staphylococci. These include survival modes that have been observed in clinical specimens and animal models:

- Microcolonies
- Abscesses
- Adoption of an intracellular lifestyle
- Opportunistic survival in protected niches in the host

Each of these mechanisms may contribute to the persistence of *S aureus* infections, and it is possible that individual strains of *S aureus* can use more than one of these strategies in chronic infection.

Microcolonies have been observed in many settings where they are associated with recurrent infections. Microcolonies are not well defined, but appear to be soft-tissue-associated patches of biofilm that are clinically associated with recurrent soft-tissue infections [114, 115], and they have been observed in a mouse model of chronic osteomyelitis [116]. Little is known about their formation or stability. While we have not observed microcolonies in our osteomyelitis models, they are included in this discussion primarily as another potential reservoir of chronic infection that has been documented in laboratory and clinical settings.

Staphylococcus aureus abscesses manipulate the host's innate immune response to create short-term shelter that can be reservoirs for recurrence [117]. The formation of abscesses includes zones defined by a perimeter of fibrin deposits surrounding an infection. However, *S aureus* has developed ways to manipulate the normal host response to its advantage, possibly contributing to prolonged extension of chronic infection. Using a mouse model of bacteremia that leads to abscess formation in multiple organs, Schneewind et al have described a four-step process of abscess development and regeneration [117].

The "life cycle" of an abscess is in the order of a month, and there is little evidence that the immune response elicited by the initial infection has any protective value against reinfection [118, 119]. Consequently, successive cycles of abscess formation could be a vehicle for long-lasting chronic infections.

Further investigations in the authors' laboratory have examined the impact of antibodies selected for potential immune interference with the progress or persistence of *S aureus* infections in the model of implant-associated osteomyelitis. Immunoglobulin G antibodies that block the enzymatic activities of the bifunctional cell-wall modifying enzyme autolysin reduced the number of abscesses that formed in the bone marrow, and enable macrophage penetration of the interior of the abscess [79].

Generally considered an extracellular pathogen, *S aureus* may persist as small-colony variants (SCV) inside host cells [120]. The possibility of an intracellular lifestyle for *S aureus* is based on numerous observations of internalization of *S aureus* by nonprofessional phagocytes such as keratinocytes, epithelial cells, and osteoblasts [121–124]. In vitro, such internalization frequently leads to death or apoptosis of the host cell [125, 126], but in some instances the host cells are stably infected with SCVs of *S aureus* [127]. Small-colony variants are distinguished by the presence of mutations in menadione or hemin uptake, elevated expression of FnBpA, decreased expression of *agr* and Hla and distinctive colonies in vitro that are nonlytic (no Hla), noncolored (no staphyloxanthin), and small. The hypothesis is that these intracellular SCVs are another potential source of long-lived persistent infections and that these associated changes are adaptations to the intracellular lifestyle. Interest in SCVs has been enhanced by clinical observations of SCVs cultured from chronic osteomyelitis patients [116, 128].

Others have reported the identification of *S aureus* in osteoblasts [116], but there is no indication so far that such infections are regularly observed. The authors have examined numerous chronic infections using a transtibial pin model and have so far not observed intracellular *S aureus* in living osteoblasts or any other resident cell type.

Staphylococcus aureus can survive in protected niches in the host. As the acute infection progresses, bone near the infection site is lysed in a region ringed by new bone formation, the involucrum, that surrounds and isolates the pathogen and dead bone fragments called sequestra. Both involucra and sequestra are characteristic of osteomyelitis in humans. In principle, sequestra can serve as a reservoir for prolonged survival of *S aureus* [112]. In fact, in recent examinations of sequestra by transmission electron microscopy, the authors have observed the presence of *S aureus* in small fissures in the sequestrum, which they call microcracks. The abundance of cells with cell division septa indicates that the bacteria are alive and dividing. In a related and unexpected observation, the authors identified the presence of *S aureus* in canaliculi, the 0.2–0.5 µm channels that serve as conduits for communication between the surface of the bone and osteocytes embedded in cortical bone (**Fig 1-4**). It is probable that *S aureus* in canaliculi can survive indefinitely by dissolving bone locally to gain access to collagen, and also by consuming remnants of the resident osteocytes.

The success of these survival modes for *S aureus* and the frequency of chronic or recurrent infections are augmented by the impotent nature of the human adaptive immune response to natural infections. Each of the chronic infection modes described above provides a haven for *S aureus* for a finite time before it needs to be reformed or converted to another mode. Biofilms, and possibly microcolonies, appear to be particularly dynamic, proceeding through the entire cycle of adherence, maturation, and dispersal in weeks and possibly days. Likewise, abscesses turn over within a month or so. If SCVs in osteoblasts are to be indefinitely stable, they need to find new host cells when their resident cell turns over. Finally, *S aureus* in sequestra will ultimately consume the local nutrient supply and need some mechanism for escape and reinfection. Indeed, the need of these proposed reservoirs of long-term infection to turn over has attracted the attention of developers of antibiotics hoping to identify valuable new targets for intervention [129–136].

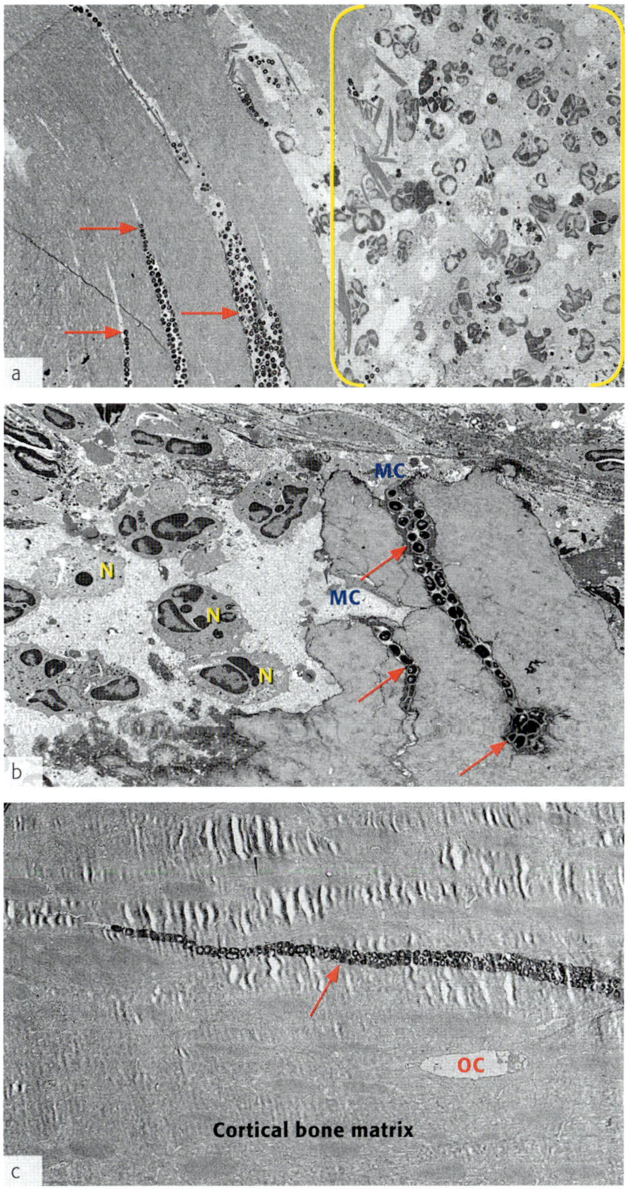

Fig 1-4a–c *Staphylococcus aureus* invades both surgically produced microcracks and bone canaliculi.

a *Staphylococcus aureus* in bone (arrows). Large cluster of dead neutrophils (inside yellow bars).

b *Staphylococcus aureus* invades (arrows) microcracks (MC) caused by surgical drilling into bone. Note several dead neutrophils (N) adjacent to the microcrack.

c *Staphylococcus aureus* invasion (arrow) into cortical bone and canaliculi adjacent to an osteocyte (OC) [137].

6 Conclusion

- The clinical challenges surgeons face in implant-associated infections are due to the growth of bacteria in biofilms.
- Even though the concept of biofilms is new to humans, biofilms are ancient lifestyles for essentially all bacteria.
- In vitro, biofilms are the products from genetically programmed steps and cooperative behavior among bacteria that construct a matrix of self-made, extracellular polymeric substances on a living or nonliving surface.
- In vivo, biofilms are mosaic matrices comprising both bacterial and host components.
- Bacteria benefit from biofilms by acquiring resistance to antibiotics and to host immune responses.
- Biofilms are not static fortresses. They are dynamic incubators spawning fast-growing, virulent bacteria that disperse to populate new surfaces, as well as slow-growing antibiotic-resistant persister cells.
- Implants including TJRs, plates, nails, screws, and sutures are excellent foreign bodies that can dramatically favor the local growth of bacteria at the expense of the host.
- The immune response is not very effective against *S aureus* biofilm infections because of its capabilities of modulating the host immune response.
- The management of chronic *S aureus* infections may be made more difficult because *S aureus* has additional lifestyle options that may also be protective and how they interact with biofilms is unknown.
- Treatment of implant surfaces and intervention in every step in the biofilm lifestyle are areas of active inquiry for therapeutic intervention.

7 References

1. **Kurtz S, Ong K, Lau E, et al.** Projections of primary and revision hip and knee arthroplasty in the United States from 2005 to 2030. *J Bone Joint Surg Am.* 2007 Apr;89(4):780–785.
2. **Darouiche RO.** Treatment of infections associated with surgical implants. *N Engl J Med.* 2004 Apr 1;350(14):1422–1429.
3. **Haenle M, Skripitz C, Mittelmeier W, et al.** Economic impact of infected total knee arthroplasty. *ScientificWorldJournal.* 2012;2012:196515.
4. **Kurtz SM, Lau E, Schmier J, et al.** Infection burden for hip and knee arthroplasty in the United States. *J Arthroplasty.* 2008 Oct;23(7):984–991.
5. **Kurtz SM, Lau E, Watson H, et al.** Economic burden of periprosthetic joint infection in the United States. *J Arthroplasty.* 2012 Sep;27(8 Suppl):61–65 e61.
6. **Kurtz SM, Ong KL, Schmier J, et al.** Future clinical and economic impact of revision total hip and knee arthroplasty. *J Bone Joint Surg Am.* 2007 Oct;89 Suppl 3:144–151.
7. **Murray CK, Hsu JR, Solomkin JS, et al.** Prevention and management of infections associated with combat-related extremity injuries. *J Trauma.* 2008 Mar;64(3 Suppl):S239–251.
8. **Ong KL, Kurtz SM, Lau E, et al.** Prosthetic joint infection risk after total hip arthroplasty in the Medicare population. *J Arthroplasty.* 2009 Sep;24(6 Suppl):105–109.
9. **Parvizi J, Azzam K, Ghanem E, et al.** Periprosthetic infection due to resistant staphylococci: serious problems on the horizon. *Clin Orthop Relat Res.* 2009 Jul;467(7):1732–1739.
10. **Parvizi J, Zmistowski B, Berbari EF, et al.** New definition for periprosthetic joint infection: from the Workgroup of the Musculoskeletal Infection Society. *Clin Orthop Relat Res.* 2011 Nov;469(11):2992–2994.
11. **Pulido L, Ghanem E, Joshi A, et al.** Periprosthetic joint infection: the incidence, timing, and predisposing factors. *Clin Orthop Relat Res.* 2008 Jul;466(7):1710–1715.
12. **Stoodley P, Ehrlich GD, Sedghizadeh PP, et al.** Orthopaedic biofilm infections. *Curr Orthop Pract.* 2011 Nov;22(6):558–563.
13. **Toms AD, Davidson D, Masri BA, et al.** The management of peri-prosthetic infection in total joint arthroplasty. *J Bone Joint Surg Br.* 2006 Feb;88(2):149–155.
14. **Walls RJ, Roche SJ, O'Rourke A, et al.** Surgical site infection with methicillin-resistant Staphylococcus aureus after primary total hip replacement. *J Bone Joint Surg Br.* 2008 Mar;90(3):292–298.
15. **Costerton JW, Geesey GG, Cheng KJ.** How bacteria stick. *Sci Am.* 1978 Jan;238(1):86–95.
16. **Zobell CE.** The Effect of Solid Surfaces upon Bacterial Activity. *J Bacteriol.* 1943 Jul;46(1):39–56.
17. **McCoy WF, Bryers JD, Robbins J, et al.** Observations of fouling biofilm formation. *Can J Microbiol.* 1981 Sep;27(9):910–917.
18. **Sugarman B, Musher D.** Adherence of bacteria to suture materials. *Proc Soc Exp Biol Med.* 1980;167(2):156–160.
19. **Edmiston CE, Jr., Krepel CJ, Marks RM, et al.** Microbiology of explanted suture segments from infected and noninfected surgical patients. *J Clin Microbiol.* 2013 Feb;51(2):417–421.
20. **Jara FM, Toledo-Pereyra L, Lewis JW, Jr., et al.** The infected pacemaker pocket. *J Thorac Cardiovasc Surg.* 1979 Aug;78(2):298–300.
21. **Choo MH, Holmes DR, Jr., Gersh BJ, et al.** Permanent pacemaker infections: characterization and management. *Am J Cardiol.* 1981 Sep;48(3):559–564.
22. **Nickel JC, Ruseska I, Wright JB, et al.** Tobramycin resistance of Pseudomonas aeruginosa cells growing as a biofilm on urinary catheter material. *Antimicrob Agents Chemother.* 1985 Apr;27(4):619–624.
23. **Gristina A, Costerton JW.** Bacteria-laden biofilms: a hazard to orthopedic prostheses. *Infect Surg.* 1984;3:655–662.
24. **Costerton JW.** Cystic fibrosis pathogenesis and the role of biofilms in persistent infection. *Trends Microbiol.* 2001 Feb;9(2):50–52.
25. **Costerton JW, Stewart PS, Greenberg EP.** Bacterial biofilms: a common cause of persistent infections. *Science.* 1999 May 21;284(5418):1318–1322.
26. **Moormeier DE, Bose JL, Horswill AR, et al.** Temporal and stochastic control of Staphylococcus aureus biofilm development. *MBio.* 2014;5(5):e01341–01314.
27. **Archer NK, Mazaitis MJ, Costerton JW, et al.** Staphylococcus aureus biofilms: properties, regulation, and roles in human disease. *Virulence.* 2011 Sep-Oct;2(5):445–459.
28. **Joo HS, Otto M.** Molecular basis of in vivo biofilm formation by bacterial pathogens. *Chem Biol.* 2012 Dec 21;19(12):1503–1513.
29. **Karatan E, Watnick P.** Signals, regulatory networks, and materials that build and break bacterial biofilms. *Microbiol Mol Biol Rev.* 2009 Jun;73(2):310–347.
30. **Otto M.** Staphylococcal infections: mechanisms of biofilm maturation and detachment as critical determinants of pathogenicity. *Annu Rev Med.* 2013;64:175–188.
31. **Arciola CR, Campoccia D, Speziale P, et al.** Biofilm formation in Staphylococcus implant infections. *A review of molecular mechanisms and implications for biofilm-resistant materials. Biomaterials.* 2012 Sep;33(26):5967–5982.
32. **Corrigan RM, Abbott JC, Burhenne H, et al.** c-di-AMP is a new second messenger in Staphylococcus aureus with a role in controlling cell size and envelope stress. *PLoS Pathog.* 2011 Sep;7(9):e1002217.
33. **Valle J, Solano C, Garcia B, et al.** Biofilm switch and immune response determinants at early stages of infection. *Trends Microbiol.* 2013 Aug;21(8):364–371.
34. **Foster TJ, Geoghegan JA, Ganesh VK, et al.** Adhesion, invasion and evasion: the many functions of the surface proteins of Staphylococcus aureus. *Nat Rev Microbiol.* 2014 Jan;12(1):49–62.
35. **Kwasny SM, Opperman TJ.** Static biofilm cultures of Gram-positive pathogens grown in a microtiter format used for anti-biofilm drug discovery. *Curr Protoc Pharmacol.* 2010 Sep;Chapter 13:Unit 13A 8.
36. **Beenken KE, Dunman PM, McAleese F, et al.** Global gene expression in Staphylococcus aureus biofilms. *J Bacteriol.* 2004 Jul;186(14):4665–4684.
37. **Otto M.** Staphylococcal biofilms. *Curr Top Microbiol Immunol.* 2008;322:207–228.
38. **Geoghegan JA, Corrigan RM, Gruszka DT, et al.** Role of surface protein SasG in biofilm formation by Staphylococcus aureus. *J Bacteriol.* 2010 Nov;192(21):5663–5673.
39. **Gruszka DT, Wojdyla JA, Bingham RJ, et al.** Staphylococcal biofilm-forming protein has a contiguous rod-like structure. *Proc Natl Acad Sci U S A.* 2012 Apr 24;109(17):E1011–1018.
40. **Rohde H, Burandt EC, Siemssen N, et al.** Polysaccharide intercellular adhesin or protein factors in biofilm accumulation of Staphylococcus epidermidis and Staphylococcus aureus isolated from prosthetic hip and knee joint infections. *Biomaterials.* 2007 Mar;28(9):1711–1720.

41. **Bayles KW.** The biological role of death and lysis in biofilm development. *Nat Rev Microbiol.* 2007 Sep;5(9):721–726.
42. **Sadykov MR, Bayles KW.** The control of death and lysis in staphylococcal biofilms: a coordination of physiological signals. *Curr Opin Microbiol.* 2012 Apr;15(2):211–215.
43. **Beenken KE, Spencer H, Griffin LM, et al.** Impact of extracellular nuclease production on the biofilm phenotype of Staphylococcus aureus under in vitro and in vivo conditions. *Infect Immun.* 2012 May;80(5):1634–1638.
44. **Cassat JE, Hammer ND, Campbell JP, et al.** A secreted bacterial protease tailors the Staphylococcus aureus virulence repertoire to modulate bone remodeling during osteomyelitis. *Cell Host Microbe.* 2013 Jun 12;13(6):759–772.
45. **Chen C, Krishnan V, Macon K, et al.** Secreted proteases control autolysin-mediated biofilm growth of Staphylococcus aureus. *J Biol Chem.* 2013 Oct 11;288(41):29440–29452.
46. **Mootz JM, Malone CL, Shaw LN, et al.** Staphopains modulate Staphylococcus aureus biofilm integrity. *Infect Immun.* 2013 Sep;81(9):3227–3238.
47. **Rohde H, Burdelski C, Bartscht K, et al.** Induction of Staphylococcus epidermidis biofilm formation via proteolytic processing of the accumulation-associated protein by staphylococcal and host proteases. *Mol Microbiol.* 2005 Mar;55(6):1883–1895.
48. **Iwase T, Uehara Y, Shinji H, et al.** Staphylococcus epidermidis Esp inhibits Staphylococcus aureus biofilm formation and nasal colonization. *Nature.* 2010 May 20;465(7296):346–349.
49. **Sugimoto S, Iwamoto T, Takada K, et al.** Staphylococcus epidermidis Esp degrades specific proteins associated with Staphylococcus aureus biofilm formation and host-pathogen interaction. *J Bacteriol.* 2013 Apr;195(8):1645–1655.
50. **Park JH, Lee JH, Cho MH, et al.** Acceleration of protease effect on Staphylococcus aureus biofilm dispersal. *FEMS Microbiol Lett.* 2012 Oct;335(1):31–38.
51. **Chen M, Yu Q, Sun H.** Novel strategies for the prevention and treatment of biofilm related infections. *Int J Mol Sci.* 2013;14(9):18488–18501.
52. **Savage VJ, Chopra I, O'Neill AJ.** Population diversification in Staphylococcus aureus biofilms may promote dissemination and persistence. *PLoS One.* 2013;8(4):e62513.
53. **Singh R, Ray P, Das A, et al.** Role of persisters and small-colony variants in antibiotic resistance of planktonic and biofilm-associated Staphylococcus aureus: an in vitro study. *J Med Microbiol.* 2009 Aug;58(Pt 8):1067–1073.
54. **Conlon BP.** Staphylococcus aureus chronic and relapsing infections: Evidence of a role for persister cells: An investigation of persister cells, their formation and their role in S aureus disease. *Bioessays.* 2014 Oct;36(10):991–996.
55. **Prax M, Bertram R.** Metabolic aspects of bacterial persisters. *Front Cell Infect Microbiol.* 2014 Oct 22;4:148.
56. **Boles BR, Horswill AR.** Agr-mediated dispersal of Staphylococcus aureus biofilms. *PLoS Pathog.* 2008 Apr 25;4(4):e1000052
57. **Boles BR, Horswill AR.** Staphylococcal biofilm disassembly. *Trends Microbiol.* 2011 Sep;19(9):449–455.
58. **Periasamy S, Joo HS, Duong AC, et al.** How Staphylococcus aureus biofilms develop their characteristic structure. *Proc Natl Acad Sci U S A.* 2012 Jan 24;109(4):1281–1286.
59. **Bjarnsholt T, Alhede M, Alhede M, et al.** The in vivo biofilm. *Trends Microbiol.* 2013 Sep;21(9):466–474.
60. **Stoodley P, Nistico L, Johnson S, et al.** Direct demonstration of viable Staphylococcus aureus biofilms in an infected total joint arthroplasty. A case report. *J Bone Joint Surg Am.* 2008 Aug;90(8):1751–1758.
61. **Li D, Gromov K, Soballe K, et al.** Quantitative mouse model of implant-associated osteomyelitis and the kinetics of microbial growth, osteolysis, and humoral immunity. *J Orthop Res.* 2008 Jan;26(1):96–105.
62. **Lin MH, Shu JC, Huang HY, et al.** Involvement of iron in biofilm formation by Staphylococcus aureus. *PLoS One.* 2012;7(3):e34388.
63. **McAdow M, DeDent AC, Emolo C, et al.** Coagulases as determinants of protective immune responses against Staphylococcus aureus. *Infect Immun.* 2012 Oct;80(10):3389–3398.
64. **McAdow M, Kim HK, Dedent AC, et al.** Preventing Staphylococcus aureus sepsis through the inhibition of its agglutination in blood. *PLoS Pathog.* 2011 Oct;7(10):e1002307.
65. **McAdow M, Missiakas DM, Schneewind O.** Staphylococcus aureus secretes coagulase and von Willebrand factor binding protein to modify the coagulation cascade and establish host infections. *J Innate Immun.* 2012;4(2):141–148.
66. **DuMont AL, Yoong P, Surewaard BG, et al.** Staphylococcus aureus elaborates leukocidin AB to mediate escape from within human neutrophils. *Infect Immun.* 2013 May;81(5):1830–1841.
67. **Kim HK, Thammavongsa V, Schneewind O, et al.** Recurrent infections and immune evasion strategies of Staphylococcus aureus. *Curr Opin Microbiol.* 2012 Feb;15(1):92–99.
68. **Kubica M, Guzik K, Koziel J, et al.** A potential new pathway for Staphylococcus aureus dissemination: the silent survival of S aureus phagocytosed by human monocyte-derived macrophages. *PLoS One.* 2008;3(1):e1409.
69. **Veerachamy S, Yarlagadda T, Manivasagam G, et al.** Bacterial adherence and biofilm formation on medical implants: a review. *Proc Inst Mech Eng H.* 2014 Oct;228(10):1083–1099.
70. **Elek SD.** Experimental staphylococcal infections in the skin of man. *Ann N Y Acad Sci.* 1956 Aug 31;65(3):85–90.
71. **Lew DP, Waldvogel FA.** Osteomyelitis. *Lancet.* 2004 Jul 24-30;364(9431):369–379.
72. **Peltola H, Paakkonen M.** Acute osteomyelitis in children. *N Engl J Med.* 2014 Jan 23;370(4):352–360.
73. **Zimmerli W.** Clinical practice. Vertebral osteomyelitis. *N Engl J Med.* 2010 Mar 18;362(11):1022–1029.
74. **Del Pozo JL, Patel R.** Clinical practice. Infection associated with prosthetic joints. *N Engl J Med.* 2009 Aug 20;361(8):787–794.
75. **Nishitani K, Sutipornpalangkul W, de Mesy Bentley KL, et al.** Quantifying the natural history of biofilm formation in vivo during the establishment of chronic implant-associated Staphlyococcus aureus osteomyelitis in mice to identify critical pathogen and host factors. *J Orthop Res.* 2015 Mar 26.
76. **Ha KY, Chung YG, Ryoo SJ.** Adherence and biofilm formation of Staphylococcus epidermidis and Mycobacterium tuberculosis on various spinal implants. *Spine.* 2005 Jan 1;30(1):38–43.
77. **Gracia E, Fernandez A, Conchello P, et al.** Adherence of Staphylococcus aureus slime-producing strain variants to biomaterials used in orthopaedic surgery. *Int Orthop.* 1997;21(1):46–51.
78. **Koseki H, Yonekura A, Shida T, et al.** Early staphylococcal biofilm formation on solid orthopaedic implant materials: in vitro study. *PLoS One.* 2014;9(10):e107588.

79. **Varrone JJ, de Mesy Bentley KL, Bello-Irizarry SN, et al.** Passive Immunization with Anti-Glucosaminidase Monoclonal Antibodies Protects Mice from Implant-Associated Osteomyelitis by Mediating Opsonophagocytosis of Staphylococcus aureus Megaclusters. *J Orthop Res.* 2014 Oct;32(10):1389–1396.
80. **Harris LG, Meredith DO, Eschbach L, et al.** Staphylococcus aureus adhesion to standard micro-rough and electropolished implant materials. *J Mater Sci Mater Med.* 2007 Jun;18(6):1151–1156.
81. **Schmidlin PR, Muller P, Attin T, et al.** Polyspecies biofilm formation on implant surfaces with different surface characteristics. *J Appl Oral Sci.* 2013 Jan-Feb;21(1):48–55.
82. **Teughels W, Van Assche N, Sliepen I, et al.** Effect of material characteristics and/or surface topography on biofilm development. *Clin Oral Implants Res.* 2006 Oct;17 Suppl 2:68–81.
83. **Arens S, Schlegel U, Printzen G, et al.** Influence of materials for fixation implants on local infection. An experimental study of steel versus titanium DCP in rabbits. *J Bone Joint Surg Br.* 1996 Jul;78(4):647–651.
84. **Schlegel U, Perren SM.** Surgical aspects of infection involving osteosynthesis implants: implant design and resistance to local infection. *Injury.* 2006 May;37 Suppl 2:S67–73.
85. **Harris LG, Richards RG.** Staphylococci and implant surfaces: a review. *Injury.* 2006 May;37 Suppl 2:S3–14.
86. **Pieske O, Geleng P, Zaspel J, et al.** Titanium alloy pins versus stainless steel pins in external fixation at the wrist: a randomized prospective study. *J Trauma.* 2008 May;64(5):1275–1280.
87. **Clauss M, Graf S, Gersbach S, et al.** Material and biofilm load of K wires in toe surgery: titanium versus stainless steel. *Clin Orthop Relat Res.* 2013 Jul;471(7):2312–2317.
88. **Meredith DO, Eschbach L, Wood MA, et al.** Human fibroblast reactions to standard and electropolished titanium and Ti-6Al-7Nb, and electropolished stainless steel. *J Biomed Mater Res A.* 2005 Dec 1;75(3):541–555.
89. **Petrini P, Arciola CR, Pezzali I, et al.** Antibacterial activity of zinc modified titanium oxide surface. *Int J Artif Organs.* 2006 Apr;29(4):434–442.
90. **Wu Y, Yu J, Liu HM, et al.** One-dimensional TiO2 nanomaterials: preparation and catalytic applications. *J Nanosci Nanotechnol.* 2010 Oct;10(10):6707–6719.
91. **Singh P, Cameotra SS.** Potential applications of microbial surfactants in biomedical sciences. *Trends Biotechnol.* 2004 Mar;22(3):142–146.
92. **Kinnari TJ, Peltonen LI, Kuusela P, et al.** Bacterial adherence to titanium surface coated with human serum albumin. *Otol Neurotol.* 2005 May;26(3):380–384.
93. **Arciola CR, Montanaro L, Moroni A, et al.** Hydroxyapatite-coated orthopaedic screws as infection resistant materials: in vitro study. *Biomaterials.* 1999 Feb;20(4):323–327.
94. **Di Martino A, Sittinger M, Risbud MV.** Chitosan: a versatile biopolymer for orthopaedic tissue-engineering. *Biomaterials.* 2005 Oct;26(30):5983–5990.
95. **Alt V, Bechert T, Steinrucke P, et al.** An in vitro assessment of the antibacterial properties and cytotoxicity of nanoparticulate silver bone cement. *Biomaterials.* 2004 Aug;25(18):4383–4391.
96. **Bosetti M, Masse A, Tobin E, et al.** Silver coated materials for external fixation devices: in vitro biocompatibility and genotoxicity. *Biomaterials.* 2002 Feb;23(3):887–892.
97. **Shirai T, Tsuchiya H, Nishida H, et al.** Antimicrobial megaprostheses supported with iodine. *J Biomater Appl.* 2014 Oct;29(4):617–623.
98. **Cochis A, Azzimonti B, Della Valle C, et al.** Biofilm formation on titanium implants counteracted by grafting gallium and silver ions. *J Biomed Mater Res A.* 2015 Mar;103(3):1176–1187.
99. **Dinauer MC.** Disorders of neutrophil function: an overview. *Methods Mol Biol.* 2007;412:489–504.
100. **Kang D, Liu G, Lundstrom A, et al.** A peptidoglycan recognition protein in innate immunity conserved from insects to humans. *Proc Natl Acad Sci U S A.* 1998 Aug 18;95(17):10078–10082.
101. **Hänsch GM.** Host defence against bacterial biofilms: "Mission impossible"? *ISRN Immunology.* 2012;2012:1.
102. **Hirschfeld J.** Dynamic interactions of neutrophils and biofilms. *J Oral Microbiol.* 2014;6:26102.
103. **Amcheslavsky A, Hemmi H, Akira S, et al.** Differential contribution of osteoclast- and osteoblast-lineage cells to CpG-oligodeoxynucleotide (CpG-ODN) modulation of osteoclastogenesis. *J Bone Miner Res.* 2005 Sep;20(9):1692–1699.
104. **Varoga D, Wruck CJ, Tohidnezhad M, et al.** Osteoblasts participate in the innate immunity of the bone by producing human beta defensin-3. *Histochem Cell Biol.* 2009 Feb;131(2):207–218.
105. **O'Keefe RJ, Teot LA, Singh D, et al.** Osteoclasts constitutively express regulators of bone resorption: an immunohistochemical and in situ hybridization study. *Lab Invest.* 1997 Apr;76(4):457–465.
106. **Yu X, Huang Y, Collin-Osdoby P, et al.** CCR1 chemokines promote the chemotactic recruitment, RANKL development, and motility of osteoclasts and are induced by inflammatory cytokines in osteoblasts. *J Bone Miner Res.* 2004 Dec;19(12):2065–2077.
107. **Montonen M, Li TF, Lukinmaa PL, et al.** RANKL and cathepsin K in diffuse sclerosing osteomyelitis of the mandible. *J Oral Pathol Med.* 2006 Nov;35(10):620–625.
108. **Puzas JE, Hicks DG, Reynolds SD, et al.** Regulation of osteoclastic activity in infection. *Methods Enzymol.* 1994;236:47–58.
109. **Sanchez CJ, Jr., Ward CL, Romano DR, et al.** Staphylococcus aureus biofilms decrease osteoblast viability, inhibits osteogenic differentiation, and increases bone resorption in vitro. *BMC Musculoskelet Disord.* 2013;14:187.
110. **Pineda C, Espinosa R, Pena A.** Radiographic imaging in osteomyelitis: the role of plain radiography, computed tomography, ultrasonography, magnetic resonance imaging, and scintigraphy. *Semin Plast Surg.* 2009 May;23(2):80–89.
111. **Huang SS, Diekema DJ, Warren DK, et al.** Strain-relatedness of methicillin-resistant Staphylococcus aureus isolates recovered from patients with repeated infection. *Clin Infect Dis.* 2008 Apr 15;46(8):1241–1247.
112. **Ciampolini J, Harding KG.** Pathophysiology of chronic bacterial osteomyelitis. Why do antibiotics fail so often? *Postgrad Med J.* 2000 Aug;76(898):479–483.
113. **Libraty DH, Patkar C, Torres B.** Staphylococcus aureus reactivation osteomyelitis after 75 years. *N Engl J Med.* 2012 Feb 2;366(5):481–482.
114. **Alasil SM, Omar R, Ismail S, et al.** Evidence of Bacterial Biofilms among Infected and Hypertrophied Tonsils in Correlation with the Microbiology, Histopathology, and Clinical Symptoms of Tonsillar Diseases. *Int J Otolaryngol.* 2013;2013:408238.
115. **Kania RE, Lamers GE, Vonk MJ, et al.** Demonstration of bacterial cells and glycocalyx in biofilms on human tonsils. *Arch Otolaryngol Head Neck Surg.* 2007 Feb;133(2):115–121.

116. **Horst SA, Hoerr V, Beineke A, et al.** A novel mouse model of Staphylococcus aureus chronic osteomyelitis that closely mimics the human infection: an integrated view of disease pathogenesis. *Am J Pathol.* 2012 Oct;181(4):1206–1214.
117. **Cheng AG, DeDent AC, Schneewind O, et al.** A play in four acts: Staphylococcus aureus abscess formation. *Trends Microbiol.* 2011 May;19(5):225–232.
118. **Fowler VG, Jr., Proctor RA.** Where does a Staphylococcus aureus vaccine stand? *Clin Microbiol Infect.* 2014 May;20 Suppl 5:66–75.
119. **Spellberg B, Daum R.** Development of a vaccine against Staphylococcus aureus. *Semin Immunopathol.* 2012 Mar;34(2):335–348.
120. **Loffler B, Tuchscherr L, Niemann S, et al.** Staphylococcus aureus persistence in non-professional phagocytes. *Int J Med Microbiol.* 2014 Mar;304(2):170–176.
121. **Clement S, Vaudaux P, Francois P, et al.** Evidence of an intracellular reservoir in the nasal mucosa of patients with recurrent Staphylococcus aureus rhinosinusitis. *J Infect Dis.* 2005 Sep 15;192(6):1023–1028.
122. **Tan NW, Turvey SE, Byrne AT, et al.** Staphylococcus aureus nasal septal abscess complicated by extradural abscess in an infant. *J Otolaryngol Head Neck Surg.* 2012 Feb;41(1):E7–12.
123. **Zautner AE, Krause M, Stropahl G, et al.** Intracellular persisting Staphylococcus aureus is the major pathogen in recurrent tonsillitis. *PLoS One.* 2010;5(3):e9452.
124. **von Eiff C, Becker K, Metze D, et al.** Intracellular persistence of Staphylococcus aureus small-colony variants within keratinocytes: a cause for antibiotic treatment failure in a patient with darier's disease. *Clin Infect Dis.* 2001 Jun 1;32(11):1643–1647.
125. **Shi S, Zhang X.** Interaction of Staphylococcus aureus with osteoblasts (Review). *Exp Ther Med.* 2012 Mar;3(3):367–370.
126. **Wright JA, Nair SP.** Interaction of staphylococci with bone. *Int J Med Microbiol.* 2010 Feb;300(2-3):193–204.
127. **Tuchscherr L, Medina E, Hussain M, et al.** Staphylococcus aureus phenotype switching: an effective bacterial strategy to escape host immune response and establish a chronic infection. *EMBO Mol Med.* 2011 Mar;3(3):129–141.
128. **von Eiff C, Bettin D, Proctor RA, et al.** Recovery of small colony variants of Staphylococcus aureus following gentamicin bead placement for osteomyelitis. *Clin Infect Dis.* 1997 Nov;25(5):1250–1251.
129. **Blanco AR, Sudano-Roccaro A, Spoto GC, et al.** Epigallocatechin gallate inhibits biofilm formation by ocular staphylococcal isolates. *Antimicrob Agents Chemother.* 2005 Oct;49(10):4339–4343.
130. **Bordi C, de Bentzmann S.** Hacking into bacterial biofilms: a new therapeutic challenge. *Ann Intensive Care.* 2011;1(1):19.
131. **Conlon BP, Nakayasu ES, Fleck LE, et al.** Activated ClpP kills persisters and eradicates a chronic biofilm infection. *Nature.* 2013 Nov 21;503(7476):365–370.
132. **Karaolis DK, Rashid MH, Chythanya R, et al.** c-di-GMP (3'-5'-cyclic diguanylic acid) inhibits Staphylococcus aureus cell-cell interactions and biofilm formation. *Antimicrob Agents Chemother.* 2005 Mar;49(3):1029–1038.
133. **Lu J, Turnbull L, Burke CM, et al.** Manuka-type honeys can eradicate biofilms produced by Staphylococcus aureus strains with different biofilm-forming abilities. *PeerJ.* 2014 Mar 25;2:e326.
134. **Manner S, Skogman M, Goeres D, et al.** Systematic exploration of natural and synthetic flavonoids for the inhibition of Staphylococcus aureus biofilms. *Int J Mol Sci.* 2013;14(10).19434–19451.
135. **Okuda K, Zendo T, Sugimoto S, et al.** Effects of bacteriocins on methicillin-resistant Staphylococcus aureus biofilm. *Antimicrob Agents Chemother.* 2013 Nov;57(11):5572–5579.
136. **Su Z, Yeagley AA, Su R, et al.** Structural studies on 4,5-disubstituted 2-aminoimidazole-based biofilm modulators that suppress bacterial resistance to beta-lactams. *ChemMedChem.* 2012 Nov;7(11):2030–2039.
137. **Inzana JA, Schwarz EM, Kates SL, et al.** A novel murine model of established Staphylococcal bone infection in the presence of a fracture fixation plate to study therapies utilizing antibiotic-laden spacers after revision surgery. *Bone.* 2015 Mar;72:128–136.

2 Host immunity

John L Daiss, Edward M Schwarz

1 Basics

1.1 Role of the immune system

Bacteria, both commensals and pathogens, obtain food and shelter from humans. One of the fundamental differences between prokaryotic and eukaryotic organisms is the time it takes to make a new cell. Mammalian cells divide in about 24 hours compared to bacteria which can divide in as little as 20 minutes in a nutrient-rich environment. In the time a mammalian cell divides once, a single bacterium could go through 72 generations and produce about 10^{30} progeny. Of course this is unlikely, but the point is that in order to provide a robust defense, our immune system has to efficiently destroy such rapidly growing invaders. The human immune system is designed to totally degrade invading microorganisms by combining:

- Soluble components in the blood that recognize and lyse the microbe (humoral immunity)
- Microbe-eating cells that carry degradative machinery within them (cellular immunity)

Thus, fundamental concepts to understand host immunity in this brief chapter are:

- The main elements of the immune system
- Their mechanisms for recognition and action against bacteria

1.2 Limitations of this chapter

We limit our considerations of the host immune response to bacterial pathogens, the primary causes of orthopedic infections. Although similar rules apply, immunity against fungi, viruses, Protista, and worms are not specifically addressed. Assuming that orthopedic infections generally result from a significant breach of the skin or mucosa, our discussion will be limited to the systemic immune response; the mucosal immune response will not be addressed.

1.3 Two systems that interact

The mammalian immune response has come to be perceived as two distinct and interacting systems [1]. Historically, investigators and physicians have thought in terms of humoral immunity and cellular immunity, a distinction first made in the 1890s by scientists including Emil von Behring, Jules Bordet, and Paul Ehrlich, who discovered the protective powers of sera from infected animals [2]. They also discovered the presence of heat-stable, infection-inducible factors in the sera (antibodies), and of a second heat-labile, noninducible factor that worked with the antibodies to kill bacteria (complement). Considering that scientists went on to save millions of children from a cruel death from diphtheria using serum alone, one can respect their perception that humoral immunity was most important. At the same time, Ilya Metchnikoff discovered that immunity could be mediated by phagocytic cells that engulfed and killed bacteria [3]. Logically, he concluded that immunity was mediated by these specialized cells and called them phagocytes. While cellular and humoral immunity were initially perceived to be somehow in opposition, it has been clear for over a century that humoral and cellular elements of immunity work together to prevent and cure infection [3].

A more contemporary distinction is based on the identification of two distinct evolutionary strategies for defense against bacterial infections: the innate immune response and the adaptive immune response. The two systems are complementary and interactive (**Fig 2-1**). The innate immune system is always at the ready and can be engaged within minutes of a nascent infection. In contrast, the adaptive immune system takes weeks to become fully engaged and provides enhanced defense in the event of re-exposure to the same pathogen.

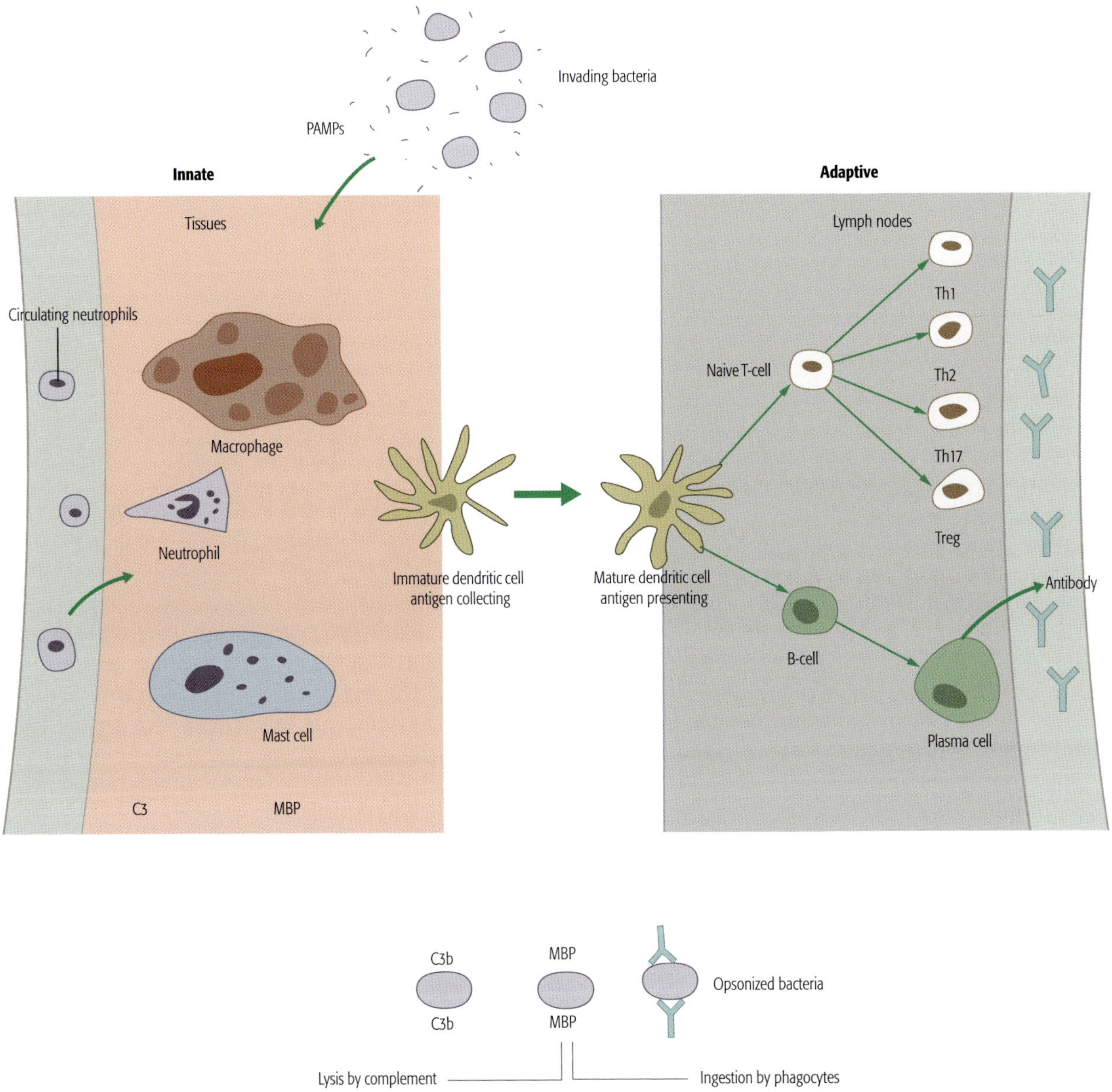

Fig 2-1 Schematic depiction of the main elements of the innate and adaptive immune systems. Invading bacteria produce PAMPs which elicit the secretion of cytokines and vasodilators from tissue-resident macrophages and mast cells and recruitment of neutrophils from the circulation. Bacteria coated with complement or MBP are ingested by phagocytes or lysed by complement. Immature dendritic cells collect antigens from the bacteria and mature into antigen-presenting cells that migrate to the lymph nodes where they engage and activate antigen-specific T and B cells. Activated T cells secrete cytokines that further activate macrophages (Th1), neutrophils (Th17), and B cells (Th2); regulatory T cells (Treg) produce immunosuppressive molecules. Activated B cells mature into antibody-producing plasma cells or memory B cells. Antibody binding to bacteria further promotes complement activation and phagocytosis by macrophages and neutrophils. Abbreviations: PAMPs, pathogen-associated molecular patterns; MBP, mannose-binding protein.

2 The innate immune system: conserved, dispersed, rapid, at the ready

The evolution of multicellular organisms required the development of mechanisms to defend against constant attack by pathogenic microbes seeking food and shelter. As a result, all invertebrate and vertebrate animals from fruit flies to man share a remarkably conserved array of cellular and humoral components, which collectively are referred to as innate immunity. Importantly, many of these components are not specific for immune defense, but serve additional vital functions. For example, the exoskeleton, or skin and mucosae, constitute a difficult-to-penetrate barrier for most pathogens. Beyond physical barriers, we are endowed with cells that produce antibacterial agents including microbicidal peptides [4, 5] and lipids [6]. Should bacteria breach the primary skin barrier by puncture, insect bite, or wound, they will immediately be faced with two elements of the immune system: a humoral component called complement and a cellular component that are macrophages dispersed throughout the connective tissues [7]. In mammals, complement is the primary humoral lytic agent of the innate immune system. It comprises a family of abundant serum proteins that promote defensive action by:

1. Identifying invading bacteria
2. Recruiting and activating immune cells like macrophages and neutrophils
3. Self-assembling into a lytic pore that directly kills certain gram-negative bacteria

In the absence of antibodies (see part 3 of this chapter) one of the complement proteins, C3, has the special property of containing an internal thioester bond that is spontaneously broken at a low rate generating a highly reactive enzyme (C3b), which can react with any cell surface. On normal host tissues the reactive C3b is rapidly inactivated, but most bacteria cannot inactivate C3b, which can covalently attach itself to the cell wall and initiate a self-amplifying series of proteolytic events that set three processes in motion. Firstly, proteolytic products called anaphylatoxins are released and act as chemotactic signals for nearby phagocytes. Secondly, the phagocytes bear cell surface receptors which bind to the microbe-bound C3b, promoting ingestion and internal degradation. Finally, activated C3b initiates a chain reaction with additional complement components, and ultimately produces a macromolecular assembly that creates a pore in the cell membranes of certain types of bacteria leading to osmotic lysis. This process of complement activation is called the alternative pathway, and it is one of the three ways that the lytic power of this protein system can be targeted against pathogenic bacteria.

The cellular components in most tissues are long-lived, resident cells of the immune system called macrophages, mast cells, and dendritic cells. As the name implies, macrophages are "big eaters": phagocytes that internalize and degrade bacteria and other organic materials. Macrophages are present mostly in connective tissues where they serve multiple roles. Firstly, they clear host cells that normally turnover by apoptosis [8], so they have a housekeeping function separate from their role in immunity. Secondly, they recognize and kill invading bacteria through receptors on their cell membranes that are specific for surfaces laden with the products of activated complement. Bacteria coated with phagocytosis-promoting proteins like complement are said to be "opsonized", based on a Greek word loosely translated as "to prepare for dining". Thirdly, they act as sentinels, and secrete biochemical signals called cytokines, such as tumor necrosis factor (TNF) and interleukins-1, -6, and -8 (IL-1, -6, -8). These secreted products amplify both local and systemic elements of the innate immune response resulting in inflammation (heat and swelling) at the site of infection.

Inflammatory cytokines also induce cell-surface changes in the local endothelia, which are recognized by blood-borne neutrophils. The neutrophils literally migrate through the endothelium (extravasation) and follow the biochemical trail consisting of cytokines, anaphylatoxins, and bacterial debris to the site of infection (chemotaxis). Along with macrophages, neutrophils destroy the invading bacteria. Macrophages are initially present as relatively few, long-lived, metabolically active phagocytes already positioned in the tissues. In contrast, neutrophils are recruited in great numbers from the bloodstream, where they are the most abundant white blood cells [9]. Distinguished by their relatively small size, distinctive heterochromatic, multilobed nuclei, and granular cytoplasm, neutrophils are mobile vehicles containing presynthesized antibacterial agents including small antimicrobial peptides, degradative enzymes, and generators of toxic reactive oxygen species. They can deliver their toxic payload either by degranulation (releasing their antimicrobial contents to the immediate environment) or they can ingest the bacteria and kill them by degrading them internally. Additionally, these cells can also kill bacteria in a suicidal process called NETosis, in which they combine their DNA with lysosomal proteins to catch and destroy microbes in neutrophil extracellular traps [10, 11].

Mast cells contain abundant histamine-rich granules that are released upon stimulation by, among other things, C5a, one of the anaphylatoxins noted above. Histamine release leads to local vasodilation accelerating the influx of neutrophils, rapidly manifested as erythema and swelling. This rapid cascade leads to systemic responses that direct additional lytic activity to the infection site, and attempt to restrict bacterial proliferation and spread. For example, within a few hours, secreted signals, notably tumor necrosis factor-α (TNF-α) and interleukin-6 (IL-6), stimulate the production of acute-phase proteins in the liver, including opsonins such as the complement protein C3, and C-reactive protein (CRP), and proteins such as ferritin, hepcidin, and ceruloplasmin that limit the availability of metal ions, particularly Fe^{++} which is essential for bacterial growth. A second example of a systemic response is the elevation of temperature. Interleukins-6 and TNF-α, among other signaling molecules, stimulate the secretion of prostaglandin E2 (PGE2) by cells in the hypothalamus which governs body temperature. Elevated temperature slows bacterial division rates and enhances some immune responses [7].

Since the innate immune response is mostly derived from preexisting resources that can be applied immediately to generate a robust local and systemic response, it is essential that rigorous controls limit the initiation and extent of the response to prevent serious tissue damage or death (eg, toxic shock syndrome). For the most part, this control lies with evolutionarily conserved receptors in macrophages and dendritic cells, referred to as pattern-recognition receptors (PRR), which specifically recognize pathogen-associated molecular patterns (PAMPs) and biochemical structures that are unique to pathogens and absent in metazoan hosts. There are three classes of PRRs:

- Toll-like receptors (TLR)
- NOD-like receptors (NLR)
- Lectin-like receptors

Discovered initially in *Drosophila*, TLRs are cell membrane-associated PRRs that recognize PAMPs from many potential pathogens including bacteria, viruses, and fungi in the extracellular environment [12]. Bacteria-specific PAMPs include peptidoglycan and phenol-soluble modulins (TLR2); lipopolysaccharide (LPS; TLR4); lipoteichoic acid (LTA; TLR6); and CpG-containing DNA (TLR9). Toll-like receptors do not directly drive phagocytosis by macrophages or neutrophils; they promote secretion of cytokines and interleukins that activate other immune cells. NOD-like receptors are intracellular receptors that stimulate the secretion of immune activators when bacteria have successfully invaded host cells. It is worth noting that one of the receptors in this family (NOD2/CARD15) has been identified as a susceptibility gene in Crohn's disease [13, 14] highlighting the dangers of a dysregulated innate immune system.

Finally, a soluble receptor mannose-binding protein (MBP, also called mannan-binding lectin) that binds sugars frequently present on bacterial cell walls but not on human cells, activates complement which coats the bacterial surface with opsonizing complement products [15].

3 Adaptive immunity: centralized, slow, custom-made

3.1 The challenge

Innate immunity has evolved to manage constant exposure to the most abundant pathogens. This approach to host defense has major limitations for vertebrates that have long life spans, including the means to defend against a new pathogenic toxins, strains, or species that never existed before. To achieve this, the adaptive immune response has developed the ability to recognize any molecular structure, while maintaining self-tolerance to prevent severe autoimmunity that Paul Ehrlich originally described as horror autotoxicus. As a result, this second recognition system adds powerful molecules and cell types to the host's defenses, and synergizes with the innate immune system to enhance the activity of both complement and phagocytes to recognize and destroy extracellular bacteria. In addition, the adaptive immune system adds two new capabilities to host immunity:

- The ability to identify and destroy host cells with pathogens inside of them
- Immunological memory, the ability to maintain a population of long-lived cells ready to respond to a second challenge by a previous invader

Antibodies are the most well-known aspect of adaptive immunity. Each antibody is a protein molecule that binds with exquisite specificity to a discrete molecular structure introduced by an invading bacterium. The bacterial protein or carbohydrate structure targeted by the antibody is called its antigen. Upon antigen binding, antibodies activate complement (complement fixation) and promote the ingestion of bacteria by phagocytes (opsonization). This dual nature of antibodies was discovered over a century ago by Paul Ehrlich who called them *Zwischenkörper* or connecting bodies [16]. The modular structure of the antibody molecule reveals how the connecting function is achieved.

The most widely studied type of antibodies is called immunoglobulin G (IgG). They share a common structure composed of two types of polypeptide chains; 25 kDa light chains and 50 kDa heavy chains (**Fig 2-2**). Each heavy chain pairs with one light chain and the heavy chains are paired to yield a four-polypeptide, 150 kDa molecule that assembles in a Y-shape familiar in most images of IgG. The arms of the Y are called the Fab (fragment with antigen-binding activity); the stem of the Y is called the Fc (fragment that crystallizes or is constant), and the short segment between them is called the hinge region.

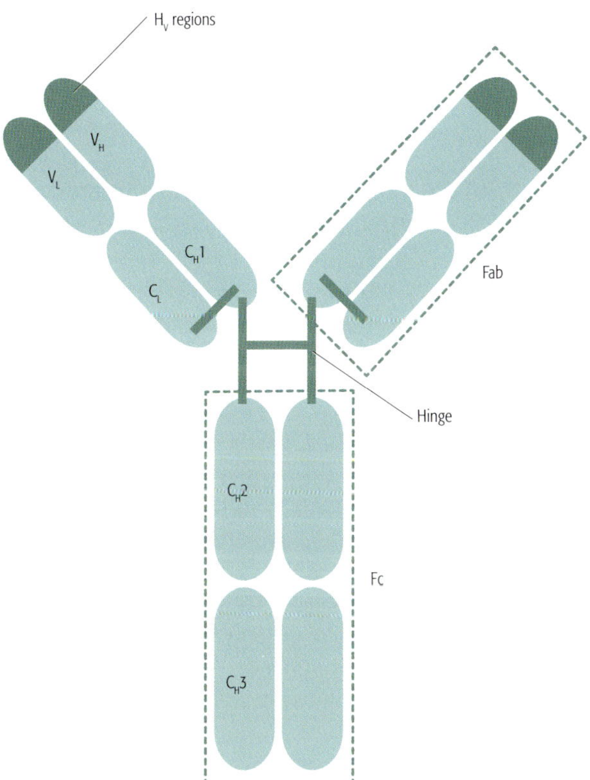

Fig 2-2 The anatomy of an immunoglobulin G antibody molecule. Antibodies are bivalent 150 kDa proteins consisting of two identical 25 kDa light chains and two identical 50 kDa heavy chains that assemble into a Y-shaped molecule. Each light chain is folded into two 12.5 kDa globular domains designated the V_L (variable region of the light chain) and the C_L (constant region of the light chain). Similarly, the heavy chain is folded into four 12.5 kDa globular domains: VH, C_H1, C_H2, and C_H3; C_H1 and C_H2 are separated by a short extended segment called the hinge region. The two heavy chains are associated through the hinge region and the C_H2 and C_H3 domains constitute the Fc (fragment that crystallizes or is constant) region of the molecule that mediates interaction with complement and phagocytes. Each light chain is paired with one heavy chain through interactions between the C_L and the C_H1 domains and the V_H and V_L domains. Together these form the Fab region which is the antigen-binding part of the antibody with the antigen-specific Hv regions presented at the ends of the arms of the Y.

The light chain consists of two 12.5 kDa globular domains: one near the end of the top of the Y called the V_L or variable region of the light chain and one near the neck of the Y (ie, the hinge) called the C_L or constant region of the light chain. The C_L is identical in sequence for all the antibodies of the same class and does not change with binding specificity. The sequence of the V_L varies among antibodies with different antigen-binding specificities. A close look at the light-chain amino acid sequences of a diverse selection of antibodies reveals that there are numerous sequence differences between any two V_L domains and that these differences are clustered in three segments called hypervariable (Hv) regions. The Hv regions fold in the finished molecule at the outermost end of the Fab arm creating part of a unique antigen-specific binding site. The heavy chain is constructed along similar lines; the V_H domain nearest to the outermost end of the Fab arm contains the three Hv regions that fold so that they form a continuous surface with the Hv regions of the V_L, making a composite surface that maximizes sequence diversity at the tips of the Fab arms. The heavy chain has three constant regions designated C_H1, C_H2, and C_H3. The C_H1 combines with the C_L completing the Fab; the hinge, C_H2, and C_H3 domains of two heavy chains align with each other to form the Fc.

Antibodies are custom-made, shape recognition molecules that can be selected to specifically bind to almost any antigen structural element of an invading pathogen, although proteins and carbohydrates predominate. B-cells produce the antibodies and each B-cell is committed to the production of a single type of antibody molecule, a key distinction from the innate system where each macrophage or neutrophil expresses many or all of the innate recognition molecules including TLR and receptors for multiple-complement products.

The diversity of the Hv regions, and consequently the range of structures that can be recognized, is based on two fascinating genetic mechanisms. First, V_H and V_L domains are created by the combinatorial assembly of multiple discrete genetic segments from an extensive repertoire of genomically-encoded V-region fragments during B-cell ontogeny in the bone marrow. Each B cell is committed to a single assembled V_H/V_L pair, which functions as the B-cell receptor (BCR). Importantly, B cells that assemble a BCR that recognize host factors in the bone marrow are killed off in a process call clonal deletion. Then further BCR specificity can be achieved via V_H and V_L targeted somatic hypermutation in the V-region genes under the influence of other adaptive system cells called T cells. This process, called affinity maturation, leads to the creation of antibodies that bind more tightly to their antigens.

3.2 Antibodies enhance the activity of innate immune effectors

The two main effectors of bactericidal activity of the innate immune system are complement and phagocytes. Antibodies augment the impact of each by increasing the number pathogen-specific antigens the immune system can target and they achieve this by cooperation with antibody-specific adapter molecules. We have already described the activation of complement by the alternative and mannose pathways; antibodies are the third way to focus the activity of complement onto a pathogen. Just as MBP is an adapter molecule that connects complement to mannose-rich structures on bacteria, so antibodies recruit complement through interaction with soluble complement factors, the first of which is called C1. C1 binds to the Fc regions of IgG when they are present in a closely-packed array as might be found when many are IgG molecules bound to the surface of a bacterium by their Fab arms. Just as Ehrlich's *Zwischenkörper* model predicts, the Fab provides the specificity while the Fc connects to the effector mechanisms.

The interaction of IgG, bacteria, and phagocytes is similar except that the adapter molecule is a receptor protein in the plasma membrane of the phagocyte. As in the case for complement C1, the receptor is specific for the Fc part of IgG, so it is called the Fc-receptor. Encountering IgG molecules densely arrayed on a bacterial surface a macrophage or neutrophil will ingest and destroy the bacterium.

3.3 For certain bacteria, antibodies alone can protect against infection

Many bacteria secrete toxins that promote infection by damaging host cells and causing severe pathology. Antibodies can be elicited that neutralize these toxins, reduce the tissue damage and allow the immune system to more readily defeat the invading pathogen. Well-known cases include pertussis, tetanus, and diphtheria [2].

3.4 There are multiple types or classes of antibodies

In addition to IgG antibodies, there are multiple other types of antibodies that differ in the constant regions and mediate other functions. Immunoglobulin M is the first antibody made in response to infection and a potent activator of complement; IgA antibodies are made primarily in response to mucosal infections; IgE antibodies are associated with worm infections and allergy.

3.5 The innate and adaptive immune systems are connected by specialized antigen-presenting cells called dendritic cells

Like mast cells and macrophages, immature dendritic cells are prepositioned in the tissues where they monitor and collect the array of antigens present in that vicinity. Upon stimulation by the presence of pathogens, they transform into antigen-presenting mature dendritic cells and migrate to lymph nodes or other secondary lymphoid tissues where they interact with T cells. Depending on the pathogen and the constellation of antigenic signals the dendritic cell has processed, naïve T cells will differentiate into one of several types: Th1 cells that stimulate macrophage activity, Th2 cells that stimulate B-cell activity, Th17 cells that promote neutrophil and osteoclast activity, or regulatory T cells (Treg) that limit potential immunological over-reaction.

3.6 Cells of the adaptive immune system interact by both secreted signals and direct cell-to-cell contact

Unlike the innate immune system, cells of the adaptive immune system communicate through a family of cell-surface receptors that incorporate and display peptide fragments of the pathogen. This will not be developed further here except to say that each B cell and each T cell expresses only one antigen receptor, which for B cells is a cell surface-bound antibody (BCR), and for T cells is the T-cell receptor (TCR). There are millions of T-cell and B-cell clones available, but only a tiny fraction of each type are likely to react with any given antigen during an immune response, in part due to the processes of negative selection and peripheral tolerance that eliminate autoreactive lymphocytes by inducing anergy and apoptosis. Uniting antigen-presenting dendritic cells with antigen-specific T cells and B cells requires a place where intensive sorting can occur until productive combinations are identified, resulting in the production of more antigen-specific cells and antigen-specific antibodies. Lymph nodes are the places where this sorting and selective growth of activated B cells and T cells occurs.

3.7 Adaptive immune system has memory

During an active infection, pathogen-specific B cells and T cells that have connected in the lymph node proliferate rapidly. Some of the daughter cells become immediately engaged in the ongoing immune response. For example, most B cells become the prodigious and short-lived producers of antibody molecules called plasma cells. However, a subpopulation enters the circulation and travels to other lymphoid tissues and the bone marrow, where they become long-lived memory B cells available for activation upon reinfection.

3.8 Harmonizing the discoveries of Ehrlich and Metchnikoff

Viewed through the lens of this chapter, we can see that Metchnikoff, the advocate of cellular immunology, and Ehrlich, the advocate of humoral immunology, each made crucially important observations about how immunity works in humans. In fact, they shared the Nobel Prize for Medicine in 1908 [3]. It is also clear that each was looking at a very limited aspect of the whole system. Ehrlich was focused on antibodies primarily in a disease, diphtheria, where most of the pathology was caused by a secreted toxin. The removal of the bacteria that secreted the toxin was invisible to him, and was probably performed by macrophages and neutrophils. Metchnikoff had discovered the role of phagocytes in many species including water fleas and starfish. He was observing innate immunity in action, and unaware of the opsonins that guided the ingestion of invading bacteria. Over a century later, we now have the privilege of understanding how elements of immunity, cellular and humoral, innate and adaptive, work together. A summary of the innate and adaptive immune systems is presented in **Table 2-1**.

4 Impaired immunity

Protection from infection by the immune system requires that each element works properly and interacts efficiently with the other elements. There are at least three classes of factors that impair the immune system leading to enhanced risk for bacterial infections.

First, some patients have primary immunodeficiencies in major elements of the immune system [1]. The most popularly known cases are the "bubble boys" who have X-linked severe combined immunodeficiency resulting from mutations in a gene essential for T-cell development. Lacking T cells, they have aberrant B-cell function and essentially no adaptive immunity. However, deficiencies in the central innate immune components, complement, and phagocytes also have severe consequences. For example, mutations in C3 or in the proteins that lead to its activation like MBL and C1 lead to increased risk of bacterial infections. Likewise, phagocyte deficiencies, notably severe congenital neutropenia which causes dramatic reductions in the abundance

Attribute	Innate	Adaptive
Response time	**Minutes to hours**	**Days to weeks**
Distribution vs centralization	Distributed, already positioned, with circulating cells in support	Centralized, circulating cells interact in lymph nodes and spleen
Range of specificities	Narrow	Vast
Principle structures recognized	PAMPs: mannans, cell-wall components, DNA	Peptidoglycan, proteins, capsule polysaccharides
Time of synthesis	Preexisting	Custom-made
Major cell types	Myeloid cells: • Macrophages • Neutrophils • Mast cells • Dendritic cells	Lymphocytes: • B cells • Th1 cells • Th2 cells • Th17 cells • Treg cells
Major cytokines	TNF-α IL-1 IL-6 IL-8 IFN-α	IL-2 IL-5 IL-6 IL-4 IL-10 IFN-γ
Major receptors	Complement receptors TLR Mannose-binding protein	T-cell receptors Membrane Ig (B-cell receptor) MHC I and II FcR
Memory	No	Yes, memory cells
Receptor distribution	Each effector cell possesses many receptors from a limited set	Each B cell or T cell expresses one antigen receptor; but a vast repertoire is expressed by the billions of cells
Effectors	Phagocytes Complement Natural killer cells	Phagocytes Complement Cytotoxic T cells

Table 2-1 Summary of the attributes of the innate and adaptive immune systems.
Abbreviations: PAMPs, pathogen-associated molecular patterns; TNF-α, tumor necrosis factor-α; IL, interleukin; IFN-α, interferon-α; MHC, major histocompatibility complex; FcR, Fc receptor; Treg, regulatory T cells.

of neutrophils, or chronic granulomatous disease which renders phagocytosis-competent macrophages and neutrophils incapable of killing internalized bacteria, and leaves patients vulnerable to frequent and severe bacterial infections.

Secondary or acquired immunodeficiencies are familiar primarily because of the prevalence of acquired immunodeficiency syndrome and human immunodeficiency virus, which eliminates essential T-cell populations. However, less dramatic but more common conditions, specifically type II diabetes mellitus and aging, may be more important factors in clinical practice. The precise mechanisms have not been fully determined, but these patients suffer increased frequency and persistence of bacterial infections [17, 18].

A third category of immune impairment is that caused by infecting pathogens. Many bacteria secrete products that directly alter the immune system. *Staphylococcus aureus*, a major cause of orthopedic infections, is a compelling example. It has developed an impressive array of secreted factors that interfere with essentially every major element of both innate and adaptive immunity. It secretes proteins that alter or inhibit the functions of T cells (secreted exotoxin A) [19], B cells (protein A) [20], neutrophils (α-hemolysin [21, 22], CHIPS), macrophages (adenosine synthase) [23], and complement (SCIN). In many patients, the immune response is minimally effective due to these immunosuppressive factors [24, 25]. Even though antibodies are made against these bacterial proteins, they are not generally protective, and prior infection frequently does not protect against reinfection even by the same strain of *S aureus* [26, 27].

5 Outlook

The immense growth of total joint replacement and other orthopedic implant surgeries, and its remarkable outcome in most patients, represent some of medicine's greatest success stories. However, there is always a dark side, and for total joint replacement and fracture fixation surgery that has been implant-associated infection, primarily with *S aureus*. The conventional clinical intervention has been the elaborate and extensive use of antibiotics, which frequently fails, necessitating surgical intervention and sometimes explantation. While these infections are infrequent, they are serious and expensive [28–31]. Thus, new approaches are being sought to reduce the frequency of infections and to provide clinicians with better therapeutic options when they occur.

One approach has been the development of surface treatments that will prevent the adhesion of bacteria thereby reducing the "foreign body" effect [32] and preventing the establishment of nascent infections [33–35]. These include toxic metals like silver, proteins that prevent bacterial adhesion, and immobilized antibiotics. Others include injectable, biodegradable hydrogels that can serve as long-term depots for antibiotics.

With the rising frequency of antibiotic-resistant microorganisms, many observers foresee a coming era of pathogen-specific therapeutics and associated diagnostics [36]. Some target the bacteria directly, such as lytic enzymes or bacteriophage [37–39]. There are at least three classes of immunological reagents that are currently under investigation. The first is passive vaccination with IgG antibodies selected to directly focus complement and phagocytes against the bacterium. Several attempts to achieve this have failed, and others remain under development [26, 40–44]. The second is analogous to the use of antibodies against diphtheria toxin, ie, passive immunization to reduce the impact of secreted toxins and enable the immune system to operate more effectively [21, 22]. A third approach is to bypass bacterium-derived immune inhibitors by providing the cytokines that the bacteria have evolved to suppress [45].

6 Conclusion

Bacterial infection remains a serious problem in orthopedics, particularly in association with implants. Our immune system is generally adequate to identify and eliminate most bacterial infections through innate and adaptive processes described briefly above and summarized in **Fig 2-1** and **Table 2-1**. However, some patients have an elevated risk for infection, including those with hereditary immunological disorders, and, more commonly, those with type II diabetes mellitus. Confronted with microorganisms that have evolved ways to thwart many of the elements of the innate or adaptive immune responses, some patients cannot overcome early infections and progress to chronic, sometimes life-threatening infections that require extensive therapy. Immunological interventions figure prominently in the spectrum of therapeutic concepts under development for these challenging infections.

7 References

1. **Murphy K.** *Janeway's Immunobiology.* 8th Edition. Garland Science, Taylor & Francis Group, LLC; 2012.
2. **Winau F, Winau R.** Emil von Behring and serum therapy. *Microbes Infect.* 2002 Feb;4(2):185–188.
3. **Silverstein AM.** Ilya Metchnikoff, the phagocytic theory, and how things often work in science. *J Leukoc Biol.* 2011 Sep;90(3):409–410.
4. **Choi KY, Chow LN, Mookherjee N.** Cationic host defence peptides: multifaceted role in immune modulation and inflammation. *J Innate Immun.* 2012;4(4):361–370.
5. **Kopfnagel V, Harder J, Werfel T.** Expression of antimicrobial peptides in atopic dermatitis and possible immunoregulatory functions. *Curr Opin Allergy Clin Immunol.* 2013 Oct;13(5):531–536.
6. **Fischer CL, Blanchette DR, Brogden KA, et al.** The roles of cutaneous lipids in host defense. *Biochim Biophys Acta.* 2014 Mar;1841(3):319–322.
7. **Helmberg A.** Immune System and Immunology. Available from: http://www.helmberg.at/immunology.htm. Accessed February, 2016.
8. **Hochreiter-Hufford A, Ravichandran KS.** Clearing the dead: apoptotic cell sensing, recognition, engulfment, and digestion. *Cold Spring Harb Perspect Biol.* 2013 Jan 1;5(1):a008748.
9. **Amulic B, Cazalet C, Hayes GL, et al.** Neutrophil function: from mechanisms to disease. *Annu Rev Immunol.* 2012;30:459–489.
10. **Remijsen Q, Kuijpers TW, Wirawan E, et al.** Dying for a cause: NETosis, mechanisms behind an antimicrobial cell death modality. *Cell Death Differ.* 2011 Apr;18(4):581–588.
11. **Yipp BG, Petri B, Salina D, et al.** Infection-induced NETosis is a dynamic process involving neutrophil multitasking in vivo. *Nat Med.* 2012 Sep;18(9):1386–1393.
12. **O'Neill LA, Golenbock D, Bowie AG.** The history of Toll-like receptors - redefining innate immunity. *Nat Rev Immunol.* 2013 Jun;13(6):453–460.
13. **Alvarez-Lobos M, Arostegui JI, Sans M, et al.** Crohn's disease patients carrying Nod2/CARD15 gene variants have an increased and early need for first surgery due to stricturing disease and higher rate of surgical recurrence. *Ann Surg.* 2005 Nov;242(5):693–700.
14. **Laghi L, Costa S, Saibeni S, et al.** Carriage of CARD15 variants and smoking as risk factors for resective surgery in patients with Crohn's ileal disease. *Aliment Pharmacol Ther.* 2005 Sep 15;22(6):557–564.
15. **Ip WK, Takahashi K, Ezekowitz RA, et al.** Mannose-binding lectin and innate immunity. *Immunol Rev.* 2009 Jul;230(1):9–21.
16. **Prüll CR.** Part of a scientific master plan? Paul Ehrlich and the origins of his receptor concept. *Med Hist.* 2003 Jul;47(3):332–356.
17. **Geerlings SE, Hoepelman AI.** Immune dysfunction in patients with diabetes mellitus (DM). *FEMS Immunol Med Microbiol.* 1999 Dec;26(3-4):259–265.
18. **Lecube A, Pachón G, Petriz J, et al.** Phagocytic activity is impaired in type 2 diabetes mellitus and increases after metabolic improvement. *PLoS One.* 2011;6(8):e23366.
19. **Salgado-Pabón W, Breshears L, Spaulding AR, et al.** Superantigens are critical for Staphylococcus aureus infective endocarditis, sepsis, and acute kidney injury. *MBio.* 2013; Aug 20;4(4).
20. **Falugi F, Kim HK, Missiakas DM, et al.** Role of protein A in the evasion of host adaptive immune responses by Staphylococcus aureus. *MBio.* 2013; Aug 27;4(5):e00575–00513.
21. **Tkaczyk C, Hamilton MM, Datta V, et al.** Staphylococcus aureus alpha toxin suppresses effective innate and adaptive immune responses in a murine dermonecrosis model. *PLoS One.* 2013; Oct 2;8(10):e75103.
22. **Tkaczyk C, Hua L, Varkey R, et al.** Identification of anti-alpha toxin monoclonal antibodies that reduce the severity of Staphylococcus aureus dermonecrosis and exhibit a correlation between affinity and potency. *Clin Vaccine Immunol.* 2012 Mar;19(3):377–385.
23. **Thammavongsa V, Kern JW, Missiakas DM, et al.** Staphylococcus aureus synthesizes adenosine to escape host immune responses. *J Exp Med.* 2009 Oct 26;206(11):2417–2427.

24. **Proctor RA.** Challenges for a universal Staphylococcus aureus vaccine. *Clin Infect Dis.* 2012 Apr;54(8):1179–1186.
25. **Spellberg B, Daum R.** Development of a vaccine against Staphylococcus aureus. *Semin Immunopathol.* 2012 Mar;34(2):335–348.
26. **Bröker BM, Holtfreter S, Bekeredjian-Ding I.** Immune control of Staphylococcus aureus - regulation and counter-regulation of the adaptive immune response. *Int J Med Microbiol.* 2014 Mar;304(2):204–214.
27. **Bröker BM, van Belkum A.** Immune proteomics of Staphylococcus aureus. *Proteomics.* 2011 Aug;11(15):3221–3231.
28. **Klevens RM, Morrison MA, Nadle J, et al.** Invasive methicillin-resistant Staphylococcus aureus infections in the United States. *JAMA.* 2007 Oct 17;298(15):1763–1771.
29. **Kurtz S, Ong K, Lau E, et al.** Projections of primary and revision hip and knee arthroplasty in the United States from 2005 to 2030. *J Bone Joint Surg Am.* 2007 Apr;89(4):780–785.
30. **Ong KL, Kurtz SM, Lau E, et al.** Prosthetic joint infection risk after total hip arthroplasty in the Medicare population. *J Arthroplasty.* 2009 Sep;24(6 Suppl):105–109.
31. **Parvizi J, Azzam K, Ghanem E, et al.** Periprosthetic infection due to resistant staphylococci: serious problems on the horizon. *Clin Orthop Relat Res.* 2009 Jul;467(7):1732–1739.
32. **Elek SD.** Experimental staphylococcal infections in the skin of man. *Ann N Y Acad Sci.* 1956 Aug 31;65(3):85–90.
33. **Ciampolini J, Harding KG.** Pathophysiology of chronic bacterial osteomyelitis. Why do antibiotics fail so often? *Postgrad Med J.* 2000 Aug;76(898):479–483.
34. **Ribeiro M, Monteiro FJ, Ferraz MP.** Infection of orthopedic implants with emphasis on bacterial adhesion process and techniques used in studying bacterial-material interactions. *Biomatter.* 2012 Oct-Dec;2(4):176–194.
35. **Zimmerli W, Lew PD, Waldvogel FA.** Pathogenesis of foreign body infection. Evidence for a local granulocyte defect. *J Clin Invest.* 1984 Apr;73(4):1191–1200.
36 **Centers from Disease Control and Prevention.** Antibiotic Resistance Threats in the United States, 2013. Centers for Disease Control and Prevention [Internet]. 2013 Sept 16. Available from http://www.cdc.gov/drugresistance/threat-report-2013/. Accessed February, 2016.
37. **Becker SC, Dong S, Baker JR, et al.** LysK CHAP endopeptidase domain is required for lysis of live staphylococcal cells. *FEMS Microbiol Lett.* 2009 May;294(1):52–60.
38. **Becker SC, Foster-Frey J, Donovan DM.** The phage K lytic enzyme LysK and lysostaphin act synergistically to kill MRSA. *FEMS Microbiol Lett.* 2008 Oct;287(2):185–191.
39. **Fenton M, Ross P, McAuliffe O, et al.** Recombinant bacteriophage lysins as antibacterials. *Bioeng Bugs.* 2010 Jan-Feb;1(1):9–16.
40. **Fowler VG, Jr.**, Proctor RA. Where does a Staphylococcus aureus vaccine stand? *Clin Microbiol Infect.* 2014 May;20 Suppl 5:66–75.
41. **Kim HK, Missiakas D, Schneewind O.** Mouse models for infectious diseases caused by Staphylococcus aureus. *J Immunol Methods.* 2014 Aug,410:88–99.
42. **Otto M.** Targeted immunotherapy for staphylococcal infections: focus on anti-MSCRAMM antibodies. *BioDrugs.* 2008;22(1):27–36.
43. **Proctor RA.** Is there a future for a Staphylococcus aureus vaccine? *Vaccine.* 2012 Apr 19;30(19):2921–2927.
44. **Projan SJ, Nesin M, Dunman PM.** Staphylococcal vaccines and immunotherapy: to dream the impossible dream? *Curr Opin Pharmacol.* 2006 Oct;6(5):473–479.
45. **Liu Y, Egilmez NK, Russell MW.** Enhancement of adaptive immunity to Neisseria gonorrhoeae by local intravaginal administration of microencapsulated interleukin 12. *J Infect Dis.* 2013 Dec 1;208(11):1821–1829.

3 Microbiology

Virginia Post, R Geoff Richards, T Fintan Moriarty

1 Basics

The confirmed presence of viable bacteria in any intraoperative tissue specimen is a critical point in the treatment of orthopedic patients. Culture-positive biopsies define the course of treatment for the patient, and it is therefore vitally important that culture results are available rapidly and are reliable [1, 2]. Inadvertent contamination of tissue biopsies may divert the treatment path and compromise patient care. One of the most crucial issues in the microbiological diagnosis of a bone infection, therefore, is to differentiate infecting pathogens from innocuous contaminants. By definition, infection is described as the invasion and multiplication of bacteria within a tissue, while contamination is the presence of bacteria in a sample but does not imply an invasive infection. The most common sources of contamination of intraoperative samples are from unfiltered air, skin flakes, or unsterile sample handling. Unfortunately, the microbiological laboratory is unable to differentiate with any certainty contaminants from infecting bacteria. This is primarily due to the fact that many of the microorganisms commonly associated with bone infections are also readily cultured from personnel and materials in the operating room and the laboratory.

The bacteria most commonly isolated from bone and joint infections are shown in **Fig 3-1**. These bacterial species are not considered professional pathogens, and all are regularly present in the normal human microbiome or ubiquitous inhabitants of the environment. The natural habitat of bacteria varies depending upon the species, although many of the most common microorganisms, such as *Staphylococcus aureus* and *Staphylococcus epidermidis*, are commonly present on human skin. In fact, *S epidermidis* is ubiquitously present on the human skin and resides there commensally, ie, without any interference in the normal healthy skin. Approximately 30% of the human population also harbor *S aureus*, which is the most prominent and possibly most virulent pathogen encountered in bone and joint infections [1].

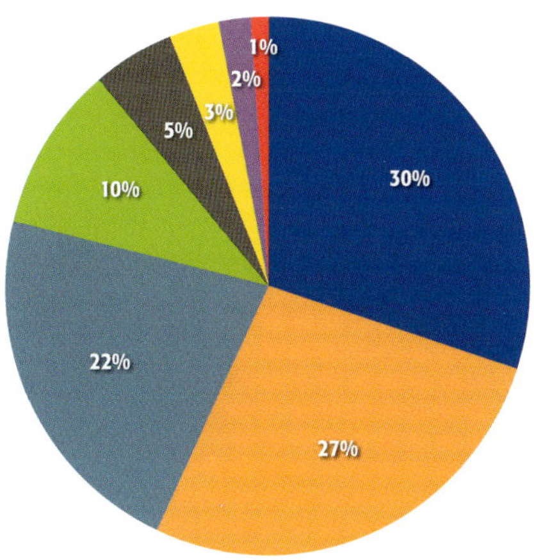

Microorganism	Frequency (%)
Staphylococcus aureus	30
Polymicrobial	27
Coagulase-negative staphylococci	22
Gram-negative bacilli	10
Anaerobes	5
Enterococci	3
Unknown	2
Streptococci	1

Fig 3-1 Prevalence of bacterial pathogens in bone and joint infections [1].

Staphylococcus aureus may also reside commensally on human skin but is also capable of causing skin infections in otherwise healthy individuals. Other potential pathogens are also commonly present on or in the human body: *Propionibacterium acnes* colonizes the human skin (particularly moist areas such as the armpit); enterococci (*Enterococcus faecalis* and *Enterococcus faecium*) and *Escherichia coli* are normally found in the gastrointestinal tract; and numerous streptococci may be found in the human oral cavity and respiratory tract. Many other potential pathogens may be found in the environment, including *Pseudomonas aeruginosa*, which is commonly found in water systems and many of the more rarely encountered species such as *Acinetobacter baumannii*, mycobacteria, and *Candida albicans*.

Each of these bacterial species poses a unique combination of challenges to treating physicians including the clinical presentation of the disease, the bacteriological culture conditions required to recover the responsible pathogens, and the antibiotics that may be effective against them. The aim of this chapter is to provide an overview of the most critical features that define the most common pathogens in bone infection.

1.1 Virulence and pathogenicity

In the terminology of bacterial infection, pathogenicity is a term that describes the ability of a microorganism to cause a disease in a host organism. The mechanisms or tools used by a pathogen to do so are termed its virulence factors. The reason only a limited number of bacterial species regularly appear in bone infection patients is due to the fact that only those bacteria possess sufficient virulence factors enabling them to evade one or more of the host defenses to establish an infection. The most significant virulence factors include biofilm formation, adhesion to host-tissue components in a specific (ie, nonrandom) manner and inactivation of host defense molecules such as antibodies, or host defense cells such as polymorphonuclear neutrophils. In the absence of a skin breach, infection of the underlying tissue by opportunistic pathogens that lack potent virulence factors is unlikely. However, low-virulence microorganisms may be afforded assistance in establishing an infection by the surgical incision and placement of an implant as occurs in trauma and orthopedic surgery. Many bacteria retain the ability to adhere and attach to the surface of implanted materials, which provides a surface to which the bacteria attach or adhere. Once adherent on the implanted device, many bacteria will rapidly form a complex biofilm (**Fig 3-2**) and also adapt their metabolism and gene expression profile to take advantage of the protection offered by this inanimate object in the host. In this way, low-virulence microorganisms may gain entry to the deep tissues and successfully establish infection.

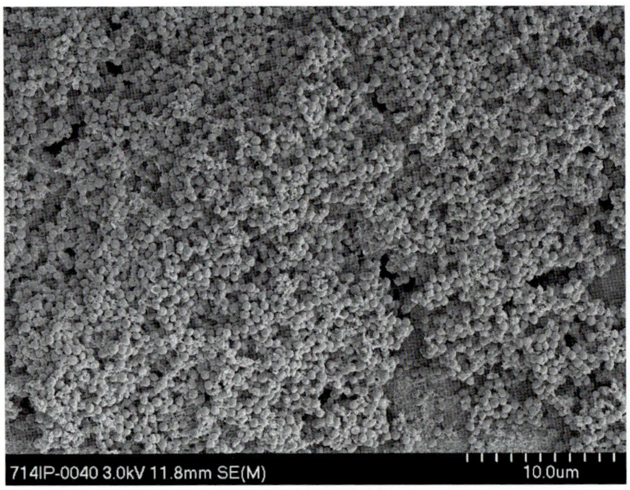

Fig 3-2 Bacterial biofilm formed by *Staphylococcus aureus* on the surface of a titanium substrate. In this mode of growth, bacteria are much more resistant to antibiotics and host defenses.

The clinical presentation of any particular patient with a bone infection may range from an acute infection characterized by swelling, pus formation, and pain at one end of the spectrum, to a subtle, subclinical, and pain-free infection at the other end. The variability in clinical presentation results from a combination of the host response and the virulence of the infecting bacteria. The extent to which bacterial virulence may influence the presentation of an infection is probably best illustrated by comparing *S aureus* and *S epidermidis*. On a genetic basis, these two species belong to the same genus and considerable genetic information is shared between the species. However, *S aureus* has acquired a significant amount of additional genetic information that has endowed it with many more virulence factors, including one of the definitive tests for *S aureus*: coagulase (**Fig 3-3**). The ability to coagulate human plasma, for example, is believed to enable the bacteria to avoid phagocytosis at the center of the plasma "clot". Such virulence factors allow *S aureus* to cause, in most cases, an acute infection. In contrast, *S epidermidis* has not acquired these virulence factors and is typically unable to induce an aggressive acute infection.

The primary reason *S epidermidis* is capable of causing an infection is primarily due to biofilm formation. Due to its ability to rapidly form dense biofilms and its ubiquitous presence on human skin, *S epidermidis* has emerged as an important opportunistic pathogen in device-related bone infections. Other than biofilm formation, *S epidermidis* does not retain many virulence factors, which accounts for the typical appearance of a subacute or chronic infection, lacking in the aggressive features associated with *S aureus* infection. A similar finding has been observed for *P acnes*, another ubiquitous skin colonizer, which can cause bone destruction and retains some virulence factors, but which typically causes a localized infection without an aggressive systemic response. These generalizations often hold true, although exceptions to the rules are of course possible. Deviations from this standard manifestation may be largely explained by the variability in host response to the infection.

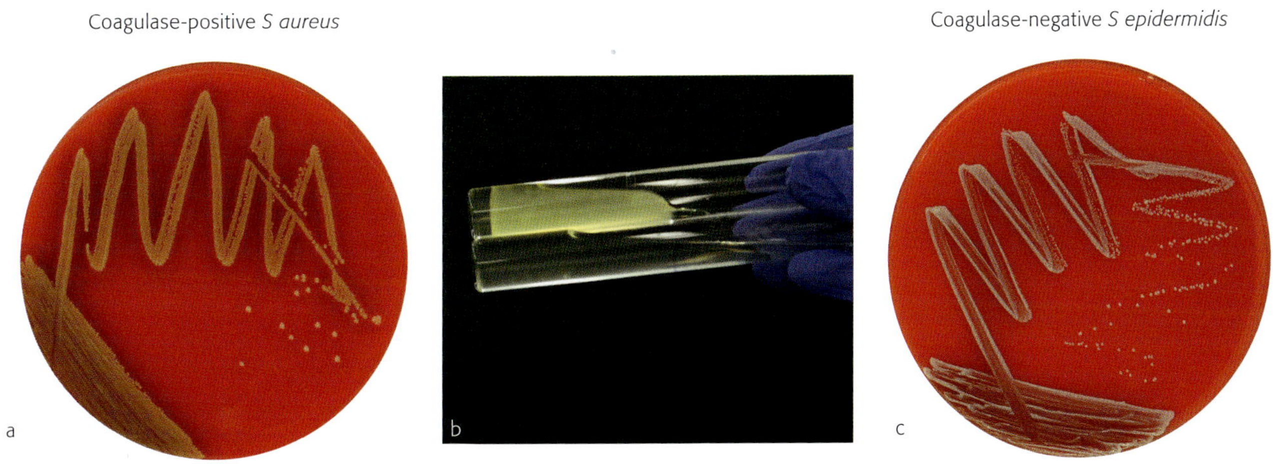

Fig 3-3a–c Differentiation between two related staphylococci: *Staphylococcus aureus* and *Staphylococcus epidermidis*. Colonies of *S aureus* appear yellow (**a**), and those of *S epidermidis* are typically smaller and whiter in color (**c**). Coagulase is produced by *S aureus* leading to coagulation of human plasma (upper tube, (**b**)). Coagulation is believed to assist these bacteria in avoiding the host defense mechanisms such as phagocytosis. *Staphylococcus epidermidis*, on the other hand, is coagulase negative and is unable to coagulate human plasma (lower tube (**b**)).

1.2 Endogenous and exogenous infections

Identifying the source of the infecting bacteria and the means through which the bacteria arrived at the site of infection is often an impossible task. Determining the source of the bacteria is not necessary to perform an identification or diagnosis, although an understanding of this concept is important. In general terms, the infecting bacteria are considered to arrive at the site of infection via one of two proposed means: either from an endogenous source (ie, a source from within the host and is normally considered to involve hematogenous spread as may occur during bacteremia) or an exogenous source (ie, via iatrogenic inoculation during surgery). This concept is clearly described by Trampuz and colleagues who have provided extensive description in the published literature [1]. According to this classification, endogenous infections typically include arthritis, spondylodiscitis, or prosthetic joint infection with a hematogenous source of bacteria. Since there is no requirement for a surgical incision, or necessarily an implant, these infections usually require a virulent pathogen to create the infection, and therefore often result in an acute infection. Exogenous infections, on the other hand, may be caused by low-virulence organisms, as already described, or more virulent organisms that happen to be present at the wound or introduced during the wound-healing process. As such, these infections may be either acute or subacute/chronic in nature.

1.3 Resistant microbes

Bacterial resistance to antibiotics is one of the most challenging aspects of treating bone infection. Numerous factors may account for bacterial resistance to antibiotics (**Table 3-1**). The majority of antibiotic agents on the market were originally purified from soil bacteria that evolved to produce these antibiotics to compete with other bacterial species for food or other resources. As such, many bacterial populations have coevolved with these bacteria and attained mechanisms of resistance to these antibiotics. An example is the intrinsic resistance of enterococci to β-lactam antibiotics due to the fact that enterococci modify the proteins to which penicillin binds [3]. A second means of achieving antibiotic resistance is by acquiring the genetic information required to resist an antibiotic. A small number of genes may confer the genetic information required to resist some antibiotics, and it has emerged that many of these small collections of genes may be easily shared between different bacterial species. A prominent example of such an acquired resistance mechanism is the spread of methicillin resistance amongst staphylococci. The genes necessary for methicillin resistance are carried on a mobile genetic element named the staphylococcal cassette chromosome "mec". This "package" of DNA is thought to have originated in *S epidermidis*, was transferred to *S aureus*, and has since emerged as a primary pathogen of global significance, including as a pathogen in bone infection. A somewhat similar story has been described for the emergence of vancomycin resistance in the enterococci [4].

Resistance feature	Example species	Antibiotic	Reference
Intrinsic resistance	Enterococci	β-lactam	[3]
Altered metabolism	*Escherichia coli*	Penicillin	[5]
Reduced penetration	*Pseudomonas aeruginosa* biofilm	Tobramycin	[6]
Intracellular survival	Staphylococci	Gentamicin	[7]
Small-colony variants	Staphylococci	Gentamicin	[8]

Table 3-1 Resistance mechanisms of bacteria*.
*Selected and simplified examples: the same feature may be valid for other bacterial species and other antibiotics.

Another important means of resisting antibiotic therapy is via growth as a biofilm. Bacterial biofilms have been described to resist antibiotic concentrations over 1,000 times higher than that described for nonbiofilm-growing (so-called planktonic or free floating) bacteria. This antibiotic resistance may be due to one or more reasons, which is discussed in more detail in chapter 1 Implant-associated biofilm. In brief, biofilm growth offers bacteria protection against antibiotics by features such as reduced metabolic activity within the biofilm, reduced penetration of antibiotics due to the extracellular polymeric substances that surround the bacterial cell, and the generation of phenotypically distinct populations with distinct metabolic activity with the biofilm [9]. Different species may exploit these different features to a different extent, and, importantly, various antibiotics will be more, or less, affected by these features than others. For example, penicillins are only active against metabolically active cells since the target of the penicillins is the synthesis of macromolecules. In a biofilm, where the synthesis of such macromolecules may be extremely low, such antibiotics will not have any activity. It should be noted that there are some antibiotics with activity against biofilm, ie, rifampin against gram-positive biofilms, and quinolones against gram-negative biofilms.

Intracellular survival of bacteria has relatively recently emerged as a potential means of resisting antibiotic therapy in bone infections. Although generally considered extracellular pathogens, the staphylococci have been described and shown to be internalized within osteoblasts, where they may survive, multiply, and eventually kill osteoblasts [10]. This can indirectly lead to antibiotic resistance, or perhaps may be better described as an antibiotic avoidance strategy as many of the antibiotics used to treat infections do not penetrate inside human cells. For example, gentamicin is one of the most widely used antibiotics in local delivery using bone cement. However, this antibiotic is unable to penetrate human cells unless exceedingly high local concentrations are achieved. Therefore, any tissue-resident bacteria may be protected from gentamicin activity by virtue of their localization inside a host cell.

A final group of bacteria that display increased resistance to antibiotics are the small-colony variants (SCVs) [8]. Small-colony variants are bacteria that display altered phenotype of small, slow-growing colonies and have been described most often for staphylococci but are also described for *P aeruginosa*, *E coli*, and salmonella species. Due to the slow growing nature and atypical appearance, SCVs may be overlooked in the clinical microbiology lab. Small-colony variants also pose further treatment challenges as they typically display resistance against quite a wide range of antibiotics and also display intracellular survival. The prevalence of SCVs may be increased in device-associated infections after failed antibiotic therapy, but true incidence is likely underestimated due to the difficulty in culturing and identifying SCVs.

1.4 Diagnosis

Isolation and culture followed by antibiotic susceptibility testing are the core functions of the microbiology laboratory. The gold standard in diagnosis is still bacterial culture, and antibiotic susceptibility testing is also required to ensure an appropriate therapy is selected.

Under most circumstances, bacterial species commonly implicated in bone infections grow quite well on the conventional agars. Certain bacterial species require particular culture conditions to be met in order to grow in the lab. The most obvious is the requirement for extended culture time for slow-growing microorganisms (eg, SCVs) [11] and anaerobic or microaerophilic conditions (eg, for *P acnes*) [12]. A growing body of evidence is now emerging in the research literature indicating that bacteria growing within a biofilm may not be culturable by conventional means, but presence is confirmed by modern molecular methods such as polymerase chain reaction (PCR) and fluorescent in situ hybridization (FISH) [13, 14]. These modern techniques are not routinely available in clinical hospitals, but this observation may explain the rather high rate of culture-negative infections observed in many clinical studies. Further details of the procedures for microbiological diagnoses will be described in chapter 7 Diagnostics.

2 Microorganism profiles

The following section will describe the basic features of a range of the most commonly encountered bacteria causing bone infections. The bacteria will be grouped based upon gram staining character (**Fig 3-4**), aerobic or anaerobic respiration, and a brief mention will be given to fungi and mycobacteria, which are less frequently encountered, but pose unique challenges for successful treatment.

2.1 Gram-positive bacteria

Gram-positive bacteria in general contain a thick layer of peptidoglycan in the cell wall that encases the cell membrane (**Fig 3-4**). This thick layer retains the crystal violet that forms part of the gram staining procedure. Since these bacteria retain the stain, they are described as gram positive. Prominent gram-positive bacteria include staphylococci, streptococci, and enterococci.

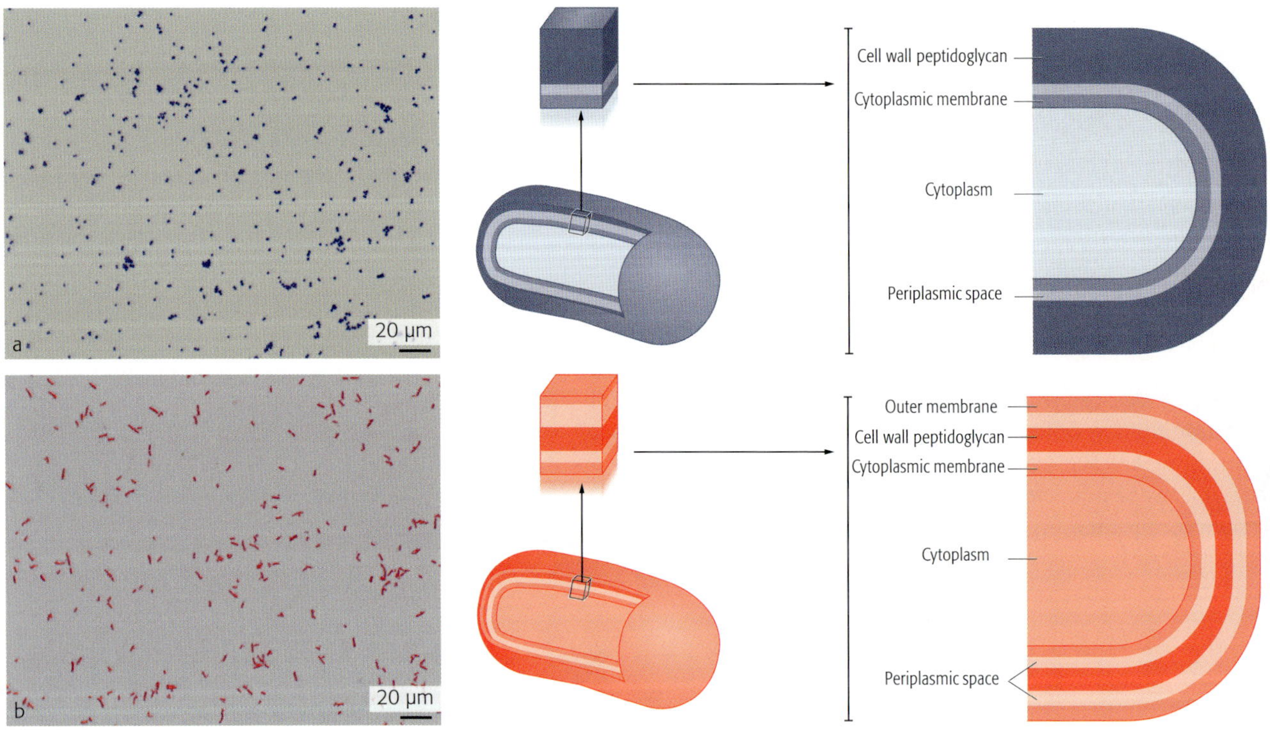

Fig 3-4a–b Gram-positive (**a**) and gram-negative (**b**) bacterial cell walls.
The difference in cell wall structure accounts for the difference in cell staining which either retains crystal violet and is blue (**a**) or loses the stain and is counterstained red (**b**).

2.1.1 Staphylococci

Morphology: Gram-positive cocci (spherical cells); cell division occurs along multiple axes and thus form grape-like clusters in planktonic growth; small white to yellow circular colonies on conventional agars (**Fig 3-5**).

Habitat: Skin and mucosa (*S epidermidis* 100%, *S aureus* 30%).

Prominent members: *S epidermidis; S aureus; Staphylococcus lugdunensis.*

Identification and differentiation: Differentiation may be assisted by the coagulase reaction. Coagulase is an enzyme that enables the conversion of fibrinogen to fibrin resulting in blood clotting. The enzyme is considered to facilitate infection by protecting the bacteria from phagocytosis. *Staphylococcus aureus* possesses this enzyme and is thus a coagulase-positive staphylococcus. *Staphylococcus epidermidis* does not possess this enzyme and is thus known as a coagulase-negative staphylococcus.

Characteristics: *S aureus* is one of the most common opportunistic pathogens, and can cause relatively simple skin infections, but also life-threatening sepsis and endocarditis. As a more virulent pathogen, *S aureus* may cause early infections after placement of a device, or late hematogenous, acute infections, or primary nonimplant-related osteomyelitis [1].

Most non-*S aureus* staphylococcal infections are caused by the coagulase-negative staphylococci (CoNS) in particular *S epidermidis*. As low-virulence microorganisms, the CoNS may historically have been considered contaminants in intraoperative biopsies. The CoNS are highly likely contaminants if biopsies are not taken in an aseptic manner, however, there is now widespread acknowledgment that the CoNS are responsible for a significant proportion of implant- related infections. As low-virulence microorganisms, the CoNS typically cause late developing subacute infections and are thus amongst the most challenging to diagnose.

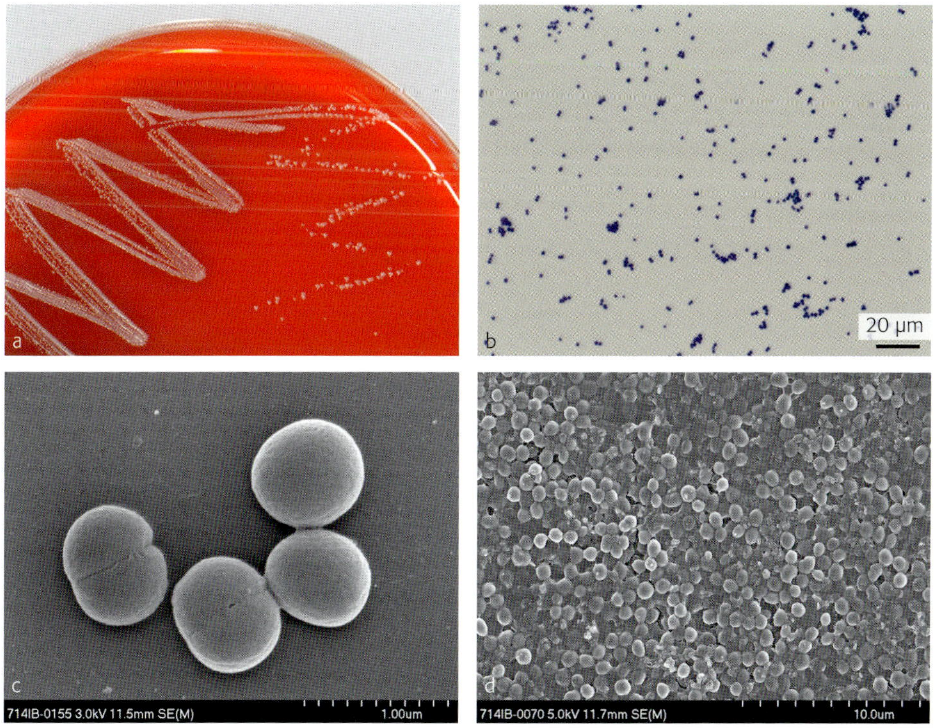

Fig 3-5a–d *Staphylococcus epidermidis.*

a *Staphylococcus epidermidis* forms small white colonies on blood agar.

b–c It is a gram-positive coccoid cell (**b**) and tends to form small clusters due to cell division along two axes (**c**).

d *Staphylococcus epidermidis* readily forms biofilms, which is its primary virulence mechanism.

Biofilm formation is the primary virulence factor of CoNS and they are amongst the most prolific biofilm forming bacteria across medical specialties, not only in orthopedics and traumatology.

Another CoNS worthy of mention is *S lugdunensis*, which is a rather unusual CoNS in that it retains quite a repertoire of virulence factors enabling it to cause infections more resembling an acute *S aureus* infection than a subclinical stereotype infection of a CoNS.

Most staphylococci are capable of forming a biofilm, and when growing as biofilm, these bacteria do not respond to antibiotic therapy. New antimicrobials targeting staphylococcal biofilms are investigated, however, at present, rifampin is the only antibiotic with significant antibiofilm activity. Rifampin should be only used in the proper clinical context and always in combination with another antibiotic to minimize the risk of developing rifampin resistance. Antibiotic selection for different bacterial pathogens will be fully discussed in chapter 5 Systemic antibiotics.

2.1.2 Streptococci

Morphology: Gram-positive cocci, cell division occurs along a single axis and thus often occur as chains or pairs of cells (**Fig 3-6**).

Habitat: Normal flora of gastrointestinal tract and mucosa.

Prominent members: *Streptococcus agalactiae; Streptococcus pyogenes; Streptococcus pneumoniae; Streptococcus viridans.*

Identification and differentiation: Streptococci can be differentiated based upon their hemolytic activity on sheep-blood agar plates. Alpha (α)-streptococci result in incomplete hemolysis leading to a green coloration on agar plates. Beta (β)-hemolysis, which is a complete hemolysis, leads to a complete lysis of red blood cells and clear zone of hemolysis on agar plates. Finally, gamma (γ)-hemolysis is in fact a lack of hemolysis.

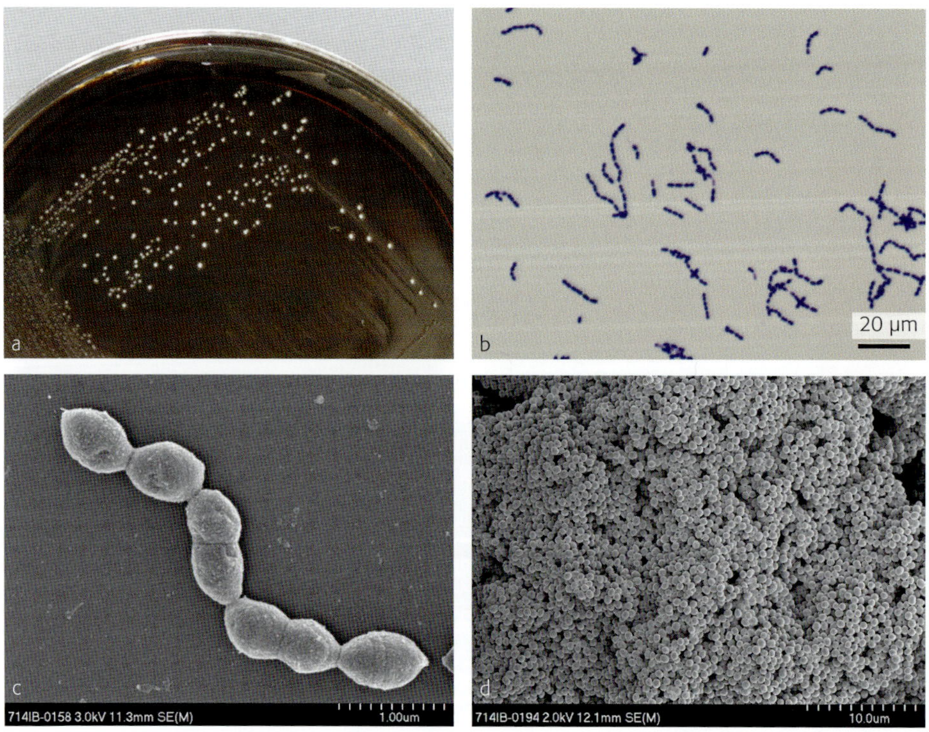

Fig 3-6a–d *Streptococcus* species.
a *Streptococcus mutans* growing on blood agar.
b–c Streptococci usually divide in a single axis and thus appear as long chains of gram-positive cocci (**b**).
d Streptococci also are capable of forming biofilm.

Characteristics: β-hemolytic streptococci can be subdivided into so-called Lancefield groups (A–G) based on the carbohydrate composition in their cell walls. In general, streptococcal bone and joint infections respond well to treatment, although large-scale studies focused on this pathogen are needed [15]. Streptococci are capable of biofilm formation, which is particularly well described in dental applications, where these streptococcal biofilms are implicated in dental caries.

2.1.3 Enterococci

Morphology: Gram-positive cocci growing in pairs or short chains. Cocci may elongate under certain growth conditions to a coccobacillus structure (**Fig 3-7**).

Habitat: Normal flora of the gastrointestinal tract.

Prominent members: Most clinically relevant species is *E faecalis* followed by the less prevalent *E faecium*.

Identification and differentiation: Enterococci are catalase-negative and α-hemolytic.

Characteristics: Enterococci are robust bacteria capable of surviving relatively extreme environmental conditions (temperature, pH, osmolality). Enterococci are capable of forming biofilm and their tendency to display significant intrinsic and acquired antibiotic resistance makes them particularly challenging to treat [16]. Vancomycin-resistant enterococci (VRE) have emerged, rendering treatment options for these pathogens extremely limited.

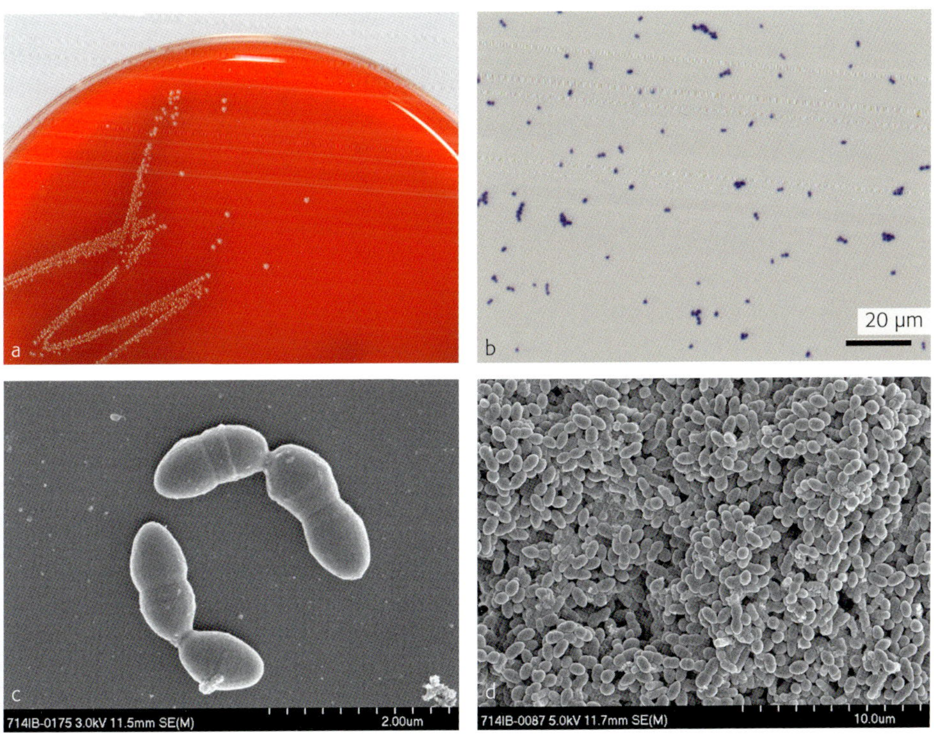

Fig 3-7a–d Enterococci.
a Enterococci such as *Enterococcus faecalis* form small white colonies on blood agar.
b–c They are usually seen as pairs or short chains of gram-positive bacteria (**b**). The cells are usually coccoid, but tend to display an elongated structure (**b**, **c**).
d Enterococci also develop biofilms.

2.1.4 *Bacillus* species

Morphology: Gram-positive, rod-shaped, endospore-producing bacteria (**Fig 3-8**).

Habitat: Widespread in nature.

Prominent members: *Bacillus subtilis*; *Bacillus anthracis*; *Bacillus cereus*.

Identification and differentiation: *Bacillus* species (spp.) can be obligate aerobes or facultative anaerobes. *Bacillus* includes both free-living (nonparasitic) and parasitic pathogenic species. Under stressful environmental conditions, the bacteria can produce oval endospores. These characteristics originally defined the genus.

Characteristics: Due to their widespread prevalence in nature, Bacillus spp. can sometimes be detected in open wounds and may be responsible for infection of open fractures.

2.2 Gram-negative bacteria

In contrast to gram-positive bacteria, gram-negative bacteria in general possess a cytoplasmic membrane and an outer cell membrane, and only a thin peptidoglycan layer that which lies between these membranes. This structure does not retain crystal violet in the Gram stain and so stains gram negative (**Fig 3-4**).

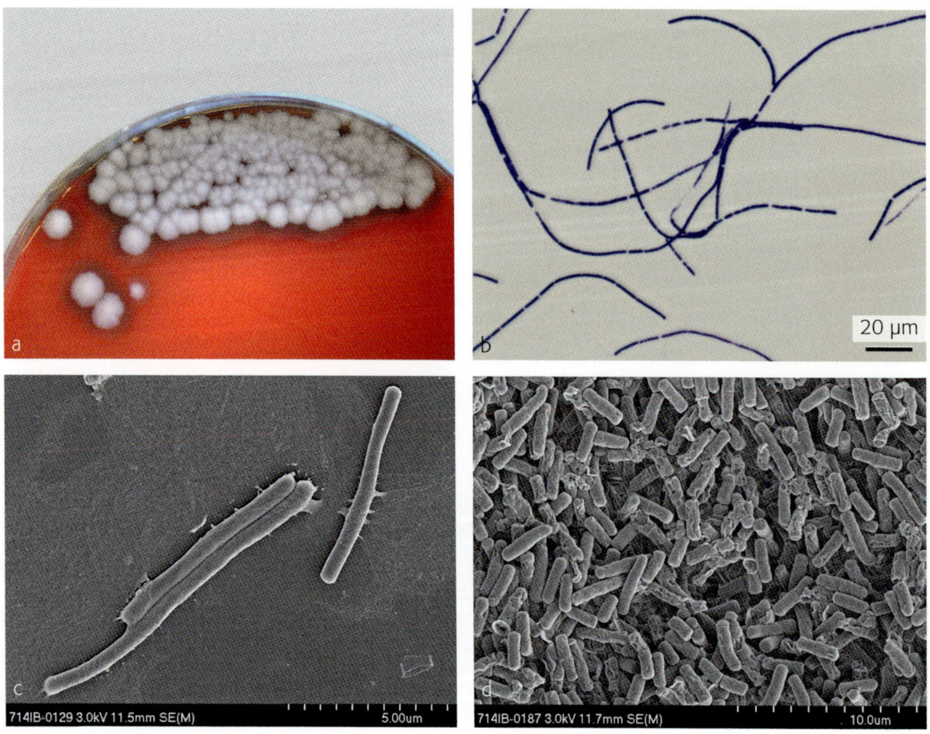

Fig 3-8a–d *Bacillus* species.
a *Bacillus cereus* on sheep blood agar plates are typically large spreading colonies.
b–c Gram staining shows a gram-positive rod that often forms longer series of cells (**b**).
d *Bacillus* species readily forms biofilms.

2.2.1 Enterobacteria

Morphology: Gram-negative rods (**Fig 3-9**).

Habitat: Mainly normal gut flora. Enterobacteria can colonize open wounds and can cause nosocomial infections.

Prominent members: *Escherichia coli, Klebsiella spp., Proteus spp., Enterobacter spp., Citrobacter spp., Serratia spp., Morganella spp.*, and *Salmonella spp.*

Identification and differentiation: Enterobacteria appear as small grey colonies on blood agar and generally lack cytochrome C oxidase. On a chromogenic medium to aid differentiation between *E coli* and other coliforms in cultures, *E coli* can be differentiated from other coliforms. The β-galactosidase and β-glucuronidase activity of *E coli* results in purple colonies with other coliforms giving pink colonies.

Characteristics: Enterobacteria show different susceptibility against antibiotics, and the presence of different β-lactamases can lead to significant antibiotic resistance. Extended-spectrum β-lactamase (ESBL) are β-lactamases that can inactivate third- and fourth-generation cephalosporins. They can commonly be found in *E coli, Klebsiella pneumonia*, and *Klebsiella oxytoca* but also sometimes in other enterobacteria.

Enterobacteria can grow and form biofilm on implants. In vitro studies have shown that using quinolones are the most effective way to eradicate enterobacteria in biofilms, eg, ciprofloxacin. Ciprofloxacin-resistant enterobacterial infections with implanted hardware are a significant clinical challenge and may require removal of the implant [17].

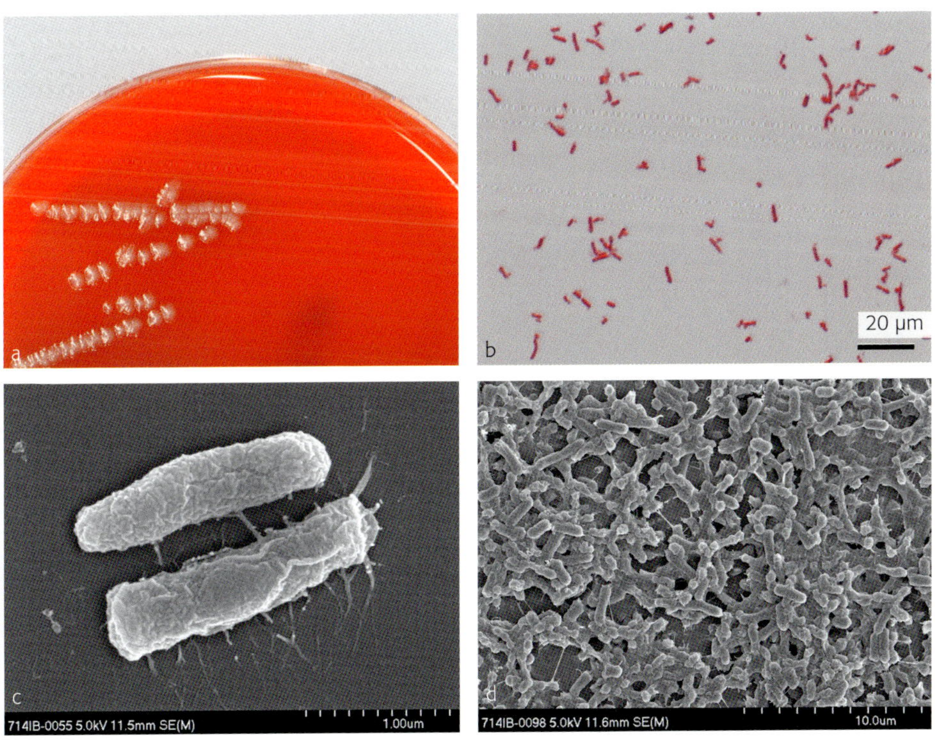

Fig 3-9a–d Enterobacteria.
- **a** Enterobacteria such as *Escherichia coli* may form medium to large colonies on blood agar.
- **b** They are consistently gram negative.
- **c** The cells appear as rods.
- **d** Enterobacteria also develop biofilms.

2.2.2 *Pseudomonas aeruginosa*

Morphology: Gram-negative rods (**Fig 3-10**).

Habitat: Soil, water, and skin flora; colonizes natural and artificial environments, open wounds, lungs, urinary tract, and kidneys. Prominent agent of nosocomial infections.

Identification and differentiation: *P aeruginosa* forms large grey/green colonies on blood agar.

Characteristics: *P aeruginosa* is naturally resistant to many antibiotics. Since it is a strong biofilm former, treatment of resistant strains is a challenge, particularly for implant-related infections.

2.3 Anaerobic bacteria

Anaerobic bacteria are bacteria that do not require oxygen for respiration. Anaerobic microorganisms present challenges to the microbiology laboratory as these microorganisms may not tolerate exposure to oxygen and may need to be rapidly transferred to an anaerobic environment as soon as a biopsy is taken. In the absence of such a rapid transfer protocol and appropriate incubation conditions, anaerobic microorganisms may lead to a false-negative result.

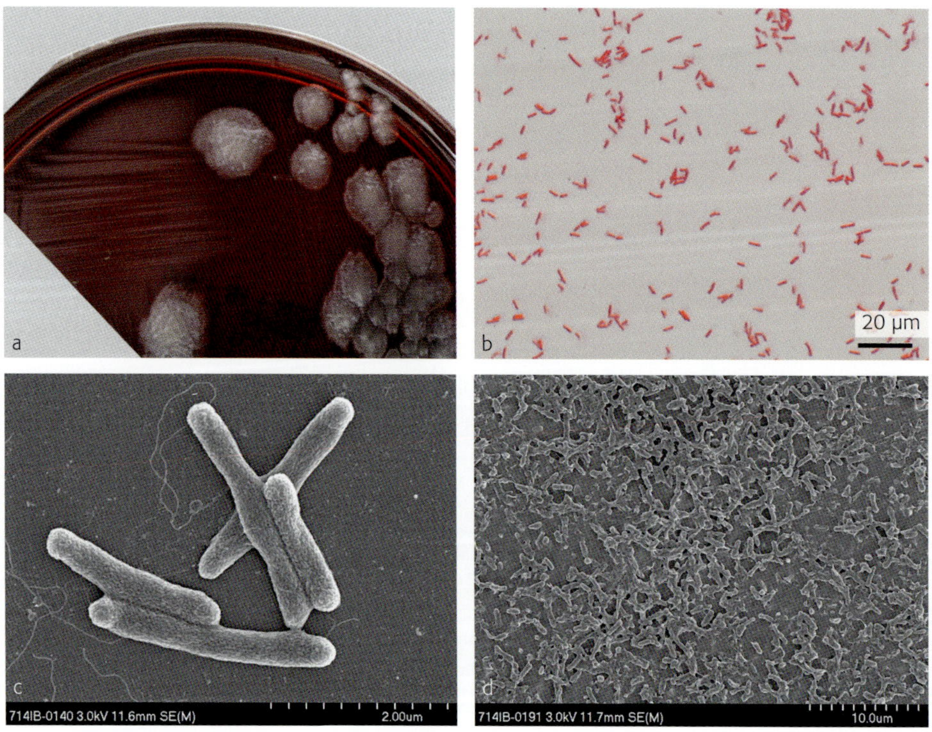

Fig 3-10a–d *Pseudomonas aeruginosa.*

- **a** *Pseudomonas aeruginosa* tends to form large grey/green colonies on blood agar.
- **b–c** They are usually seen as single gram-negative rods (**b**, **c**) with long fibrils (**c**).
- **d** *Pseudomonas aeruginosa* also develop biofilms with significant amounts of extracellular polymeric substances (EPS).

2.3.1 *Propionibacterium acnes*

Morphology: Gram-positive pleomorphic rods (**Fig 3-11**).

Habitat: Normal skin flora and mucosa.

Prominent members: *P acnes* is the most prominent propionibacterium.

Identification and differentiation: *P acnes* forms medium, raised off-white to orange colonies on blood agar. Incubation up to 2 weeks in an anaerobic environment is required for optimal cultivation.

Characteristics: Propionibacteria are most commonly interpreted as contaminants, especially in blood cultures. However, they can be the cause of endocarditis or, in orthopedic cases, prosthesis infections [18]. Since propionibacteria are slow growing, cultures need to be incubated for at least 2 weeks.

2.3.2 Clostridia

Morphology: Gram-positive rods producing spores.

Habitat: Some belonging to the normal gut flora others are found in the environment.

Prominent members: *Clostridium tetani*; *Clostridium botulinum*; *Clostridium perfringens*; *Clostridium septicum*.

Identification and differentiation: Clostridia can be distinguished from the bacilli by lacking aerobic respiration. They are obligate anaerobes, ie, oxygen is toxic to them.

Characteristics: Clostridia produce toxins such as the tetanus toxin (*C tetani*) and the botulinum toxin (*C botulinum*). *Clostridium difficile* is an important cause of intestinal disease, but infrequently associated with bone infections. The toxins produced by *C perfringens*, *C septicum*, and related clostridia are responsible for the typical appearance of gas gangrene. Clostridia are most commonly detected in open wounds such as open fractures.

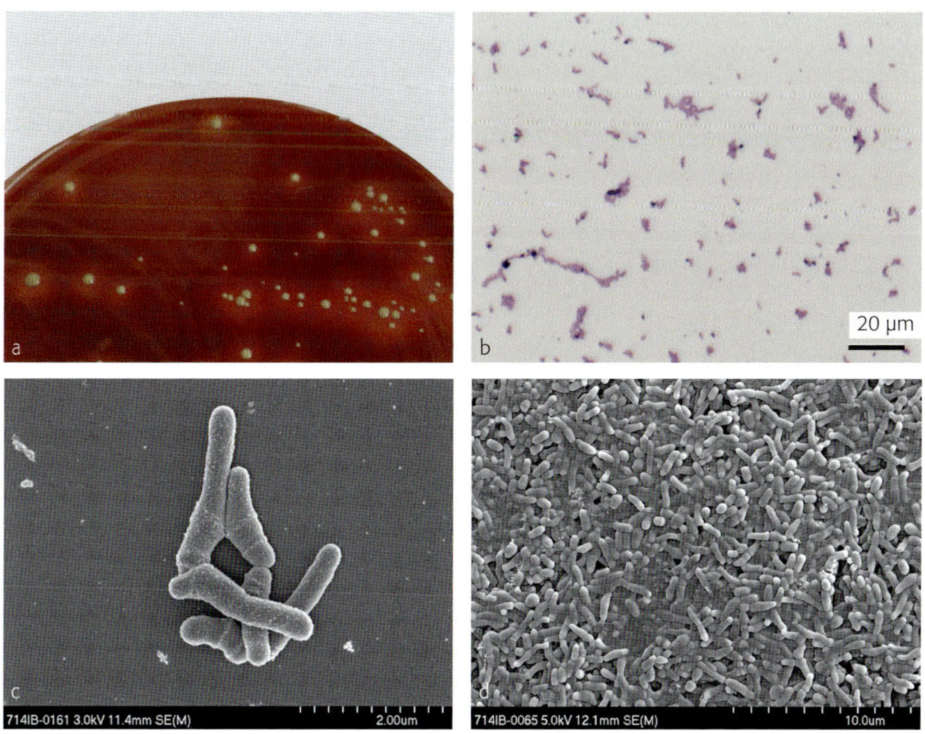

Fig 3-11a–d *Propionibacterium acnes.*
a *Propionibacterium acnes* forms medium, raised off-white to orange colonies on blood agar.
b–c They are usually seen as single pleomorphic gram-positive rods (**b**).
d *Propionibacterium acnes* also develops biofilms.

2.3.3 Peptostreptococci and Finegoldia

Morphology: Gram-positive cocci.

Habitat: Normal flora of gastrointestinal tract, oropharynx, and skin.

Prominent members: *Finegoldia magna* (previously classified as *Peptostreptococcus magnus*) is the most frequently isolated anaerobic coccus.

Identification and differentiation: *F magna* identification depends on the blood culture system used as not all routine protocols will identify it [19]. Expert clinical microbiology laboratory staff are therefore required for identification.

Characteristics: They are often regarded as contaminants in cultures. *F magna* is implicated in a range of mono- and polymicrobial infections, including skin and skin structure, bone and joint (native and prosthetic joints) [20], infective endocarditis (native and prosthetic valves), necrotizing pneumonia, mediastinitis, and meningitis.

2.4 Mycobacteria

Morphology: Acid-alcohol fast rods.

Habitat: Water and soil.

Prominent members: *Mycobacterium tuberculosis, Mycobacterium leprae.*

Identification and differentiation: The distinguishing characteristic is that the cell wall is thicker than in many other bacteria, which is hydrophobic, waxy, and rich in mycolic acids/mycolates. The cell wall consists of the hydrophobic mycolate layer and a peptidoglycan layer held together by a polysaccharide, arabinogalactan.

Characteristics: Some of them are pathogens causing severe diseases such as tuberculosis (*M tuberculosis*) and leprosy (*M leprae*). The spine (Pott's Disease) is most frequently affected in regards to musculoskeletal infections by *M tuberculosis*. Atypical mycobacteria are from the environment and are regarded as contaminants in clinical samples. Some species can cause infections in the lungs and soft tissue. Immunocompromised patients are most commonly affected, and in cases where implant-related bone infections [21] are involved, implant removal is recommended.

2.5 Fungi

The clinically most relevant fungi are either yeast such as *Candida spp*. or molds such as *Aspergillus*. Abundant biofilm formation is common amongst the fungi, and immunocompromised patients are most commonly affected. Musculoskeletal infections are rare but can happen directly after insertion of the implant. All device-related infections [22] with fungi are difficult to treat and removal of the device is required.

3 Conclusion

The microbiology laboratory is charged with providing an identification and antibiotic susceptibility of bacteria within tissue biopsy specimens. The greatest challenge is in differentiating the genuine infecting bacteria from contamination. Confidence in the result is best provided by appropriate sampling and handling in the operating room and the microbiology laboratory.

The same bacterial species may be implicated in infection or contaminant. Modern technologies may improve the detection of bacteria in tissue samples, but the most important future step that must be sought is a more confident differentiation between infection and contamination.

Understanding the basic features of bacterial pathogenicity, including biofilm formation and tissue invasion helps to understand the clinical manifestation of bone infections. Host factors are of course important, but the virulence potential of the differing bacteria accounts for a significant portion of the clinical manifestation of the infection.

Emerging threats to the treatment of patients has included the increase in antibiotic resistance within these bacteria. In general, the most difficult-to-treat infections are biofilm infections, which account for a massive increase in antibiotic resistance. Obtaining adequate numbers of uncontaminated intraoperative biopsies is therefore a key component of the proper diagnosis and the care of orthopedic and trauma patients.

4 References

1. **Trampuz A, Zimmerli W.** Diagnosis and treatment of infections associated with fracture-fixation devices. *Injury.* 2006 May;37 Suppl 2:S59–66.
2. **Eich G.** Eine mikrobiologische Orientierungshilfe [A microbiological guide]. In: Swiss Orthopaedics and the Swiss Society for Infectious Diseases Expert Group "Infections of the musculoskeletal system". *Infektionen des Bewegungsapparates.* Grandvaux: 2014: 166–181.
3. **Murray BE.** The life and times of the Enterococcus. *Clin Microbiol Rev.* 1990 Jan;3(1):46–65.
4. **Cetinkaya Y, Falk P, Mayhall CG.** Vancomycin-resistant enterococci. *Clin Microbiol Rev.* 2000 Oct;13(4):686–707.
5. **Tuomanen E, Cozens R, Tosch W, et al.** The rate of killing of Escherichia coli by beta-lactam antibiotics is strictly proportional to the rate of bacterial growth. *J Gen Microbiol.* 1986 May;132(5):1297–1304.
6. **Tseng BS, Zhang W, Harrison JJ, et al.** The extracellular matrix protects Pseudomonas aeruginosa biofilms by limiting the penetration of tobramycin. *Environ Microbiol.* 2013 Oct;15(10):2865–2878.
7. **Hess DJ, Henry-Stanley MJ, Erickson EA, et al.** Intracellular survival of Staphylococcus aureus within cultured enterocytes. *J Surg Res.* 2003 Sep;114(1):42–49.
8. **Proctor RA, von Eiff C, Kahl BC, et al.** Small colony variants: a pathogenic form of bacteria that facilitates persistent and recurrent infections. *Nat Rev Microbiol.* 2006 Apr;4(4):295–305.
9. **Hoiby N, Bjarnsholt T, Givskov M, et al.** Antibiotic resistance of bacterial biofilms. *Int J Antimicrob Agents.* 2010 Apr;35(4):322–332.
10. **Ellington JK, Reilly SS, Ramp WK, et al.** Mechanisms of Staphylococcus aureus invasion of cultured osteoblasts. *Microb Pathog.* 1999 Jun;26(6):317–323.
11. **Schafer P, Fink B, Sandow D, et al.** Prolonged bacterial culture to identify late periprosthetic joint infection: a promising strategy. *Clin Infect Dis.* 2008 Dec 1;47(11):1403–1409.
12. **Butler-Wu SM, Burns EM, Pottinger PS, et al.** Optimization of periprosthetic culture for diagnosis of Propionibacterium acnes prosthetic joint infection. *J Clin Microbiol.* 2011 Jul;49(7):2490–2495.
13. **Palmer MP, Altman DT, Altman GT, et al.** Can we trust intraoperative culture results in nonunions? *J Orthop Trauma.* 2014 Jul;28(7):384–390.
14. **Achermann Y, Vogt M, Leunig M, et al.** Improved diagnosis of periprosthetic joint infection by multiplex PCR of sonication fluid from removed implants. *J Clin Microbiol.* 2010 Apr;48(4):1208–1214.
15. **Everts RJ, Chambers ST, Murdoch DR, et al.** Successful antimicrobial therapy and implant retention for streptococcal infection of prosthetic joints. *ANZ J Surg* 2004 Apr;74(4):210–214.
16. **Yuste JR, Quesada M, Diaz-Rada P, et al.** Daptomycin in the treatment of prosthetic joint infection by Enterococcus faecalis: safety and efficacy of high-dose and prolonged therapy. *Int J Infect Dis.* 2014 Oct;27:65–66.
17. **Rodriguez-Pardo D, Pigrau C, Lora-Tamayo J, et al.** Gram-negative prosthetic joint infection: outcome of a debridement, antibiotics and implant retention approach. A large multicentre study. *Clin Microbiol Infect.* 2014 Apr 26.
18. **Zappe B, Graf S, Ochsner PE, et al.** Propionibacterium spp. in prosthetic joint infections: a diagnostic challenge. *Arch Orthop Trauma Surg.* 2008 Oct;128(10):1039–1046.
19. **Bassetti S, Laifer G, Goy G, et al.** Endocarditis caused by Finegoldia magna (formerly Peptostreptococcus magnus): diagnosis depends on the blood culture system used. *Diagn Microbiol Infect Dis.* 2003 Sep;47(1):359–360.
20. **Levy PY, Fenollar F, Stein A, et al.** Finegoldia magna: a forgotten pathogen in prosthetic joint infection rediscovered by molecular biology. *Clin Infect Dis.* 2009 Oct 15;49(8):1244–1247.
21. **Eid AJ, Berbari EF, Sia IG, et al.** Prosthetic joint infection due to rapidly growing mycobacteria: report of 8 cases and review of the literature. *Clin Infect Dis.* 2007 Sep 15;45(6):687–694.
22. **Azzam K, Parvizi J, Jungkind D, et al.** Microbiological, clinical, and surgical features of fungal prosthetic joint infections: a multi-institutional experience. *J Bone Joint Surg Am.* 2009 Nov;91 Suppl 6:142–149.

4 Prevention of intraoperative infection

Erlangga Yusuf, Olivier Borens

1 Basics

The healthcare associated infections (HCAIs) most commonly affecting surgical patients are surgical-site infections (SSIs), postoperative pneumonia, urinary tract, and bloodstream infections [1]. This chapter will focus mainly on prevention of SSIs while the prevention of other HCAIs will be discussed alongside.

Surgical-site infection was previously referred to as wound infection which would include the infection of a traumatic wound. The United States Centers for Disease Control and Prevention (CDC) therefore introduced the term SSI in 1992 [2]. Surgical-site infection is defined as an infection that occurs at or near the site of surgery within 30 days after the operation [3]. When the surgery involves a prosthetic implant, SSI can occur up to 1 year after surgery [4].

The CDC recognizes three levels of SSI based on the depth of the involved tissues [3]. The first level, ie, superficial incision, affects only the skin and subcutaneous tissue. It is characterized by localized signs such as heat, redness, pain, or pus at the incision site. The second level, ie, deep incision, involves the fascial and muscle layers. It is characterized by abscess formation, presence of pus, and fever. The third level is the infection that involves deep organ space such as the bone or joint [2].

The occurrence of SSI after orthopedic surgery depends on many variables, such as anatomical location, patient immunity, type of surgery, and where the surveillance is performed. Surgical-site infection rates in a German study showed rates of 1.4% for hip replacement and 1.0% for knee replacement [5]. One surveillance study estimated the occurrence of SSIs in orthopedic surgery at 1.5% with 9% fatality [6]. Another study showed average SSI rates of 22.7% ranging from 13.2% in clean cases to 70.0% in dirty wounds [7].

Compared to noninfected orthopedic surgery patients, orthopedic patients with SSIs stay 2 weeks longer, have double the rates of rehospitalization, and generated 300% greater health-care costs [8].

Categories of risk factors for SSI include: patient (host), surgical, and environment-related risk factors in the operating room (**Table 4-1**); and organism-related risk factors (covered in chapters 1 Implant-associated biofilm, 2 Host immunity, and 3 Microbiology) [3, 9, 10]. Some patient-related risk factors are modifiable. Modification of the patient-related and surgery-related risks can reduce rates of SSI. Evidence for prevention of SSI originates from orthopedics and other surgical disciplines [3, 9, 10].

Patient-related	Surgical	Operating room environment
Older age	Improper patient preparation prior to surgery	High operating room traffic
Active infection in other body site	Insufficient hygiene measures of surgical personnel	Frequency and duration of open door
History of previous surgery	Insufficient surgical personnel preparation	Unclean instruments
Poorly controlled diabetes mellitus	Long surgical duration	Defective ventilation
Malnutrition	Tissue damage from surgical technique	Inadequate room cleanliness
Morbid obesity	Talking	Poorly designed operating rooms
Smoking	Changing gloves	
Immunodeficiency	Antibiotic infused within 1 hour of incision	
Alcoholism	Normothermia	
Intravenous drug use	Surgical personnel not wearing clean, appropriate attire	
Chronic carrier of *Staphylococcus*		

Table 4-1 Factors associated with surgical-site infections [3, 9, 10].

2 Preoperative measures

2.1 Modifying patient-related risk factors

Some patient-related risk factors for SSI are modifiable, including diabetes, morbid obesity, malnutrition, and smoking. However, there is limited evidence that shows whether modification of these factors will lead to lower SSI rates.

Assessment of diabetic patients is done by measuring glycoslyated hemoglobin (HbA1c), a reliable indicator of diabetic control. HbA1c was used in a study to compare the SSIs in patients undergoing various noncardiac surgical procedures. It was shown that patients with HbA1c level less than 7% had a two-fold lower infection rate than patients with HbA1c higher than 7% [11].

Elective surgery in patients with morbid obesity (body mass index (BMI) > 40 kg/m^2) should be considered carefully balancing the risks and benefits [9]. It has been clearly shown that this population has a much higher SSI risk than populations with normal weight [12, 13]. The high risk of SSI is likely multifactorial including longer surgical times, too low antibiotic dosing in obese patients, and a recognized immune system compromise associated with obesity. Moreover, obese patients often have comorbidities such as diabetes and cardiovascular diseases. Malnourished patients are also at increased risk of SSI [3]. Correction of malnutrition by total parenteral nutrition has been shown to lower postoperative infections including pneumonia and urinary tract infections [14].

The effect of smoking cessation on SSIs in orthopedic procedures is readily available. In a Danish randomized controlled trial (RCT) involving patients undergoing hip and knee replacement, it was shown that patients (n = 60) having quit or reduced smoking (ie, counseling and nicotine replacement therapy) 6–8 weeks before scheduled surgery had significantly lower wound-related complications than control patients (5% vs 31%, $P = .001$) [15]. An RCT performed in Sweden reproduced these results in patients who underwent hip or knee replacement, primary hernia repair, and laparoscopic cholecystectomy [16].

Several other potentially modifiable patient-related factors have been discussed in CDC guidelines [3] and at the International Consensus Meeting on Periprosthetic Joint Infection [9] but the evidence is not clear. These risk factors are intravenous drug abuse, alcohol abuse, immunosuppressive medication, and human immunodeficiency virus (HIV) infection. The decision to perform surgery in these patients should be done on an individual basis.

The presence of active infection either in a joint or in the bloodstream is associated with increased SSI risk in joint replacement surgery [17, 18]. Screening for the presence of infection anywhere in the body is therefore recommended. There is a strong consensus among orthopedic surgeons to avoid elective arthroplasty in patients with any active infection [9]. Most orthopedic surgeons avoid elective arthroplasty in patients with active skin ulcerations. There is limited evidence that skin ulcerations pose a risk for SSI [9]. The presence of bacteria in the urine (asymptomatic bacteriuria) is another relevant issue. It has been shown that asymptomatic bacteriuria before surgery was associated with increased risk for subsequent prosthetic joint infection [19]. Interestingly, antibiotic therapy did not reduce this risk [19]. It can be inferred from this study that it is safe to perform total joint arthroplasty (TJA) in patients with asymptomatic bacteriuria without specifically eradicating the bacteria. Routine urine screening is also therefore not warranted for patients undergoing elective arthroplasty [9]. When a TJA is planned and the patient is found to have asymptomatic bacteriuria, the operation can take place as long as routine prophylactic antibiotics are given.

2.2 Nasal decolonization

As shown in chapter 3 Microbiology, the majority of SSIs result from *Staphylococcus aureus* [20] and decolonization is believed to reduce the number of SSIs. One of the main reservoirs of *S aureus* is the nares. The most extensively studied and used agent for eradication of *S aureus* since the 1980s is mupirocin [21, 22]. It is a potent decolonizing agent which is also active against other gram-positive bacteria. Nasal carriage was eliminated within 96 hours after completion of treatment in around 90% of study populations [23]. Mupirocin is usually applied to the anterior nares 2–3 times/day, for 2–5 days [24, 25]. It has been shown that mupirocin can also be used to eradicate methicillin-resistant *S aureus* (MRSA) [25]. In orthopedic surgery, use of mupirocin twice daily from the day before surgery until the day of surgery has been shown to lower rates of SSI with identical *S aureus* isolate [26]. There are several drawbacks when using mupirocin, such as recolonization, the development of resistance, and cost. In a study on healthy hospital staff, after near complete decolonization immediately following mupirocin use, the colonization was 56% and 53% after 6 months and 1 year, respectively [27]. Increased use of mupirocin correlates to the development of resistance [28]. The use of mupirocin should therefore warrant careful monitoring and alternatives should be investigated. For example, one alternative agent for nasal decolonization of *S aureus* under investigation is retapamulin [24].

2.3 Cleansing the skin

Skin is normally colonized by a range of microorganisms. The surgical skin incision can introduce the microorganisms to the exposed tissue and may result in SSI. Several studies have shown that skin cleansing can remove the microorganisms [29, 30]. However, the effect of skin cleansing on SSI rates is less clear. A systematic review including one RCT, two cohort studies, and two interventional studies, showed a significant reduction in SSI risk (pooled relative risk of 0.29 (95% confidence interval (95% CI of 0.17 to 0.49) when chlorhexidine gluconate washcloths were compared with either no intervention or other cleansing agent, such as soap-water bath, or povidone-iodine scrub [31]. Yet, many of the studies included in this systematic review were not free from bias. In contrast to this systematic review, a meta-analysis using Cochrane standards on RCTs that included 10,157 participants did not show statistically significant reduction in SSI when 4% chlorhexidine gluconate was compared with a placebo, or with using a bar of soap, or with no washing [32]. It can be concluded that skin cleansing can remove the microorganisms from the skin, but the effect of this measure on SSI is not clear. Despite the limited evidence, skin cleansing is widely used and approved of by orthopedic surgeons [9].

Skin cleansing should be performed over the whole body and not only at the surgical site [9]. A study of 1,530 operations for biliary tract disease, inguinal hernia, and breast cancer showed that the infection rate was lower for whole-body than surgical-site-specific washing [33]. Regarding the frequency and timing of skin cleansing, the CDC recommends preoperative showering on at least the night before the operative day [3]. The regimens of skin cleansing that are often described are skin cleansing twice, ie, a couple of days before and on the morning of the operation [34, 35]. Chlorhexidine should not be used excessively since this can also lead to skin irritation [36].

Many studies use chlorhexidine gluconate as an agent for skin cleansing. The CDC recommended chlorhexidine 2% as the agent of choice to reduce catheter-related bloodstream infection [37], but a specific recommendation to use chlorhexidine to reduce SSIs has not been made [3].

2.4 Hair removal

Traditionally, the preparation of a patient for surgery included removal of hair from the incision site. The published literature on the effect of hair removal on SSIs in orthopedic procedures is very limited and the knowledge is derived from other surgical fields [38]. The CDC does not recommend hair removal preoperatively unless the hair will interfere with the operation [3]. This recommendation is supported by a metaanalysis that found no statistically significant difference in SSI rates between removal of body hair by shaving, clipping, or depilatory cream, and no hair removal. Noteworthy, is that the comparison in this metaanalysis is underpowered as mentioned by the authors of this metaanalysis [38].

When hair removal is performed, clipping is preferred to use of a razor as shown in two studies performed in the 1980s [39, 40]. The authors speculate that abrasions formed due to shaving can become sites of bacterial growth which can lead to infection. There is limited data on other methods of hair removal, eg, depilatory cream. The hair removal should be performed in the hospital as close to the time of surgery as possible by either the surgical team or the nursing staff [9]. This recommendation is based more on practicality than on scientific evidence. Two studies in the 1970s and 1980s, which did not specifically look at the timing of hair removal, showed that hair removal on the morning of or immediately before surgery was associated with a lower SSI rate than shaving 24 hours or more prior to surgery [40, 41].

2.5 Antiseptic skin preparation in the operating room

The principle of aseptic surgery is one of the most important developments in surgery. This principle was described by Joseph Lister (1827–1912). He applied the advances in microbiology by another giant in the field of microbiology and infection control, Louis Pasteur, to surgery by promoting the idea of sterile surgery [42]. He used carbolic acid to clean wounds, which led to a reduction in SSI. Prior to this period, limb amputation for example, was associated with a disturbing 50% mortality due to sepsis [43].

The purpose of skin preparation in the operating room is to remove soil and transient bacteria from the skin [44]. It can be done by application of antiseptic. The antiseptic should be applied using a dedicated sterile and single-use instrument, eg, sponge, in the area that should be large enough to include any potential extension of the incision site from the main incision [3, 44]. The application should be performed in concentric circles from the incision site moving toward the periphery [44]. The reason for this movement is practical, to reduce the amount of residing microorganisms at the surgical site.

The CDC [3] and Association of Operating Room Nurses (AORN) [44] guidelines recommend only liquid products and against nonliquid products, such as powder sprays or impregnated drapes [3, 44, 45]. There are three commonly used skin antiseptics [45, 46] (**Table 4-2**).

		Povidone-iodine	Alcohol	Chlorhexidine gluconate
Efficacy	Gram-positive bacteria	Excellent	Excellent	Excellent
	Gram-negative bacteria	Excellent	Excellent	Good
	Acid-fast bacillus	Excellent	Good	Minimal
	Sporicide	Partial	No	
	Fungi	Excellent	Partial	Minimal
	Viruses	Excellent	Partial (RSV, Hepatitis B, HIV)	HIV, HSV, CMV, influenzae
Mode of action		Cell-wall penetration, oxidation, and substitution of microbial contents with iodine	Denaturation of cell-wall proteins of bacteria	Disruption of cell membranes and precipitation of cell contents
Formulation		5–10% (w/v) that contain 0.5–1% iodine	70–90% (w/v)	0.5–4% (w/v)
Major advantage			Rapid	
Major disadvantage		Possible skin irritation and damage	No residual effect	

Table 4-2 The three most commonly used skin antiseptics [45, 46].
Abbreviations: w/v, weight per volume; HIV, human immunodeficiency virus; RSV, respiratory syncytial virus; HSV, herpes simplex virus; CMV, cytomegalovirus.

The first antiseptic is iodine based. Typically, iodophors that comprise free iodine molecules are bound to a polymer such as povidone [47] to reduce the irritation effect of iodine [48]. In the majority of European hospitals, povidone-iodine is the most commonly used antiseptic [49]. Povidone-iodine is soluble in both water and alcohol. The second-most commonly used is alcohol. Its effectiveness depends mainly on its concentration [47]. The third is chlorhexidine gluconate. Like povidone-iodine, it is available in aqueous and alcohol formulations. There is limited evidence that chlorhexidine is better than the others in reducing SSI rates in clean surgery [45]. Comparison between the antiseptic agents is difficult because iodophor and chlorhexidine gluconate are available in combination with alcohol. Therefore, the efficacy of chlorhexidine gluconate cannot be attributed solely to chlorhexidine gluconate [46]. The combination of 2% chlorhexidine gluconate and 70% isopropyl alcohol is shown in a RCT involving 897 patients (no orthopedic procedures were included) to be superior to aqueous solution of 10% povidone-iodine [50]. The selection of antiseptic scrubs should consider characteristics such as costs and potential side effects. There is a limited number of studies on the agents of choice for antiseptic scrubbing in contaminated surgery [51]. In broken skin, antiseptics can also be used but not iodophor since it may have a negative effect on tissue healing [48].

2.6 Draping patients

Ideally, surgical drapes should be impermeable to liquids and impervious to tearing [52]. There are disposable and reusable surgical drapes. There is no evidence that one type is better than the other in preventing SSI according to the results of a RCT with 494 participants [53]. Surgical drapes can be kept in place by using adhesives—a transparent plastic sheet adhering to the skin. It has been shown that they prevent bacterial penetration in hip fracture surgery [54] and prevent the skin bacteria from multiplying under the drape [55] (**Fig 4-1**). Yet, there is no evidence that they reduce SSI rates [56]. The adhesive plastic drape is also available impregnated with iodine. There is no evidence that adhesive drapes are better than not using an adhesive drape [56].

2.7 Hand hygiene of surgical personnel

The Hungarian physician Ignaz Semmelweis (1818–1865) discovered that the incidence of puerperal fever could be significantly lowered by using hand disinfection in obstetrical clinics. Hand hygiene has since been recognized as the most important measure to prevent HCAIs.

Two options are available for surgical personnel for the preoperative treatment of hands, which should include nails, hands, and forearms [57]. The first option is washing of hands with antimicrobial soap and water: surgical hand-antiseptic soaps (scrub). The second option is the application of an alcohol-based hand liquid applied onto dry hands without water: surgical hand disinfection (rub) [57].

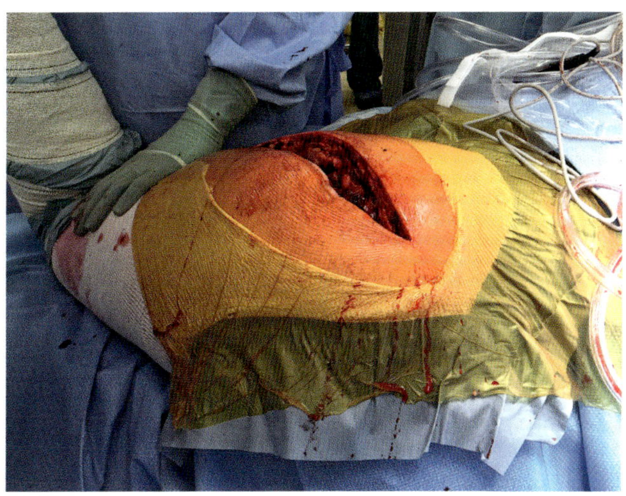

Fig 4-1 Surgical drapes.

Surgical hand scrubbing is aimed at removing transient organisms, ie, microorganisms that can be isolated from the skin but are not consistently present in the majority of personnel, such as *Escherichia coli* and *Pseudomonas aeruginosa,* and at reducing commensal flora, ie, permanent flora of the skin such as *Propionibacterium* species, *Corynebacterium* species, and coagulase-negative staphylococci [47, 58]. This is necessary because even low levels of contamination can cause infections, especially in implant surgeries [58]. Hospital guidelines often recommend the use of a sponge or brush for surgical hand scrubbing. The usual agents for this purpose are water-based solutions or soap that contain chlorhexidine or povidone-iodine [43, 61]. Chlorhexidine-gluconate based aqueous solutions seems to be more effective in reducing the number of colony-forming units on the hands than povidone-iodine-based aqueous scrubs [61]. The duration of surgical scrub is often a part of hospital recommendations. It has long been thought that longer scrubbing was more effective, but it has been shown that scrubbing for 3–5 minutes should reduce bacterial counts to acceptable levels. Longer duration of scrubbing does not give an added effect and will only increase the risk of skin damage [59, 60].

An alternative for surgical scrub is alcohol-based hand rub. Here, surgical hand disinfection is performed without using brushes or sponges. This alternative is an interesting option because it may increase compliance and is faster to perform [58]. Brushless surgical hand antiseptics can be performed using alcohol with a concentration of 60–95%. The three main alcohols used are ethanol, isopropanol, and n-propanol [61, 62]. Chlorhexidine, iodine, and other active ingredients can be added to the surgical hand disinfectant solutions. It has been shown in one trial that alcohol-based disinfectants are as effective as aqueous scrubbing in preventing SSIs [63] but there is no evidence that suggests that any particular alcohol is better than another [61].

2.8 Surgical attire for surgical personnel

Any simple movement can liberate microorganisms from the skin and from casual clothing [64]. The consensus is to wear surgical scrub clothes, masks, and surgical caps to minimize the transfer of microorganisms from surgical team members to the patients and to the operating room environment (**Fig 4-2**). However, the scientific evidence for these measures to prevent SSIs is lacking [3, 65, 66]. Masks belong to the standard surgical attire. Indeed, it has been shown that bacteria can be dispersed via talking [64, 67]. However, in an interesting study where the participants were requested to talk while a culture plate placed one meter from these volunteers, it was shown that mouth bacteria could not disperse to that distance [68]. Despite this observation, wearing masks for surgical personnel is required since they stand closer to the patient than one meter, both to protect the patient and surgical team from contamination.

Clean surgical garments should be used and they should be washed in the health facilities rather than at home. The practice of washing scrub clothing at home still occurs in several countries such as in the US. The garments should not be flammable, and should not harbor dust or droplets [69].

Gloves are the only item of attire that is scientifically shown to reduce SSI rates. When gloves are perforated during a procedure, it can lead to twice the SSI risk [70]. In about 9% of orthopedic surgeries, gloves are perforated [70] and in the majority of cases glove perforation is not recognized during surgery [71]. It is therefore advisable to use double gloves to improve the sterile barrier between surgeon and patient, even though this will reduce tactile sensation.

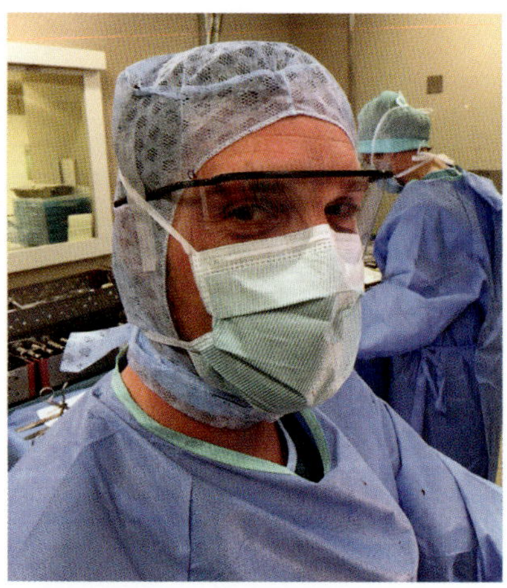

Fig 4-2 The surgeon in scrub attire.

3 Intraoperative measures

3.1 Atraumatic surgical technique

Atraumatic surgical technique is an essential clinical practice that should in theory reduce the risk of SSI. The surgeon should minimize the amount of tissue damage, handle tissue with care, while maintaining the patient's temperature, oxygenation, and perfusion. Gentle wound closure and drainage are factors that can prevent SSIs. Moreover, keeping the duration of surgery as short as possible might prevent SSIs.

Surgical incisions can be made by using scalpel and/or electrocautery. In many institutions separate blades are used for skin incision versus incision into deeper tissue for high-risk surgeries. There is limited scientific evidence for this practice. Skin blades can be contaminated up to 15% after skin incision; much of the contamination consists of coagulase-negative staphylococci, one of the causes of prosthetic-joint infection [72]. On the other hand, it is shown that even if the knife blades are contaminated, they do not lead to transfer of the bacteria to the wound edges and the deeper tissue [73]. Compared to scalpel, electrocautery is faster and causes less bleeding. The SSI rate in a small study involving 60 patients showed that the SSI rates in patients who underwent scalpel and electrocautery for skin incisions, were comparable [74].

During surgery, tissue should be handled gently and devitalized tissue and debris should be removed. Irrigation can also remove inflammatory mediators and dilute contamination [75]. There are variations in practice in terms of volume, pressure, and techniques as well as which solution should be used. Arguably, increased volume will improve wound cleansing, but no optimal volume has been recommended [9, 75]. High- or low-pressure lavage can be performed. Studies have used various definitions of high and low pressure. Pressure below 15 psi (103.4 kPa) can be considered as low pressure and over 35 psi (241.3 kPa) as high pressure [76]. In theory, high-pressure lavage can remove the debris and the necrotic tissue rapidly, and will allow better cement penetration in cancellous bone tissue in cemented arthroplasty [9]. The drawback of using high-pressure lavage is the possible damage to tissue and deeper penetration of bacteria as shown in an in vivo study [76]. Arguably, high-pressure lavage should be beneficial in severely contaminated wounds or in open injuries. However, the majority of surgeons in an international survey of 984 surgeons mainly from Canada and from an international fracture course (AO Foundation, Davos, Switzerland), favored low-pressure lavage for the initial management of open fracture wounds [77]. Saline can be used for the lavage and is preferred by many surgeons [77]. Additional information on irrigation can be found in chapter 6 Local delivery of antibiotics and antiseptics.

Maintaining adequate tissue oxygenation seems to be important in preventing SSIs. Oxygenation plays an important role in immune function, especially in oxidative killing of microorganisms by neutrophils. There are several possibilities to improve tissue oxygenation including normothermia [78], use of supplemental oxygen [79], and by maintaining cardiac output during the surgery [80]. Among these possibilities, studies have shown that normothermia [78] and supplemental oxygen [79] are associated with lower SSIs compared to hypothermia and no supplemental oxygen, respectively. However, extra fluid administration does not decrease SSI rates [80]. This evidence is based on a very limited number of studies.

When the odds of infection are low, traumatic wounds should be closed [81]. There are several possibilities for closure such as sutures and staples. Tissue adhesives are also available, but they may lack mechanical strength and perhaps should be considered as a biological sealant [9]. Closure material, like any other foreign material, can promote microorganism growth [82]. Sutures can be roughly divided into absorbable and nonabsorbable. Absorbable sutures are made from various materials such as polyglycolic acid, polyglactic acid, polydioxanone, polytrimethylene carbonate, and catgut. The absorbable sutures are completely absorbed between 60–210 days [83]. When absorbable suture cannot be used, for example, due to infection in the surrounding tissues, nonabsorbable sutures can be used [81]. Examples of nonabsorbable sutures are nylon, polypropylene, braided polyester, polybutester, and silk [83]. A study using a mouse model showed that synthetic sutures were better than natural sutures in resisting gram-positive and gram-negative bacteria [84]. Absorbable and nonabsorbable sutures can be monofilaments or braided. Compared to monofilaments, braided sutures allow easy handling, but probably at the cost of higher risk for infection. It is shown in a mouse model that braided sutures resist bacteria less than monofilament sutures [84]. Moreover, bacteria that reside in a biofilm in a braided suture are protected from phagocytosis because leukocytes cannot penetrate freely into the braided sutures [85].

To close the wound, staples can also be used. Like sutures, they are absorbable or nonabsorbable (ie, stainless steel). Contaminated wounds closed with staples are associated with fewer SSIs when compared to wounds closed with sutures [86]. There is no consensus among orthopedic surgeons on the best method of closure to prevent SSIs [9]. A metaanalysis that included six small-sized studies (five of six studies involved surgery of the hip) showed more than a three-fold increase in SSIs in stapled wounds compared with sutured wounds [87]. The results of this metaanalysis should be interpreted cautiously because of methodological limitations of the included studies, such as inadequate and varied definition of SSI [87]. Adhesives, such as 2-octylcyanoacrylate can be used to seal the wound. There are a limited number of studies that investigate the SSI rates with adhesives in comparison to staples or sutures. Khan and colleagues compared 2-octylcyanoacrylate, subcuticular suture (monocryl), and skin staples in 102 hip replacements and 85 of the knee [88]. They showed that 2-octylcyanoacrylate was associated with less wound discharge in the first 24 hours for both the hip and the knee [88].

Delayed primary closure should be performed in highly contaminated wounds [89]. Since the first randomized study on this topic published in the 1960s [90], several other studies [91–93] have shown the beneficial effect of delayed primary closure in abdominal operations. The proof of principle of the delayed primary closure was established in 1933, where it was shown that application of *S aureus* to surgical wounds in guinea pigs on day 5 to day 7 gave less infection than when the bacteria was applied earlier [94]. In patients with open fractures, delayed closure has not been shown to be more beneficial than primary closure [95]. The use of prophylactic antibiotics and preemptive antibiotic therapy in open fractures might confound this research.

The concept of delayed primary closure has been extended, for example, by using negative-pressure wound therapy [89]. It is used as a bridge to close contaminated wounds and is shown in animal studies to reduce bacterial load in the wound [96, 97]. Interestingly, in a study in patients with chronic wounds it was shown that the negative-pressure wound therapy foams were heavily colonized by bacteria, despite routine replacement of the foam [98].

A drain can be used to evacuate fluids and hematoma from wounds or body spaces. Fluids and hematomata can impair wound healing by increasing pressure. The increasing pressure can subsequently lead to problems in tissue perfusion [99]. A drain, on the other hand, is also a foreign body and can act as a conduit for infection. This dilemma has been investigated by several studies in orthopedic procedures. A systematic review of five RCTs involving 349 patients did not show significant difference in the use of closed suction drains following anterior cruciate ligament reconstruction surgery [100]. Another systematic review that included six RCTs involving 664 patients also showed that the use of closed suction drains did not increase SSI rates following hip fracture surgery [101].

The duration of surgery should be kept as short as possible to prevent SSIs. It has been shown that in total knee arthroplasty, prolonged duration of surgery is a risk factor for SSI [102, 103]. The increased duration of surgery can be confounded by the other SSI risk factors such as obesity and washout of prophylactic antibiotics.

3.2 Keeping contamination in the operating room environment as low as possible

The operating room environment can harbor pathogens. For example, staphylococci have been isolated from air samples of the operating room [104]. In prosthetic joint surgery there is a correlation between air contamination in the operating room and prosthetic joint infection [105]. The operating room should therefore be properly ventilated to minimize airborne microorganisms [106]. This can be done by applying positive pressure in the operating room with respect to corridors and adjacent areas. Positive pressure prevents airflow from less clean into more clean areas [107]. Using the same logic, airflow should go from the ceiling to the floor [3].

An interesting issue for the orthopedic field is the use of laminar airflow in joint prosthesis surgery. Joint prosthesis is a foreign material and foreign materials are prone to attachment of microorganisms [82]. The additional ventilation with laminar flow is believed to increase the removal of bacteria around the surgical field. The laminar flow should move particle-free air over the aseptic operating field at uniform velocity. The flow can be delivered horizontally or vertically. Horizontal flow is provided by wall-mounted distribution systems and vertical flow is provided by ceiling-mounted distribution systems. The size of the distribution systems varies and is usually larger than 3.2 x 3.2 m [108]. The laminar airflow facilities are used in the majority of operating rooms used for orthopedic implant surgery in many countries, such as Germany [109] and New Zealand [110]. Several early studies [106] showed that laminar air flow is beneficial in reducing SSI rates. However, this observation is challenged in more recent studies, for example, in a study from Brandt [111]. Until solid evidence is available, orthopedic surgery may be performed in operating rooms without laminar flow. This statement is supported by 85% of orthopedic surgeons in a consensus [9]. The consensus also stated that applying laminar airflow is a complex technology that must function in strict adherence to maintenance protocols.

In the operating room, many individuals are present, including the surgeon, anesthesiologist, surgeon in training, operating nurses, and sometimes students. Microorganisms residing on the hair, skin, and clothes can be dispersed to the operating room environment, including to the patients [64]. Human movement creates turbulence and disturbs the ventilation of the operating room. The dispersion can occur by simple movement or by talking [64]. A study in 1975 showed that the bacterial counts increased from 13 ± 31 CFU/ square feet/hour in an empty operating room to 447.3 ± 186.7 CFU/ square feet/hour when five people were introduced [67]. It is therefore important to limit the number of people in the operating room to as few as possible. The more personnel in the operating room the higher the number of door openings [112] which can in turn increase SSIs [113]. It was noted in a study that on average the door opening in prosthetic joint surgery occurred at the rate of 0.7/minute in primary arthroplasty and 0.8/minute in revision arthroplasty surgery [113]. Opening the doors of operating rooms has been shown to increase the number of bacteria twofold [67]. Another problem that can be caused by multiple openings of the doors is the overuse of the laminar airflow filter because of the need to increase the air passing through the filter in response to the pressure gradient drop caused by multiple door openings. Minimizing operating room door opening can be achieved simply by, for example, using the phone rather than conducting discussions in person.

3.3 Using sterilized instruments

Surgical instruments making contact with body tissues or fluids are considered critical items [52]. These instruments should be sterile when used because inadequately sterilized instruments may result in disease transmission [114]. Most surgical devices are made of heat-stable materials and can therefore undergo pressurized steam sterilization. When the instruments are not heat stable, low-temperature sterilization with, eg, ethylene oxide gas, hydrogen peroxide gas plasma, peracetic acid immersion, and ozone can be used [52]. A "sterile" instrument is defined as a probability of the presence of microorganisms on the instrument after sterilization [52]. This probability is expressed as the sterility assurance level. The sterility assurance level for scalpels, for example, is arbitrarily set at 10^{-6} [52]. The sterilized instruments are kept in instrument trays in the operating room. It is recommended that the instrument trays should be opened shortly before the start of the surgical procedure. The contamination rate of the trays increases from 4% after 30 minutes of opening to 30% 4 hours after opening [115]. Surgical instruments can also be "flash sterilized". "Flash sterilization" is performed on an unwrapped object at 132° C for 3 minutes. It should be performed only on surgical instruments for immediate use, such as to sterilize an inadvertently dropped instrument [3]. It should be avoided and not be done for convenience reasons.

4 Postoperative measures

Appropriate postoperative care of the surgical wound is important to prevent SSIs. The surgical incision that is closed primarily is usually covered with a sterile dressing for 24–48 hours [3]. There is limited evidence on best practice as to whether an incision must be covered by a dressing and whether the patient can shower after 48 hours [3]. In practice, the surgical wound is often cleansed with sterile saline solution to remove wound debris and surplus of wound exudates.

A surgical incision that is left open to heal by secondary intention can also be packed with sterile moist gauze and covered with a sterile dressing [3]. There are various types of dressing, with or without topical solutions [116, 117], but there is no evidence that one is better than the others in reducing SSI rates [118] as shown by studies involving gastrointestinal surgeries [116–118]. Arguably, topical antibiotics can be used in a wound that is left open to heal by secondary intention. The possible side effects of this action are antimicrobial resistance and possible allergic reaction. An RCT failed to show the beneficial effect of application of topical chloramphenicol on surgical wounds after hip fractures [119]. In this study, SSI rates at 30 days served as the outcome measure. In practice, antiseptics such as chlorhexidine and povidone-iodine are sometimes used in chronic wound care.

The dressing of the wound that is primarily closed or wound that is left open for secondary healing should be changed by using either "sterile" or "clean" techniques. Both techniques involve meticulous hand washing. In "sterile" technique, a sterile field is created and sterile gloves are used for application of a sterile dressing, while in "clean" technique, clean gloves are used [120]. The "sterile" technique is clearly more expensive than the "clean" technique. The scientific basis of "sterile technique" is lacking [118] but it is considered the gold standard and recommended by the CDC [3].

Patients are often discharged before incision wounds are fully healed. It is paramount to educate the patients and their family member(s) regarding proper incision care. Also, the patients and their family member(s) should be educated to recognize and report the presence of symptoms of SSI [3].

5 Antibiotic prophylaxis

5.1 The basics of antimicrobial prophylaxis

Surgical antimicrobial prophylaxis is given to prevent SSIs. Its benefit in preventing SSIs has been shown as early as the 1980s, where cefazolin prophylaxis was shown to reduce the number of prosthetic joint infections significantly from 3.3% (placebo) to 0.9% [121]. The practice of prophylaxis is a broadly accepted practice, especially in prosthetic joint surgery. The practice has evolved regarding the timing and the number of the doses that should be given. In Germany, prophylaxis is given to 98% of patients having hip and knee replacements [111]. The use of surgical antibiotic prophylaxis can lead to adverse events, such as allergy, antibiotic-associated diarrhea, and antimicrobial resistance. But these potential problems are quite uncommon. There is very limited data on other adverse events on surgical antibiotic prophylaxis and in case of allergy, alternative antibiotics can be used, as will be described below [122].

The choice of a prophylactic antibiotic depends on the microorganisms likely to cause SSI in the planned surgery. Surgical-site infections after orthopedic procedures are mainly caused by gram-positive bacteria, most frequently *S aureus*. The antibiotic used should therefore cover these microorganisms. The recommendations and characteristics of prophylactic antibiotics that can be used in orthopedic procedures are shown in **Table 4-3**. For practical reasons and due to better bioavailability, antibiotic prophylaxis is administered intravenously. Cefazolin or cefuroxime are recommended by several guidelines, such as the American Academy of Orthopedic Surgeons [123] and Scottish Intercollegiate Guidelines [122], to be used as the first choice for antibiotic prophylaxis in orthopedic surgeries. Cefazolin is a first-generation cephalosporin active against streptococci and methicillin-susceptible *S aureus*. Cefuroxime is a second-generation cephalosporin and has broader activity against gram-negative bacteria. When patients present with penicillin allergy, it should be determined whether an IgE-mediated response (anaphylaxis) has occurred previously when penicillin was administered [9]. A useful method to do this is by inquiring about the time of occurrence of the allergic reaction. Reactions starting within the first hour after administration are IgE mediated. Among the possible reactions are urticaria, pruritic rash, wheezing, and dysphagia due to laryngeal edema and bronchospasm, hypotension and local swelling. It is estimated that the rate of allergic reaction to cephalosporins in patients with penicillin allergy is 7%, and in nonpenicillin-allergic patients 1% [127]. A patient who experienced an allergic reaction to a specific cephalosporin should perhaps not receive that same cephalosporin again, but a different cephalosporin may be used [126]. There are other alternative prophylactic antibiotics which can be used when patients are allergic to β-lactam antibiotics such as clindamycin (600–900 mg intravenously) or vancomycin (1 g intravenously). Routine use of vancomycin for surgical-site infection prophylaxis is not recommended for any type of surgery because its use is associated with vancomycin-resistant *Enterococcus* colonization and infection [9, 129]. Patients allergic to β-lactam antibiotics should receive clindamycin as a first choice. Vancomycin is a second choice for those with known colonization of MRSA and with higher risk for postoperative MRSA infection, eg, patients with recent hospitalization and institutionalized patients [9]. It is important to bear in mind that the choice of antibiotic surgical prophylaxis should also consider the local epidemiology. For example, the susceptibilities of *S aureus* and *Staphylococcus epidermidis* to cefazolin in two academic hospitals in New York and Chicago in the USA were only 74% and 44%, respectively [130].

The above-mentioned surgical prophylaxis guidelines apply to clean and clean-contaminated elective and emergency surgeries. When contamination is already present before

	Primary choice		Alternative	
	Cefazolin	Cefuroxime	Clindamycin (in case of β-lactam allergies)	Vancomycin (in case of β-lactam allergies and MRSA during screening)
Dose (intravenous)	1–2 g	1.5 g	600–900 mg	1 g
Redosing interval in case of prolonged surgery	2–5 h	3–4 h	3–6 h	6–12 h
Renal half-life	1.25–2.5 h	1–2 h	2–5.1 h	3.5–5.0 h
Renal half-life in patients with end-stage renal disease	40–70 h	15–22 h	3.5–5.0 h	44.1–406.4 h
Infusion duration when dose is injected directly into vein or via running intravenous fluids	3–5 min	3–5 min	10–60 min	60 min

Table 4-3 Recommendations and characteristics of prophylactic antibiotics that can be used in orthopedic procedures, adapted from Bratzler, et al [139]. Dosing is based on a 70 kg patient but dosing should be adjusted based on the body weight in kilograms (mg/kg dosing). Abbreviation: MRSA, methicillin-resistant *Staphylococcus aureus*.

surgery, for example, in open fractures, other antibiotics should be given as treatment since gram-positive and gram-negative bacteria are found in open fracture wounds [131]. This finding suggests that in open fractures additional gram-negative coverage should be added [132]. To this end, various regimens have been used and proposed, such as amoxicillin/clavulanic acid [131], a combination of cephalosporins with aminoglycosides [132], and a combination of cephalosporins with quinolones [133].

5.2 When and for how long to administer prophylactic antibiotics

Antimicrobial prophylaxis should be given so that serum and tissue drug levels are achieved for the duration of the operation. Serum levels should be higher than the minimum inhibitory concentration of the microorganisms possibly encountered during the surgery. Minimum inhibitory concentration is the lowest antibiotic concentration that inhibits the growth of bacteria. In 1961, it was shown that when antibiotics were given before incision *S aureus* could be suppressed [134]. About 30 years later an RCT was performed on the rate of SSI in the preoperative phase (administration of antibiotics 2 hours before the surgical incision), the early phase (2–24 hours before the surgical incision), the intraoperative phase (within the 3 hours after the incision), and the postoperative phase (more than 3 but less than 24 hours after the incision) [135]. The patients in this study underwent elective-clean or "clean-contaminated" surgical procedures. The comparison showed that the lowest SSI rates occurred when the prophylactic antibiotic was given in the preoperative phase (0.6%), followed by intraoperative (1.4%), postoperative (3.3%), and early (3.8%) phase administration. A more recent study from Switzerland elaborated further on the timing of prophylactic antibiotic administration and found that administration of cefuroxime 30–59 minutes before incision is more effective than during the last 30 minutes [136]. The SSI rate was higher when the antibiotic was given within 30 minutes of incision than between 31 and 60 minutes, however, this difference was not statistically significant [137]. The consensus is thus to administer antibiotics within 1 hour prior to surgical incision. This may be extended to 2 hours for vancomycin.

A study from Germany listed the common mistakes in administration of antibiotic prophylaxis and the timing of administration is often mentioned. In some cases, antibiotics were given too early or too late after the skin incision had been made [138].

Antibiotic prophylaxis usually involves just a single dose preoperatively. In situations of significant blood loss (more than 1.5 L) and lengthy operations (beyond 3 hours), antibiotics should be redosed at intervals of 1–2 times half-life of the antibiotics. As prophylaxis, cefazolin and cefuroxime can be redosed every 3–5 hours, clindamycin every 3–6 hours, and vancomycin every 6–12 hours (**Table 4-3**) [139]. Prophylactic antibiotics should not be used longer than a 24-hour duration.

5.3 Prophylactic antibiotics in special cases

As mentioned previously, patients with asymptomatic bacteriuria planned to undergo orthopedic surgery do not need to be treated with antibiotics. Only patients presenting with symptoms of urinary tract infection need to be treated prior to elective arthroplasty [9].

In patients who have implants such as heart valves, the same prophylactic antibiotics as in patients without earlier implanted prostheses can be used [9]. Individuals with prosthetic heart valves have a higher risk for endocarditis. Endocarditis and prosthetic joint infection are both most often caused by *S aureus* and *S epidermidis* [140].

6 Conclusion

Surgical-site infection prevention has been studied for more than 150 years after being pioneered by great scholars, such as Louis Pasteur, Ignaz Semmelweis, Joseph Lister, and Alexander Fleming. We have reviewed here the best practices to prevent SSIs, such as modifying patient-related risk factors and taking appropriate preoperative, intraoperative, and postoperative measures.

The preventive measures described in this chapter can be combined into a care "bundle". A care bundle is defined by Institute for Healthcare Improvement [141] as a structured way of improving the processes of care and patient outcomes by using a small, straightforward set of evidence-based practices (generally three to five). Surgical-site infection rates are often used as hospital quality measures [142] and implementation of bundle elements: intraoperative normothermia, appropriate hair removal before surgery, the use of intraoperative antibiotic prophylaxis, and discipline in the operation room have been shown to reduce SSIs by up to 51 % in vascular procedures [143]. Such a bundle can also be implemented in orthopedic surgeries since many evidence-based measures are readily available. Additional study is required where scientific proof is limited to contribute more knowledge on the measures preventing SSIs.

7 References

1. **Wallace WC, Cinat ME, Nastanski F, et al.** New epidemiology for postoperative nosocomial infections. *Am Surg.* 2000 Sep, 66(9):874–878.
2. **Horan TC, Gaynes RP, Martone WJ, et al.** CDC definitions of nosocomial surgical site infections, 1992: A modification of CDC definitions of surgical wound infections. *Infect Control Hosp Epidemiol.* 1992 Oct;13(10):606–608.
3. **Mangram AJ, Horan TC, Pearson ML, et al.** Guideline for prevention of surgical site infection, 1999. Hospital Infection Control Practices Advisory Committee. *Infect Control Hosp Epidemiol.* 1999 Apr;20(4):250–278; quiz 279–280.
4. **Leaper D, Tanner J, Kiernan M.** Surveillance of surgical site infection: more accurate definitions and intensive recording needed. *J Hosp Infect.* 2013 Feb;83(2):83–86.
5. **Gastmeier P, Sohr D, Brandt, et al.** Reduction of orthopaedic wound infections in 21 hospitals. *Arch Orthop Trauma Surg.* 2005 Oct;125(8):526–530.
6. **Astagneau P, Rioux C, Golliot F, et al.** Morbidity and mortality associated with surgical site infections: results from the 1997-1999 INCISO surveillance. *J Hosp Infect.* 2001 Aug;48(4):267–274.
7. **Maksimović J, Marković-Denić L, Bumbasirević M, et al.** Surgical site infections in orthopedic patients: prospective cohort study. *Croat Med J.* 2008 Feb;49(1):58–65.
8. **Whitehouse JD, Friedman ND, Kirkland KB, et al.** The impact of surgical-site infections following orthopedic surgery at a community hospital and a university hospital: adverse quality of life, excess length of stay, and extra cost. *Infect Control Hosp Epidemiol.* 2002 Apr;23(4):183–189.
9. **Parvizi J, Gehrke T, Chen AF.** Proceedings of the International Consensus on Periprosthetic Joint Infection. *Bone Joint J.* 2013 Nov;95-B(11):1450–1452.
10. **Anderson DJ, Kaye KS, Classen D, et al.** Strategies to prevent surgical site infections in acute care hospitals. *Infect Control Hosp Epidemiol.* 2008 Oct;29 Suppl 1:S51-61
11. **Dronge AS, Perkal MF, Kancir S, et al.** Long-term glycemic control and postoperative infectious complications. *Arch Surg.* 2006 Apr;141(4):375–380; discussion 380.
12. **Dowsey MM, Choong PF.** Obese diabetic patients are at substantial risk for deep infection after primary TKA. *Clin Orthop Relat Res.* 2009 Jun;467(6):1577–1581.
13. **Malinzak RA, Ritter MA, Berend ME, et al.** Morbidly obese, diabetic, younger, and unilateral joint arthroplasty patients have elevated total joint arthroplasty infection rates. *J Arthroplasty.* 2009 Sep;24(6 Suppl):8488.
14. **Hu SS, Fontaine F, Kelly B, et al.** Nutritional depletion in staged spinal reconstructive surgery. The effect of total parenteral nutrition. *Spine (Phila Pa 1976).* 1998 Jun 15;23(12):1401–1405.
15. **Møller AM, Villebro N, Pedersen T, et al.** Effect of preoperative smoking intervention on postoperative complications: a randomised clinical trial. *Lancet.* 2002 Jan 12;359(9301):114–117.
16. **Lindström D, Sadr Azodi O, Wladis A, et al.** Effects of a perioperative smoking cessation intervention on postoperative complications: a randomized trial. *Ann Surg.* 2008; Nov;248(5):739–745.
17. **Schmalzried TP, Amstutz HC, Au MK, et al.** Etiology of deep sepsis in total hip arthroplasty. The significance of hematogenous and recurrent infections. *Clin Orthop Relat Res.* 1992 Jul;(280):200–207.
18. **Stinchfield FE, Bigliani LU, Neu HC, et al.** Late hematogenous infection of total joint replacement. *J Bone Joint Surg Am.* 1980 Dec; 62(8):1345–1350.
19. **Sousa R, Muñoz-Mahamud E, Quayle J, et al.** Is asymptomatic bacteriuria a risk factor for prosthetic joint infection? *Clin Infect Dis.* 2014 Jul 1;59(1):41–47.
20. **Weigelt JA, Lipsky BA, Tabak YP, et al.** Surgical site infections: Causative pathogens and associated outcomes. *Am J Infect Control.* 2010 Mar; 38(2):112–120.
21. **Coates T, Bax R, Coates A.** Nasal decolonization of Staphylococcus aureus with mupirocin: strengths, weaknesses and future prospects. *J Antimicrob Chemother.* 2009 Jul;64(1):9–15.
22. **Perl TM, Cullen JJ, Wenzel RP, et al.** Intranasal mupirocin to prevent postoperative Staphylococcus aureus infections. *N Engl J Med.* 2002 Jun 13; 346(24):1871–1877.
23. **Doebbeling BN, Breneman DL, Neu HC, et al.** Elimination of Staphylococcus aureus nasal carriage in health care workers: analysis of six clinical trials with calcium mupirocin ointment. The Mupirocin Collaborative Study Group. *Clin Infect Dis.* 1993 Sep;17(3):466–474.
24. **McConeghy KW, Mikolich DJ, LaPlante KL.** Agents for the decolonization of methicillin-resistant Staphylococcus aureus. *Pharmacotherapy.* 2009 Mar;29(3):263–280.
25. **Dupeyron C, Campillo B, Bordes M, et al.** A clinical trial of mupirocin in the eradication of methicillin-resistant Staphylococcus aureus nasal carriage in a digestive disease unit. *J Hosp Infect.* 2002 Dec; 52(4):281–287.
26. **Kalmeijer MD, Coertjens H, van Nieuwland-Bollen PM, et al.** Surgical site infections in orthopedic surgery: the effect of mupirocin nasal ointment in a double-blind, randomized, placebo-controlled study. *Clin Infect Dis.* 2002 Aug 15;35(4):353–358.
27. **Doebbeling BN, Reagan DR, Pfaller MA, et al.** Long-term efficacy of intranasal mupirocin ointment. A prospective cohort study of Staphylococcus aureus carriage. *Arch Intern Med.* 1994 Jul 11;154(13):1505–1508.
28. **Jones JC, Rogers TJ, Brookmeyer P, et al.** Mupirocin resistance in patients colonized with methicillin-resistant Staphylococcus aureus in a surgical intensive care unit. *Clin Infect Dis.* 2007 Sep 1;45(5):541–547.
29. **Garibaldi RA, Skolnick D, Lerer T, et al.** The impact of preoperative skin disinfection on preventing intraoperative wound contamination. *Infect Control Hosp Epidemiol.* 1988 Mar;9(3):109–113.
30. **Hayek L.** A placebo-controlled trial of the effect of two preoperative baths or showers with chlorhexidine detergent on postoperative wound infection rates. *J Hosp Infect.* 1989 Feb;13(2):202–204.
31. **Karki S, Cheng AC.** Impact of non-rinse skin cleansing with chlorhexidine gluconate on prevention of healthcare-associated infections and colonization with multi-resistant organisms: a systematic review. *J Hosp infect.* 2012 Oct;82(2):71–84.
32. **Webster J, Osborne S.** Preoperative bathing or showering with skin antiseptics to prevent surgical site infection. *Cochrane Database Syst Rev.* 2012 Sep 12;9: CD004985.

33. **Wihlborg O.** The effect of washing with chlorhexidine soap on wound infection rate in general surgery. A controlled clinical study. *Ann Chir Gynaecol.* 1987;76(5):263–265.
34. **Eiselt D.** Presurgical skin preparation with a novel 2% chlorhexidine gluconate cloth reduces rates of surgical site infection in orthopaedic surgical patients. *Orthop Nurs.* 2009 May-Jun;28(3):141–145.
35. **Zywiel MG, Daley JA, Delanois RE, et al.** Advance pre-operative chlorhexidine reduces the incidence of surgical site infections in knee arthroplasty. *Int Orthop.* 2011 Jul;(7):1001–1006.
36. **Lilly HA, Lowbury EJ, Wilkins MD.** Limits to progressive reduction of resident skin bacteria by disinfection. *J Clin Pathol.* 1979 Apr; 32(4): 382–385.
37. **O'Grady NP, Alexander M, Burns LA, et al.** Guidelines for the prevention of intravascular catheter-related infections. *Clin Infect Dis.* 2011 May;52(9):e162–193.
38. **Tanner J, Norrie P, Melen K.** Preoperative hair removal to reduce surgical site infection. *Cochrane database Syst Rev.* 2011 Nov 9;(11):CD004122.
39. **Balthazar ER, Colt JD, Nichols RL.** Preoperative hair removal: a random prospective study of shaving versus clipping. *South Med J.* 1982 Jul;75(7):799–801.
40. **Alexander JW, Fischer JE, Boyajian M, et al.** The influence of hair-removal methods on wound infections. *Arch Surg.* 1983 Mar; 118(3):347–352.
41. **Seropian R, Reynolds BM.** Wound infections after preoperative depilatory versus razor preparation. *Am J Surg.* 1971 Mar;121(3):251–254.
42. **Lister J.** On the Antiseptic Principle in the Practice of Surgery. *Br Med J.* 1867 Sep 21;2(351): 246–248.
43. **Hemani ML, Lepor H.** Skin preparation for the prevention of surgical site infection: which agent is best? *Rev Urol.* 2009 Fall; 11(4):190–195.
44. **Association of Operating Room Nurses.** Recommended practices for skin preparation of patients. *AORN J.* 1996 Nov;64(5):813–816.
45. **Dumville JC, McFarlane E, Edwards P, et al.** Preoperative skin antiseptics for preventing surgical wound infections after clean surgery. *Cochrane Database Syst Rev.* 2013 Mar 28;3:CD003949.
46. **Maiwald M, Chan ES.** The forgotten role of alcohol: a systematic review and meta-analysis of the clinical efficacy and perceived role of chlorhexidine in skin antisepsis. *PloS One.* 2012;7(9):e44277.
47. **Larson EL.** APIC guideline for handwashing and hand antisepsis in health care settings. *Am J Infect Control.* 1995 Aug;23(4):251–269.
48. **Rodeheaver G, Bellamy W, Kody M, et al.** Bactericidal activity and toxicity of iodine-containing solutions in wounds. *Arch Surg.* 1982 Feb;117(2):181 186.
49. **Tschudin-Sutter S, Frei R, Egli-Gany D, et al.** No risk of surgical site infections from residual bacteria after disinfection with povidone-iodine-alcohol in 1014 cases: a prospective observational study. *Ann Surg.* 2012;255(3):565–569.
50. **Darouiche RO, Wall MJ Jr, Itani KM, et al.** Chlorhexidine-Alcohol versus Povidone-Iodine for Surgical-Site Antisepsis. *N Engl J Med.* 2010 Jan 7;362(1):18–26.
51. **Noorani A, Rabey N, Walsh SR, Davies RJ.** Systematic review and meta-analysis of preoperative antisepsis with chlorhexidine versus povidone-iodine in clean-contaminated surgery. *Br J Surg.* 2010 Nov;97(11):1614–1620.
52. **Burlingame B, Denholm B, Link T, et al.** AORN Guidelines for Perioperative Practice. Vol. 1. 2016. Guideline for Sterile Technique. Available at: http://www.aornstandards.org/content/1/SEC5.extract?sid=915f30c9-0da1-4ffb-8621-254589662ac4#. Accessed April, 2016.
53. **Garibaldi RA, Maglio S, Lerer T, et al.** Comparison of nonwoven and woven gown and drape fabric to prevent intraoperative wound contamination and postoperative infection. *Am J Surg.* 1986 Nov;152(5):505 509.
54. **Chiu KY, Lau SK, Fung B, et al.** Plastic adhesive drapes and wound infection after hip fracture surgery. *Aust N Z J Surg.* 1993 Oct;63(10):798–801.
55. **French ML, Eitzen HE, Ritter MA.** The plastic surgical adhesive drape: an evaluation of its efficacy as a microbial barrier. *Ann Surg.* 1976 Jul;184(1):46–50.
56. **Webster J, Alghamdi A.** Use of plastic adhesive drapes during surgery for preventing surgical site infection. *Cochrane Database Syst Rev.* 2013 Jan 31;1:CD006353.
57. **Kampf G, Kramer A.** Epidemiologic background of hand hygiene and evaluation of the most important agents for scrubs and rubs. *Clin Microbiol Rev.* 2004 Oct;17(4):863–893, table of contents.
58. **Widmer AF.** Replace hand washing with use of a waterless alcohol hand rub? *Clin Infect Dis.* 2000 Jul;31(1):136–143.
59. **Chen CF, Han CL, Kan CP, et al.** Effect of surgical site infections with waterless and traditional hand scrubbing protocols on bacterial growth. *Am J Infect Control.* 2012 May;40(4):e15–17.
60. **Hingst V, Juditzki I, Heeg P, et al.** Evaluation of the efficacy of surgical hand disinfection following a reduced application time of 3 instead of 5 min. *J Hosp Infect.* 1992 Feb;20(2):79–86.
61. **Tanner J, Swarbrook S, Stuart J.** Surgical hand antisepsis to reduce surgical site infection. *Cochrane Database Syst Rev.* 2008 Jan 23;(1):CD004288.
62. **Boyce JM, Pittet D, Healthcare Infection Control Practices Advisory Committee, et al.** Hand Hygiene Task Force. Guideline for Hand Hygiene in Health-Care Settings: recommendations of the Healthcare Infection Control Practices Advisory Committee and the HICPAC/SHEA/APIC/IDSA Hand Hygiene Task Force. *Infect Control Hosp Epidemiol.* 2002 Dec;23(12 Suppl):S3–40.
63. **Parienti JJ, Thibon P, Heller R, et al.** Hand-rubbing with an aqueous alcoholic solution vs traditional surgical hand-scrubbing and 30-day surgical site infection rates: a randomized equivalence study. *JAMA.* 2002 Aug 14;288(6):722–727.
64. **Duguid JP, Wallace AT.** Air infection with dust liberated from clothing. *Lancet.* 1948 Nov 27;2(6535):845–849
65. **Berger SA, Kramer M, Nagar H, et al.** Effect of surgical mask position on bacterial contamination of the operative field. *J Hosp Infect.* 1993 Jan;23(1):51–54.
66. **Romney MG.** Surgical face masks in the operating theatre: re-examining the evidence. *J Hosp Infect.* 2001 Apr;47(4):251–256.
67. **Ritter MA, Eitzen H, French ML, Hart JB.** The operating room environment as affected by people and the surgical face mask. *Clin Orthop Relat Res.* 1975 Sep;(111):147–150.
68. **Mitchell NJ, Hunt S.** Surgical face masks in modern operating rooms - a costly and unnecessary ritual? *J Hosp Infect.* 1991 Jul;18(3):239–242.
69. **Braswell ML, Spruce L.** Implementing AORN recommended practices for surgical attire. *AORN J.* 2012 Jan;95(1):122-37; quiz 138–140.
70. **Misteli H, Weber WP, Reck S, et al.** Surgical glove perforation and the risk of surgical site infection. *Arch Surg.* 2009 Jun;144(6):553–558; discussion 558.

71. **Laine T, Aarnio P.** How often does glove perforation occur in surgery? Comparison between single gloves and a double-gloving system. *Am J Surg.* 2001 Jun;181(6):564–566.
72. **Schindler OS, Spencer RF, Smith MD.** Should we use a separate knife for the skin? *J Bone Joint Surg Br.* 2006 Mar;88(3):382–385.
73. **Ritter MA, French ML, Eitzen HE.** Bacterial contamination of the surgical knife. *Clin Orthop Relat Res.* 1975 May;(108):158–160.
74. **Meka PN KP, Khullar P, Anand VJ.** To compare the superiority of electrocautery over the traditional scalpel for skin incisions. *J Surg Res.* 2004 Oct;121(2):341.
75. **Anglen JO.** Wound irrigation in musculoskeletal injury. *J Am Acad Orthop Surg.* 2001 Jul-Aug;9(4):219–226.
76. **Hassinger SM, Harding G, Wongworawat MD.** High-pressure pulsatile lavage propagates bacteria into soft tissue. *Clin Orthop Relat Res.* 2005 Oct;439:27–31.
77. **Petrisor B, Jeray K, Schemitsch E, et al.** Fluid lavage in patients with open fracture wounds (FLOW): an international survey of 984 surgeons. *BMC Musculoskelet Disord.* 2008 Jan 23;9:7.
78. **Kurz A, Sessler DI, Lenhardt R.** Perioperative normothermia to reduce the incidence of surgical-wound infection and shorten hospitalization. Study of Wound Infection and Temperature Group. *N Engl J Med.* 1996 May 9;334(19):1209–1215.
79. **Greif R, Sessler DI.** Supplemental oxygen and risk of surgical site infection. *JAMA.* 2004 Apr 28;291(16):1957; author reply 1958–1959.
80. **Kabon B, Akca O, Taguchi A, et al.** Supplemental intravenous crystalloid administration does not reduce the risk of surgical wound infection. *Anesth Analg.* 2005 Nov;101(5):1546–1553.
81. **McHugh SM, Hill AD, Humphreys H.** Intraoperative technique as a factor in the prevention of surgical site infection. *J Hosp Infect.* 2011 May;78(1):1–4.
82. **Elek SD, Conen PE.** The virulence of Staphylococcus pyogenes for man; a study of the problems of wound infection. *Br J Exp Pathol.* 1957 Dec;38(6):573–586.
83. **Tajirian AL, Goldberg DJ.** A review of sutures and other skin closure materials. *J Cosmet Laser Ther.* 2010 Dec;12(6):296–302.
84. **Sharp WV, Belden TA, King PH, et al.** Suture resistance to infection. *Surgery.* 1982 Jan;91(1):61–63.
85. **Osterberg B.** Enclosure of bacteria within capillary multifilament sutures as protection against leukocytes. *Acta Chir Scand.* 1983;149(7):663–668.
86. **Gabrielli F, Potenza C, Puddu, et al.** Suture materials and other factors associated with tissue reactivity, infection, and wound dehiscence among plastic surgery outpatients. *Plast Reconstr Surg.* 2001 Jan;107(1):38–45.
87. **Smith TO, Sexton D, Mann C, et al.** Sutures versus staples for skin closure in orthopaedic surgery: meta-analysis. *BMJ.* 2010 Mar 16;340:c1199
88. **Khan RJ, Fick D, Yao F, et al.** A comparison of three methods of wound closure following arthroplasty: a prospective, randomised, controlled trial. *J Bone Joint Surg Br.* 2006 Feb;88(2):238–242.
89. **Alexander JW, Solomkin JS, Edwards MJ.** Updated recommendations for control of surgical site infections. *Ann Surg. Ann Surg.* 2011 Jun;253(6):1082–1093.
90. **Bernard HR, Cole WR.** Wound infections following potentially contaminated operations. Effect of delayed primary closure of the skin and subcutaneous tissue. *JAMA.* 1963 Apr 27;184:290–292.
91. **Duttaroy DD, Jitendra J, Duttaroy B, et al.** Management strategy for dirty abdominal incisions: primary or delayed primary closure? A randomized trial. *Surg Infect (Larchmt).* 2009 Apr;10(2):129–136.
92. **Strasen KM, Berne TV.** Wound infection in patients with traumatic small intestinal injuries. *Am Surg.* 1991 Dec;57(12):803–805.
93. **Verrier ED, Bossart KJ, Heer FW.** Reduction of infection rates in abdominal incisions by delayed wound closure techniques. *Am J Surg.* 1979 Jul;138(1):22–28.
94. **DuMortier JJ.** The resistance of healing wounds to infection. *Surg Gynecol Obstet.* 1933;56: 762–766.
95. **Weitz-Marshall AD, Bosse MJ.** Timing of closure of open fractures. *The Journal of the J Am Acad Orthop Surg.* 2002 Nov-Dec;10(6):379–384.
96. **Lalliss SJ, Stinner DJ, Waterman SM, et al.** Negative pressure wound therapy reduces pseudomonas wound contamination more than Staphylococcus aureus. *J Orthop Trauma.* 2010 Sep;24(9):598–602.
97. **Morykwas MJ, Argenta LC, Shelton-Brown EI, et al.** Vacuum-assisted closure: a new method for wound control and treatment: animal studies and basic foundation. *Ann Plast Surg.* 1997 Jun;38(6):553–562.
98. **Yusuf E, Jordan X, Clauss M, et al.** High bacterial load in negative pressure wound therapy (NPWT) foams used in the treatment of chronic wounds. *Wound Repair Regen.* 2013 Sep-Oct;21(5):677–681.
99. **Parker MJ, Roberts CP, Hay D.** Closed suction drainage for hip and knee arthroplasty. A meta-analysis. *J Bone Joint Surg Am.* 2004 Jun;86-A(6):1146–1152.
100. **Clifton R, Haleem S, McKee A, et al.** Closed suction surgical wound drainage after anterior cruciate ligament reconstruction: a systematic review of randomised controlled trials. *Knee.* 2007 Oct;14(5):348–351.
101. **Clifton R, Haleem S, McKee A, et al.** Closed suction surgical wound drainage after hip fracture surgery: a systematic review and meta-analysis of randomised controlled trials. *Int Orthop.* 2008 Dec;32(6):723–727.
102. **Leong G, Wilson J, Charlett A.** Duration of operation as a risk factor for surgical site infection: comparison of English and US data. *J Hosp Infect.* 2006 Jul;63(3):255–262.
103. **Peersman G, Laskin R, Davis J, et al.** Prolonged operative time correlates with increased infection rate after total knee arthroplasty. *HSS J.* 2006 Feb;2(1):70–72.
104. **Edmiston CE, Jr, Seabrook GR, Cambria RA, et al.** Molecular epidemiology of microbial contamination in the operating room environment: Is there a risk for infection? Surgery. *2005 Oct;138(4):573-579; discussion 579–582.*
105. **Lidwell OM, Lowbury EJ, Whyte W, et al.** Airborne contamination of wounds in joint replacement operations: the relationship to sepsis rates. *J Hosp Infect.* 1983 Jun;4(2):111–131.
106. **Friberg B.** Ultraclean laminar airflow ORs. *AORN J.* 1998 Apr;67(4):841–842, 845–851.
107. **Lidwell OM.** Clean air at operation and subsequent sepsis in the joint. *Clin Orthop Relat Res.* 1986 Oct;(211):91–102.
108. **Gastmeier P, Breier AC, Brandt C.** Influence of laminar airflow on prosthetic joint infections: a systematic review. *J Hosp Infect.* 2012 Jun;81(2):73–78.
109. **Breier AC, Brandt C, Sohr D, et al.** Laminar airflow ceiling size: no impact on infection rates following hip and knee prosthesis. *Infect Control Hosp Epidemiol.* 2011 Nov;32(11):1097–1102.

110. **Hooper G, Rothwell, A., Frampton, et al.** Does the use of laminar airflow and space suits reduce early deep infection after total hip and knee replacement? *J Bone Joint Surg Br.* 2011 Jan;93(1):85–90.
111. **Brandt C, Hott U, Sohr D, et al.** Operating room ventilation with laminar airflow shows no protective effect on the surgical site infection rate in orthopedic and abdominal surgery. *Ann Surg.* 2008 Nov;248(5):695–700.
112. **Lynch RJ, Englesbe MJ, Sturm L, et al.** Measurement of foot traffic in the operating room: implications for infection control. *Am J Med Qual.* 2009 Jan-Feb;24(1):45–52.
113. **Panahi P, Stroh M, Casper DS, et al.** Operating room traffic is a major concern during total joint arthroplasty. *Clin Orthop Relat Res.* 2012 Oct;470(10):2690–2694.
114. **Soto LE, Bobadilla M, Villalobos Y, et al.** Post-surgical nasal cellulitis outbreak due to Mycobacterium chelonae. *J Hosp Infect.* 1991 Oct;19(2):99–106.
115. **Dalstrom DJ, Venkatarayappa I, Manternach AL, et al.** Time-dependent contamination of opened sterile operating-room trays. *J Bone Joint Surg Am.* 2008 May;90(5):1022–1025.
116. **Macfie J, McMahon MJ.** The management of the open perineal wound using a foam elastomer dressing: a prospective clinical trial. *Br J Surg.* 1980 Feb;67(2):85–89.
117. **Cannavo M, Fairbrother G, Owen D, et al.** A comparison of dressings in the management of surgical abdominal wounds. *J Wound Care.* 1998 Feb;7(2):57–62.
118. **National Collaborating Centre for Women's and Children's Health (UK).** Surgical site infection prevention and treatment of surgical site infection. *RCOG Press.* London; 2008 Oct.
119. **Kamath S, Sinha S, Shaari E, et al.** Role of topical antibiotics in hip surgery. A prospective randomised study. *Injury.* 2005 Jun;36(6):783–787.
120. **Wound, Ostomy and Continence Nurses Society (WOCN) Wound Committee, Association for Professionals in Infection Control and Epidemiology, Inc. (APIC) 2000 Guidelines Committee.** Clean vs. sterile dressing techniques for management of chronic wounds: a fact sheet. *J Wound Ostomy Continence Nurs.* 2012 Mar-Apr;39(2 Suppl):S30–34.
121. **Hill C, Flamant R, Mazas F, et al.** Prophylactic cefazolin versus placebo in total hip replacement. Report of a multicentre double-blind randomised trial. *Lancet.* 1981 Apr 11;1(8224):795–796.
122. **Scottish Intercollegiate Guidelines Network.** Antibiotic prophylaxis in surgery (SIGN publication no.104). Edinburgh, 2008, updated April, 2014.
123. **American Association of Orthopaedic Surgeons.** Recommendations for the Use of Intravenous Antibiotic Prophylaxis in Primary Total Joint Arthroplasty, 2004. Information Statement 1027, revised March, 2014.
124. **Kalman D, Barriere SL.** Review of the pharmacology, pharmacokinetics, and clinical use of cephalosporins. *Tex Heart Inst J.* 1990;17(3):203–215.
125. **Legendre DP, Muzny CA, Marshall GD, et al.** Antibiotic hypersensitivity reactions and approaches to desensitization. *Clin Infect Dis.* 2014 Apr;58(8):1140–1148.
126. **Pichichero ME.** A review of evidence supporting the American Academy of Pediatrics recommendation for prescribing cephalosporin antibiotics for penicillin-allergic patients. *Pediatrics.* 2005 Apr;115(4):1048–1057.
127. **Dash CH.** Penicillin allergy and the cephalosporins. *J Antimicrob Chemother.* 1975;1(3 Suppl):107–118.
128. **Koch CG, Nowicki ER, Rajeswaran J, et al.** When the timing is right: Antibiotic timing and infection after cardiac surgery. *J Thorac Cardiovasc Surg.* 2012 Oct;144(4):931–937.e4.
129. **French GL.** Enterococci and vancomycin resistance. *Clin Infect Dis.* 1998 Aug;27 Suppl 1:S75–83.
130. **Fulkerson E, Valle CJ, Wise B, et al.** Antibiotic susceptibility of bacteria infecting total joint arthroplasty sites. *J Bone Joint Surg Am.* 2006 Jun;88(6):1231–1237.
131. **Yusuf E, Steinrücken J, Buchegger T, et al.** A descriptive study on the surgery and the microbiology of Gustilo type III fractures in an university hospital in Switzerland. *Acta Orthop Belgica.*2015 Jun;81(2):327–332.
132. **Hoff WS, Bonadies JA, Cachecho R, et al.** East Practice Management Guidelines Work Group: update to practice management guidelines for prophylactic antibiotic use in open fractures. *J Trauma.* 2011 Mar;70(3):751–754.
133. **Patzakis MJ, Bains RS, Lee J, et al.** Prospective, randomized, double-blind study comparing single-agent antibiotic therapy, ciprofloxacin, to combination antibiotic therapy in open fracture wounds. *J Orthop Trauma.* 2000 Nov;14(8):529–533.
134. **Burke JF.** The effective period of preventive antibiotic action in experimental incisions and dermal lesions. *Surgery.* 1961 Jul;50:161–168.
135. **Classen DC, Evans RS, Pestotnik SL, et al.** The timing of prophylactic administration of antibiotics and the risk of surgical-wound infection. *N Engl J Med.* 1992 Jan 30;326(5):281–286.
136. **Weber WP, Marti WR, Zwahlen M, et al.** The timing of surgical antimicrobial prophylaxis. *Ann Surg.* 2008 Jun;247(6):918–926
137. **Steinberg JP, Braun BI, Hellinger WC, et al.** Timing of antimicrobial prophylaxis and the risk of surgical site infections: results from the Trial to Reduce Antimicrobial Prophylaxis Errors. *Ann Surg.* 2009 Jul;250(1):10–16.
138. **Dettenkofer M, Forster DH, Ebner W, et al.** The practice of perioperative antibiotic prophylaxis in eight German hospitals. *Infection.* 2002 Jun;30(3):164–167.
139. **Bratzler DW, Houck PM, Surgical Infection Prevention Guidelines Writers Workgroup, et al.** Antimicrobial prophylaxis for surgery: an advisory statement from the National Surgical Infection Prevention Project. *Clin Infect Dis.* 2004 Jun 15;38(12):1706–1715.
140. **Dajani AS, Taubert KA, Wilson W, et al.** Prevention of bacterial endocarditis. Recommendations by the American Heart Association. *JAMA.* 1997 Jun 11;277(22):1794–1801.
141. **Institute for Healthcare Improvement.** Evidence-based care bundles. Available at: http://www.ihi.org/topics/bundles/Pages/default.aspx. Accessed April, 2016.
142. **Kao LS, Ghaferi AA, Ko CY, et al.** Reliability of superficial surgical site infections as a hospital quality measure. *J Am Coll Surg.* 2011 Aug;213(2):231–235.
143. **van der Slegt J, van der Laan L, Veen EJ, et al.** Implementation of a bundle of care to reduce surgical site infections in patients undergoing vascular surgery. *PLoS One.* 2013 Aug 13;8(8):e71566.

5 Systemic antibiotics

Werner Zimmerli, Parham Sendi

1 Basics

The introduction of antimicrobial drugs has been one of the biggest success stories in clinical medicine. *Staphylococcus aureus* sepsis or bacterial meningitis, which led to a lethal outcome in more than 50% of the patients, became treatable, and mortality dropped to less than 20% with appropriate antimicrobial therapy [1, 2]. In the field of bone and joint infections, surgical treatment alone, besides amputations, cannot completely eliminate microorganisms [3–6]. In the preantibiotic era, arthrodesis was often required after staphylococcal arthritis. Similarly, after open fracture, chronic osteomyelitis was commonplace. Such infections often required dozens of surgical interventions over several decades [7]. Likewise, antibiotic therapy alone is insufficient for curing implant-associated bone and joint infections [8, 9]. As an exception, therapeutic surgery is generally not required in patients with acute hematogenous osteomyelitis not involving implants, as long as antibiotic therapy is rapidly started [10]. For an optimal outcome, most bone and joint infections are best managed by a team of different specialists (see part 5 of this chapter). In comparison to historical care, loss of joint function and chronic osteomyelitis have become uncommon with adequate management. More than 80% of patients with osteomyelitis or periprosthetic joint infection can now be cured with the first treatment attempt if the correct multidisciplinary approach is chosen [8, 11, 12].

During the last decade, the postantibiotic era has been repeatedly heralded [13]. The reason for this unfortunate evolution is the misuse of antimicrobial agents. The most common misconception is the idea that giving antibiotics more frequently and/or for a longer time decreases the risk for infection. Another error is treatment with antibiotics alone in a case actually requiring surgery. The fact is that prolonged antibiotic prophylaxis does not decrease the rate of infection in any type of surgery, and treatment without surgery increases the risk for chronic persistence of the biofilm [12, 14]. In addition, if a febrile patient gets empiric antibiotics without suffering from a bacterial infection, the change of his/her microbiome endangers him/her for an infection with more resistant microorganisms [15]. Therefore, the correct use of antibiotics should be understood well by all physicians. In contrast to other drugs such as antihypertensive agents, the liberal use of antibiotics has an unfavorable impact on future patients, ie, it may decrease the susceptibility of bacteria in a whole population [16, 17]. This is illustrated by different rates of multiresistant bacteria in different geographical areas with different antibiotic prescribing patterns. Therefore, antibiotic stewardship has become an important task for the infectious diseases specialist, who should not only consider the infectious problem of the individual patient but also the epidemiological situation for future patients.

The appropriate use of an antimicrobial agent depends on the type of infection, the species, and susceptibility of the microorganism. If an infection is difficult to diagnose, an experienced microbiologist should be consulted prior to the intervention. This allows adequate sampling and appropriate identification procedures. Correct identification and knowledge of the susceptibility pattern allows antimicrobial therapy with the optimal drug.

The choice of an antimicrobial agent should consider both special properties of the microorganism and the host. The issue of antibiotics and special properties of the microorganism are discussed below (see parts 2 and 3 of this chapter). Host factors should also be considered when treating patients with antibiotics. These include previous antimicrobial therapy, recent hospitalization or travels to regions with a high prevalence of multiresistant microorganisms [18, 19]. These patients potentially have an altered skin flora, which is a risk factor for more difficult-to-treat surgical-site infections [15]. The immunocompetence of the host is also a crucial factor. In the field of bone and joint infection, this plays a special role in patients with malignant bone tumors undergoing chemotherapy as well as bone replacement by tumor prosthesis [20]. If these patients suffer from implant-associated infection, long-term bactericidal therapy is required. If complete eradication of infection is not possible, lifelong antibiotic suppression is needed. It has been shown that the presence of an implant leads to an impaired elimination of even a low number of microorganisms due to a local granulocyte defect [21, 22]. This is caused by so-called frustrated phagocytosis [22]. In addition, microorganisms forming a biofilm are partially resistant to intact granulocytes [23].

2 Definition of the use of antibiotics

In order to use antimicrobial agents in a rational way, the type of use should be defined before starting treatment. Antibiotic therapy is often inappropriately prolonged. This error is based on the misconception that infection can be prevented by antibiotics during the early postoperative period. Unfortunately, the opposite is true. The altered skin microbiome around the wound increases the risk for infection with a multiresistant microorganism [15].

The following terms and definitions are commonly used.

2.1 Antimicrobial prophylaxis

Prophylaxis means that the antibiotic is present in the wound before appearance of microorganisms. Since penetration of the antimicrobial drug in tissue requires time, application at least 30 minutes before starting surgery is needed for optimal efficacy of surgical prophylaxis [24, 25]. A single dose is generally enough. Prolongation of prophylaxis beyond 24 hours has never been shown to decrease the rate of surgical-site infection [26–28].

2.2 Preemptive therapy

In preemptive therapy, the antibiotic penetrates the wound after the microorganisms, but before the establishment of overt infection. This situation is observed in patients with open fracture undergoing internal fixation within a few hours. A short course of antibiotics, not longer than a few days, is suggested for prevention of surgical-site infection [28–30].

2.3 Empiric therapy

Empiric therapy is defined as administration of an antibiotic in a patient with signs and symptoms of a bacterial infection but without identification of the microorganism. This procedure is also called an "educated guess". This indicates that the treating physician should consider the type of infection, epidemiology, and the probable resistance pattern of the most probable microorganism(s), when choosing an antibiotic. As a rule, empiric therapy should be optimized as soon as the microorganism and its susceptibility are known, which generally requires not more than a few days.

2.4 Targeted therapy

Targeted therapy means that antibiotics are chosen according to a known microorganism and its confirmed antibiotic susceptibility. The length of therapy and the time of transition from intravenous (IV) to oral therapy depend on the type of infection.

2.5 Suppressive therapy

If bacterial elimination (microbiological cure) is not a realistic option, long-term antibiotic treatment with an oral drug may suppress symptoms of infection [31]. In general, this treatment is only palliative. However, periodic stopping of suppressive therapy by an experienced team at a predefined point in time allows identification of patients who do not require lifelong suppression.

2.6 Special considerations regarding antimicrobial therapy of bone and joint infections, including pharmacokinetics in bone

Antibiotic therapy of septic native joint arthritis is generally not more demanding than treatment of pneumonia or bacteremia, because all antibiotics have a good penetration in synovial tissues [32, 33]. Therefore, local therapy is not required and potentially harmful due to possible cartilage damage. However, rapid initiation of antibiotics as well as prompt and often repetitive removal of purulent synovial membranes is important. In contrast, osteomyelitis requires a prolonged antimicrobial therapy with the highest doses to prevent recurrence. As in each type of infection, penetration of the antibiotic to the site of infection is a prerequisite for the elimination of microbes [34, 35]. Limited antibiotic penetration in bone and sequestra (ie, bone fragments devoid of blood supply) at the site of infection jeopardize treatment success. However, it is important to stress that surgery is a prerequisite for the success of antimicrobial treatment. Therefore, it is a clinical commonplace that pus must be drained or removed to cure the patient (ubi pus, ibi evacua). There are several reasons for this statement. Some antibiotics such as β-lactams have a significantly higher minimal inhibitory concentration (MIC) when the number of bacteria is increased. This phenomenon is called inoculum effect and plays a considerable role if β-lactams are used. Since microorganisms are tested at a density of 10^5 colony-forming units (CFU) in vitro, susceptibility may not predict their effect on an abscess where the bacterial density is at 10^6–10^8 CFU [36]. Pus not only contains a high number of bacteria, but also numerous granulocytes either still active with ingested bacteria, or apoptotic or necrotic.

Bony penetration among different groups of antimicrobial agents is variable. However, antibiotic concentration in bone cannot be simply extrapolated to efficacy of treatment for various reasons. Firstly, usually only a single dose is given, which does not reflect equilibrium. Secondly, the drug concentration is measured in sterile bone, which is different from the clinical situation. Thirdly, various time intervals between drug application and harvesting are used, resulting in noncomparable bone or serum concentrations. Fourthly, variable techniques of sample preparation are used. Finally, variable drug determination methods (HPLC, bioassay, etc) preclude direct comparison of results from different studies. However, the following statements can be made for clinical practice. Fluoroquinolones, clindamycin, linezolid, and rifampin have good bone penetration with bone or serum concentration ratios between 0.3–1.1. Penicillin derivatives and cephalosporins have a lower penetration ratio of only 0.1–0.3, and 0.1–0.5, respectively [34].

2.7 Treatment studies

Unfortunately, good clinical studies on the role of defined antibiotics in bone and joint infection are scarce. End of-treatment analysis (eg, after 3 months) is meaningless, because cure cannot yet be definitively judged at this time. A minimum follow-up of 1 year and 2 years, respectively, for bone and implant-associated infection is required. In addition, concomitant-adequate surgical management is as important as antimicrobial therapy in chronic osteomyelitis and periprosthetic joint infection. In the metaanalysis by Stengel et al [37], only 22 of 167 studies were eligible for primary outcome. They found no difference between different antibiotic groups, except for rifampin, which has shown a higher clinical success rate in implant-associated infection than it did in control treatment [38]. Since treatment of bone and joint infection cannot be based on controlled trials, the lack of evidence has been replaced by expert opinions [39]. Indeed, there are several guidelines dealing with bone and joint infection. The Infectious Diseases Society of America (IDSA) published guidelines on the management of diabetic foot infection [40], periprosthetic joint infection [41], and vertebral osteomyelitis [42].

3 What to do if there is a failure?

If treatment fails, possible surgical and medical reasons for failure must both be evaluated. Adherence to recommended surgical treatment concepts should be assessed. Surgical management of different types of bone and joint infections is described in chapters 8 Open fractures, 9.1 Infection after fracture, 9.2 Infected nonunion, 10 Infection after joint arthroplasty, 11.1 Septic arthritis, 11.2 Septic arthritis after anterior cruciate ligament surgery, and 12 Spondylodiscitis. The possibility of a secondary infection (also called superinfection) must also be considered. From the perspective of an infectious diseases specialist, it is crucial to reanalyze the organism(s) causing the failure for its antimicrobial susceptibility, and the potential reasons for emergence of resistance. Medical reasons for failure include inadequate antimicrobial treatment during the first episode, noncompliance of the patient, drug-drug interactions, reduced absorption of orally administered antibiotics (eg, due to drug-drug interaction in the gastrointestinal tract), and inconsistent use because of underreported adverse events and intolerance of the drug.

3.1 Microbiological reasons for failure

Generally, susceptible microorganisms do not become resistant during therapy. However, there are a few exceptions, such as staphylococci, which can develop resistance by mutation against fluoroquinolones, rifampin, or fusidic acid [43–45]. Similarly, by selection of a resistant subpopulation, *Pseudomonas aeruginosa* can become resistant to any known antibiotic during therapy [46, 47]. The risk for emergence of resistance is highest when the bacterial load is high or a biofilm persists. Adherent bacteria forming a biofilm cannot be eliminated with antibiotics exclusively, such as β-lactams.

Characteristic	Example
Intracellular persistence of microorganism	Mycobacteria, *Legionella* species, *Neisseria* species, *S aureus*, *S pneumonia*
Small-colony variants	*S aureus*, *Escherichia coli*, etc.
Biofilm formation	Presence of an implant or bony sequestrum
High bacterial density	Abscess (inoculum effect)
Emergence of resistance during therapy	Staphylococci to fluoroquinolones, rifampin; *P aeruginosa* to fluoroquinolones

Table 5-1 Properties of microorganisms influencing their elimination by antimicrobial agents.
Abbreviations: *S aureus, Staphylococcus aureus; S pneumonia, Streptococcus pneumonia; P aeruginosa, Pseudomonas aeruginosa.*

Other factors leading to persistence of bacteria in the host are summarized in **Table 5-1**. For example, if intracellular bacteria are treated with antibiotics, which are not able to penetrate into the cell, treatment generally fails [48, 49]. Some microorganisms are obligatorily intracellular, others such as *S aureus* or *Streptococcus pneumonia* are localized intra- and extracellularly. Small-colony variants of bacteria typically survive antimicrobial therapy because this phenotype is resistant to many antibiotics, and because it is able to persist in nonprofessional phagocytes, such as fibroblasts [50, 51]. Intracellular microorganisms are protected against β-lactams or aminoglycosides [48].

3.2 Medical reasons for failure—inadequate antimicrobial treatment

The principles of appropriate antimicrobial treatment are described above (see part 2 of this chapter), and the specific choice of antibiotics elsewhere [8]. Despite choosing the correct compound, the timing of its administration may be inadequate. For example, rifampin resistance of staphylococci may emerge if administered before debridement surgery, ie, at a time when there is still a high bacterial load [52]. Thus, if treatment of staphylococcal infection fails in a patient previously exposed to rifampin, thorough susceptibility testing is essential for the evaluation of further treatment options. Fluoroquinolones are not sufficiently effective in an acid environment (eg, large amount of pus) [53]. Similarly, aminoglycosides are bound and inactivated by free DNA, which is abundant in the abscess fluid [54]. In infections caused by gram-negative bacteria, it is important to recognize microorganisms displaying a false susceptibility result in vitro, eg, *Enterobacter* species. Although phenotypically susceptible to third-generation cephalosporins, these pathogens are genotypically resistant, eg, AmpC producers [55]. In other words, for some bacteria the susceptibility pattern in vitro does not reliably predict the treatment success in vivo. Therefore, good collaboration with a specialized microbiological laboratory must be initiated in these cases, in particular, in the event of treatment failure.

3.3 Medical reasons for failure—noncompliance of the patient

In some cases, the importance of drug adherence is not obvious to the patient for social, mental, economic, or intellectual reasons. In addition, the possibility of adverse events or intolerance without obvious side effects must be actively evaluated (see part 3.6 in this chapter). If poor drug adherence is not rapidly recognized by the responsible physician, treatment failure may occur. In these cases, directly observed treatment or outpatient IV treatment are important options.

3.4 Medical reasons for failure—drug-drug interactions

Most patients with an osteoarticular infection have several comorbidities, and hence must be treated with other medications in addition to antibiotics. Therefore, drug-drug interactions must be evaluated prior to prescribing antimicrobial treatment. In addition, each new drug, which is added in a patient already taking antibiotics, must be checked for possible interaction. Importantly, the possibility that the patient's comedication reduces the serum concentrations of the antibiotics must be evaluated. Consideration must be given to substances that may reduce the absorption of orally administered antibiotics. **Table 5-2** provides an overview of commonly administered compounds in osteoarticular infections and of substances that can potentially reduce their serum concentrations.

3.5 Medical reasons for failure—reduced absorption of orally administered antibiotics

Antacids, food (eg, milk products), and chelators (eg, substances containing iron, calcium or magnesium) decrease the absorption of several antibiotics (**Table 5-2**). The patient's history must be carefully evaluated in this respect, because many patients do not consider supplements, such as magnesium or calcium, as true drugs. The clinical relevance of a reduced serum concentration of antibiotics is difficult to estimate in a broad population, but cases of treatment failure have been observed [56, 57]. Consequently, the intake of these supplements should be evaluated and adequately scheduled (eg, 1 hour before or 2 hours after intake of another drug or meal). Counseling of the patient and family by a hospital-based pharmacist prior to discharge can be useful.

3.6 Medical reasons for failure—intolerance of antibiotics

Adverse events and intolerance without obvious measurable drug toxicity must be evaluated during the follow-up of patients treated with antibiotics. Nausea and vomiting must be rapidly recognized and adequately managed. If administration of antiemetics is not helpful, alternative treatment options should be evaluated. In case of rifampin treatment of implant-associated staphylococcal infection, however, maintenance of rifampin therapy is important. The authors recommend 450 mg twice daily on an empty stomach with a glass of water, preferentially 1 hour prior to meals or 2 hours after. Others have recommended 900 mg daily, 600 mg daily, or 300 mg twice daily (reviewed in [39]). In the authors' experience, 900 mg is often not well tolerated. If 450 mg twice daily causes nausea or vomiting, intake with meals is a first step. If symptoms persist, a dose reduction to 300 mg twice daily is the second step.

Agent	Other drug → antibiotic[*]		Antibiotic → other drug[†]		Avoid combination with[‡]	Intake[§]	Proposed mechanism for reduced absorption	Common side effects[‖] / Comments
	Antibiotic serum concentration ↑ by	Antibiotic serum concentration ↓ by	May ↑ serum concentration of	May ↓ serum concentration of				
Penicillin, amoxicillin, ampicillin, amoxicillin/clavulanic acid	Probenecid, salicylate,[¶] indometacin,[¶] sulfinpyrazon[¶]	Chloroquine,[#] lanthanum[#]	Methotrexate, vitamin K antagonists, digoxin,[#] allopurinol[**]	Mycophenolate, hormonal contraceptives, atenolol[#]	Bacteriostatic acting antimicrobial agents, eg, tetracycline derivates	Without food	Acid liability	–Diarrhea, hypersensitivity reaction Only for selected OAI cases after sufficiently long IV treatment[††]
Ciprofloxacin, levofloxacin	Metoclopramide (faster resorption)	Cations (eg, aluminium, calcium, iron, magnesium), antacids (eg, omeprazole)	Inhibition of isoenzymes of cytochrome P450 1A2 and 3A4[‡‡] Sildenafil, vitamin K antagonists, methotrexate	----	Cations, antiarrhythmic drugs of class IA or III (QT time prolongation)	Without milk products	Chelation	Nausea, diarrhea, fatigue, neurotoxicity, tendinopathy, arthralgia
Rifampin	Probenecid, cotrimoxazole.[***]	Antacids, opium derivates, anticholinergic compounds, ketoconazole	----	Strong induction of isoenzymes of cytochrome P450,[‡‡] vitamin K antagonists, hormonal contraceptives	Compounds enhancing side effects	Without food	Food increases first-pass metabolism	Nausea, vomitus, abdominal pain, elevation of liver values, hypersensitivity reaction, vasculitis
Doxycycline, minocycline	----	Cations (eg, aluminium, calcium, iron, magnesium), antacids, rifampin, alcohol	Vitamin K antagonists, methotrexate, cyclosporine	Hormonal contraceptives	Methoxyflurane	Without milk products	Chelation	Nausea, phototoxicity

Table 5-2 Oral formulations of antimicrobial agents commonly used in osteoarticular infections, and compounds influencing their enteral absorption and/or serum concentration. The list is not exhaustive.

Abbreviations: OAI, osteoarticular infection; HIV, human immunodeficiency virus.

[*] Other drugs influencing the serum concentration or effects of antimicrobial agent or its metabolites.

[†] Antimicrobial agent influencing the serum concentration or effects of other drugs or its metabolites.

[‡] Avoid live vaccines susceptible to antibiotics (eg, typhoid vaccine, Bacille de Calmette et Guérin [BCG]). The consultation of a pharmacologists or computer-based drug interaction program is always recommended. All combinations that point towards increased serum levels, enhanced side effects, or toxicity of one or the other drug must be closely monitored or avoided.

[§] Preferred dietary recommendations.

[‖] All antibiotics can cause diarrhea. In case of diarrhea, resorption of antibiotics may be impaired. Only common side effects are listed. For more detail consult your local pharmacopoeia.

[¶] Mainly described for penicillin.

[#] Mainly described with compounds containing ampicillin and amoxicillin.

[**] May enhance the potential for hypersensitivity reactions to ampicillin and amoxicillin.

[††] The authors recommend these against osteoarticular infections due to bacteria with low-penicillin minimal-inhibition concentration (eg, *Priopionibacterium acnes*, β-hemolytic streptococci or amoxicillin for amoxicillin-susceptible enterococci), and if the patient has no evidence of impaired enteral absorption. The bioavailability of amoxicillin and ampicillin are higher and more predictable than the one for penicillin V.

[‡‡] Due to the large variety of possible interactions, the consultation of a pharmacologist or computer-based drug interaction program is strongly recommended.

[***] The clinical significance of this interaction in the treatment of osteoarticular infections is unknown. Monitor treatment success and potential side effects of the drug.

Information from references [65–67].

Agent	Other drug → antibiotic*		Antibiotic → other drug†		Avoid combination with‡	Intake§	Proposed mechanism for reduced absorption	Common side effects‖ / Comments
	Antibiotic serum concentration ↑ by	Antibiotic serum concentration ↓ by	May ↑ serum concentration of	May ↓ serum concentration of				
Fusidic acid	Statins, ritonavir	----	Vitamin K antagonists, statins, ritonavir, cyclosporine	----	HIV protease inhibitors, statins	----	----	Nausea, fatigue
Cotrimoxazole	Indomethacin	Rifampin***	Digoxin, phenytoin, methotrexate, dofetilid	Tricyclic antidepressants, hormonal contraceptives	Dofetilid, compounds enhancing side effects (eg, linezolid and hematotoxicity)	After a meal	----	Hypersensitivity reaction, hematotoxicity, increased creatinine, hyperkalemia
Linezolid	----	----	Sympathomimetics, vasopressors, dopaminergic compounds, serotonin-uptake inhibitors	----	Compounds enhancing adverse events (eg, cotrimoxazole and hematotoxicity)	----	----	Hyperglycemia, headache, diarrhea, vomitus, nausea, elevated liver values, reversible hematotoxicity, irreversible neurotoxicity
Clindamycin	----	----	Neuromuscular blocking agents	----	Erythromycin (antagonisms)	----	----	Nausea, vomitus, diarrhea
Metronidazole	Cimetidine	Phenobarbital, phenytoin	Alcohol, vitamin K antagonists, disulfiram, lithium, cyclosporine 5-fluoruracil, busulfan	----	Busulfan	----	----	Nausea, abdominal pain, headache, rarely neurotoxicity

Table 5-2 Oral formulations of antimicrobial agents commonly used in osteoarticular infections, and compounds influencing their enteral absorption and/or serum concentration. The list is not exhaustive. (cont).

Abbreviations: OAI, osteoarticular infection; HIV, human immunodeficiency virus.

* Other drugs influencing the serum concentration or effects of antimicrobial agent or its metabolites.

† Antimicrobial agent influencing the serum concentration or effects of other drugs or its metabolites.

‡ Avoid live vaccines susceptible to antibiotics (eg, typhoid vaccine, Bacille de Calmette et Guérin [BCG]). The consultation of a pharmacologists or computer-based drug interaction program is always recommended. All combinations that point towards increased serum levels, enhanced side effects, or toxicity of one or the other drug must be closely monitored or avoided.

§ Preferred dietary recommendations.

‖ All antibiotics can cause diarrhea. In case of diarrhea, resorption of antibiotics may be impaired. Only common side effects are listed. For more detail consult your local pharmacopoeia.

¶ Mainly described for penicillin.

\# Mainly described with compounds containing ampicillin and amoxicillin.

** May enhance the potential for hypersensitivity reactions to ampicillin and amoxicillin.

†† The authors recommend these against osteoarticular infections due to bacteria with low-penicillin minimal-inhibition concentration (eg, *Priopionibacterium acnes*, β-hemolytic streptococci or amoxicillin for amoxicillin-susceptible enterococci), and if the patient has no evidence of impaired enteral absorption. The bioavailability of amoxicillin and ampicillin are higher and more predictable than the one for penicillin V.

‡‡ Due to the large variety of possible interactions, the consultation of a pharmacologist or computer-based drug interaction program is strongly recommended.

*** The clinical significance of this interaction in the treatment of osteoarticular infections is unknown. Monitor treatment success and potential side effects of the drug.

Information from references [65–67].

	Mechanisms of action and comments		
Class: β-lactams	Growth inhibition by inactivating enzymes located in the bacterial cell membrane, which are involved in cell wall synthesis. They are generally bactericidal.		
Compounds	**Spectrum**	**Dose***	**Comment**
Penicillin G	*Propionibacterium acnes,* streptococci, staphylococci (penicillin-susceptible)	3–5 million units every 4–6 hr	The authors recommend determining MIC prior to treatment
Amoxicillin (Europe) Ampicillin (USA)	See Penicillin G, *Enterococcus* species (amoxicillin-susceptible)	2 g every 4 to 6 hr 2 g every 4 hr	Typically used for targeted therapy: OAI due to *Enterococcus* species
Amoxicillin / clavulante (Europe) Ampicillin / sulbactam (USA)	Staphylococci (oxacillin-susceptible), streptococci, anaerobes, *Enterococcus* species (amoxicillin-susceptible), *Haemophilus influenzae*, susceptible enteroacteriaceae	2.2 g every 6 hr 3 g every 6 hr	Commonly used as empiric therapy in regions with low prevalence of MRSA and ESBL-producing enterobacteriaceae
Flucloxacillin (Europe) Nafcillin (USA)	Staphylococci (oxacillin-susceptible)†	2 g every 6 hr 1.5 to 2 g every 4 to 6 hr	Targeted therapy with narrow staphylococcal spectrum
Cefazolin	Staphylococci (oxacillin-susceptible)†, streptococci	1.5 to 2 g every 6 hr	Treatment option in case of cutaneous hypersensitivity reaction to penicillin derivates
Ceftriaxone	Streptococci, *Haemophilus influenzae*, susceptible enterobacteriaceae	2 g every 24 hr	Target therapy often used for outpatient IV treatment
Ceftazidime	See ceftriaxone‡	2 g every 8 hr	
Cefepime	See ceftazidime, higher in vitro activity against staphylococci (oxacillin-susceptible), streptococci, and *Enterobacter* species	2 g every 8 hr	For the treatment of *Enterobacter* species, the authors recommend determining MIC. Monitor neurotoxicity, in particular in patients with impaired renal function.
Class: Carbapenems	Have a β-lactam ring (potential for allergic cross-reactivity). Carbapenems are generally resistant to cleavage by most plasmid and chromosomal β-lactamases. Given their broad spectrum, their use should be strictly limited both to duration of therapy and isolated pathogen.		
Compounds	**Spectrum**	**Dose***	**Comment**
Imipenem	See cefepime, plus Gram-negative bacteria, including *Enterobacter* species, and nonfermenters, eg, *P aeruginosa*	0.5 g every 6 hr	Treatment of possible or proven presence of multidrug-resistant Gram-negative bacteria
Meropenem		1 to 2 g every 8 hr	
Ertapenem	See imipenem and meropenem, but no activity against *P aeruginosa*	1 g every 24 hr	See imipenem or meropenem but often applied for outpatient IV treatment
Class: Glycopeptides	Inhibition of the cell wall formation by blocking peptidoglycan synthesis. They bind to the amino acids within the cell wall, thereby interfering with new units of the peptidoglycan chain.		
Compounds	**Spectrum**	**Dose***	**Comment**
Vancomycin	Gram-positive bacteria, staphylococci, streptococci, *Propionibacterium* species, *Enterococcus* species	15 mg / kg every 12 hr	Treatment of possible or proven staphylococci (oxacillin-resistant), *Enterococcus* species (amoxicillin-resistant)
Teicoplanin (Europe)		0.8 g loading dose on day 1, followed by 0.4 g every 24 hr	
Class: Lipopeptide	Inserts into to the cell membrane, alters the curvature, and thereby, creates holes in the membrane. Ions leak and cause a rapid depolarization, leading to inhibition of essential bacterial products, and eventually to cell death.		
Compounds	**Spectrum**	**Dose***	**Comment**
Daptomycin	Gram-positive bacteria, staphylococci, streptococci, *Enterococcus* species	6–10 mg / kg every 24 hr	MIC of *Enterococcus* species must be tested prior to treatment.

Table 5-3 Most important antibiotics for intravenous use in bone and joint infection **[41, 68]**.
Abbreviations: MIC, minimal inhibition concentration; OAI, osteoarticular infection; MRSA, methicillin-resistant *S aureus*; ESBL, extended-spectrum β-lactamase; IV, intravenous.

* Antimicrobial dosage recommendations are based on normal renal and hepatic function. Adaptations are required in case of renal or hepatic dysfunction.

† In coagulase-negative staphylococci oxacillin-susceptibility must be reliably tested.

‡ When using it for *Pseudomonas* species, consult a microbiologist because of AmpC induction and resistance development.

4 Which drugs are important in systemic antibiotics?

Table 5-3 and **Table 5-4** present a list of the most common drugs that orthopedic surgeons should be aware of. The list is not exhaustive, since not every antibiotic is available in every region of the world. The doses are recommended for patients with normal renal and liver function. If these organs are impaired, doses must be adapted accordingly. Whether the dose for septic arthritis, osteomyelitis, and implant-associated infections should differ from one another has not been sufficiently investigated. Most antibiotics have a good serum/synovial fluid concentration ratio [33]. Therefore, recommendations with lower doses and/or longer intervals of antimicrobial administration exist for septic arthritis. Nevertheless, for IV β-lactams, it is meaningful to administer the same dose for all three entities.

4.1 Drugs for empiric therapy

Orthopedic surgeons should know which empiric therapy is the most appropriate for a given patient. Empiric should cover the most common pathogens causing osteoarticular infections, including staphylococci, streptococci, and enterobacteriaceae (see chapter 3 Microbiology). Second, the concept for empiric therapy should be established from local resistance patterns. Thus, constant epidemiological surveillance of bacterial resistance patterns, and close collaboration with microbiologists and hospital epidemiologists are necessary. In addition, adaptations must be evaluated if a trend or change occurs in resistance patterns. In areas with a low

Compound	Spectrum*	Bioavailability (%)†	Dose‡	Comments
Amoxicillin	*P acnes*, β-hemolytic streptococci	70–80§	1 g every 8 hr§	Bone penetration after a single dose 10–20%. Therefore, restricted to pathogens with low MIC‖
Amoxicillin/clavulanate	*P acnes*, β-hemolytic streptococci, anaerobes	70–80§	1 g every 8 hr§	
Clindamycin	Staphylococci, streptococci, *P acnes*, anaerobes	90	0.3–0.45 g every 6–8 hr	Determination of MIC and inducible clindamycin resistance recommended
Ciprofloxacin	Gram-negative bacteria, staphylococci when treated in combination with rifampin	80	0.75 g every 12 hr	Monitor side effects (**Table 5-2**), in particular in elderly patients
Levofloxacin	Gram-negative bacteria, staphylococci when treated in combination with rifampin	> 90	0.5 g every 12 hr or 0.75 g every 24 hr	Staphylococci have discreet lower MICs for levofloxacin than for ciprofloxacin
Moxifloxacin	Gram-negative bacteria, staphylococci when treated in combination with rifampin	90	0.4 g every 24 hr	According to manufacture activity also against anaerobes
Minocycline	Staphylococci, *P acnes*	> 90	0.1 g every 12 hr	For staphylococcal infection as suppressive therapy or curative in combination with rifampin
Doxycycline	Staphylococci, *P acnes*	> 90	0.1 g every 12 hr	
Cotrimoxazole	Gram-negative bacteria¶, staphylococci when treated in combination with rifampin	> 90	1 double dose table every 8 hr	Monitor side effects (**Table 5-2**), in particular in elderly patients
Fusidic acid	Staphylococci	90	0.5 g every 8 hr	Monitor compliance because high number of tablets required
Rifampin	Staphylococci when treated in combination with other active antistaphylococcal antibiotic	> 90	0.3 to 0.45 g every 12 hr	Never use rifampin as monotherapy
Linezolid	Gram-positive bacteria, staphylococci, enterococci	> 90	0.6 g every 12 hr	Monitor side effects (**Table 5-2**), in particular in elderly patients
Metronidazole	Anaerobes, Clostridium species	>80	0.5 g every 8 hr	Monitor neurotoxic side effects in case of long-term treatment

Table 5-4 Most important antibiotics for oral use in bone and joint infection [41, 68].
Abbreviations: MIC, minimal inhibition concentration.

* Antimicrobials must be chosen on in vitro susceptibility and after consultation of a microbiologists or infectious diseases specialist.

† The bioavailability data are presented in rounded percentages.

‡ Antimicrobial dosage recommendations are based on normal renal and hepatic function. Adaptations are required in case of renal or hepatic dysfunction.

§ The dosages of IV (**Table 5-3**) and oral formulation vary significantly. However, higher dosages of the oral formulation cannot be administered.

‖ The authors only recommend these against osteoarticular infections due to bacteria with low minimal-inhibition concentration (eg, *P acnes*, β-hemolytic streptococci), and if the patient has no evidence of impaired enteral absorption. The bioavailability of amoxicillin and ampicillin are higher and more predictable than the one for penicillin V.

¶ In gram-negative infections, the curative effect in the presence of a foreign body material is unproven.

prevalence of oxacillin-resistant staphylococci and extended spectrum β-lactamase (ESBL)-producing enterobacteriaceae, amoxicillin/clavulanate or cefuroxime are commonly used drugs for empiric IV treatment. In contrast, in areas with a high prevalence of oxacillin-resistant staphylococci and ESBL-producing enterobacteriaceae, a glycopeptide (eg, vancomycin) and a carbapenem (eg, meropenem) are often used.

4.2 Risk factors influencing empiric therapy

Risk factors for the presence of multidrug-resistant bacteria influence the choice of empiric therapy. Therefore, it is important to screen the patient's history for previous microbiological results, indicating the resistance pattern of the patient's microbiome. In IV drug users, the involvement of *P aeruginosa* species or methicillin-resistant *S aureus* (MRSA) should be considered [58]. Hospital tourism should also be considered. If patients from countries with endemic multidrug-resistant bacteria (eg, the Middle East) are transferred to countries with a low prevalence of ESBL-producing enterobacteriaceae and MRSA, empiric treatment should be adapted accordingly.

4.3 Drugs not to use for oral treatment

Oral formulations of a rifamycin (rifampin, rifabutin), fluoroquinolones, clindamycin, cotrimoxazole, and tetracyclines have excellent bioavailability (**Table 5-4**). Cephalosporins, in contrast, do not. Therefore, although used in IV formulations, these compounds should not be used in oral applications in bone and joint infections. Oral formulations of penicillin derivates generally have a low bioavailability and should only be administered in selected cases (eg, *Propipionibacterium acnes*, β-hemolytic streptococci) after previously having been treated sufficiently long with IV formulation, and after consultation with a microbiologist or infectious diseases specialist.

4.4 Drugs for multidrug-resistant gram-negative bacteria

Worrisome epidemiological observations are showing an increase in carbapenemase-producing bacteria: implant-associated osteoarticular infections with these bacteria have been reported [59]. In these cases, the choice of possible antimicrobial agents is limited. Fosfomycin, nitrofurantoin, and colistin are currently used in these cases. Other compounds are currently in trial evaluations (ceftazidime/avibactam) [60, 61]. Experience from other types of infections (eg, urinary tract infection) should not be indiscriminately extrapolated to osteoarticular infections. Given the complexity of these infections and the limited active antimicrobial agents available, infectious diseases specialists, microbiologists, and pharmacologists should be involved in the treatment planning as soon as possible.

4.5 When to use rifampin

Rifampin is an established compound in the treatment of staphylococcal bone and joint treatment [62]. It must be administered only in combination with another compound, and current data support its role only in infections due to rifampin-susceptible staphylococci. Before evaluating when to use rifampin, it is important to determine the indications of the compound. An algorithm is proposed in **Fig 5-1**.

4.5.1 Osteoarticular infections without foreign body material

The rationale for using rifampin in patients without biofilm infection is its excellent bioavailability. In this concept, only the combination with a fluorquinolone has been analysed in clinical studies [63]. Because β-lactams must be given intravenously, the use of the rifampin/fluorquinolone combination allows an early transition from parenteral to oral therapy. However, to avoid superinfection with rifampin-resistant bacteria, rifampin combination therapy should only be started when wounds are dry and enteral absorption is reliable.

4.5.2 Osteoarticular infections associated with implants

The rationale for the use of rifampin in these cases is its activity against bacteria adhering to an implant. Such infections are called biofilm infections. Thus, rifampin should be administered as soon as possible when the implant is retained. There are, however, important issues to consider prior to administering the compound. It is prudent not to use rifampin too early in the course of infection for two reasons. Firstly, perioperative rifampin therapy increases the risk of superinfection with rifampin-resistant staphylococci by selection pressure on the local flora [52]. Secondly, emergence of resistance is highest when the bacterial load is high [44, 64]. The authors recommend not starting rifampin combination therapy until after all drains are removed, the wound is dry, and the bacterial load is lowered by surgical treatment and initial IV antimicrobial therapy. When this situation has been achieved, rifampin can be added to the established antistaphylococcal IV treatment (eg, IV flucloxacillin plus oral rifampin). The tolerability of rifampin can thereby be observed during hospitalization. On discharge, the IV component can be replaced by an antistaphylococcal compound with good bioavailability. As a first option, the authors recommend a fluoroquinolone if bacteria are susceptible to it. Alternatives in the case of fluoroquinolone-resistant bacteria are cotrimoxazole, tetracycline (eg, minocycline), or clindamycin [39].

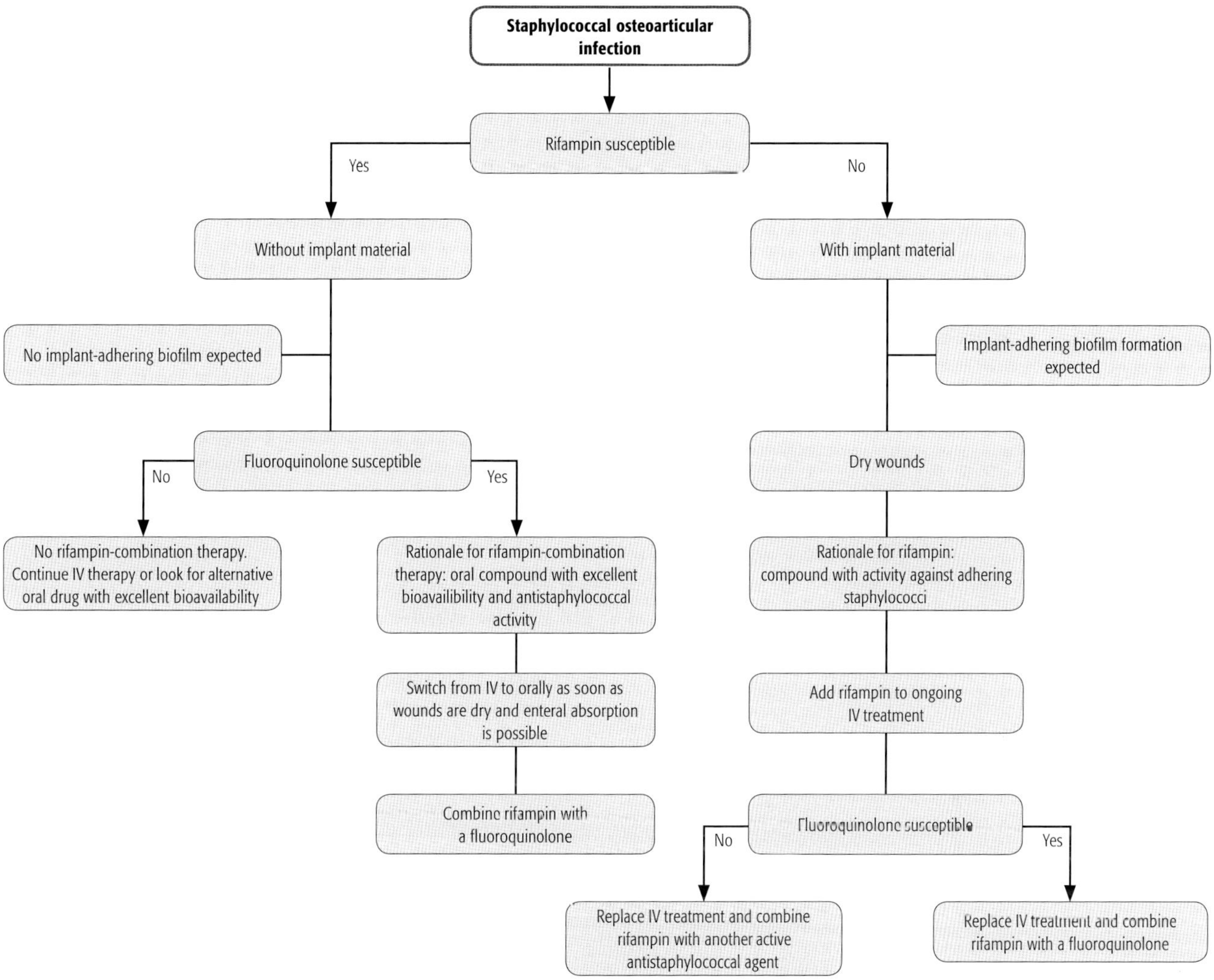

Fig 5-1 Proposed algorithm for the use of rifampin in osteoarticular infections.
Abbreviation: IV, intravenous.

5 Teamwork

The treatment of osteoarticular infections requires integrated and coordinated teamwork between orthopedic surgeons and infectious diseases specialists. Often other specialists such as plastic surgeons, pharmacologists, microbiologists, pathologists, and radiologists complete the team. When a patient suffers from a complex bone and joint infection, referral to a specialized center must be considered. Most specialized centers have established either an interdisciplinary unit for bone and joint infections, or clinical rounds and regular case discussions that are performed with an interdisciplinary team. Those who are not surgeons thereby improve their knowledge and experience in the judgement and management of intraoperative findings and pre- and postoperative wounds, as well as their skills in interpreting clinical and radiological images in the field of osteoarticular infections. On the other hand, surgeons are able to associate clinical presentation with a specific microorganism (eg, virulent versus low-grade) and are involved in the most important issues of hygiene precautions, in improving microbiological preanalysis to optimize sampling results, and in correcting antimicrobial treatment and potential side effects. The interdisciplinary treatment concept contributes to the collegial atmosphere and improves further interdisciplinary work. The authors are convinced that through such an interdisciplinary team effort, patients will truly benefit from treatment, and more importantly, inadequate treatment events will be avoided.

6 Conclusion

Inappropriate use of antimicrobial agents may damage the patient's health. The most frequent errors are prolonged antibiotic prophylaxis and empiric therapy without confirmed evidence of infection. Unintended implications of antimicrobial therapy are change of the patient's microbiome, superinfection with more difficult-to-treat microorganisms, and emergence of resistance during therapy. Therefore, good knowledge about antibiotics is needed for the whole team involved in the management of patients with osteoarticular infections. The knowledge of bone penetration for most antibiotics is based on investigations after a single dose, and hence, limited after prolonged treatment. Therefore, high doses and a prolonged treatment are recommended. However, for oral formulations of antibiotics, bone penetration is better for fluoroquinolones, clindamycin, linezolid, and rifampin, than for penicillins and cephalosporins. In addition, most bone and joint infections require antibiotics combined with surgical treatment. Therefore, a team of specialized physicians, namely orthopedic surgeons and infectious diseases specialists, is needed. Other specialists, such as plastic surgeons, pharmacologists, microbiologists, pathologists, and radiologists can be involved if needed. Failure of therapy may occur for many different reasons. Before changing antibiotic therapy, the reason for failure must be analyzed. Among other causes, it may be related to inadequate surgery, missing or inappropriate microbiological work-up, drug-drug interaction, inadequate dose or duration of antimicrobial therapy, emergence of resistance, or noncompliance of the patient.

7 References

1. **McGowan JE Jr, Barnes MW, Finland M.** Bacteremia at Boston City Hospital: Occurrence and mortality during 12 selected years (1935-1972), with special reference to hospital-acquired cases. *J Infect Dis.* 1975 Sep;132(3):316–335.
2. **Kaech C, Elzi L, Sendi P, et al.** Course and outcome of Staphylococcus aureus bacteraemia: a retrospective analysis of 308 episodes in a Swiss tertiary-care centre. *Clin Microbiol Infect.* 2006 Apr;12(4):345–352.
3. **McWilliams CA.** Central bone abscess: Brodie's abscess. Chronic suppurative osteomyelitis. *Ann Surg.* 1921 Nov;74(5):568–578.
4. **O'Connell JG.** Cases of chronic suppurative osteomyelitis. *Proc R Soc Med.* 1945 Oct;38(12):687–688.
5. **Keir DM.** Penicillin in chronic osteomyelitis. *Lancet.* 1946 Jun 8;1(6406):848.
6. **Widmer A, Barraud GE, Zimmerli W.** [Reactivation of Staphylococcus aureus osteomyelitis after 49 years]. *Schweiz Med Wochenschr.* 1988 Jan 9;118(1): 23–26. German.
7. **Zweifel-Schlatter M, Haug M, Schaefer DJ, et al.** Free fasciocutaneous flaps in the treatment of chronic osteomyelitis of the tibia: a retrospective study. *J Reconstr Microsurg.* 2006 Jan;22(1): 41–47.
8. **Zimmerli W, Trampuz A, Ochsner PE.** Prosthetic-joint infections. *N Engl J Med.* 2004 Oct 14;351(16):1645–1654.
9. **Kowalski TJ, Berbari EF, Huddleston PM, et al.** The management and outcome of spinal implant infections: contemporary retrospective cohort study. *Clin Infect Dis.* 2007 Apr 1;44(7):913–920.
10. **Zimmerli W.** Clinical practice. *Vertebral osteomyelitis. N Engl J Med.* 2010 Mar 18;362(11):1022–1029.
11. **Conterno LO, Turchi MD.** Antibiotics for treating chronic osteomyelitis in adults. *Cochrane Database Syst Rev.* 2013 Sep 6;9:CD004439.
12. **Zimmerli W.** Clinical presentation and treatment of orthopaedic implant-associated infection. *J Intern Med.* 2014 Aug;276(2):111–119.
13. **Livermore DM.** Has the era of untreatable infections arrived? *J Antimicrob Chemother.* 2009 Sep;64 Suppl 1:i29–36.
14. **Andy UU, Harvie HS, Ackenbom MF, et al.** Single versus multi-dose antibiotic prophylaxis for pelvic organ prolapse surgery with graft/mesh. *Eur J Obstet Gynecol Reprod Biol.* 2014 Jul 30;181C:37–40.
15. **Morgan XC, Huttenhower C.** Chapter 12: Human microbiome analysis. *PLoS Comput Biol.* 2012;8(12):e1002808.
16. **Tamma PD, Holmes A, Ashley ED.** Antimicrobial stewardship: another focus for patient safety? *Curr Opin Infect Dis.* 2014 Aug;27(4):348–355.
17. **Tamma PD, Turnbull AE, Milstone AM, et al.** Ventilator-associated tracheitis in children: does antibiotic duration matter? *Clin Infect Dis.* 2011 Jun;52(11):1324–1331.
18. **Jain A, Hopkins KL, Turton J, et al.** NDM carbapenemases in the United Kingdom: an analysis of the first 250 cases. *J Antimicrob Chemother.* 2014 Jul;69(7):1777–1784.
19. **Biswal I, Arora BS, Kasana D, et al.** Incidence of multidrug resistant pseudomonas aeruginosa isolated from burn patients and environment of teaching institution. *J Clin Diagn Res.* 2014 May;8(5):DC26–29.
20. **Pala E, Henderson ER, Calabro T, et al.** Survival of current production tumor endoprostheses: complications, functional results, and a comparative statistical analysis. *J Surg Oncol.* 2013 Nov;108(6):403–408.
21. **Zimmerli W, Waldvogel FA, Vaudaux P, et al.** Pathogenesis of foreign body infection: description and characteristics of an animal model. *J Infect Dis.* 1982 Oct;146(4):487–497.
22. **Zimmerli W, Lew PD, Waldvogel FA.** Pathogenesis of foreign body infection. Evidence for a local granulocyte defect. *J Clin Invest.* 1984 Apr;73(4):1191–1200.
23. **Kristian SA, Birkenstock TA, Sauder U, et al.** Biofilm formation induces C3a release and protects Staphylococcus epidermidis from IgG and complement deposition and from neutrophil-dependent killing. *J Infect Dis.* 2008 Apr 1;197(7):1028–1035.
24. **Classen DC, Evans RS, Pestotnik SL, et al.** The timing of prophylactic administration of antibiotics and the risk of surgical-wound infection. *N Engl J Med.* 1992 Jan 30;326(5):281–286.
25. **Weber WP, Marti WR, Zwahlen M, et al.** The timing of surgical antimicrobial prophylaxis. *Ann Surg.* 2008 Jun;247(6):918–926.
26. **Dellinger EP, Gross PA, Barrett TL, et al.** Quality standard for antimicrobial prophylaxis in surgical procedures. *The Infectious Diseases Society of America. Infect Control Hosp Epidemiol.* 1994 Mar;15(3):182–188.
27. **Anderson DJ, Podgorny K, Berrios-Torres SI, et al.** Strategies to prevent surgical site infections in acute care hospitals: 2014 update. *Infect Control Hosp Epidemiol.* 2014 Jun;35(6): 605–627.
28. **Bratzler DW, Dellinger EP, Olsen KM, et al.** Clinical practice guidelines for antimicrobial prophylaxis in surgery. *Surg Infect (Larchmt).* 2013 Feb;14(1): 73–156.
29. **Hauser CJ, Adams CA, Jr., Eachempati SR, et al.** Surgical Infection Society guideline: prophylactic antibiotic use in open fractures: an evidence-based guideline. *Surg Infect (Larchmt).* 2006 Aug;7(4):379–405.
30. **Dellinger EP, Caplan ES, Weaver LD, et al.** Duration of preventive antibiotic administration for open extremity fractures. *Arch Surg.* 1988 Mar;123(3):333–339.
31. **Hoiby N, Ciofu O, Johansen HK, et al.** The clinical impact of bacterial biofilms. *Int J Oral Sci.* 2011 Apr;3(2):55–65.
32. **Somekh E, Golan T, Tanay A, et al.** Concentration and bactericidal activity of fusidic acid and cloxacillin in serum and synovial fluid. *J Antimicrob Chemother.* 1999 Apr;43(4):593–596.
33. **Bamberger DM, Foxworth JW, Bridwell DL, et al.** Extravascular antimicrobial distribution and the respective blood and urine concentrations in humans. In: Lorian V, ed. *Antibiotics in laboratory medicine.* 5th ed. Philadelphia: Lippincott Williams & Wilkins; 2005: 719–814.
34. **Landersdorfer CB, Bulitta JB, Kinzig M, et al.** Penetration of antibacterials into bone: pharmacokinetic, pharmacodynamic and bioanalytical considerations. *Clin Pharmacokinet.* 2009;48(2):89–124.
35. **Landersdorfer CB, Kinzig M, Hennig FF, et al.** Penetration of moxifloxacin into bone evaluated by Monte Carlo simulation. *Antimicrob Agents Chemother.* 2009 May;53(5):2074–2081.
36. **Tshefu K, Zimmerli W, Waldvogel FA.** Short-term administration of rifampicin in the prevention or eradication of infection due to foreign bodies. *Rev Infect Dis.* 1983 Jul-Aug;5 Suppl 3:S474–480.
37. **Stengel D, Bauwens K, Sehouli J, et al.** Systematic review and meta-analysis of antibiotic therapy for bone and joint infections. *Lancet Infect Dis.* 2001 Oct;1(3):175–188.
38. **Zimmerli W, Widmer AF, Blatter M, et al.** Role of rifampicin for treatment of orthopedic implant-related staphylococcal infections: a randomized controlled trial. Foreign-Body Infection (FBI) Study Group. *JAMA.* 1998 May 20;279(19):1537–1541.
39. **Sendi P, Zimmerli W.** Antimicrobial treatment concepts for orthopaedic device-related infection. *Clin Microbiol Infect.* 2012 Dec;18(12):1176–1184.

40. **Lipsky BA, Berendt AR, Cornia PB, et al.** 2012 Infectious Diseases Society of America clinical practice guideline for the diagnosis and treatment of diabetic foot infections. *Clin Infect Dis.* 2012 Jun;54(12):e132–173.
41. **Osmon DR, Berbari EF, Berendt AR, et al.** Diagnosis and management of prosthetic joint infection: clinical practice guidelines by the Infectious Diseases Society of America. *Clin Infect Dis.* 2013 Jan;56(1):e1–e25.
42. **Berbari EF, Kanj SS, Kowalski TJ, et al.** 2015 Infectious Diseases Society of America (IDSA) Clinical Practice Guidelines for the Diagnosis and Treatment of Native Vertebral Osteomyelitis in Adults. *Clin Infect Dis.* 2015 Sep;61(6):e26–46.
43. **de Lastours V, Chau F, Roy C, et al.** Emergence of quinolone resistance in the microbiota of hospitalized patients treated or not with a fluoroquinolone. *J Antimicrob Chemother.* 2014 Dec;69(12):3393–400.
44. **John AK, Baldoni D, Haschke M, et al.** Efficacy of daptomycin in implant-associated infection due to methicillin-resistant Staphylococcus aureus: importance of combination with rifampicin. *Antimicrob Agents Chemother.* 2009 Jul;53(7):2719–2724.
45. **Howden BP, Grayson ML.** Dumb and dumber-the potential waste of a useful antistaphylococcal agent: emerging fusidic acid resistance in Staphylococcus aureus. *Clin Infect Dis.* 2006 Feb 1;42(3):394–400.
46. **Sriramulu D.** Evolution and impact of bacterial drug resistance in the context of cystic fibrosis disease and nosocomial settings. *Microbiol Insights.* 2013 Apr 14;6:29–36.
47. **Giwercman B, Lambert PA, Rosdahl VT, et al.** Rapid emergence of resistance in Pseudomonas aeruginosa in cystic fibrosis patients due to in-vivo selection of stable partially derepressed beta-lactamase producing strains. *J Antimicrob Chemother.* 1990 Aug;26(2):247–259.
48. **Vaudaux P, Waldvogel FA.** Gentamicin antibacterial activity in the presence of human polymorphonuclear leukocytes. *Antimicrob Agents Chemother.* 1979 Dec;16(6):743–749.
49. **Hohl P, Buser U, Frei R.** Fatal Legionella pneumophila pneumonia: treatment failure despite early sequential oral-parenteral amoxicillin-clavulanic acid therapy. *Infection.* 1992 Mar-Apr;20(2):99–100.
50. **von Eiff C, Becker K, Metze D, et al.** Intracellular persistence of Staphylococcus aureus small-colony variants within keratinocytes: a cause for antibiotic treatment failure in a patient with darier's disease. *Clin Infect Dis.* 2001 Jun 1;32(11):1643–1647.
51. **Sendi P, Rohrbach M, Graber P, et al.** Staphylococcus aureus small colony variants in prosthetic joint infection. *Clin Infect Dis.* 2006 Oct 15;43(8):961–967.
52. **Achermann Y, Eigenmann K, Ledergerber B, et al.** Factors associated with rifampicin resistance in staphylococcal periprosthetic joint infections (PJI): a matched case-control study. *Infection.* 2013 Apr;41(2):431–437.
53. **Iravani A, Welty GS, Newton BR, et al.** Effects of changes in pH, medium, and inoculum size on the in vitro activity of amifloxacin against urinary isolates of Staphylococcus saprophyticus and Escherichia coli. *Antimicrob Agents Chemother.* 1985 Apr;27(4):449–451.
54. **Vaudaux P, Waldvogel FA.** Gentamicin inactivation in purulent exudates: role of cell lysis. *J Infect Dis.* 1980 Oct;142(4):586–593.
55. **Jacoby GA.** AmpC beta-lactamases. *Clin Microbiol Rev.* 2009 Jan;22(1):161-182.
56. **Noyes M, Polk RE.** Norfloxacin and absorption of magnesium-aluminum. *Ann Intern Med.* 1988 Jul 15;109(2):168–169.
57. **Radandt JM, Marchbanks CR, Dudley MN.** Interactions of fluoroquinolones with other drugs: mechanisms, variability, clinical significance, and management. *Clin Infect Dis.* 1992 Jan;14(1):272–284.
58. **Allison DC, Holtom PD, Patzakis MJ, et al.** Microbiology of bone and joint infections in injecting drug abusers. *Clin Orthop Relat Res.* 2010 Aug;468(8):2107–2112.
59. **de Sanctis J, Teixeira L, van Duin D, et al.** Complex prosthetic joint infections due to carbapenemase-producing Klebsiella pneumoniae: a unique challenge in the era of untreatable infections. *Int J Infect Dis.* 2014 Aug;25:73–78.
60. **Sader HS, Farrell DJ, Castanheira M, et al.** Antimicrobial activity of ceftolozane/tazobactam tested against Pseudomonas aeruginosa and Enterobacteriaceae with various resistance patterns isolated in European hospitals (2011-12). *J Antimicrob Chemother.* 2014 Oct;69(10):2713–2722.
61. **Farrell DJ, Sader HS, Flamm RK, et al.** Ceftolozane/tazobactam activity tested against Gram-negative bacterial isolates from hospitalised patients with pneumonia in US and European medical centres (2012). *Int J Antimicrob Agents.* 2014 Jun;43(6):533–539.
62. **Kim BN, Kim ES, Oh MD.** Oral antibiotic treatment of staphylococcal bone and joint infections in adults. *J Antimicrob Chemother.* 2014 Feb;69(2):309–322.
63. **Schrenzel J, Harbarth S, Schockmel G, et al.** A randomized clinical trial to compare fleroxacin-rifampicin with flucloxacillin or vancomycin for the treatment of staphylococcal infection. *Clin Infect Dis.* 2004 Nov 1;39(9):1285–1292.
64. **Widmer AF, Frei R, Rajacic Z, et al.** Correlation between in vivo and in vitro efficacy of antimicrobial agents against foreign body infections. *J Infect Dis.* 1990 Jul;162(1):96–102.
65. **UpToDate.** Available at: http://www.uptodate.com. Accessed May, 2016.
66. **Drugs compendium.** Available at: http://www.pdr.net/browse-by-drug-name. Accessed June, 2016.
67. **Rosin D, Henschler D.** Antibiotika und Chemotherapeutika–Antiinfektiöse Therapie [Antibiotics and chemotherapy—noninfective therapies]. In: Forth W, Henschler D, Rummel W, et al., eds. *Allgemeine und spezielle Pharmakologie und Toxikologie.* 7. Heidelberg: Spektrum Akademischer Verlag; 1996: 677–787.
68. **Zimmerli W, Sendi P.** Orthopedic Implant-Associated Infections. In: Bennett JE, Dolin R, Blaser MJ, eds. *Mandell, Douglas, and Bennett's Principles and Practice of Infectious Diseases.* 8th ed. Philadelphia:Elsevier;2015:1328–1340.

6 Local delivery of antibiotics and antiseptics

Volker Alt

1 Basics

The treatment and prevention of bone and implant-associated infections is based on two principles: thorough surgical debridement and intelligent use of antibiotics and antiseptics. The goal of local use of antibiotics and antiseptics is to deliver high local concentrations of the antimicrobial agents to eradicate bacteria with low systemic levels of the antibiotic to reduce the likelihood of adverse systemic effects. Local administration of antibiotics achieve high concentrations where needed with reduced risks for systemic adverse events. Furthermore, local antimicrobial therapy enables access of the agents to poorly vascularized infected bone, which cannot be achieved by intravenous therapy alone.

The surgeon requires detailed knowledge of the different antibiotic administration methods for the successful management of open fractures, bone- and implant-associated infection cases. The use of antimicrobial agents does not replace proper surgical debridement and should be considered an adjunctive tool in the armamentarium of the surgeon.

The goal of this chapter is to give an overview of the different antiseptics, antibiotics, and delivery systems to provide a practical guideline for their successful intraoperative use. Furthermore, the clinical aspects of antimicrobial-coated implants will be elucidated.

2 Antiseptics

Antiseptics are antimicrobial substances that can be applied to wounds to eradicate bacteria. In contrast to antibiotics, antiseptics cannot be administered systemically and can only be used locally to manage infected or contaminated tissue. Disinfectants also exhibit antimicrobial properties but can only be used on inanimate objects.

In orthopedic and trauma surgery, polyhexanide, octenidine dihydrochloride, and povidone-iodine are the most frequently used antiseptics.

2.1 Polyhexanide

Polyhexanide is a commonly used antiseptic agent for infected or critically colonized wounds, including poorly healing and chronic wounds. It is also used in antiseptic wound dressings [1]. It is the antiseptic of choice for contaminated acute traumatic wounds. It is fungicidal and bactericidal including activity against methicillin-resistant *Staphylococcus aureus* (MRSA) and vancomycin-intermediate sensitivity *S aureus* (VISA). Gaps in effectiveness are not known and effectiveness against biofilm-dwelling organisms has been reported [1]. Polyhexanide has a relatively slow onset of antibacterial activity of 5–20 minutes in quantitative suspension test for a concentration of 0.04%. It has selective activity against acidic lipids of bacterial cell membranes with only a minor effect on the neutral lipids of human cell membranes. This is the reason for its excellent biocompatibility. It has been found to promote wound healing. These properties distinguish polyhexanide from most other antiseptics. Contraindications include:

- Peritoneal lavage
- Intravenous application
- Joint lavage on hyaline cartilage (> 0.005%) due to cartilage toxicity
- Use in any part of the central nervous system, middle or inner ear
- Intraocular applications [1]

2.2 Octenidine dihydrochloride

Octenidine dihydrochloride (OCT) can be considered as an excellent antiseptic for acute contaminated traumatic wounds and as an antiseptic of choice for chronic wounds. It has a broad antibacterial spectrum on gram-positive and gram-negative bacteria. It also exhibits antifungal activity and antiviral activity against enveloped viruses such as herpes simplex and hepatitis B [1]. During surgery, no pressurized irrigation of cavities without adequate outflow should be performed. Octenidine dihydrochloride exhibits toxicity to hyaline cartilage and is contraindicated for use in peritoneal lavage.

2.3 Povidone-iodine

Indications for povidone-iodine are limited to stab, cut, and bite wounds [1]. This is mainly related to the systemic toxicity with negative effects on thyroid function and deleterious effects on wound healing compared to polyhexanide. In vivo results have shown inhibition of wound healing by povidone-iodine even at low concentrations of 0.75%. It has microbicidal properties against gram-positive and gram-negative bacteria, fungi, and protozoa. It is effective against hepatitis B virus, hepatitis C virus, and human immunodeficiency virus. It exhibits a rapid onset of activity.

2.4 Chlorhexidine (gluconate/digluconate)

Chlorhexidine should not be used as a wound antiseptic. It possesses low effectiveness against gram-negative clinical isolates combined with a decrease of activity in the presence of proteins and blood. Chlorhexidine is cytotoxic, which results in wound healing problems; possible allergic reactions and potentially a mutagenic potential have also been described [1].

2.5 Antiseptic use in open fractures

The principles of initial management of open fractures include intravenous antibiotics, meticulous wound debridement, and irrigation followed by stabilization of the fracture. A variety of different additives, such as povidone-iodone, chlorhexidine, or castile soap solution, and different pressures at which fluid is delivered to the wound have been described in the literature [2–4].

In a recent randomized control trial of fluid lavage of open wounds (FLOW) on 111 patients, the potential differences in outcome between irrigation with castile soap versus irrigation with normal saline was performed. An irrigation volume of at least 3 L and 6 L was used for Gustilo-Anderson type I and type II/III open fractures, respectively. In the castile soap group, 80 mL of castile soap solution was added to each 3 L of normal saline. Furthermore, low (6–10 psi) versus high pressure (25–30 psi) for the delivery of the irrigation fluid was assessed. There was no statistically significant difference noted between the use of castile soap und normal saline for irrigation in open fractures with the primary composite outcome of reoperation procedures for infection, wound healing problems, and nonunion, measured at 12 months after initial operative procedure [2]. There was an apparent increase in the infection rate in the castile soap group compared to normal saline. The authors discussed a potential rebound effect in bacterial growth after initial irrigation of an open wound in the castile soap group which was previously found to be worse with castile soap compared to saline alone or to saline with other additives [3]. An alternative explanation is that the soap acts as local irritant for the skin leading to local erythema and subsequent infection. Another previous randomized controlled study with 400 patients with 458 open fractures also showed no advantages of the irrigation of open fracture wounds with antibiotic solution over the use of a nonsterile soap solution [5]. In an open fracture experiment using an animal, there was no statistically significant difference noted between saline and chlorhexidine gluconate regarding the subsequent presence or quantity of bacteria after irrigation [4]. This study also discouraged the use of chlorhexidine gluconate in open fractures. Regarding irrigation pressure, the fluid lavage of open wounds investigators found no statistically significant difference between low and high pressure, but the results revealed a strong trend in favor of low-pressure pulsatile lavage [2].

3 Antibiotics and carriers

In general, many different antibiotics can be used with different carriers for local administration. The most frequently used local antibiotics are gentamicin, tobramycin, and vancomycin. Carriers can be distinguished into nondegradable versus biodegradable materials. The most frequently used nondegradable carrier is polymethylmethacrylate (PMMA). Calcium sulfate or collagen-based carriers are also used as biodegradable materials. Rifampin cannot be used with PMMA but can be used with resorbable carriers. Recently, bioactive glass with its combination of antimicrobial and osteoconductive properties has become an additional option.

3.1 Local antibiotics

Antibiotics that can be used for local administration in orthopedic and orthopedic trauma surgery must fulfill several preconditions. They have to be effective against the infection-causing microorganism. Bactericidal antibiotics are preferred over bacteriostatic antibiotics. Bioavailability from the carrier of the antibiotic must be ensured. Antibiotic heat stability is of high importance when PMMA is used as carrier, as the exothermic polymerization procedure can lead to temperatures of 80° C [6]. For PMMA loading, the antibiotic must be used in powder form because liquid antibiotics dramatically weaken the strength of PMMA [7]. Liquid antibiotics are more favorable for the loading of degradable carriers. For facilitation of antibiotic release, water solubility and hydrophilic properties are important. Furthermore, the antibiotic should not be cytotoxic to eukaryotic cells and should not interfere with fracture healing. General systemic side effects and allergic profile must also be considered.

The most frequently used local antibiotics are: gentamicin, tobramycin, and vancomycin. Rifampin cannot be used in combination with PMMA as it interferes with its polymerization [8]. Rifampin can be used with a calcium sulfate-hydroxyapatite carrier [9].

Despite generally accepted excellent biocompatibility [10], case reports have been published documenting acute renal failure as systemic complication in patients caused by gentamicin-, tobramycin-, or vancomycin-loaded spacers [11–13]. This emphasizes the need for carefully considered dosage, increased vigilance, and prudent monitoring in patients at increased risk for nephrotoxicity.

3.1.1 Gentamicin and tobramycin

Gentamicin and tobramycin are bactericidal aminoglycoside antibiotics that bind to the 30S subunit of the bacterial ribosome with subsequent interruption of protein synthesis. Infections with *S aureus* or gram-negative bacteria such as *Pseudomonas*, *Proteus*, or *Serratia* can be treated with gentamicin or tobramycin. The high heat resistance and favorable release kinetics make gentamicin and tobramycin suitable for loading with PMMA and their use with PMMA has been well established and proven clinically effective [10]. Gentamicin and tobramycin at concentrations up to 400 µg/mL did not demonstrate negative effects on the metabolic activity on human osteoblasts [14].

3.1.2 Vancomycin

Vancomycin is an antibiotic of the glycopeptide class. It shows high antimicrobial activity against most gram-positive bacteria, eg, *S aureus*, including MRSA, which is the rationale for its use in many cases with documented or suspected infections with MRSA. Vancomycin is the second most frequently used antibiotic in PMMA after aminoglycosides although its high molecular weight of > 600 Daltons results in less favorable but acceptable release kinetics [15]. Vancomycin was shown at concentrations of < 1,000 µg/mL to have no or only minimal effects on the replication of osteoblasts. In very high concentrations > 10,000 µg/mL vancomycin can lead to eukaryotic cell death [16].

3.1.3 Rifampin

Rifampin belongs to the rifamycin group and exhibits bactericidal activity by inhibiting bacterial deoxyribonucleic acid-dependent ribonucleic acid synthesis. In bone and implant-associated infections, rifampin is a cornerstone of the antibiotic treatment due to its excellent activity against *S aureus* including MRSA but also against enterococci [17, 18]. Another major advantage is its almost unique ability to eradicate bacteria in biofilms that has been demonstrated in several experimental and clinical studies [19, 20]. Rifampin shows good biocompatibility with bone cells with intracellular antibiotic activity in osteoblasts fighting intracellular bacteria such as *S aureus* [21]. Monotherapy with rifampin should be avoided due to rapid development of resistance. Major adverse events are hepatotoxicity, allergic reactions, reversible neutropenia, and thrombocytopenia. Rifampin can cause an orange coloring of body fluids such as urine, tears, sweat, and stools without any negative clinical impact. As mentioned above, the interference with the polymerization of PMMA prevents its use in bone cement [8] but it is suitable for the loading of a degradable carrier [9].

3.1.4 Daptomycin

Daptomycin has recently been shown to be usable in PMMA cement. It is less effective than vancomycin when used as monotherapy but is more effective if used in combination with an aminoglycoside in the PMMA cement [22, 23].

3.2 Carriers

The most commonly used nonresorbable antibiotic carrier is PMMA. Different commercially available antibiotic-loaded PMMA bone cements and antibiotic-loaded PMMA bead chains are available. There are only a few biodegradable delivery biomaterials based on collagen, calcium sulfate, calcium phosphate, or antibiotic-loaded cancellous bone allografts.

3.2.1 Polymethylmethacrylate

The idea of local delivery of antibiotics via PMMA as a carrier and drug delivery system was introduced in the 1970s by Buchholz and Engelbrecht in the treatment of infected total joint replacements [24]. Klemm [25] adapted this principle to the treatment of chronic osteomyelitis to achieve high local antibiotic concentration with the use of antibiotic-loaded PMMA beads that could be directly applied into the infected bone tissue.

There are different forms and indications for antibiotic-loaded PMMA carriers. First, the prophylactic use of low-dose PMMA bone cement for infection prophylaxis in primary total joint arthroplasty. Second, there is a therapeutic use of antibiotic PMMA devices as antibiotic-loaded PMMA beads in osteomyelitis and infected nonunion cases, or spacers after removal of a joint prosthesis in the two-stage revision concept for periprosthetic joint infections. The last is explained further in chapter 10 Infection after joint arthroplasty. A new concept was introduced by Masquelet and colleagues [26] using solid antibiotic-loaded PMMA spacers after resection of infected bone tissue for both local delivery of antibiotics and induction of an osteogenic membrane that stimulates new bone formation in the course of bone reconstruction of the defect in this two-stage treatment concept.

Commercially available gentamicin-loaded PMMA beads

Commercially available gentamicin-loaded PMMA beads must be distinguished from handmade PMMA beads. One commonly used product is a gentamicin-loaded PMMA bead chain which is available with different lengths (**Fig 6-1**). The beads have a diameter of 7 mm, a weight of 200 mg and consist of PMMA with 7.5 mg gentamicin sulfate corresponding to 4.5 mg gentamicin, a small amount of glycine for improvement of release kinetics and 20 mg of the radio-opaque zirconium. Also, there are so-called "minichains" with 10 or 20 beads with a size of 3 x 5 mm with 2.8 mg of gentamicin sulfate corresponding to 1.7 mg of gentamicin, available for smaller bone defects. The beads are strung on a thin chromium-nickel wire. Official indications of these beads are their temporary use in surgically treated bone and soft-tissue infections with gentamicin-susceptible strains. Contraindications are allergies to gentamicin and the carrier material. In case of nickel or other metal allergies, tissue reactions could occur to the chromium and nickel content in the metal wire.

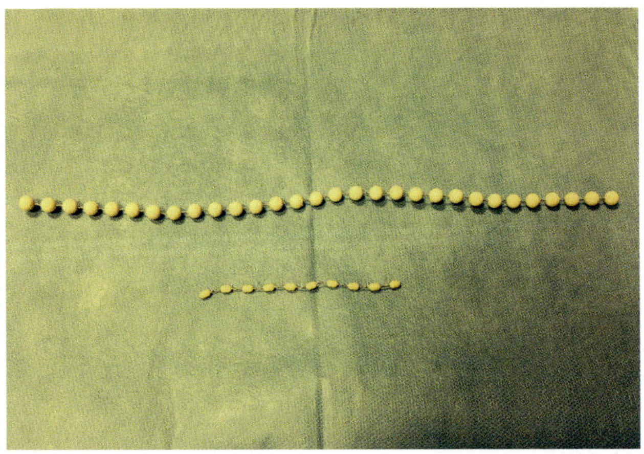

Fig 6-1 Commercially available polymethylmethacrylate (PMMA) beads. Chain with 30 PMMA beads with a bead diameter of 7 mm consisting of 7.5 mg gentamicin sulfate and "minichain" with 10 beads of 3 x 5 mm with 2.8 mg of gentamicin sulfate.

Elution kinetics of commercially available gentamicin-loaded PMMA beads

Elution of antibiotics from PMMA generally depends on the surface and porosity of PMMA which can be increased by the incorporation of glycine or cefazolin as "porogens". This is one of the principles in gentamicin-loaded PMMA beads. Both the total quantity of antibiotics and the composition of the bone cement components affect the elution kinetics [27].

The release process of gentamicin from PMMA is a diffusion process as in all antibiotic-loaded PMMA devices [28] through which gentamicin is exchanged with the surrounding body fluid. The antibiotic is then transported to the adjacent tissue following a concentration gradient. Clinical data show high local concentrations of gentamicin in the first days in the wound fluid up to 200–300 µg/mL after application of 360 gentamicin beads in a two-stage hip infection treatment [29]. This is much higher than the minimal inhibitory concentration that kills 90% of the strains (MIC_{90}) of 1 µg/mL of *S aureus* [30]. In contrast, gentamicin concentrations reached only 0.4 µg/mL in serum and only 10–30 µg/mL in urine. The total released amount of gentamicin after a treatment of 9–14 days was 20–70% of the incorporated gentamicin. Jenny et al [31] published clinical data on gentamicin concentrations in the drainage fluid on postoperative day one in 188 patients treated with 3–390 gentamicin-loaded PMMA beads. Mean concentrations of 16 µg/mL for a treatment with 17 beads and of 420 µg/mL for a treatment with 156 beads was found confirming high local gentamicin concentrations that is above the MIC_{90} of 1 µg/mL of *S aureus*. However, no correlation between the number of implanted beads and mean gentamicin concentrations could be demonstrated, which makes it impossible to reliably predict the actual achievable local antibiotic concentration for an individual patient impossible. After an initial relatively high-burst release, a consequently subtherapeutic release is most likely [32, 33].

Serum concentrations of 0.03–0.4 µg/mL and a renal excretion rate of 3–40 µg/min were measured in five patients treated with 48–360 beads [29]. No signs of nephrotoxicity or other systemic adverse effects were detected. To the author's best knowledge, only one clinical case report on a patient exists that developed end-stage renal dysfunction after being treated with a combination of 210 beads and cement containing 2 g gentamicin in 240 g cement powder. After removal of the materials containing gentamicin, renal function normalized. In summary, the use of commercially available gentamicin beads is typically safe. However, the above-mentioned contraindications should be considered.

Commercially available PMMA beads offer the advantage of reliable release behavior of gentamicin, whereas handmade beads carry the risk of an uneven distribution of the antibiotic in the PMMA with subsequent unpredictable release behavior [34].

Surgical handling of commercially available gentamicin-loaded PMMA beads

Regarding the surgical handling of gentamicin-loaded PMMA beads, the following should be considered. First, a thorough surgical debridement of the infected site must be performed. The local antibiotics are not a substitute for an appropriate surgical procedure. Only when all infected and compromised tissue has been debrided and the wound has been sufficiently irrigated, the application of the antibiotic beads into the debrided bone or soft-tissue area is performed (**Fig 6-2**) [35] at the end of the procedure. A drain without suction may be placed as negative-wound pressure could lead to washout of the antibiotics via the drain. The drain can be removed routinely after 1–3 days depending on the amount of drainage and surgeon's preference. Polymethylmethacrylate beads should be removed after 2–4 weeks due to the decreased amount of released antibiotic which carries the risk of the presence of subinhibitory antibiotic concentrations with development of resistance and subsequent colonization of the beads with resistant bacteria. This could serve as a reservoir of the infection [32, 33].

Antibiotic-loaded PMMA beads are commercially available only in Europe, therefore in most parts of the world PMMA beads are handmade for local antibiotic therapy.

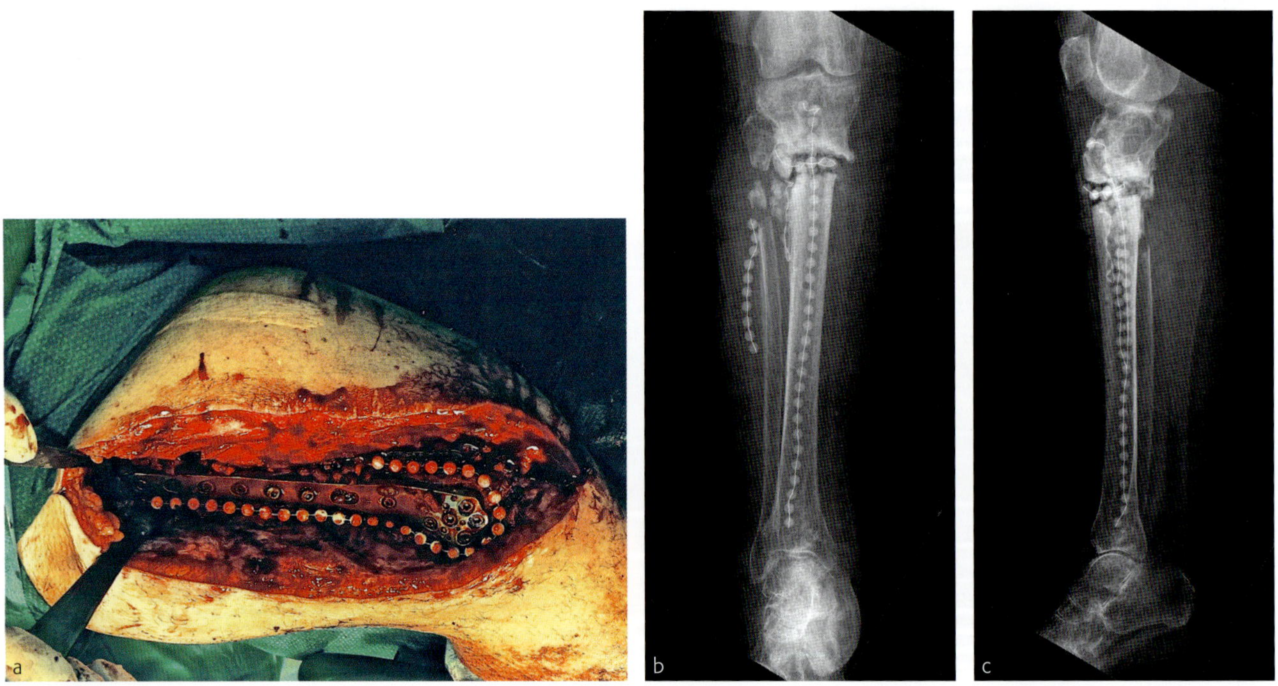

Fig 6-2a–c Application of antibiotic beads.
a Intraoperative use of a commercially available polymethylmethacrylate (PMMA) beads.
b–c Placement of a chain with 30 PMMA beads around an acutely infected locking plate at the distal femur. X-ray controls after intramedullary placement of 30 beads into the tibia, 10 beads into the infected tibial nonunion site, and extramedullary placement of 10 beads beside the infected proximal fibula (**b** AP view; **c** lateral view).

Handmade antibiotic-loaded PMMA beads

The advantage of handmade antibiotic-loaded PMMA beads is that not only gentamicin but a variety of other antibiotics can be used depending on the antibiotic susceptibility of the infection-causing microorganism, particularly if there is gentamicin resistance. Hand-mixed antibiotic beads are generally less expensive than commercially available beads. Furthermore, the synergistic effect between aminoglycosides and vancomycin for elution kinetics from PMMA and antimicrobial effectivity can be leveraged when both antibiotics are incorporated in hand-mixed bone cement (**Table 6-1**) [36, 37].

Elution kinetics of handmade PMMA beads

Anagnostakos et al [36] analysed the elution kinetics of 40 handmade PMMA beads loaded with 0.5 g of gentamicin and 2 g of vancomycin per 40 g of PMMA in the wound drainage of 11 patients over 7–13 days. Peak mean concentrations of 116 µg/mL of gentamicin with a range of 12–371 µg/mL and mean concentrations of 80 µg/mL of vancomycin with a range of 21–198 µg/mL were measured on day 1 (**Fig 6.3**). Lowest concentrations of 3.7 µg/mL and 23 µg/mL were found on day 13 for gentamicin and vancomycin, respectively. The authors attributed the high intersubject variability of the release of both antibiotics to the manual incorporation of vancomycin into the cement powder. However, in all cases the concentrations on day 13 are still above the MIC_{90} of *S aureus* for gentamicin and vancomycin. No hepatic or renal dysfunction was observed and, therefore, this dosage appeared safe for handmade PMMA beads.

Rasyid et al [38] presented a method to improve release kinetics from handmade gentamicin PMMA beads, ie, 1 g of gentamicin sulfate and 40 g of PMMA powder, with addition of only 50% of monomer to create a less dense polymer matrix. The addition of 15% by weight of polyvinylpyrrolidone (PVP) 17 as gel-forming polymeric filler was found to further optimize release kinetics which was even better than the one of commercially available beads for 14 days in vitro. This is a cheap and effective method to improve release behavior of gentamicin in handmade PMMA beads.

Besides this study, there is limited clinical information on the elution kinetics of other handmade antibiotic-loaded PMMA beads in patients and, therefore, no further recommendation on specific antibiotic combinations and dosages can be made. Citak et al [10] published in the Proceedings of the International Consensus Meeting on Periprosthetic Joint Infection a table with all clinically reported antibiotic loadings for spacers in patients for treatment of periprosthetic joint infections. However, it must be stated that this information is only valid for PMMA block spacers and not for PMMA beads as the latter have a higher surface with the theoretical risk of undesirable release kinetics if high spacer dosage is used for beads.

Antibiotic	Dosage	Potential side effects
Gentamicin	1 g per 40 mg PMMA powder	Allergic reactions Nephrotoxicity
Tobramycin	1 g per 40 mg PMMA powder	Allergic reactions Nephrotoxicity
Gentamicin and vancomycin	0.5 g gentamicin and 2 g vancomycin per 40 mg PMMA	Allergic reactions Nephrotoxicity

Table 6-1 Suitable antibiotics and dosages for handmade polymethylmethacrylate (PMMA) beads.

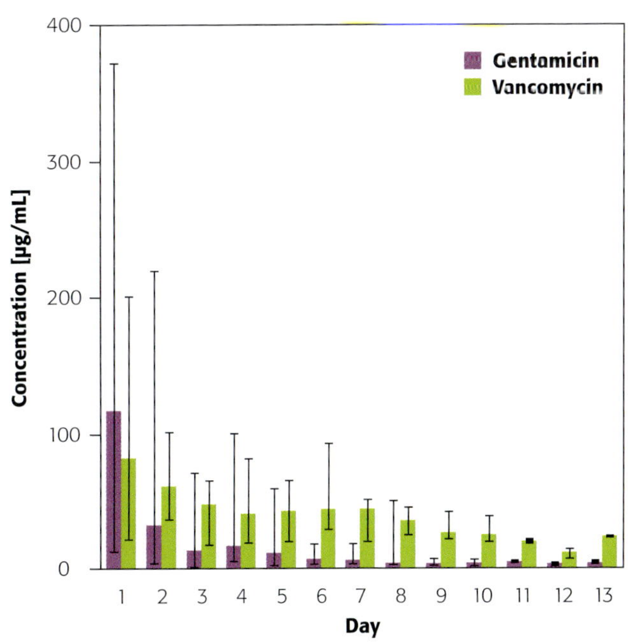

Fig 6-3 Release kinetics of gentamicin and vancomycin of 40 handmade polymethylmethacrylate (PMMA) beads loaded with 0.5 g of gentamicin and 2 g of vancomycin per 40 g of PMMA in the wound drainage of 11 patients over the first 13 days (with permission from Anagnostakos et al [39], Taylor & Francis Ltd. www.tandfonline.com).

Practical tips for manufacture of handmade PMMA beads

For practical aspects in hand mixing, the antibiotic powder should be placed in a mixing container under sterile conditions and then the same amount of PMMA as the antibiotic powder should be added corresponding to mixture principles in pharmacy to achieve homogenous distribution of the antibiotic in the PMMA beads [40]. After mixing with a spatula, another PMMA amount equal to the antibiotic PMMA powder mixture in the container is added and mixed. This is continued until the PMMA polymer powder is used up. After addition of the monomer the hardening antibiotic-loaded cement is then used to form the beads. For the manufacturing of the beads, molds can be produced or purchased [41, 42] that help to standardize the size and form of the beads.

Handmade antibiotic-loaded spacers for Masquelet technique

The philosophy of the Masquelet technique is based on a two-stage surgical procedure with placement of an antibiotic-loaded PMMA in a resected bone defect after debridement in a first stage [26] (**Fig 6-4a–b**). This stage is intended both to eradicate remaining bacteria by released antibiotics and induction of a biological active membrane on the surface of the PMMA spacer. After 6–8 weeks, the second step is performed with careful removal of the spacer in which the PMMA-induced membrane is incised carefully and left in place followed by filling of the space that was initially occupied by the PMMA spacer with autograft and/or bone substitutes for bony consolidation (**Fig 6-4c–d**). The membrane that is induced by PMMA over 6–8 weeks is vascularized and contains a certain amount of growth factors such as vascular endothelial growth factor (VEGF), transforming-growth factor β-1 (TGF β -1), and bone morphogenetic protein-2 (BMP-2) providing a positive biological environment for the bony consolidation of the defect [43].

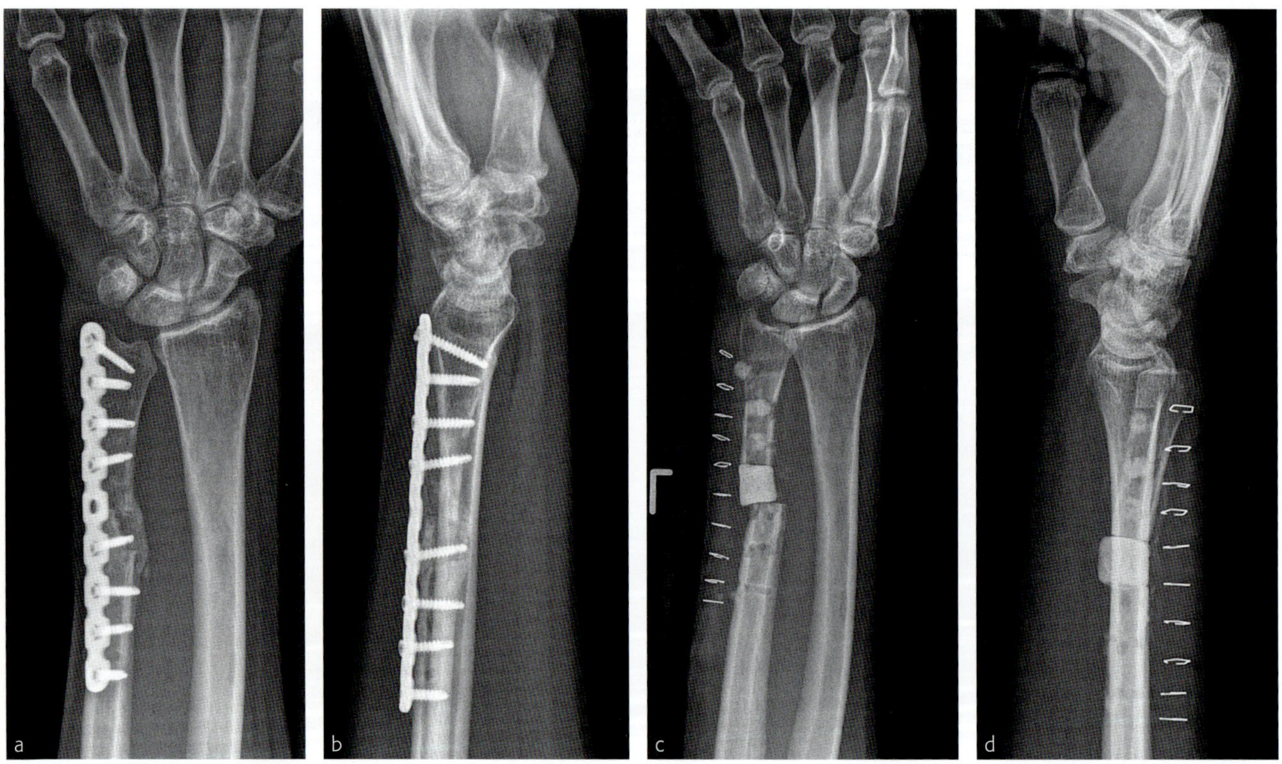

Fig 6-4a–d Masquelet technique.

a–b X-ray series of a *Staphylococcus aureus*-infected distal ulnar shaft nonunion and two-stage Masquelet technique treatment. Resection of the infected nonunion and placement of a gentamicin-loaded polymethylmethacrylate spacer into the defect (stage one).

c–d Stage two procedure with removal of the spacer and corticocancellous autogenous bone graft from the iliac crest and locking plate fixation 6 weeks after stage one.

Practical tips for the Masquelet technique

Hand mixing of the antibiotic-loaded PMMA is performed as described above and the spacer is then introduced into the bone defect between the bone edges. It should surround the proximal and distal two bone ends of the defect to create a "wrap" for the bone graft in the second procedure [44]. For stage two, the membrane surrounding the PMMA spacer should be incised carefully followed by removal of the spacer. The medullary cavity should be debrided and opened and the cortical bone should also be decorticated. The defect is then filled with cancellous bone graft with small pieces of 1–2 mm^3 and/or bone substitutes within the membrane and the membrane should then be closed again. For reconstruction of the tibia, the PMMA spacer may be placed in contact with the fibula if a construct for the graft-tibia-fibula is desired.

In a series of 84 patients with large diaphyseal long bone defects, consolidation was achieved in 90%, and bone defects of up to 230 mm in the tibial diaphysis were successfully treated with this technique [44].

3.2.2 Collagen

Collagen has been studied extensively as a degradable carrier due to its biocompatibility, low cost, and availability [45]. Antibiotic-loaded collagen fleeces are based on collagen from bovine or equine skin or soft tendon and can also act as hemostatic agents [6]. There are several products commercially available. Both products are loaded with gentamicin which is released relatively quickly over the first few days with a burst release directly after implantation in the body. In vitro studies showed that more than 95% of gentamicin was released from collagen fleeces within the first 1.5 hours [45]. The clinical application of the devices is easy as they can be implanted into bone and soft tissue without difficulty. They do not have to be removed because they are biodegradable within the first 8 weeks. However, the degradation process can be associated with seroma formation which is most likely attributable to the tissue reaction to collagen [45, 46]. In smaller wounds, the fleece can be cut into small pieces to reduce the amount of the implanted antibiotic carriers.

3.2.3 Calcium sulfate

Resorbable bone substitute materials as antibiotic carriers are ideal for cases in which infected bone defects need to be filled. Those materials combine antibiotic-releasing and osteoconductive properties for the eradication of bacteria and support of new bone formation. Calcium sulfate and in particular the hemihydrate ($CaSO_4$ $0.5H_2O$), commonly known as "plaster of Paris", has been widely used in this context since 1892 [47]. Despite theoretical osteoconductive properties, the capability of new bone formation by calcium sulfate is limited and degradation products must be considered mildly cytotoxic leading to prolonged and persistent drainage from the wound [48]. Water-soluble antibiotics such as aminoglycosides, vancomycin, daptomycin, and teicoplanin are suitable antibiotics for the loading of calcium sulfate carriers [49]. A high range of the release kinetics of antibiotics from calcium sulfate was reported with a delivery of approximately 45–80% of the antibiotic content within the first 24 hours [48].

There are two commercially available products with medical-grade calcium sulfate containing 4% tobramycin sulfate. The pellets are 3.3 x 4.4 mm. They can be used to fill bone defects and do not have to be removed. Another product consists of biconvex cylinders with a diameter of 6 mm and with a loading of 2.5 mg of gentamicin per bead (**Fig 6-5**).

The combination of calcium sulfate with nanoparticulate hydroxyapatite is another option for a degradable antibiotic carrier. This material was shown to have reliable release kinetics after handloading of the pellets with gentamicin or vancomycin [9]. The material exhibited remarkably improved biocompatibility compared to calcium sulfate alone. The pellets are solid and can be loaded with different antibiotics according to the antibiotic susceptibility of the bacteria before its implantation.

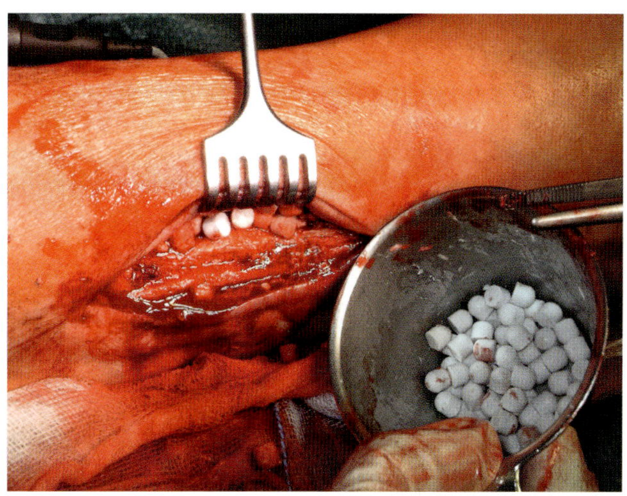

Fig 6-5 Intraoperative use of degradable and osteoconductive pellets of calcium sulfate and nanoparticulate hydroxyapatite loaded with vancomycin for the filling of a defect in a tibial midshaft osteomyelitis.

3.2.4 Bioglass

Bioactive glasses have become of interest in this field due to the combination of antibacterial, osteoinductive, and angiogenic properties within one material that does not have to be removed after implantation [50, 51].

The antimicrobial effects of bioactive glasses are mainly related to the creation of a hostile environment for the bacterial adhesion and proliferation due to calcium and sodium ions as well as phosphorous salts combined with an increase of local pH and osmotic pressure [52].

Particularly, the SiO_2, Na_2O, CaO, P_2O_5—called BAG-S53P4 composition was shown to have good antimicrobial and new bone formation activity [53] and is now commercially available as a biomaterial. Recently, activity against MRSA, *Staphylococcus epidermidis, Pseudomonas aeruginosa,* and *Acinetobacter baumanii* isolates was shown for this material [54].

After thorough debridement of the bone, the biomaterial is simply introduced either as granules or as putty into the bone defect. A first clinical series on patients with chronic osteomyelitis show healing rates of 88.9% in 24 cases treated with the BAG-S53P4 granules [54].

3.3 Coated implants

Implants and all foreign bodies are prone to bacterial adherence, colonization, and subsequent biofilm formation which are the crucial pathophysiological steps in implant-associated infections. Biofilm formation is of major importance as bacteria become embedded within this biofilm substance. Biofilm is a barrier to host immune cells and antibiotic therapy (see chapter 1 Implant-associated biofilm for a detailed explanation). Therefore, the purpose of implant coatings is to prevent bacterial colonization and biofilm formation. There are different strategies, eg, antibiotic coatings or surface modifications with other antiinfective agents. Technologies based on gentamicin or silver are commercially available for fracture fixation devices and endoprostheses.

3.3.1 Gentamicin coating for tibial nails

Polylactic acid (PLA)-gentamicin coating is the first coating that has been commercially available for tibial nails [55]. The initial product has now been replaced by a newer version.

The PLA-gentamicin coating has a thickness of approximately 50 µm with approximately 10–50 g of gentamicin sulfate depending on the size of the nail. In vitro studies have shown an initial burst release of gentamicin within the first minutes [56]. The coating can withstand the forces during insertion of the nail due to its abrasion resistance and is completely resorbed after approximately 6 months. These gentamicin-coated nails are mainly indicated in cases with an increased risk of infection such as open fractures, revision surgery, in patients with systemic immune deficiency (eg, uncontrolled diabetes, morbid obesity), or polytrauma patients. Contraindications are only related to allergies against gentamicin or polylactides. Fuchs et al [55] have published the first study on 21 patients treated with the gentamicin-coated nail in prospective nonrandomized trial with complex tibial fractures and revision cases. The use of this nail showed good clinical, laboratory, and x-ray outcomes. No implant-related infections occurred and no patient showed any systemic or local adverse reaction to the implant coating.

3.3.2 Silver coatings

The broad antimicrobial effect of silver has been known for centuries and is mainly related to the availability of free silver ions that bind to cellular components such as enzymes and structural proteins, particularly to their SH-groups, leading to altered functions of the respective molecules [57]. Another advantage of silver is its activity against multiresistant strains such as MRSA, and that resistance against silver has only rarely been reported in clinical isolates. A major point for silver-coated implants is to ensure biocompatibility as silver can be toxic to eukaryotic cells.

Combined gold-silver coating of megaendoprostheses for orthopedic tumor surgery has already been reported in a clinical setting. The gold substrate on top of the titanium prosthesis is intended to induce silver release from a 10–15 µm elementary silver overcoating layer [58]. In a consecutive case series with 20 patients undergoing bone tumor resection and reconstruction by megaendoprostheses, silver serum levels < 56.4 ppb were measured, which is considered to be nontoxic, and no adverse systemic events from the silver were detected such as argyria, although up to 2.89 g of silver was used on the prosthesis. In a further prospective study with 51 patients with silver-coated megaendoprostheses, infection rates were reported to be 5.9% showing convincing results in this special field of high-risk surgery [59].

Another technology for fracture fixation devices based on silver microparticles embedded in a siloxane-coated layer has already been reported in the literature but is not yet commercially available [60].

4 Conclusion

Local treatment options are of major interest for bone and implant-associated infections. Antiseptics are mainly intended for eradication of bacteria from contaminated and infected wounds.

Gentamicin, tobramycin, and vancomycin are the most important antibiotics for local antibiotic treatment in bone and implant infections. Polymethylmethacrylate is the most commonly used carrier for antibiotic-loaded beads and spacers. In general, commercially available products offer the option of more reproducible release kinetics. In comparison, handmade implants offer the surgeon freedom in antibiotic choice. The use of PMMA-loaded beads and spacers can be considered to be clinically safe, however, dosage recommendations for the individual patient with an allergic profile and problematic kidney function should always be considered. For the Masquelet technique the PMMA-loaded antibiotic spacer serves two purposes: the eradication of bacteria via the released antibiotic and induction of a biologically active membrane to facilitate further bone reconstruction in a two-stage procedure. Degradable carriers such as collagen, calcium sulfate, and bioglass do not require removal. Bioglass has osteoconductive properties and is a filler for bone defects after resection of infected bone fragments. Rifampin cannot be used in combination with PMMA but can be used with degradable carriers such as calcium sulfate-hydroxyapatite. There are only two commercially available antimicrobial implant coatings available which are a PLA-gentamicin coating for tibial nails and a silver coating for megaendoprostheses. These and other coatings together with all other strategies in local antibiotic treatment may help to improve outcomes in bone and implant-associated infections in the future.

5 References

1. **Kramer A, Assadian O, Below H, et al.** Wound antiseptics today—an overview. In: Willy C, ed. *Antiseptics in surgery—update 2013*. Berlin: Lindqvist Book Publishing; 2013:85–111.
2. **FLOW Investigators, Petrisor B, Sun X, et al.** Fluid lavage of open wounds (FLOW): a multicenter, blinded, factorial pilot trial comparing alternative irrigating solutions and pressures in patients with open fractures. *J Trauma*. 2011 Sep;71(3):596–606.
3. **Owens BD, White DW, Wenke JC.** Comparison of irrigation solutions and devices in a contaminated musculoskeletal wound survival model. *J Bone Joint Surg Am*. 2009 Jan;91(1):92–98.
4. **Anglen JO.** Comparison of soap and antibiotic solutions for irrigation of lower-limb open fracture wounds. A prospective, randomized study. *J Bone Joint Surg Am*. 2005 Jul;87(7):1415–1422.
5. **Penn-Barwell JG, Murray CK, Wenke JC.** Comparison of the antimicrobial effect of chlorhexidine and saline for irrigating a contaminated open fracture model. *J Orthop Trauma*. 2012 Dec;26(12):728–732.
6. **Kluin OS, van der Mei HC, Busscher HJ, et al.** Biodegradable vs non-biodegradable antibiotic delivery devices in the treatment of osteomyelitis. *Expert Opin Drug Deliv*. 2013 Mar;10(3):341–351.
7. **Seldes RM, Winiarsky R, Jordan LC, et al.** Liquid gentamicin in bone cement: a laboratory study of a potentially more cost-effective cement spacer. *J Bone Joint Surg Am*. 2005 Feb;87(2):268–272.
8. **Anguita-Alonso P, Rouse MS, Piper KE, et al.** Comparative study of antimicrobial release kinetics from polymethylmethacrylate. *Clin Orthop Relat Res*. 2006 Apr;445:239–244.
9. **Inzana JA, Trombetta RP, Schwarz EM, et al.** 3D printed bioceramics for dual antibiotic delivery to treat implant-associated bone infection. *Eur Cell Mater*. 2015 Nov 4;30:232–247.
10. **Citak M, Argenson JN, Masri B, et al.** Spacers. *J Orthop Res*. 2014 Jan;32 Suppl 1:S120–129.
11. **Patrick BN, Rivey MP, Allington DR.** Acute renal failure associated with vancomycin- and tobramycin-laden cement in total hip arthroplasty. *Ann Pharmacother*. 2006 Nov;40(11):2037–2042.
12. **Curtis JM, Sternhagen V, Batts D.** Acute renal failure after placement of tobramycin-impregnated bone cement in an infected total knee arthroplasty. *Pharmacotherapy*. 2005 Jun;25(6):876–880.
13. **van Raaij TM, Visser LE, Vulto AG, et al.** Acute renal failure after local gentamicin treatment in an infected total knee arthroplasty. *J Arthroplasty*. 2002;17:948–950.
14. **Düwelhenke N, Krut O, Eysel P.** Influence on mitochondria and cytotoxicity of different antibiotics administered in high concentrations on primary human osteoblasts and cell lines. *Antimicrob Agents Chemother*. 2007 Jan;51(1):54–63.
15. **Mader JT, Calhoun J, Cobos J.** In vitro evaluation of antibiotic diffusion from antibiotic-impregnated biodegradable beads and polymethylmethacrylate beads. *Antimicrob Agents Chemother*. 1997 Feb;41(2):415–418.
16. **Edin ML, Miclau T, Lester GE, et al.** Effect of cefazolin and vancomycin on osteoblasts in vitro. *Clin Orthop Relat Res*. 1996 Dec;(333):245–251.
17. **Pankey G, Ashcraft D, Patel N.** In vitro synergy of daptomycin plus rifampin against Enterococcus faecium resistant to both linezolid and vancomycin. *Antimicrob Agents Chemother*. 2005 Dec;49(12):5166–5168.
18. **Giron KP, Gross ME, Musher DM, et al.** In vitro antimicrobial effect against Streptococcus pneumoniae of adding rifampin to penicillin, ceftriaxone, or 1-ofloxacin. *Antimicrob Agents Chemother*. 1995 Dec; 39(12):2798–2800.
19. **Baldoni D, Haschke M, Rajacic Z, et al.** Linezolid alone or combined with rifampin against methicillin-resistant Staphylococcus aureus in experimental foreign-body infection. *Antimicrob Agents Chemother*. 2009 Mar; 53(3):1142–1148.
20. **Trampuz A, Widmer AF.** 2006. Infections associated with orthopedic implants. *Curr Opin Infect Dis*. 2006 Aug;19(4):349–356.
21. **Mohamed W, Sommer U, Sethi S, et al.** Intracellular proliferation of S. aureus in osteoblasts and effects of rifampicin and gentamicin on S. aureus intracellular proliferation and survival. *Eur Cell Mater*. 2014 Oct 23;28:258–268.
22. **Yusuf E, Perrottet N, Orasch C, et al.** Daptomycin-associated eosinophilic pneumonia in two patients with prosthetic joint infection. *Surg Infect (Larchmt)*. 2014 Dec;15(6):834–837.
23. **Peñalba Arias P, Furustrand Tafin U, Bétrisey B, et al.** Activity of bone cement loaded with daptomycin alone or in combination with gentamicin or PEG600 against Staphylococcus epidermidis biofilms. *Injury*. 2015 Feb;46(2):249–253.
24. **Buchholz HW, Engelbrecht H.** [Depot effects of various antibiotics mixed with Palacos resins]. *Chirurg*. 1970 Nov;41(11):511–515. German.
25. **Klemm K.** Gentamicin-PMMA-Kugeln in der Behandlung abszedierender Knochen- und Weichteilinfektionen [Gentamicin-PMMA-beads in treating bone and soft tissue infections (author's transl.)]. *Zentralbl Chir*. 1979;104(14):934–942. German.
26. **Masquelet AC, Fitoussi F, Begue T, et al.** Reconstruction des os longs par membrane induite et autogreffe spongieuse. [Reconstruction of the long bones by the induced membrane and spongy autograft]. *Ann Chir Plast Esthet*. 2000 Jun;45(3):346–353. French.
27. **Baker AS, Greenham LW.** Release of gentamicin from acrylic bone cement. Elution and diffusion studies. *J Bone Joint Surg Am*. 1988 Dec;70(10):1551–1557.
28. **Wahlig H.** Experimentelle Grundlagen für die Anwendung von antibiotika-haltigem Polymethymetharylat. In: Burri C and Rüter A, eds. *Lokalbehandlung chirurgischer Infektionen. Aktuelle Probleme in Chirurgie und Orthopädie, Vol. 12*. Bern: Huber, 1979:103.
29. **Wahlenkamp GH, Vree TB, van Rens TJ.** Gentamicin-PMMA beads. Pharmacokinetic and nephrotoxicological study. *Clin Orthop Relat Res*. 1986 Apr;(205):171–183.
30. **Fluit AC, Jones ME, Schmitz FJ, et al.** Antimicrobial susceptibility and frequency of occurrence of clinical blood isolates in Europe from the SENTRY antimicrobial surveillance program, 1997 and 1998. *Clin Infect Dis*. 2000 Mar;30(3):454–460.
31. **Jenny JY, Jenny G, Lambert J, et al.** Utility of measurement of gentamicin release from PMMA beads in wound drainage fluid after in-vivo implantation. *Acta Orthop Belg*. 1995;61(1):10–13.
32. **Diefenbeck M, Mückley T, Hofmann GO.** Prophylaxis and treatment of implant-related infections by local application of antibiotics. *Injury*. 2006 May;37 Suppl 2:S95–104. Review.

33. **Neut D, van de Belt H, van Horn JR, et al.** Residual gentamicin-release from antibiotic-loaded polymethylmethacrylate beads after 5 years of implantation. *Biomaterials.* 2003. May;24(10):1829–1831.
34. **Neut D, van de Belt H, van Horn JR, et al.** The effect of mixing on gentamicin release from polymethylmethacrylate bone cements. *Acta Orthop Scand.* 2003. Dec;74(6):670–676.
35. **Schnettler R.** Surgical treatment of osteomyelitis. Acute and chronic post-traumatic osteomyelitis. In: Schnettler R and Stein U, eds. *Septic bone and joint surgery.* New York: Thieme; 2010:94–125.
36. **Anagnostakos K, Kelm J, Regitz T, et al.** In vitro evaluation of antibiotic release from and bacteria growth inhibition by antibiotic-loaded acrylic bone cement spacers. *J Biomed Mater Res B Appl Biomater.* 2005 Feb 15;72(2):373–378.
37. **Cui Q, Mihalko WM, Shields JS, et al.** Antibiotic-impregnated cement spacers for the treatment of infection associated with total hip or knee arthroplasty. *J Bone Joint Surg Am.* 2007 Apr;89(4):871–882.
38. **Rasyid HN, van der Mei HC, Frijlink HW, et al.** Concepts for increasing gentamicin release from handmade bone cement beads. *Acta Orthop.* 2009 Oct;80(5):508–513.
39. **Anagnostakos K, Wilmes P, Schmitt E, et al.** Elution of gentamicin and vancomycin from polymethylmethacrylate beads and hip spacers in vivo. *Acta Orthop.* 2009 Apr;80(2):193–197.
40. **Frommelt L.** Local antibiotic therapy. *In:* Schnettler R and Stein U, eds. *Septic bone and joint surgery.* New York: Thieme; 2010:78–86.
41. **Decoster TA, Bozorgnia S.** Antibiotic beads. *J Am Acad Orthop Surg.* 2008 Nov;16(11):674–678.
42. **Kelm J, Anagnostakos K, Regitz T, et al.** MRSA-Infektionen des Bewegungsapparats Behandlung mit intraoperativ herstellbaren Gentamicin-Vancomycin-PMMA-Ketten [MRSA-infections-treatment with intraoperatively produced gentamycin-vancomycin PMMA beads]. *Chirurg.* 2004 Oct;75(10):988–995. German.
43. **Viateau V, Guillemin G, Calando Y, et al.** Induction of a barrier membrane to facilitate reconstruction of massive segmental diaphyseal bone defects: an ovine model. *Vet Surg.* 2006 Jul;35(5):445–452.
44. **Karger C, Kishi T, Schneider L, et al.** Treatment of posttraumatic bone defects by the induced membrane technique. *Orthop Traumatol Surg Res.* 2012 Feb;98(1):97–102.
45. **Sørensen TS, Sørensen AI, Merser S.** Rapid release of gentamicin from collagen sponge. In vitro comparison with plastic beads. *Acta Orthop Scand.* 1990 Aug;61(4):353–356.
46. **Zilberman M, Elsner JJ.** Antibiotic-eluting medical devices for various applications. *J Control Release.* 2008 Sep 24;130(3):202–215.
47. **Dressmann H.** Über Knochenplombierung bei Hohlenformigen Defekten des Knochens. [Filling cave-shaped bone defects.] *Beitr Klin Chir.* 1892;9:804–810. German.
48. **El-Husseiny M, Patel S, MacFarlane RJ, et al.** Biodegradable antibiotic delivery systems. *J Bone Joint Surg Br.* 2011 Feb;93(2):151–157.
49. **Wichelhaus TA, Dingeldein E, Rauschmann M, et al.** Elution characteristics of vancomycin, teicoplanin, gentamicin and clindamycin from calcium sulphate beads. *J Antimicrob Chemother.* 2001 Jul;48(1):117–119.
50. **Arkudas A, Balzer A, Buehrer G, et al.** Evaluation of angiogenesis of bioactive glass in the arteriovenous loop model. *Tissue Eng.* Part C: Methods. 2013 Jun;19(6):479–486.
51. **Hu S, Chang J, Liu M, Ning C.** Study on antibacterial effect of 45S5 Bioglass. *J Mater Sci Mater Med.* 2009 Jan;20(1):281–286.
52. **Munukka E, Leppäranta O, Korkeamäki M, et al.** Bactericidal effects of bioactive glasses on clinically important aerobic bacteria. *J Mater Sci Mater Med.* 2008 Jan;19(1):27–32.
53. **Lindfors NC, Hyvönen P, Nyyssönen M, et al.** Bioactive glass S53P4 as bone graft substitute in treatment of osteomyelitis. *Bone.* 2010 Aug;47(2):212–218.
54. **Drago L, Romanò D, De Vecchi E, et al.** Bioactive glass BAG-S53P4 for the adjunctive treatment of chronic osteomyelitis of the long bones: an in vitro and prospective clinical study. *BMC Inf Dis.* 2013 Dec 10(13):584–592.
55. **Fuchs T, Stange R, Schmidmaier G, et al.** The use of gentamicin-coated nails in the tibia: preliminary results of a prospective study. *Arch Orthop Trauma Surg.* 2011 Oct;131(10):1419–1425.
56. **Schmidmaier G, Wildemann B, Stemberger A, et al.** Biodegradable poly(D,L-lactide) coating of implants for continuous release of growth factors. *J Biomed Mater Res.* 2001;58(4):449–455.
57. **Petering HG.** Pharmacology and toxicology of heavy metals: Silver. *Pharmacol Ther.* 1976;1:127–130.
58. **Hardes J, Ahrens H, Gebert C, et al.** Lack of toxicological side-effects in silver-coated megaprostheses in humans. *Biomaterials.* 2007 Jun;28(18):2869–2875.
59. **Hardes J, von Eiff C, Streitbuerger A, et al.** Reduction of periprosthetic infection with silver-coated megaprostheses in patients with bone sarcoma. *J Surg Oncol.* 2010 Apr 1;101(5):389–395.
60. **Khalilpour P, Lampe K, Wagener M, et al.** Ag/SiO(x)C(y) plasma polymer coating for antimicrobial protection of fracture fixation devices. *J Biomed Mater Res B Appl Biomater.* 2010 Jul;94(1):196–120.

7 Diagnostics

Stéphane Corvec, María Eugenia Portillo, Josephina A Vossen, Andrej Trampuz, Peter J Haar

1 Basics

The management of prosthetic joint infection (PJI) is often guided by tradition, personal experience, and liability aspects, and consequently differs substantially between institutions and countries. Various specialists with different points of view are involved in the management of PJI, such as orthopedic surgeons, infectious disease specialists, and microbiologists. In fact, no gold standard definition of bone and joint infection exists that is accepted by everyone. Although the definitions vary, a consensus group of experts from around the world contributed to the International Consensus Meeting on Prosthetic Joint Infection in an attempt to refine an international consensus definition of PJI [1].

An interdisciplinary team is crucial for successful bone and joint infection management. A correct diagnosis, including the identification of the infecting microorganism(s) and its antimicrobial susceptibility remains the first step for successful treatment (**Fig 7-1**).

A combination of laboratory, histopathology, microbiology, and imaging studies is usually necessary to prove the diagnosis of PJI (**Table 7-1**). To take advantage of an early antimicrobial therapy or to plan an appropriate surgical treatment, an accurate preoperative diagnosis of an infection is essential.

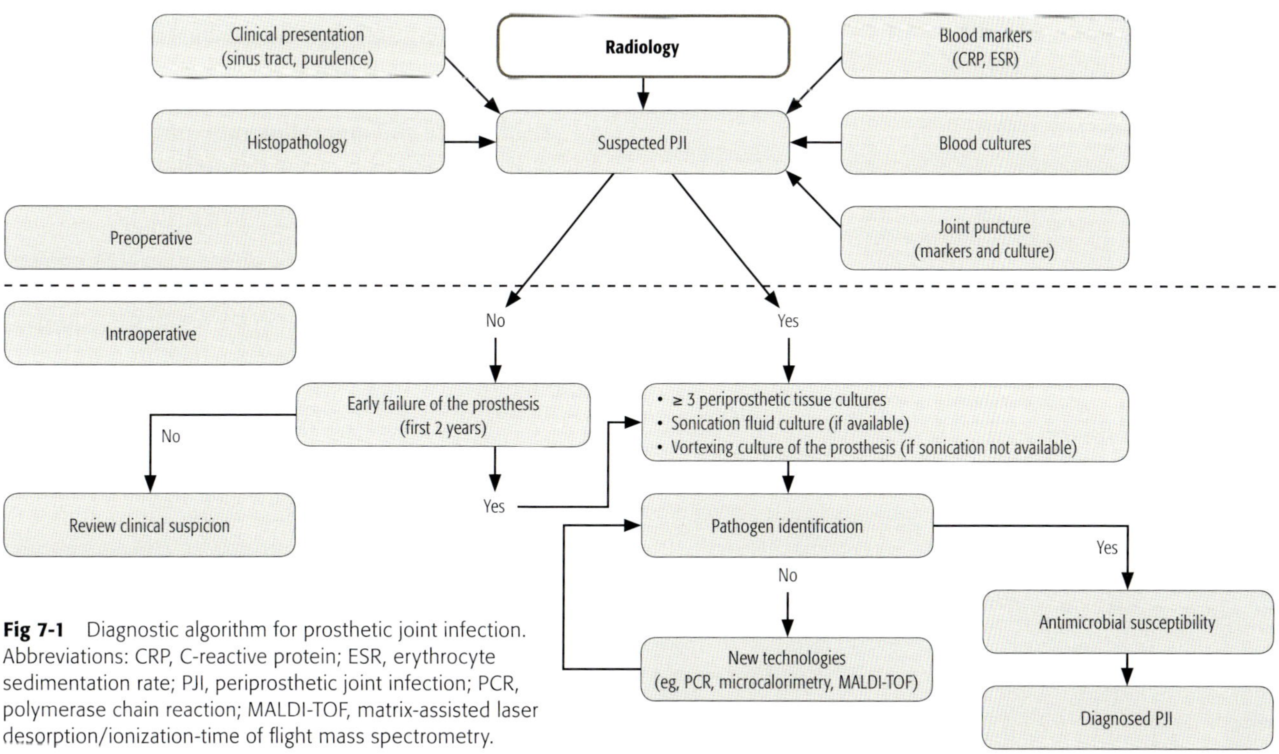

Fig 7-1 Diagnostic algorithm for prosthetic joint infection. Abbreviations: CRP, C-reactive protein; ESR, erythrocyte sedimentation rate; PJI, periprosthetic joint infection; PCR, polymerase chain reaction; MALDI-TOF, matrix-assisted laser desorption/ionization-time of flight mass spectrometry.

2 Blood

For the diagnosis of bone/joint infection, routine peripheral blood tests depend on the host's response to the infecting pathogen. The characteristics of the most available serum inflammatory markers are summarized in **Table 7-2.**

Type of sample	Diagnostic test
Blood	Leukocytes with diff, CRP, ESR, PCT, and TNF-α, IL-6, immunology
Joint puncture	Cell count, diff, Gram stain, arthrography, leukocyte esterase test, culture, new biomarkers (α-defensin)
Radiology	X-ray, CT scan, MRI, sonography, nuclear medicine, PET-CT scan, scintigraphy
Intraoperative samples (eg, biopsy, synovial fluid, sonication fluid)	Culture, PCR, ESI MALDI-TOF, histology, calorimetry, antibodies, sonication

Table 7-1 Tests for diagnosis of prosthetic joint infection.
Abbreviations: diff, differential; CRP, C-reactive protein; ESR, erythrocyte sedimentation rate; PCT, procalcitonin; TNF-α, tumor necrosis factor-α; IL-6, interleukin-6; CT, computed tomography; MRI, magnetic resonance imaging; PET-CT, positron-emission tomography computed tomography; PCR, polymerase chain reaction; ESI, electrospray ionization time of flight; MALDI-TOF, matrix-assisted laser desorption/ionization-time of flight mass spectrometry.

Marker	Cut-off	Sensitivity (%)	Specificity (%)	References
WBC	11,000 x 10^9 cells/L	45	87	**[2]**
CRP	10 mg/L	88	74	**[2]**
ESR	30 mm/h	75	70	**[2]**
PCT	0.3 ng/mL	33	98	**[3]**
TNF-α	40 ng/mL	43	97	**[3,4]**
IL-6	10 pg/mL	97	91	**[2]**

Table 7-2 Serum inflammatory markers for the diagnosis of prosthetic joint infection.
Abbreviations: WBC, white blood cell count; CRP, C-reactive protein; ESR, erythrocyte sedimentation rate; PCT, procalcitonin; TNF-α, tumor necrosis factor-α; IL-6, interleukin-6.

2.1 Leukocyte count and differential

The blood leukocyte count or white blood cell (WBC) count is typically ordered as part of routine blood analysis. Many problems can result in an elevated WBC count. Nevertheless, bacterial infections remain a frequent cause. However, its sensitivity is limited (45%), although its reported specificity (87%) may be useful in some situations [2]. Systemic inflammatory markers do not discriminate whether an infection is of bacterial or fungal origin [5].

2.2 C-reactive protein

C-reactive protein (CRP) is one of the most frequently used inflammatory markers because it is readily available, inexpensive, and easy to perform. The CRP level is independent of age, sex, blood loss, or kind of surgery. Its use has been supported by the Infectious Diseases Society of America [6] and the American Academy of Orthopedic Surgeons (AAOS) [7]. However, alone, this marker is not sufficiently sensitive or specific enough to diagnose or exclude infection with a high accuracy [8]. The CRP level increases within 6–24 hours in response to inflammatory circumstances and has a half-life of one day. Normal values of CRP do not exclude infection, especially in case of low-grade infections. Moreover, CRP levels are increased normally after surgery (peak after 3–4 days), reflect postintervention inflammation, and are limited by underlying inflammatory diseases. Therefore, serial postoperative measurements are essential for accurate interpretation rather than a single value [9]. C-reactive protein has a slightly better sensitivity and specificity than erythrocyte sedimentation rate (ESR) [2, 10].

2.3 Erythrocyte sedimentation rate

Together with CRP, ESR is one of the most used inflammatory markers. However, ESR has neither enough sensitivity nor specificity to correctly detect PJI. Furthermore, ESR levels are also increased normally after surgery. Moreover, it is recognized that determinations of ESR and CRP levels are less accurate for shoulder than for hip or knee arthroplasty infections [11]. Receiver operating characteristic curves were different between ESR and CRP analyzing early versus late chronic infections [12]. This observation may be related to the higher proportion of *Propionibacterium acnes* infections in shoulder infections, reflecting that normal values of CRP and/or ESR levels do not exclude low-grade infections [13]. Therefore, a number of authors consider ESR as obsolete for diagnosing PJI [2, 14].

2.4 Procalcitonin and tumor necrosis factor-α

Procalcitonin (PCT) determination in blood has been shown to be useful in other infections but has been studied in only a small number of patients for diagnosis of PJI. It seems that serum PCT level is specific (98%) but not sensitive (33%) [3]. However, CRP combined with PCT leads to 83% sensitivity and 83% specificity revealing a positive predictive value and a negative predictive value of 89% and 74%, respectively [10]. At a cut-off level of 0.4 ng/mL, PCT seems to be a sensitive and specific marker in the diagnosis of septic arthritis and acute osteomyelitis [15]. According to a recent systematic review and metaanalysis, PCT may be more suitable as an aid for rule-in diagnosis rather than for exclusion of septic arthritis or osteomyelitis and the use of a lower cut-off value may improve its diagnostic performance [16].

Tumor necrosis factor (TNF)-α is elevated in patients with osteolysis compared to matched controls. The role of TNF-α and its potential as a target of nonsurgical therapy to prevent osteolysis warrant further investigation in larger, prospective studies [17]. Patients that had cemented implants have significantly higher levels of TNF-α than patients with cementless varieties ($P = .042$) [18]. Further studies are needed to demonstrate the real advantage of this new marker in PJI and infection.

2.5 Interleukin-6

Interleukin-6 (IL-6) is produced by macrophages and stimulated monocytes. Monocytes can also respond to polyethylene particles by secreting IL-6 but high concentrations of IL-6 have also been detected in the interface membrane surrounding loosened implants [18, 19]. Interleukin-6 returns to baseline level as early as a few hours postoperatively during healing processes leading to normal value after an arthroplasty in 2–3 days, making it a useful marker for early postoperative PJI [20]. A recent systematic review and metaanalysis demonstrates that IL-6 and CRP had a significantly higher diagnostic odds ratio than the leukocyte count and ESR for discriminating infectious from noninfectious causes in revision arthroplasty [2]. Despite these theoretical advantages, given the lack of consistent data and that it is less available and more expensive than other inflammatory markers, the IL-6 test is not, at present, part of standard clinical practice.

To summarize, a systematic review and metaanalysis was performed in 2010 on inflammatory blood laboratory levels as markers for PJI but as with any blood biomarkers, it must be remembered that an infection may be present even if the values are normal [2]. Additional diagnostic tools must be developed in the future.

2.6 Immunology

Staphylococcus aureus remains the leading microorganism responsible for PJI and implant-associated infections. Staphylococcal infections can be challenging to diagnose for many reasons (eg, negative culture, antibiotic treatment, or small-colony variant), and there is no clinically available diagnostic test for host immunity. A cost-effective assay for determining the antiglucosaminidase titer, which can be readily combined with conventional serology to improve diagnosis and to assess host immunity against *S aureus* has been developed [21]. Like for other biomarkers, further studies on immunology, serum markers, and inflammation disequilibrium are needed to better understand the role and the impact on the osteogenesis during an implant-associated infection linked to low concentrations of metal particles. For example, the role of leptin in bone and cartilage function and its implication in inflammatory and degenerative joint diseases have been recently reported. Leptin is an adipokine with pleiotropic actions that regulates food intake, energy metabolism, inflammation, and immunity, and also participates in the complex mechanism that regulates skeleton biology, both at bone and cartilage level [22].

2.7 Outlook on blood markers

Multidisciplinary teams involved in PJI management perform a wide spectrum of tests in an attempt to diagnose PJI [23], including:

- Local measures of synovial inflammation: synovial fluid WBC count and differential, synovial tissue histology
- Systemic measures of inflammation: serum CRP level, ESR, IL-6
- Radiographic tests: x-rays, bone scan, magnetic resonance imaging, computed tomography, positron-emission tomography
- Bacterial isolation techniques: Gram stain, culture

Facing the challenge of accurately diagnosing infection, despite the lack of a clear definition of PJI/implant-associated infection with different criteria, several societies, such as Infectious Diseases Society of America [6], the Musculoskeletal Infection Society [7] and in France *La Société de Pathologie Infectieuse de Langue Française* (SPILF) [24], recently published different definitions of PJI using a combination of clinical data and six of the above tests. Recently, a revival of biomarkers has occurred. Therefore, a recent study chose to screen 43 biomarkers that demonstrated an elevation in the setting of PJI and could potentially be diagnostic for PJI (**Table 7-3**). Among them, 16 evaluated biomarkers demonstrated the greatest and most consistent elevations in the screening process: human α-defensin 1–3 (α-defensin), IL-1a, IL-1, IL-6, IL-8, IL-10, IL-17, granulocyte colony-stimulating factor (G-CSF), vascular endothelial growth factor (VEGF), CRP, neutrophil elastase 2 (ELA-2), lactoferrin, neutrophil gelatinase-associated lipocalin (NGAL), resistin, thrombospondin, and bactericidal/permeability-increasing protein (BPI). Only five biomarkers, including human α-defensin 1-3, neutrophil elastase 2, bactericidal/permeability-increasing protein, neutrophil gelatinase-associated lipocalin, and lactoferrin, correctly predicted the Musculoskeletal Infection Society classification of all patients, with 100% sensitivity and specificity for the diagnosis of PJI.

Despite the fact that only a limited number of patients (46) were included, the last study reveals that the synovial fluid α-defensin immunoassay correctly predicted the Musculoskeletal Infection Society's classification of all patients, demonstrating a sensitivity and specificity of 100% for the diagnosis of PJI [25].

	Native joints		Prosthetic joints	References
	Normal	**Septic arthritis**	**PJI**	
Leukocytes ($\times 10^9$/L)	< 0.2	> 50	> 1.7 (knee), > 4.2 (hip)	**[27, 33]**
Neutrophils (%)	< 25	> 90	> 65 (knee), > 80 (hip)	**[27, 33]**

Table 7-3 Cut-off values for the diagnosis of prosthetic joint infection compared with septic arthritis.
Abbreviation: PJI, prosthetic joint infection.

3 Joint puncture

3.1 How to perform joint puncture

Arthrocentesis, ie, synovial fluid aspiration, can be performed either diagnostically or therapeutically on native or prosthetic joints. Whereas the synovial fluid aspiration of a knee is easy to perform in the office, the aspiration of a hip arthroplasty frequently requires ultrasound or radiographic guidance. Nevertheless, especially when performed preoperatively, this type of sampling requires maximum care to avoid contamination either of the sample or the joint itself.

Synovial fluid is usually sent for cell count, differentiation, and microbiological culture. Furthermore, inflammatory markers may also be investigated although currently they are not widely used.

3.2 Cell count, differentiation, Gram stain test

The detection of leukocytes in the synovial fluid, ie, cell count and differential, is an effective and simple way to distinguish between PJI and aseptic failure. Despite cut-off values for positive tests being similar although not equal in different study populations and different joint types, guidelines do not include a specific cut-off value in their diagnostic criteria [6, 26]. It is significant that the cut-off values for diagnosing PJI are considerably lower than the ones for septic arthritis in native joints (**Table 7-3**). The optimal cut-off values appear to be higher in hip than in knee arthroplasties, probably related to the higher frequency of *S aureus* infections in hip PJI, reflecting that infections caused by highly virulent microorganisms are associated with a higher total leukocyte count [27]. In the majority of these studies, patients with inflammatory diseases were excluded. For these patients, a higher baseline nucleated cell count would be expected, and accordingly, the cut-off values mentioned above would be expected to be less specific [1]. In contrast to prosthetic joints, there are no precisely defined thresholds for native joints because the cell count alone does not provide sufficient evidence of an infection. Therefore, it is usually necessary to wait for the bacteriology results for an accurate diagnosis (> 10 days). In the presence of a high leukocyte count, urgent surgical intervention may be undertaken prior to a definitive diagnosis.

For determination of leukocyte count and differential, vials should contain ethylene-diamine-tetraacetic acid (EDTA), citrate, or heparin to prevent coagulation of the aspirate. The cell count can be determined by automated hematology or by manual cell counters. Metal-on-metal hip arthroplasties can give a falsely elevated synovial fluid cell count when using automated cell counters. This can be overcome by manually counting cell counters. Importantly, the neutrophil percentage remains accurate for this group of patients, given that it is determined manually [1]. Clotted specimens are treated before analysis with hyaluronidase for 10 minutes at room temperature.

Additional tests in synovial fluid, such as glucose, lactate, or CRP have not been shown to bring additional information regarding the diagnosis of infection [28–31].

Crystal analysis provides information about crystal-induced arthropathy. The gross appearance of synovial fluid can provide useful diagnostic information in terms of the degree of joint inflammation and presence of hemarthrosis. Microbiological studies of synovial fluid are the key test to provide confirmation of an infectious condition. Joint inflammation is associated with increased synovial fluid volume, reduced viscosity, increasing turbidity and cell count, and increasing ratio of polymorphonuclear to mononuclear cells, but such changes are nonspecific and must be interpreted in the clinical setting. However, detection of synovial fluid monosodium urate and calcium pyrophosphate dihydrate crystals, even from uninflamed joints during clinically quiet periods, allows a precise diagnosis of gout and calcium pyrophosphate crystal-related arthritis [32].

One aliquot of native fluid should be conserved for direct microscopic Gram stain examination. Direct bacteriological examination after Gram stain can visualize bacteria, especially after a cytocentrifugation step and investigation of the pellet. The specificity of Gram stain is high (up to 97%) but it has poor sensitivity (< 25%) [27, 34, 35]. Therefore, Gram staining is not routinely recommended [36].

3.3 Arthrography

Imaging using contrast agent administered once the puncture is complete via the in situ needle is especially useful in the case of prosthetic hip joints. It reveals protrusions from the joint cavity, abscess cavities, and fistulous tracts, even if no external fistula is visible. These signs are often criteria for two-stage revision. Improved resolution through digital subtraction technique is possible. In 2005, a metaanalysis found that the subtraction arthrography was a sensitive technique for detection of loosening of total hip prosthesis, offering added value over contrast arthrography, especially for evaluation of the femoral component [37].

3.4 Leukocyte esterase test

Leukocyte esterase is an enzyme present in neutrophils, which is frequently measured by a colorimetric strip to determine pyuria for the diagnosis of urinary tract infection (**Fig 7-2**). This test strip has recently been tested in two studies in synovial fluid to evaluate PJI [38, 39]. Limitations of this test are that it is semiquantitative (results are read by comparison with colors printed on the product label with a colorfast printing method colorimetric) and that presence of blood in synovial fluid may promote false-positive results. In fact, in one of these studies, patients with excessive blood in synovial fluids (10%) were excluded [38] and in the other study, almost 30% of the tests were not valid because they were unreadable due to blood, debris, or were indeterminate results [22].

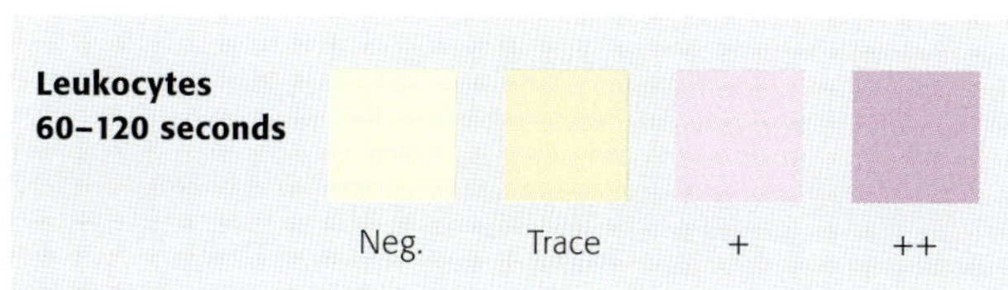

Fig 7-2 Leukocyte esterase strip test results.

3.5 Outlook on markers

Other markers, including those used in blood, show some promise for the diagnosis of PJI. C-reactive protein determination in synovial fluid appears to have a sensitivity ranging from 85 to 87%, but the specificities varied widely [14, 30, 40].

Determination of synovial fluid IL-6 levels showed high specificity (93–100%) but variable sensitivity (69–100%) and specificity [14, 40, 41]. A recent study also investigated the value of PCT in synovial fluid, and authors concluded that this marker had a high negative predictive value that could exclude infection in both native and prosthetic joints. However, only 14 subjects with PJI were included [42]. Therefore, further studies are needed to confirm these findings.

Other interleukins, such as interleukin-1 β (IL-1 β) have been studied in synovial fluid. Its sensitivity and specificity were lower than for IL-6 [40]. Recently, the role of antimicrobial peptides, such as α- and β-defensins, has been assessed. Cells of the immune system contain these peptides to assist in killing phagocytized bacteria and almost all epithelial cells. Most defensins function by binding to the microbial cell membrane and, once embedded, forming pore-like membrane defects that allow efflux of essential ions and nutrients. This study showed promising results but only 15 patients with staphylococcal PJI were included [4]. Currently, these new biomarkers may be considered as promising tools for diagnosis or follow-up, but robust data are still missing, and until further data become available and costs reduced, a recommendation for clinical use cannot be made [1].

3.6 Culture-negative infection

Culture of preoperative synovial fluid is priceless for early identification of the infecting pathogen and determination of antimicrobial susceptibility. Although some surgeons inoculate the aspirated fluid obtained by arthrocentesis at the time of collection into blood-bottle culture, an aliquot of aspirated synovial fluid should be conserved and sent to the microbiology laboratories for cell count, differentiation, and conventional cultures on agar plates and enrichment broth. Sensitivity of aspirated fluid culture is between 65–100% and may be further improved by inoculation into blood-culture bottles [43, 44]. Widely varied sensitivity may be related to low-grade microorganism-related infection or antimicrobial treatment prior to arthrocentesis, where sensitivity is lower if patients received antibiotics 2–3 weeks prior to aspiration [45–47], and type of infection, where sensitivity is higher in acute infections. This may be due also to the virulence of the pathogen [46]. Nevertheless, prolonged cultures are always recommended to avoid a false-negative culture. Therefore, antibiotics should be stopped at least 2 weeks prior to aspiration whenever possible, synovial fluid should be inoculated directly into blood-culture bottles, and an aliquot of native synovial fluid should be plated. To reduce the rate of culture-negative infection, aerobic agar plates should be incubated at least 5–7 days and anaerobic agar plates at least 10 days to detect slower growing microorganisms, such as small-colony variants or anaerobic organisms [48]. In fact, in a recent study, false-negative rates of preoperative aspiration relative to intra-operative culture were 56% and 46% in hip and knee PJI, respectively, with discordance rates of 25% and 21.4%, respectively. Rates of negative intraoperative cultures were 15% in hip PJI and 20.7% in knee PJI [49].

Today, accurate preanalytical conditions for preoperative, intraoperative, or postoperative sampling are necessary to isolate the infecting microorganism in PJI. Several techniques will be discussed in topic 5.2 of this chapter.

For other implant-associated infections, aspiration of the implant area can be performed with ultrasound guidance as needed to obtain fluid. Fluid should be cultured as described above, and if possible, a cell count performed for diagnosis.

4 Radiology of musculoskeletal infection

4.1 Introduction

Early diagnosis of musculoskeletal infection is imperative to initiate timely treatment and prevent potential complications. Musculoskeletal imaging is an essential diagnostic tool needed by physicians to diagnose musculoskeletal conditions including infection. Baseline studies should include at a minimum plain x-ray examinations. These x-ray examinations are helpful to detect subtle changes over time. Because each imaging modality has specific strengths and limitations, a multimodality approach is commonly used. This part of the chapter will help to define which radiological studies are beneficial to clinicians and surgeons in diagnosing musculoskeletal infection and following progress of treatment. In this part of the chapter, numerous medical images from varied clinical scenarios will be used to illustrate advantages and disadvantages of each modality. In cases of musculoskeletal infection, the radiologist is an important member of the patient care team, along with the infectious disease physician and surgeon. Treating physicians should confer with the radiologist to determine the most appropriate examinations to request so as to provide appropriate diagnosis and treatment information that will best facilitate patient care.

4.2 Standard x-ray

Conventional x-rays are often the initial imaging examination obtained and can be helpful in suggesting the correct diagnosis and to exclude other etiologies, such as tumor or trauma. Plain x-ray is often insensitive during the early stages of bone infection since at least 30–50% of bone needs to be destroyed before abnormalities are seen on x-rays [50, 51]. Initial subtle radiographic findings include focal soft-tissue swelling, periosteal elevation or thickening, osteopenia, and osteolysis (**Fig 7-3**, **Fig 7-4**). During the subacute or chronic stage of osteomyelitis, radiographic findings can include a radiolucent abscess, sequestrum, ie, dead sclerotic bone; involucrum, ie, periosteal new bone surrounding a sequestrum; and sinus tracts (**Fig 7-5**). Organization in the intramedullary space of a cystic cavity represents an intraosseous abscess or Brodie's abscess (**Fig 7-6**). In patients with orthopedic implants, infection can be seen as implant loosening with or without pathological fractures or dislocation (**Fig 7-7**, **Fig 7-8**, **Fig 7-9**). These radiographic findings are often similar to those seen in aseptic loosening, and the diagnosis is based on a combination of history, laboratory values, and aspiration of periprosthetic fluid.

Septic arthritis is a medical emergency associated with a significant morbidity and needs urgent diagnosis and management. X-rays may show periarticular osteopenia, effusion, soft-tissue swelling, and loss of joint space. Progression of the infection can cause erosions, periosteal reaction, joint malalignment, and ankylosis.

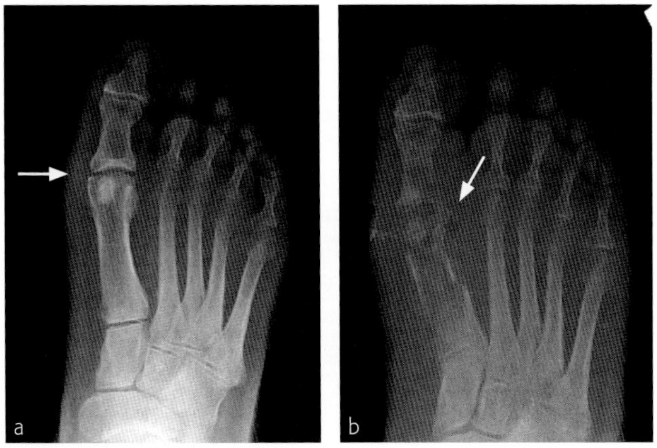

Fig 7-3a–b Foot infection in a 63-year-old woman with diabetes mellitus.

a Initial x-ray shows soft-tissue swelling at the medial aspect of the first metatarsal head (arrow).

b X-ray 4 weeks later demonstrates soft-tissue defect, osteolysis, osteosclerosis, and fragmentation. Radiolucent areas within the soft tissues are related to the presence of gas (arrow).

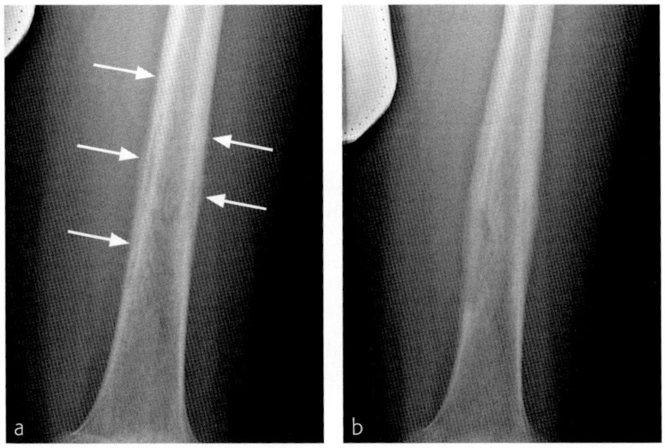

Fig 7-4a–b Periosteal reaction in a 24-year-old man with methicillin-resistant *Staphylococcus aureus* infection of the femur.

a Initial x-ray demonstrates periosteal reaction (arrows).

b X-ray 3 weeks later shows increasing periosteal reaction and erosion of cortical bone.

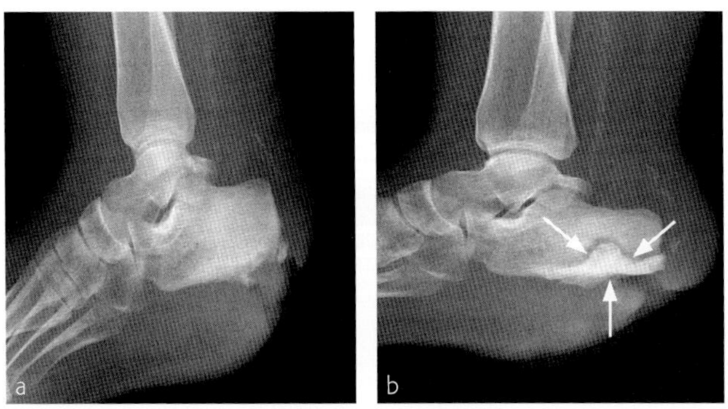

Fig 7-5a–b Heel ulcer and sequestrum formation in a 35-year-old immunocompromised woman.

a X-ray reveals a large heel ulcer with underlying osseous erosions.

b Subsequent x-ray with a large sequestrum (arrows).

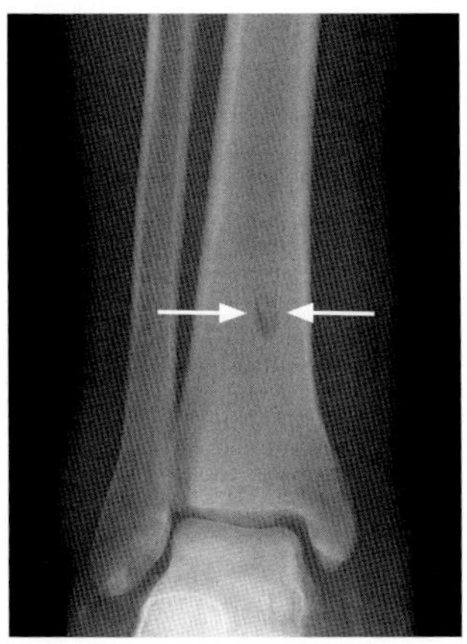

Fig 7-6 A 15-year-old boy with Brodie's abscess. AP x-ray of the tibia shows an elongated radiolucent lesion (arrows).

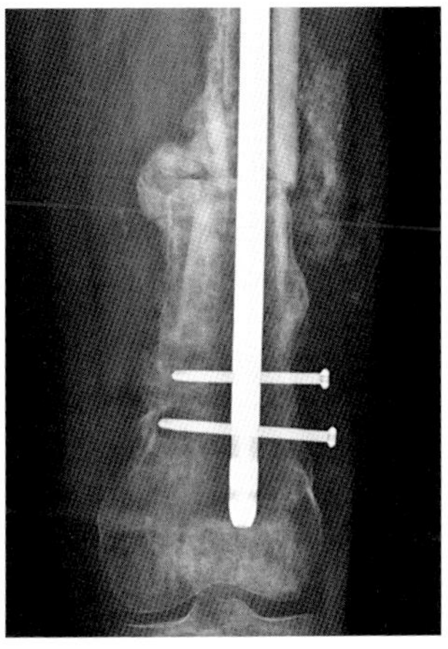

Fig 7-7 Extensive posttraumatic and postsurgical changes including an intramedullary rod and distal interlocking screws in the left femur. Lucency surrounding the screws and motion of the screws is seen. Subsequent surgery demonstrated implant-associated infection.

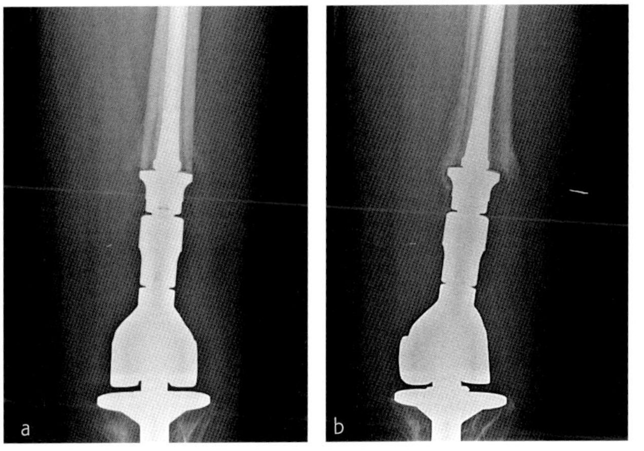

Fig 7-8a–b Long-stem custom femoral prosthesis in a 42-year-old man after osteosarcoma resection.

a Initial x-ray with prosthesis in good position.

b Follow-up imaging demonstrates loosening of the prosthesis with associated periosteal reaction. The diagnosis of infection was made based on the combination of history, laboratory values, and aspiration of periprosthetic fluid. Subsequent surgery confirmed prosthetic joint infection.

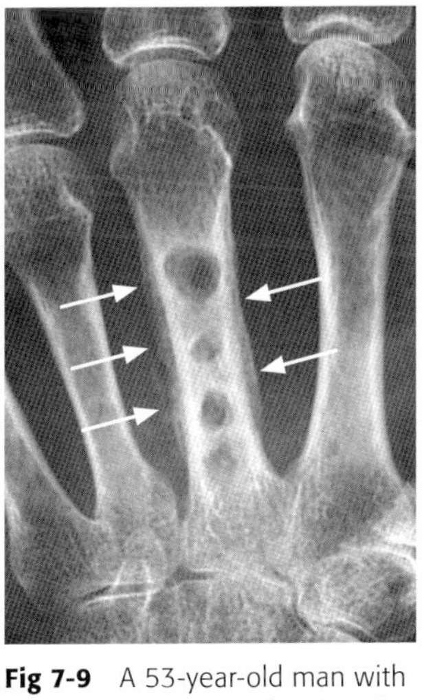

Fig 7-9 A 53-year-old man with drainage and pain at the site of the plate and screw construct. The hardware was removed. X-ray shows enlarged screw tracts and periostitis (arrows), compatible with the operative diagnosis of implant-associated infection.

4.3 Computed tomography

Computed tomographic (CT) imaging provides good spatial and contrast resolution of bone and surrounding soft tissue. The major use of intravenous contrast during CT examination is to demonstrate the extent of the infection, localize soft-tissue changes, and determine involvement of surrounding fascial compartments. Additionally, CT is the modality of choice for the detection of gas in the soft tissue and osseous structures [52]. Computed tomographic features of acute osteomyelitis include increased density of the normal fatty medullary canal as it is replaced by infectious edema, blurring of fat planes, and periosteal reaction [53]. In patients with chronic infection, CT imaging can demonstrate abnormal thickening of the affected cortical bone, encroachment of the medullary cavity, sequestrum formation and chronic draining sinus (**Fig 7-10**) [54], [55]. Computed tomography is an important modality in guiding biopsies, in evaluating the need for surgery, and in planning the surgical approach.

4.4 Magnetic resonance imaging

Magnetic resonance imaging (MRI) is useful for many aspects of diagnosis and treatment planning in musculoskeletal infection. The high spatial resolution has the ability to delineate the extent of the infection, evaluate for abscess cavity formation, and plan treatment. Magnetic resonance imaging is highly sensitive for detecting osteomyelitis as early as 3–5 days (**Fig 7-11**, **Fig 7-12**, **Fig 7-13**). In the acute phase of osteomyelitis, the edema and exudates within the medullary space produce a decreased signal on the T1-weighted images and an increased signal on T2-weighted and inversion recovery sequences. Often the surrounding soft tissues are also abnormal, and often the tract of the skin ulcer can be followed to the bone. The cortical bone may be disrupted and can have abnormally increased signal intensity. Cortical thickening can be seen in chronic infection of bone but is absent in the acute phase. The use of gadolinium enhancement can aid in identifying sinus tracts and distinguishing cellulitis from abscess [56]. Osteomyelitis should not be confused with reactive marrow changes secondary to an adjacent infection. On T2-weighted images, reactive marrow appears as hyperintense marrow. On T1-weighted images there is no low signal that illustrates osteomyelitis [57].

An increasing number of joint replacements are being performed to deal with the aging population. The use of MRI in patients with metallic implants is limited by the presence of artifacts, which can obscure signs of infection. Standard MRI techniques to reduce metal artifact include scanning on a lower field strength magnet, and using high bandwidth parameters, smaller voxel size, and appropriate sequences. Advanced MRI techniques to further reduce metal artifact include the use of specialized sequences, such as slice-encoding for metal artifact correction (SEMAC), and multiacquisition variable-resonance image combination (MAVRIC). The use of these metal artifact suppression algorithms in patients with hardware and suspected infection can improve the quality of images [58]. Specific MRI sequences to order as well as the potential need for contrast material should be discussed in advance with the radiologist to improve the yield of this imaging modality.

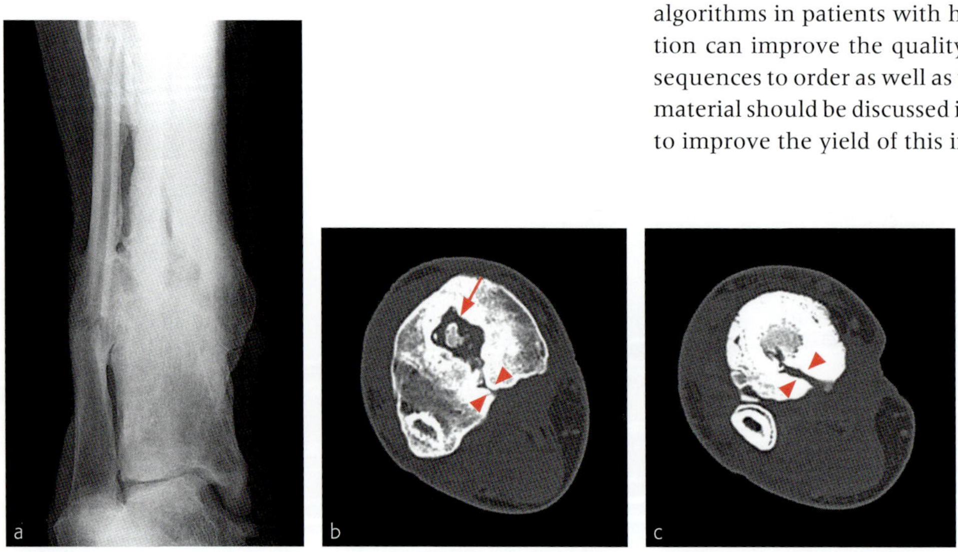

Fig 7-10a–c A 47-year-old man with a history of distal tibial and fibular fractures, open reduction and internal fixation, and subsequent removal of infected hardware.
a X-ray demonstrates extensive posttraumatic and postsurgical changes as well as periosteal thickening.
b–c Axial computed tomographic images demonstrate a sequestrum (arrow) and a sinus tract (arrowheads).

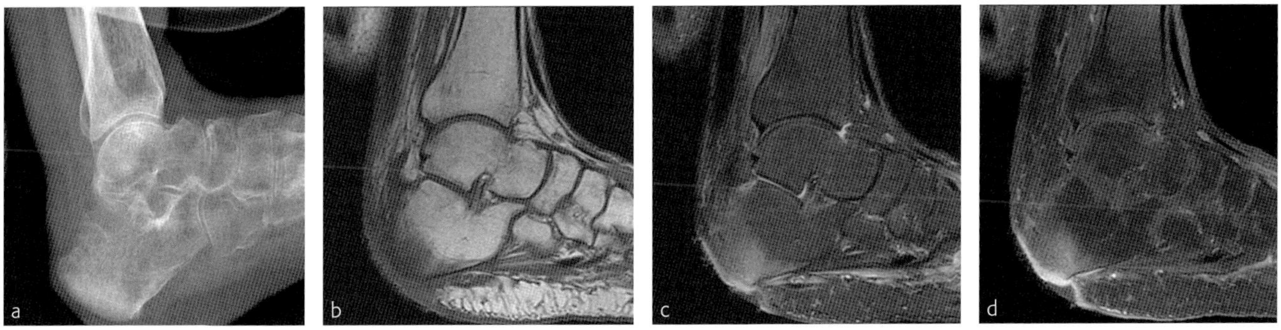

Fig 7-11a–d Heel ulcer and osteomyelitis in a 42-year-old paraplegic man.

a Lateral x-ray demonstrates loss of heel soft tissue and sclerosis of the underlying calcaneus.

b–d Sagittal T1-weighted (repetition time (TR)/echo time (TE) TR/TE = 719/9.9 ms), fluid-attenuated inversion recovery-weighted (TR/TE/TI = 6783/28/130 ms) and postgadolinium (TR/TE = 812/9.9 ms) magnetic resonance images show abnormal ill-defined decreased T1 and increased fluid-attenuated inversion recovery (FLAIR) signal in the posterior calcaneus. Enhancement on postcontrast images is seen in this area. Subsequent surgery confirmed osteomyelitis.

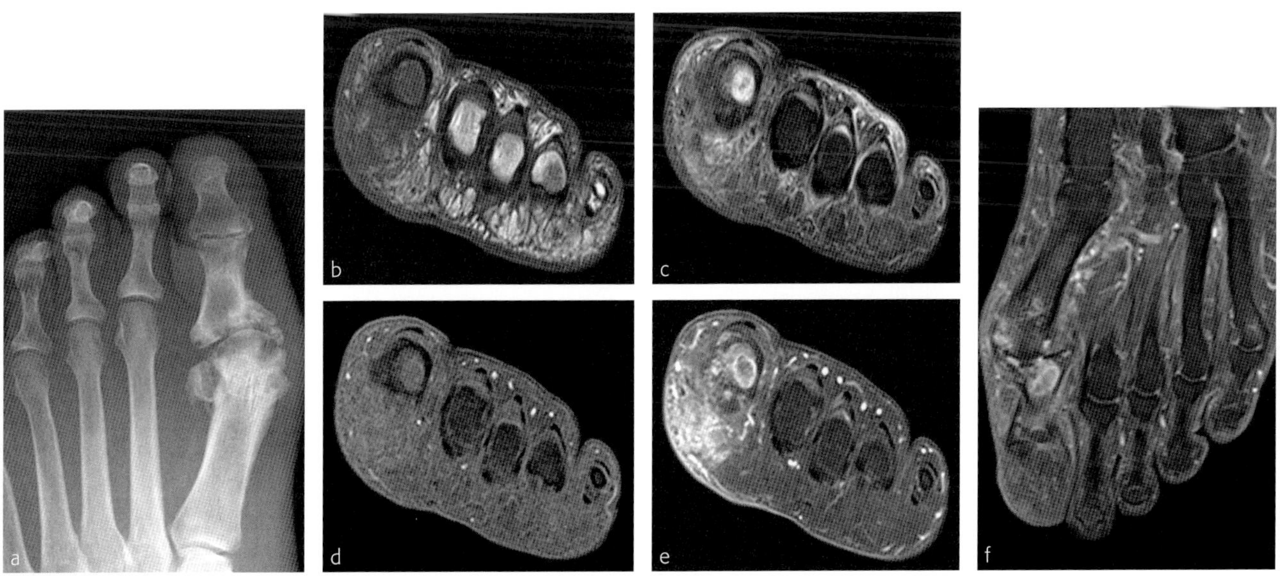

Fig 7-12a–f A 61-year-old woman with diabetic foot ulcer.

a X-ray demonstrates juxtaarticular osteoporosis, severe narrowing of the joint space due to cartilage damage and destruction of the subchondral bone on both sides of the first metatarsophalengeal joint. Adjacent soft-tissue swelling is also seen.

b–e Coronal T1-weighted (TR/TE = 615/11 ms), fat-suppressed T2-weighted (TR/TE = 3821/46 ms), and pre- and postgadolinium (TR/TE = 630/11 ms) magnetic resonance images show abnormal ill-defined decreased T1 and increased T2 signal in the first metatarsal head and proximal phalanx at the metatarsophalangeal joint. Enhancement on postcontrast images is present in this area.

f Axial and postgadolinium image demonstrates involvement of the first metatarsophalangeal joint with osseous destruction, compatible with septic arthritis. Extensive soft-tissue swelling surrounds the joint with a small fluid collection suspicious for abscess. Septic arthritis in the diabetic foot is typically a result of direct spread from adjacent bone or soft-tissue infection.

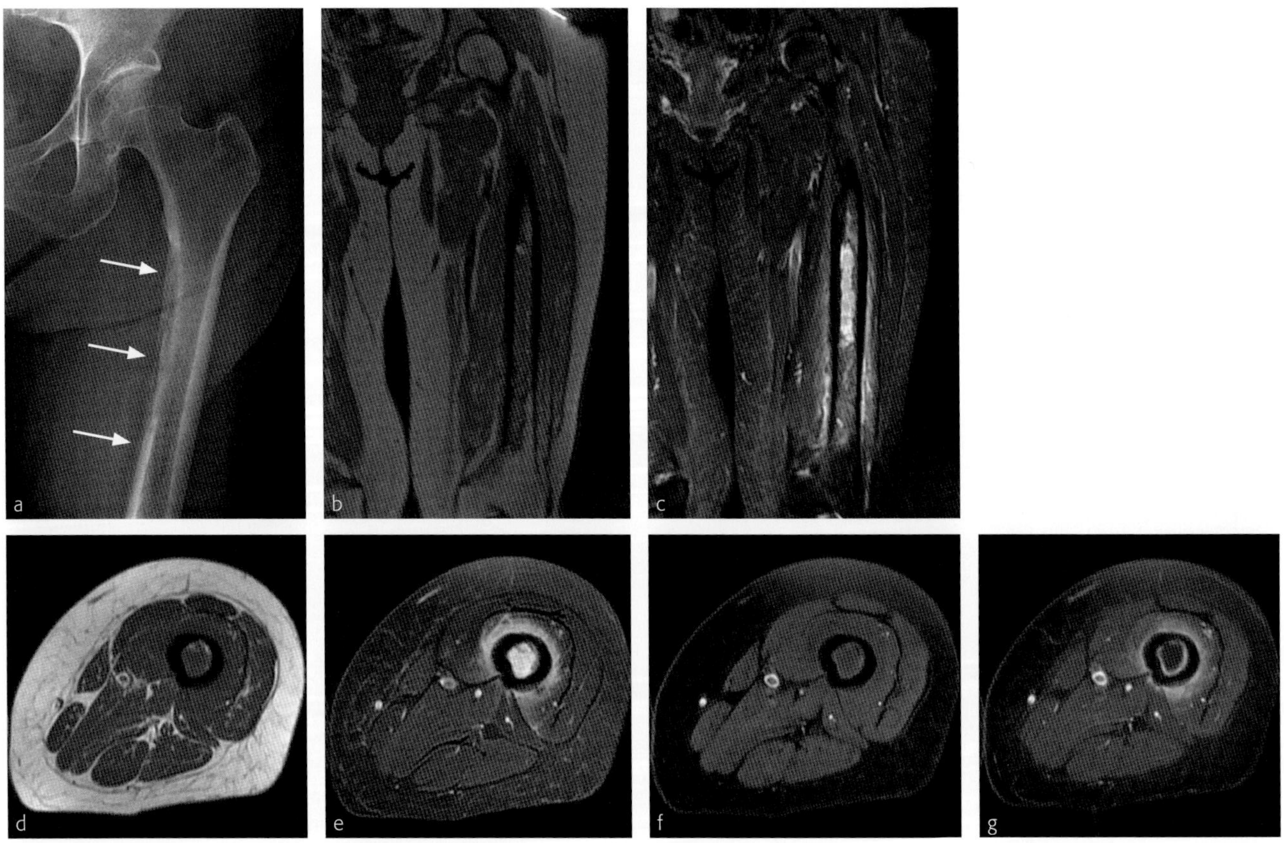

Fig 7-13a–g Methicillin-resistant *Staphylococcus aureus* osteomyelitis in a 47-year-old woman.

a X-ray shows periosteal reaction and cortical irregularity along the medial aspect of the proximal femur (arrows).

b–c Coronal T1-weighted (TR/TE = 717/14 ms) and fluid-attenuated inversion recovery-weighted (TR/TE/TI = 4600/55/145 ms) magnetic resonance images show abnormal decreased T1 and increased T2 signal within the medullary cavity. Surrounding edema is also in the surrounding soft tissues.

d–g Axial T1-weighted (TR/TE = 517/8 ms), fat-suppressed T2-weighted (TR/TE = 3300/60 ms), pre- and postgadolinium (TR/TE = 583/8 ms) magnetic resonance images demonstrate abnormal decreased T1 and increased T2 signal as well as enhancement on postcontrast images.

4.5 Sonography

Sonography is a useful technique for infection diagnosis. In particular, sonography can be used to determine size, extent, and location of abscess cavities or fluid collections. Power Doppler sonography can show increased vasculature and hyperemia in the wall of abscesses. Additionally, sonography can differentiate infection from other pathological conditions with a similar clinical presentation. Furthermore, in regions that are complicated by orthopedic hardware, ultrasound might have improved visualization when compared to CT and MRI. In children, ultrasound can be used to identify joint effusions or subperiosteal fluid associated with early septic arthritis or osteomyelitis [59]. Ultrasound has proven to be a useful method to guide the radiologist when performing a diagnostic or therapeutic aspiration, drainage, or biopsy (**Fig 7-14**) [60].

4.6 Nuclear medicine

Nuclear imaging studies can detect musculoskeletal infections in an early stage, 10–14 days before changes are visible on plain x-rays. Studies include technetium-99m labeled methylene diphosphonate (Tc-99m MDP), gallium-67 citrate, and indium-111–labeled WBCs. These studies are particularly useful in patients with multiple sites of infection and in patients with metallic hardware. The sensitivity is typically noted to be high for these studies; however, the specificity is low. The use of fluorine-18 fluorodeoxyglucose positron-emission tomography computed tomography (FDG PET-CT) is relatively novel for the detection of infection and provides a relatively high diagnostic accuracy and good spatial resolution.

4.6.1 Positron-emission tomography computed tomography

Fluorine-18 fluorodeoxyglucose positron-emission tomography-computed tomography is useful in specific cases for musculoskeletal infection. The use of FDG PET-CT is helpful for localization of the infection and discrimination between infection and other processes that affect the musculoskeletal system. When trying to understand multifocal cases of bone infection FDG PET-CT can be particularly useful [61]. Potential future applications for FDG PET-CT include development of contrast media that will label biofilm or antimicrobial peptides to enable surgeons to understand the full extent of the infectious process [62].

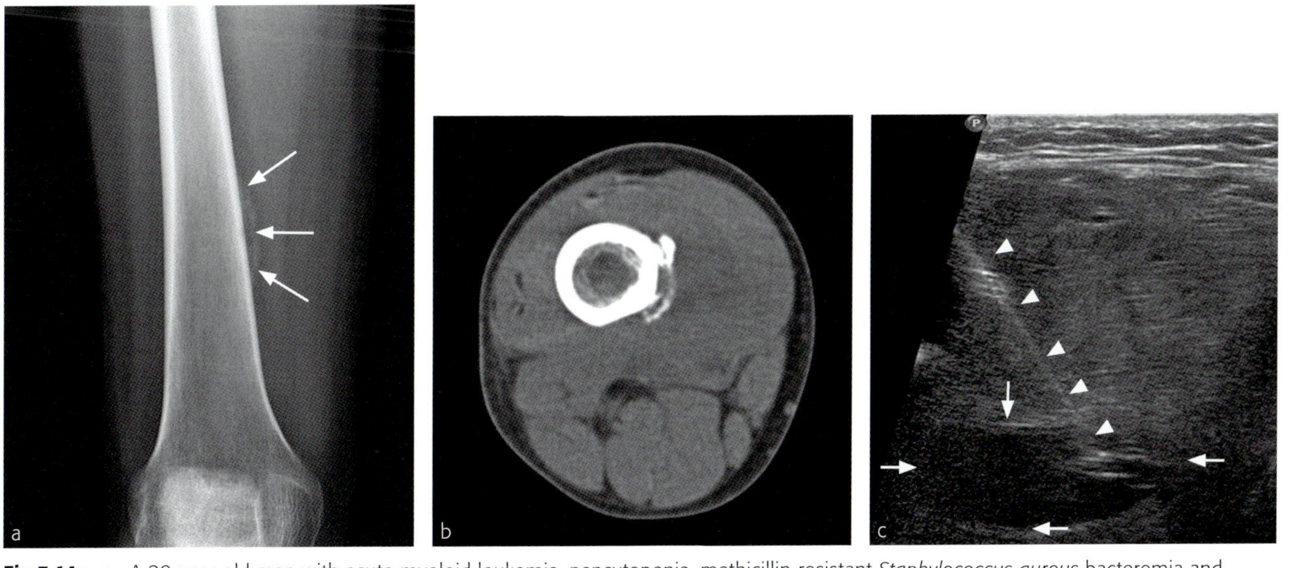

Fig 7-14a–c A 29-year-old man with acute myeloid leukemia, pancytopenia, methicillin-resistant *Staphylococcus aureus* bacteremia and abscess collection adjacent to the right femur.
a–b X-ray and computed tomographic scan demonstrate periosteal reaction along the medial aspect of the right distal femoral diaphysis (arrows).
c Ultrasound-guided aspiration of the abscess along the right femur was performed. Image demonstrates the needle (arrowheads) within the abscess collection (arrows).

4.6.2 Scintigraphy

The basic bone scintigraphy study is the Tc-99m methylene diphosphonate bone scan. The first phase of imaging is obtained 60 seconds after tracer injection (flow study or angiogram) and consists of a dynamic study of the region of interest. The second phase (blood pool) consists of static images performed a few minutes after injection. The third phase is performed 2–4 hours after injection and demonstrates the bone structures and shows increased activity in the affected bone. The three-phase bone scan offers many diagnostic possibilities including localization of an infection, discrimination between cellulitis and osteomyelitis, and delineation of the extent of a bony infection [63]. Abnormal findings for osteomyelitis on Tc-99m bone scan typically include increased flow activity, blood pool activity, and positive uptake on 3-hour images (**Fig 7-15**). The three-phase bone scan can become positive within 24–48 hours after onset of symptoms of acute osteomyelitis [64]. Bone scintigraphy has a sensitivity of greater than 90%, but has a limited specificity, only up to 50%.

A WBC scan done with indium-111-tagged leukocytes and more recently with Tc-99m hexamethyl-propyleneamine oxime (HMPAO)-labeled white cells has an increased specificity compared with bone scans, particularly when complicating conditions, such as prior trauma, prior surgery, or diabetes are superimposed. An overall sensitivity of 88% and specificity of 91% are reported for osteomyelitis [65].

Technetium-99m sulfur colloid scanning can be added to the WBC scan protocol to improve specificity for infection in complicated cases such as postarthroplasty infections. Infection is confirmed when there is less or no bone marrow activity on the sulfur colloid scan in areas with increased uptake on the labeled WBC scan. Activity present on bone marrow scans equal to or greater than that of the WBC scan indicates physiological bone marrow activity and rules out infection.

Infection can also be identified by injection of gallium-67 citrate, which leaks from the bloodstream into areas of inflammation. Although more specific than a three-phase bone scan, image quality suffers slightly compared with a three-phase bone scan and imaging takes longer (18–72 hours) [66]. Gallium-67 activity returns to baseline approximately 6 weeks after successful treatment of osteomyelitis and can therefore be used to monitor the clinical course of the disease [67].

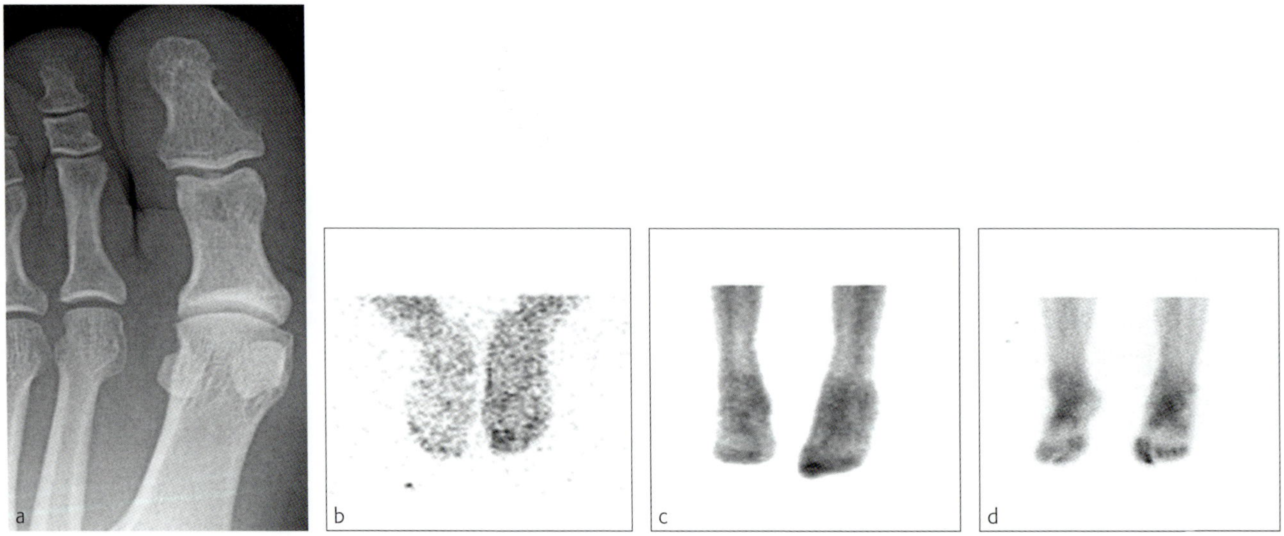

Fig 7-15a–d Osteomyelitis of the first toe in a 56-year-old man.
a X-ray demonstrates mild periosteal reaction at the medial aspect of the first distal phalanx. There is surrounding soft-tissue swelling.
b–d Three-phase bone scan with focal hyperperfusion on the blood-flow phase (**b**), focal hyperemia on the blood-pool phase (**c**), and focal increased bone activity on the delayed images (**d**). Findings are compatible with osteomyelitis.

5 Biopsy

5.1 Introduction

Intraoperative tissue samples provide accurate specimens for detecting the infecting microorganism(s), ranging from 65 to 95% [48, 68]. At least three to five intraoperative tissue specimens from different anatomical sites should be sampled for culture [69, 70]. The lower the grade of inflammation, the more samples should be collected to randomly detect organisms, which are distributed in patches around the implant/prosthesis and the burden is low. A lower number of samples may create interpretation difficulties and a higher number leads to an increased probability of contamination without evidence of improved sensitivity of the examination and extra cost for the microbiology laboratory. Swabs have a low sensitivity and should be avoided [48]. The specificity of tissue Gram stain is very high (98%) but its sensitivity is low (0–27%) [69, 71–74], so tissue Gram stain is not routinely recommended.

Intraoperative samples should be cultured on agar plates and inoculated into enrichment broths. They should be incubated aerobically in the presence of 5% of CO_2 and anaerobically. Some authors recommend inoculating synovial fluid in blood-culture bottle to improve the culture sensitivity [70]. Aerobic cultures should be incubated for up to 7 days and anaerobic cultures (especially broth) for at least 2 weeks [75, 76]. Importantly, a systemic seeding from the anaerobic broth on aerobic and anaerobic agar plates should be performed after 2 weeks to detect mixed infections, anaerobes, or low-growing bacteria [77]. Rare microorganisms such as *Mycobacteria* or *Candida* species (spp.) may be examined from the samples conserved at -80° C if all cultures remain sterile but clinically an infection is suspected. Each different colony and morphotype should be identified and susceptibility tested to avoid missing an infection with different resistance patterns.

Semiautomated techniques for homogenization (**Fig 7-16**) have been investigated to improve the diagnostic yield of microorganisms [78, 79].

Conditions for disruption, such as duration, speed, liquid volume, bead size, or amount of beads are important to avoid microbial destruction. The homogenized samples can be cultured on solid and in liquid media and also be investigated regarding neutrophils (after May Grunewald-Giemsa staining) and bacteria (after Gram stain) despite the low sensitivity of direct examination (less than 10%) [24]. This sample can be used also for 16S rDNA PCR, multiplex polymerase chain reaction (PCR) or microarray. Some authors suggested introducing the bead-mill suspension in blood-culture bottle. Thus, automated system detection can be used to reduce time to bacterial detection [44, 80]. Nevertheless, some mixed infections can be missed with the recovery of only the fastest growing bacteria.

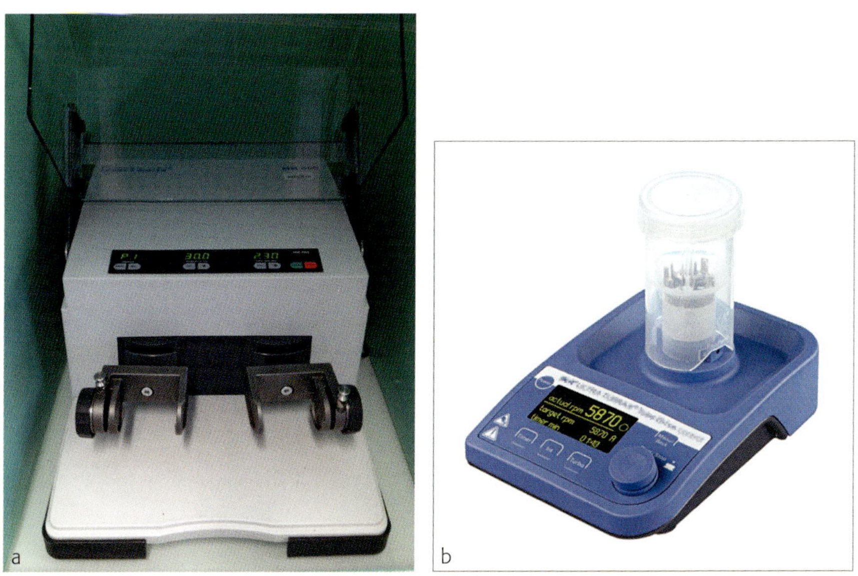

Fig 7-16a–b Two semiautomated devices for homogenization of intraoperative specimens collected in sterile vials. After the addition of 10 mL sterile water and 10 sterile stainless-steel beads (4 mm diameter), the vials are shaken on a bead mill for 2 minutes and 30 seconds, or 30 Hz per minute.

The microorganisms isolated from sinus tracts usually represent microbial colonization of the wound or surrounding skin, rather than the pathogen of the deep-tissue infection. Since these results are misleading, culture of the sinus tract should be avoided [81, 82]. Only isolation of *S aureus* from sinus tracts is predictive of the causative pathogen of the bone or implant-associated infection [83]. Two pairs of blood cultures should always be collected in case of fever or chills to detect bloodstream-borne organisms [6, 48].

5.2 Antibiotics interference with diagnosis

5.2.1 When to stop antibiotics?

Sensitivity of periprosthetic tissue culture is reduced in patients receiving antimicrobial therapy from 77% to 48% to 41% as the antimicrobial-free interval before surgery decreases from greater than 14 days, to 4 to 14 days, to 0 to 3 days, respectively [70]. Therefore, antimicrobial therapy should be discontinued at least 3 weeks prior to collecting intraoperative culture specimens, when possible. This longer interval will improve the likelihood of diagnosis [6, 79, 84].

Prophylactic antibiotics—when to administer the dose?

Despite a clear suspicion of implant-associated infection, the infecting pathogen is not always successfully isolated from the intraoperative cultures. Some authors postulate that prophylactic antibiotics could interfere with the isolation of the pathogen from the intraoperative cultures [43, 81, 85]. As a result, prophylactic antibiotics are often withheld until intraoperative cultures are obtained. Nevertheless, one should be aware of the adverse consequences of this practice that may result in systemic dissemination of infection [86–88]. For intraoperative prophylaxis, a first- or second-generation cephalosporin is recommended, which should be administered 30–60 minutes before incision. The duration of prophylaxis should not exceed 24 hours. In centers with a low incidence of infection, a single dose is sufficient [86].

5.2.2 Transport to the laboratory

Tissue biopsies, synovial fluid, bone, and other microbiologic specimens should reach the microbiology laboratory correctly identified, numbered, and at room temperature, as quickly as possible, ideally within 4 hours in sterile containers. If this deadline cannot be met, transport medium must be used to keep fragile bacteria and anaerobes alive. It is essential that samples are accompanied by clinical information such as antibiotic treatment, infectious history, and type of implant. Any delay in delivery must be mentioned to the microbiology laboratory. Samples must be handled in a class 2 biosafety cabinet by a technician wearing disposable overalls and gloves and using sterile equipment.

5.2.3 Microbiological examinations

Biopsies, synovial fluid, bone, and tissues in contact with implants are used for histology, microscopic examination, and microbiological culture. Microscopic examination may include a Gram stain (ie, specific but not sensitive, see topic 4 of this chapter) and quantification of leukocytes and semiquantitative assessment of neutrophils. The use of swabs for culture is not recommended [1, 36].

Clinical samples are usually inoculated on general agar plates, such as blood agar and incubated aerobically or/and a supplemented chocolate agar incubated in 5–10% of CO_2 for at least 7 days); agar for anaerobic bacteria, such as blood agar or Schaedler agar plates incubated anaerobically for preferably 1 week; and into a liquid medium, such as Schaedler broth, or thioglycollate broth, which can be used in difficult-to-culture cases (when suspicion of growth, even 10–14 days after incubation) on different well-selected agar plates in different atmospheres.

The use of blood culture vials (particularly with antibiotic absorbent in the case of antibiotic treatment) in automated microbial system detection could be considered. Other media could be added depending on the particular clinical context.

When reading the plates it is important to look for the different appearances of colonies, such as different morphotypes including small-colony variants [89, 90].

Some investigators have suggested that culture plates may be contaminated during the sampling procedure and/or by prolonging the time of incubation of plates [91–93]. A recent study showed that by following some important basic microbiological recommendations, such as to perform the procedures in sterile conditions or to follow the interpretive criteria of positivity [84, 94], they did not observe any increase in the rate of contamination by incubating the plates for up to 2 weeks [68].

Identification and antibiotic susceptibility testing must be performed on all isolated colonies (**Fig 7-17**).

Determination of the minimum inhibitory concentration for the typically used antibiotics is recommended. Microbiologists must be cautious with identifications obtained from previously identified organisms from other laboratories, particularly for coagulase-negative staphylococci for which the reproducibility of identification is sometimes limited. In case of doubt, use of molecular identification, such as16S rRNA, *sodA*, *tuf*, *rpoB* gene sequencing, for the different strains can be justified. The isolated bacterial strains should be systematically preserved by freezing for clinical considerations. Molecular biology methods can complement conventional techniques of culture without substituting for them. Therefore, periimplant-tissue cultures can, however, be falsely negative because of previous antimicrobial therapy, low inoculum of microorganism, a biofilm state of the infection, inadequate tissue specimens, inappropriate culture medium, inadequate culture incubation time, or a prolonged time to transport the specimen to the laboratory [36].

Culturing of multiple samples has been shown to increase diagnostic accuracy and there is growing evidence to support the utility of new preparatory techniques. A Danish team developed an "all-in-box concept sampling" to avoid missing or unsuitable transport medium from the operating room [95]. In the future, this concept could be used to provide and implement standardized sampling procedures based on international guidelines [95].

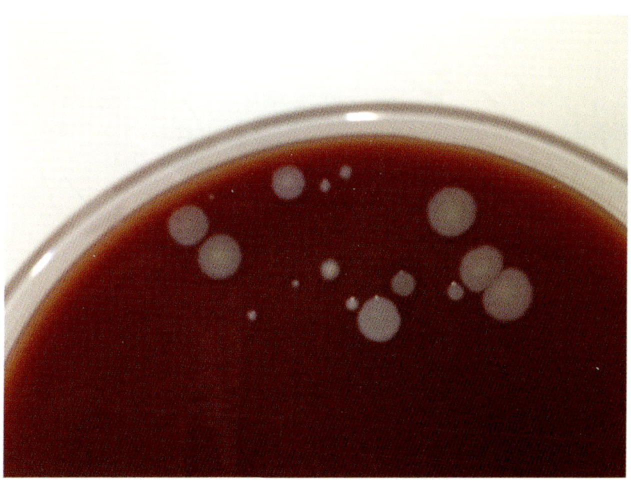

Fig 7-17 Different morphotypes of *S aureus* in hip infection with the same antibiotic susceptibility pattern (personal data, Nantes University hospital).

5.2.4 Polymerase chain reaction test

Molecular methods have been developed to improve the diagnosis of infection, despite its use being controversial [96]. Although molecular methods have proved to be helpful, strict conditions with specifically trained personnel to avoid any contamination are needed [97–99].

Polymerase chain reaction is a relatively simple technique that can detect a nucleic acid fragment and amplify this sequence. In recent years, modifications have been developed from the basic PCR method to improve performance and specificity, and to achieve the amplification of other molecules of interest in research, such as ribonucleic acid (RNA) [100]. Some of these variants are:

- Multiplex PCR: simultaneously detects several deoxyribonucleic acid (DNA) sequences by adding the sets of primers of interest.
- Nested PCR: increases the specificity by adding a second PCR with new primers that hybridize within the amplified fragment in the first PCR.
- Semiquantitative PCR: allows an approximation to the relative amount of nucleic acids present in a sample.
- Reverse transcriptase-polymerase chain (RT-PCR): generates amplification of RNA by synthesis of cDNA (DNA complementary to RNA) that is then amplified by PCR.
- Real-time PCR: performs quantification of nucleic acid copies obtained by PCR.

Polymerase chain reaction techniques can detect a specific bacteria (or a group of bacteria by multiplex PCR), or a range of bacteria, by targeting the 16S rRNA gene with sequencing of the amplified product as this target is universally present in bacteria (broad-range PCR) [101]. Therefore, although less sensitive compared with multiplex genus-oriented PCR [47], broad-range PCR allows the identification of bacteria previously not thought to cause infection whereas specific PCR (including multiplex PCR) are limited to those organisms for which targeted primers are included.

The main disadvantages of broad-range PCR are lack of sensitivity, false-positive results stemming from contamination, need of subsequent sequencing, and challenge of result interpretation [96, 102]. Also, this approach does not indicate whether a polymicrobial or solitary microbial infection is present; in the former circumstance, sequence analysis may be uninformative (ie, due to overlapping electrophoregram peaks) or misleading (ie, due to missed detection of minority species). Nevertheless, a subcloning step is the only way to reveal the mixed bacteria implicated in the PJI, but it is not available in all microbiology laboratories and it is not applicable in daily practice routine [103].

The value of PCR was mainly investigated in synovial fluid or periprosthetic tissue specimens [79, 104, 105], whereas sonication fluid was evaluated more recently [102, 106, 107]. Several commercial multiplex PCR kits are available to detect the most commonly involved bacteria, especially in bloodstream infections. The combination of two complementary diagnostic methods, sonication of removed implants, and multiplex real-time PCR of the resulting sonication fluid can improve the diagnostic accuracy of PJI and peri-implant infection, particularly among patients that had received antibiotic treatment prior to surgery and in polymicrobial infections [102, 107]. In a recent study, the pathogen detection was improved by multiplex PCR compared to culture-based techniques. The detection rate of polymicrobial infections was 29% by multiplex PCR versus 13–17% by culture. Moreover, about one-third of PJI cases were negative by culture, whereas multiplex PCR missed only one case of PJI. This PJI was caused by *P acnes*, for which specific primers were not included in the multiplex primer set and can therefore not be detected by this PCR kit [107]. These results were in agreement with another study, which demonstrated that sensitivity of sonication fluid cultures was reduced to 42% in patients that had received antimicrobial treatment, whereas multiplex PCR of sonication fluid remained at 100% [102, 108].

Further studies are probably needed to optimize the processing procedure with modified specific primers including low-virulence bacteria involved in chronic or delayed PJI like *P acnes*, *Corynebacterium* spp. or anaerobes, but also hematogenously acquired bacteria such as *Salmonella* spp. or *Campylobacter* spp. In fact, a recent study proposed a panel of 10 real-time PCR assays specifically targeting the bacteria that most frequently cause PJI [47]. The authors concluded that PCR of sonication fluids is more sensitive than tissue culture for the microbiological diagnosis of PJI and provides same-day PJI diagnosis.

5.2.5 IBIS T5000 or electrospray ionization mass spectrometry technology

This latest technique is based on nucleic-acid amplification with high-performance electrospray ionization mass spectrometry (ESI-MS) and base-composition analysis. This technology combines two well-known methods: PCR and matrix-assisted laser desorption/ionization (MALDI-TOF). The latter was introduced eight years ago in microbiology laboratories to identify quickly the bacteria and fungi. Matrix-assisted laser desorption/ionization can be used as a fast tracking identification method from synovial fluid or bead-mill samples directly introduced into blood-culture bottles to reduce the time to detection and identification [109]. This innovative but costly system enables the identification and quantification of a broad set of pathogens, including all known bacteria, all major groups of pathogenic fungi (3400 bacteria, 40 *Candida* spp.) and the major families of viruses that cause disease in humans and animals, together with the detection of virulence factors and antibiotic resistance markers [110, 111]. The IBIS T5000 can also detect bacterial genes that control antibiotic resistance, so that both species' identity and antibiotic susceptibility can be reported in a few hours. However, a recent study showed that many of the revision arthroplasty cases had positive results by this technique, showing a very low specificity and making the result interpretation very difficult [112].

The IBIS T5000 Biosensor Plex-ID PCR-electrospray ionization mass spectrometry (PCR-ESI/MS) system, although no longer marketed for routine use, with some developments, may be a promising tool. However, the technology was recently evaluated with sonication fluid and synovial fluid for the detection of PJI [1, 112]. They found that the sensitivity for the Plex-ID system to be around 80%; the specificity, and therefore the interpretation, remains difficult. The latest studies were performed comparing PCR-ESI/MS to culture with sonication fluids. The sensitivities for detecting PJI were 77.6% for PCR-ESI/MS and 69.7% for culture ($P = .0105$). The specificities were 93.5 and 99.3%, respectively ($P = .0002$). PCR-ESI/MS was more sensitive but less specific than culture for PJI diagnosis when performed on material dislodged from the surfaces of explanted orthopedic prostheses. This method may be a useful tool for the rapid detection of implant-associated infection and/or as an adjunctive method for select cases of arthroplasty failure, especially in case of slow-growing bacteria, low inoculum or antibiotic treatment prior to surgery [113]. Applied to synovial fluid, PCR-ESI/MS of synovial fluid has a similar sensitivity to culture albeit a lower specificity. PCR-ESI/MS can be performed in approximately 12–16 hours and provides not just accurate microbial identification, even in mixed infection, but also information on selected antimicrobial resistance markers. Nevertheless, due to some limitations of those studies, further prospective studies with fresh samples (not frozen) will need to be performed [114].

5.2.6 Histology

Standard

Histopathological examination demonstrating acute inflammation, evidenced by a neutrophilic infiltrate in areas contiguous to the implant that appear to be infected, has a sensitivity of > 80% and a specificity of > 90% for diagnosing PJI [115]. This examination can be performed on fixed tissue (standard), or in fresh-frozen sections for immediate intraoperative confirmation of acute inflammation, guiding intraoperative decision making [116].

The classic definition of acute inflammation in the periprosthetic tissue varies between the authors from 1 to 10 or more neutrophils per high-power field at a magnification of 400x [117]. A few years ago, Morawietz and colleagues introduced clearly defined histopathological criteria for a standardized evaluation of the periprosthetic membrane, which can appear in cases of total joint arthroplasty revision surgery [118]. Thus, based on histomorphological criteria, four types of periprosthetic membranes were defined:

- Wear-particle induced type (detection of foreign body particles; macrophages and multinucleated giant cells occupy at least 20% of the area: type I)
- Infectious type (granulation tissue with neutrophils, plasma cells, and few, if any, wear particles: type II)
- Combined type (aspects of type I and type II occur simultaneously: type III)
- Indeterminate type (neither criteria for type I nor type II are fulfilled: type IV) [119]

Although often forgotten, the histological analysis remains an important method to rule out infection since the negative predictive value ranges between 90% and 100% in most studies. This finding makes it a very important investigation complementary to most other markers that are mainly helpful to consider the possibility of PJI. If there is no clinical suspicion of infection and there are less than five neutrophils per high-power field, there is 91% chance of absence of infection [120].

The advantage of histology is that it is unlikely to be modified by the previous use of antibiotics. On the other hand, the disadvantage of this technique is the inability to identify the causative pathogen. The antimicrobial therapy cannot be directed by this method. The degree of infiltration with inflammatory cells varies among specimens even within individual tissue sections, the interobserver variability, the interpretation when a patient suffers an inflammatory joint disorder may be tricky, and false negative cases caused by low-virulent pathogens, such as *P acnes*, *Actinomyces* spp., or coagulase-negative staphylococci [121]. The results are available within several days so the histological examination of fresh-frozen tissues may be a fast alternative to support the diagnosis of infection.

Fresh-frozen sections

Fresh-frozen section analysis is a quick alternative tool to support the diagnosis of infection because the results are available while the surgeon is still in the operating room. When the potential for infection remains after a thorough preoperative evaluation, a positive result of this technique supports the diagnosis of infection, whereas the absence of acute inflammation doesn't completely exclude a diagnosis of infection. In a recent study, using current histopathology grading systems, frozen sections were specific but showed low sensitivity with respect to the *P acnes* infection. A new threshold value of a total of ten or more polymorphonuclear leukocytes in five high-power fields may increase the sensitivity of frozen section, with minimal impact on specificity [122].

In another study, intraoperative histology had also a high specificity and negative predictive value, but a low sensitivity and positive predictive value for predicting infection in the setting of revision elbow arthroplasty. Therefore, intraoperative histology should be used in conjunction with other studies to definitively establish the diagnosis of infection in the setting of revision elbow arthroplasty [123].

Consequently, this technique should be considered as a valuable part of the diagnostic workup for patients undergoing revision arthroplasty [124].

5.2.7 Outlook on microbiological examinations

The failure to isolate the causative bacterium in cases of implant infection often leads to the diagnostic conclusion of aseptic failure, even in cases in which clinical signs of infection clearly exist, thus leading to grave consequences for the patient—the therapy for infection is not pursued. In recent years, a variety of new technologies have been proposed that allow a more accurate microbiological diagnosis [125].

Calorimetry

Microcalorimetry measuring heat from replicating microorganisms in culture was first evaluated as a rapid, accurate, and simple screening method for platelet concentrates. Thereafter, the potential of microcalorimetry for detection of bacterial growth in cerebrospinal fluid (CSF) in a rat model of bacterial meningitis was also tested allowing rapid and accurate diagnosis of bacterial meningitis from a small volume of CSF with low detectable bacterial density [126]. Interestingly, the shape of the power-time curve was species-specific and independent from the initial concentration of microorganisms. The heat flow (µW) indicates an increase of the heat production due to the bacterial metabolism during replication [127]. This technique was recently evaluated in a prospective study of 90 patients with acute arthritis, in whom arthrocentesis was performed (unpublished data). A comparison between synovial fluid cultures and microcalorimetric detection was performed (detection limit 0.25 µW, positive defined as heat-flow > 10 µW). In patients with septic arthritis, the causative organism was detected by microcalorimetry in all cases after a mean of 4.3 hours (range, 2.8–7.5 hours) instead of 24–48 hours with conventional cultures. Microcalorimetry of synovial fluid allowed accurate discrimination between septic and nonseptic arthritis within 8 hours. In a recent study, the sensitivity and specificity of microcalorimetry of sonication fluid were 100% and 97%, respectively. The mean time to detection, defined as time to reach a rising heat flow signal of 20 µW, was 10.9 hours, measured after equilibration needed to get accurate measurement. Microcalorimetry of sonication fluid seems to be a reliable and a fast method to detect the presence of microorganisms in orthopedic implant-related infection (**Fig 7-18**) [128]. In the future, a combination of methods would allow better and quicker diagnosis of infection when rapid diagnosis of infection is important [129].

Early diagnosis of septic arthritis or implant-related infections might prompt earlier treatment and improve patient outcome, reducing hospital stay and saving money. In addition to synovial fluid, other patient samples can be investigated, such as sonication fluid or bead-mill suspension.

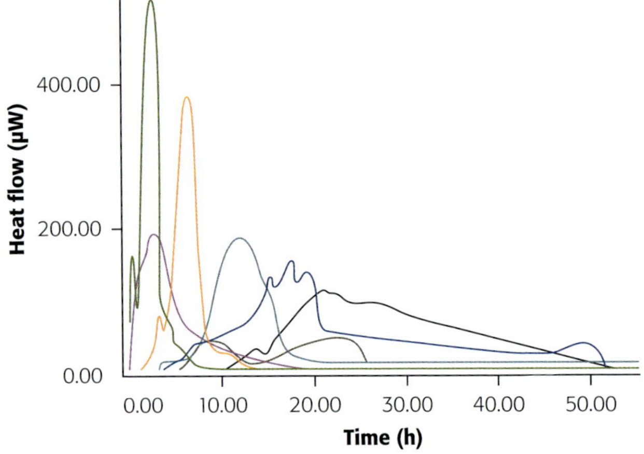

Fig 7-18 Seven different curve measurements with heat-flow calorimetry from sonication liquid after implant explantation.

Antibodies

Due to the complexity of the pathogenesis of implant-associated infection, the interest in serological tests in this field was low. For detecting antibodies, appropriate antigens need to be defined [130, 131]. Serological tests could be particularly useful in cases of false-negative cultures, relapse of infection or for the follow-up evaluation during and after antimicrobial treatment. In 2011, a new staphylococcal IgM enzyme-linked immunosorbent assay (ELISA) was adapted for the diagnosis of delayed PJI, commonly diagnosed at advanced stages of disease. This test, previously described to detect serum antibodies to staphylococcal biofilm polysaccharide antigens in late onset infections of synthetic vascular grafts, was applied to bone and joint infections. The researchers found a statistical difference between the group with delayed PJI (> 1 year after implantation) and the group with joint prostheses without infection and the control group, ie, subjects without prosthesis and infection. The test showed a sensitivity of 90% and specificity of 95%, when a cut-off of 0.35 ELISA unit were applied. The IgG group was not evaluated because the response is maintained as long as the antigenic stimulus is present. This test could be used to evaluate the response of infection to treatment [132]. Other candidate antigens should be screened to improve the sensitivity and specificity of this test, perhaps in combination with other tests. More recently, a study showed that there were significantly higher levels of antiextracellular protein IgG in sera of infected animals than in controls by using an enzyme-linked immunosorbent assay. Significantly higher antiextracellular protein IgG levels in infected patients compared to the controls were found; however, receiver operating characteristic curves did not aid in diagnosing infection. Further studies are needed to separate these proteins and investigate their antigenicity for the diagnosis of periprosthetic infection in humans [133].

Recently, InGen BioSciences developed a new serological test called BJI Inoplex adapted with the Luminex technology. Luminex technology is backed up by colored polystyrene microspheres on which the antigens are fixed. This system uses a set of several recombinant antigens to detect IgG anti-*S aureus* and *Staphylococcus epidermidis*. The BJI InoPlex test is a noninvasive and fast (2 hours) serology test. This method should be tested in the near future to evaluate its ability to accurately aid in the diagnosis of the infection, and in the biological monitoring of antibiotic treatment.

5.2.8 Sonication

Microorganisms on the implant surface form biofilms, which makes them difficult to detect by conventional methods such as periprosthetic tissue cultures. Sonication of explanted prosthesis is designed to dislodge microorganisms from the biofilms on the surface of explanted devices. The microorganisms in biofilm exist in a low metabolic or stationary growth state. Free-living bacteria (ie, planktonic bacteria) are killed by antibiotics and the host defense system, whereas adherent bacteria (ie, biofilm bacteria) can survive and persist in the extracellular matrix of the biofilm [115] (**Fig 7-19**).

Sonication works by the introduction of low-intensity ultrasound, so as not to cause bacterial cell destruction, which produces microbubble formation (cavitation). Microbubbles attach to the surface of the prosthesis and implode, releasing energy. Then, bacteria disaggregate into the liquid surrounding the prosthesis, enabling culture of viable microorganisms from this sonication fluid.

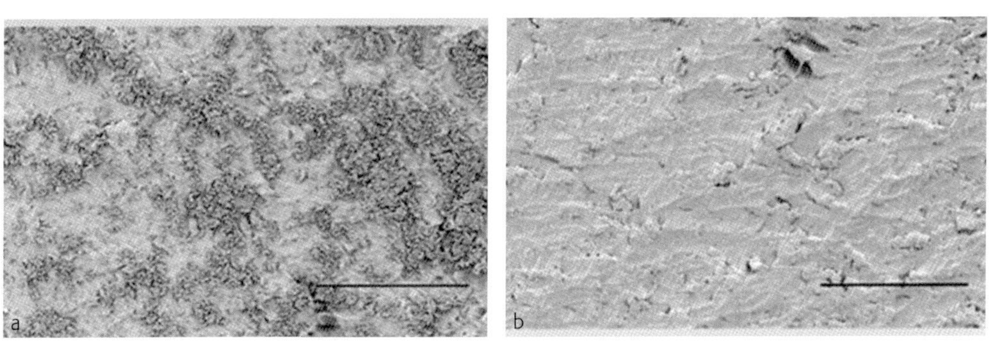

Fig 7-19a–b Electron microscopy of a *Staphylococcus epidermidis* biofilm on a polyethylene surface.

Implants should be aseptically removed in the operating room, placed in airtight solid containers and transported to the microbiology laboratory. Sonication in plastic bags should be avoided because of risk of contamination due to puncture of bags [84]. Several studies have demonstrated the higher sensitivity and specificity of sonication fluid culture than periprosthetic tissue culture [68, 70, 94, 102, 134, 135]. In addition to the improvement of sensitivity and specificity, other advantages of sonication are:

- Improved diagnosis in patients that received prior antimicrobial therapy
- A quantitative result, which is helpful to distinguish between contamination and infection
- Higher detection of mixed infections, ie, polymicrobial infections
- Difficult-to-treat microorganisms and different morphotypes
- Faster results than periprosthetic tissue cultures [68]

The removed implant should be transported to the microbiology laboratory in a sterile container. After addition of Ringer's solution or normal saline covering about 80% of the implant, the container should be vortexed for 30 seconds and sonicated (40 kHz) for 1 minute, and finally a last vortex step of 30 seconds before plating the sonication fluid (**Fig 7-20**). Some authors add a concentration centrifugation step after sonication procedure to concentrate the bacterial load [136].

Prolonged incubation, for as long as 2 weeks, is still recommended for periprosthetic tissue cultures to detect slow-growing pathogens, such as *P acnes* [75, 76, 137]. A recent study showed that a prolonged incubation (2 weeks) is also recommended for sonication fluid cultures, especially to detect anaerobes [68].

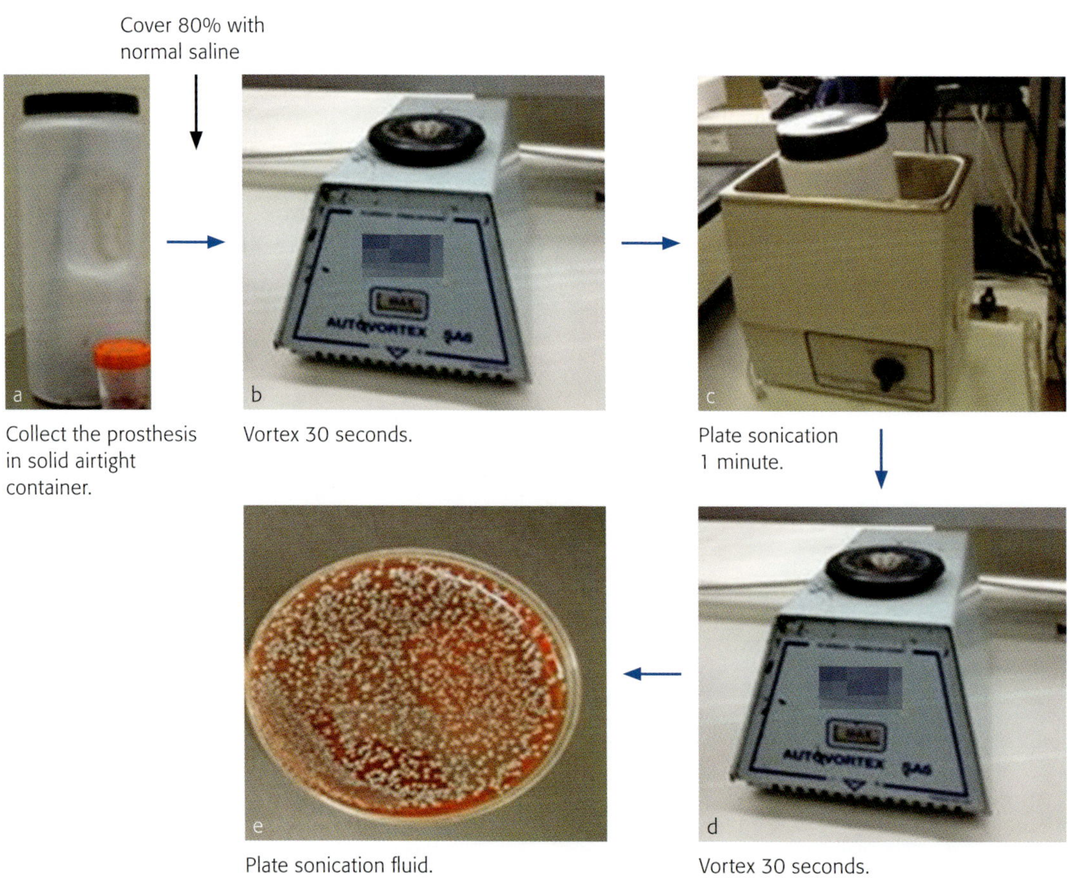

Fig 7-20a–e Sonication procedure.

The optimal cut-off value to determine a positive sonication fluid culture depends on whether or not a centrifugation concentration step is added after sonication. When using a concentration step, the most frequently used cut-off value was 200 CFU/mL [47, 135, 138], while when not using it, the reported cut-off values ranged from 1 to 50 CFU/mL [70, 94, 139]. Despite this range of cut-off values, culture of sonication fluid usually yields an uncountable number of CFU/plate. Usually, few colonies per plate grow in sonication fluid culture when patients had received antibiotics prior to surgery (**Fig 7-21**), or when only implant liners have been subjected to sonication corresponding with acute PJI, so high suspicion of previous antibiotics usage. It has been reported that any growth should be considered significant in patients receiving antibiotics [94].

The role of sonication of liners and polymethylmethacrylate spacers is uncertain. Regarding the inlays, a recent study reported that 17% of PJI cases had a microbiological growth in sonication fluid cultures < 50 CFU/mL. In all these cases, debridement with implant retention was performed, so only liners were exchanged and subjected to sonication procedure [68]. This observation was also noted in a previous study [94]. Possible reasons include the smaller surface area implant compared to the total prosthesis [94], previous antibiotic usage, or the presence of newer biofilm seen in acute infections [16, 94, 140]

Interpretation of sonication fluid culture of polymethylmethacrylate spacers during a two-stage exchange may be challenging because the spacers are frequently antibiotic-loaded, making it difficult to distinguish between persistent infection or reinfection during the second-stage exchange and lack of cut-off values for investigations [141, 142].

Interestingly, the sensitivity of sonication fluid culture was higher in patients with chronic PJI than with acute PJI [94]. These findings suggest that biofilms in acute PJI involve immature biofilm layers and the bacteria are only loosely attached to the surface, ie, "immature" biofilm. In contrast, biofilm in chronic PJI usually consists of several layers of firmly attached bacteria requiring a more efficient removal procedure, such as sonication. A recent article demonstrates the in vivo natural history of implant-associated biofilm formation [140].

Vortexing is a traditional technique for mixing widely used in routine microbiology laboratories. It was also introduced as a preparatory step before sonication to generate microbubbles, which increase the cavitation effect [70]. Vortexing alone is an easy and simple procedure, which has demonstrated an acceptable sensitivity and specificity, especially in acute PJI, and may be used for the diagnosis of PJI in laboratories where sonication is not available [94]. In addition, vortexing fluid represents a single clinical sample, reaching comparable sensitivity to multiple periprosthetic tissue cultures (~70%). Furthermore, sonication may kill bacteria, especially Gram-negative bacilli and anaerobes, whereas vortexing has not been shown to be harmful to bacteria.

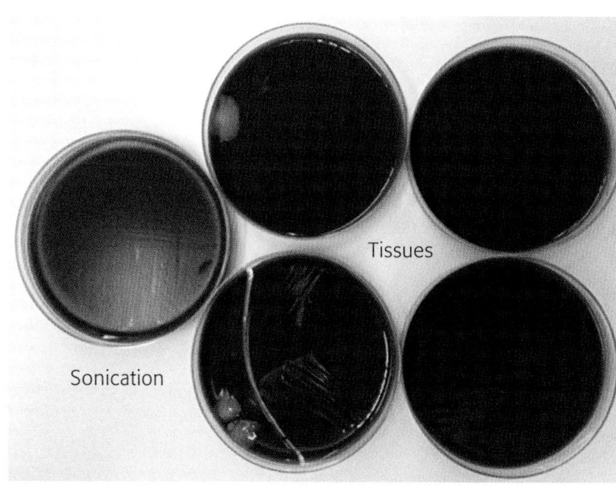

Fig 7-21 Antimicrobial effect on cultures. Sonication fluid culture remains negative and only two of four periprosthetic tissue cultures have microbiological growth.

Despite the use of sonication, culture-negative cases of PJI still remain. Possible reasons include case misclassification and microorganisms that do not grow under the conditions studied (eg, due to inappropriate media, inadequate incubation time, loss of viability during specimen transport) or earlier antimicrobial therapy [143–146]. A research group evaluated the BacT/Alert FAN aerobic and anaerobic blood-culture bottles inoculated with sonication fluid for the diagnosis of implant-associated infection and compared it with periprosthetic tissue culture and sonication fluid culture. They detected all implant-associated infection cases including those in whom patients had previously received antibiotics with a specificity of 100%. Moreover, the detection of pathogens by this system significantly reduced the time to a positive result compared with the other techniques. This may be a promising and easy-to-perform method that may improve the diagnosis of PJI.

Finally, sonication fluid contains a high quantity of bacteria, making this sample suitable for further advanced microbial and immunological analyses (eg, PCR, MALDI-TOF, microcalorimetry, biomarker determination, gene expression).

6 Conclusion

Some implants may be colonized by biofilm-dwelling bacteria, with the bacteria not being clinically apparent [147, 148]. The proportion of such asymptomatically colonized devices is unknown and largely depends on the diagnostic method employed. The results of highly sensitive diagnostic techniques such as sonication, PCR, or newer molecular techniques are difficult to interpret and further long-term studies are needed to distinguish contamination during sample processing from real-device colonization. It is also unclear whether all asymptomatic colonization becomes, at some point, clinically apparent as infection. Some colonized implants may remain asymptomatic long-term, where the host keeps the biofilm microorganisms permanently suppressed. It is also unclear what triggers asymptomatic biofilm bacteria to start detaching, replicating, and causing a clinical infection.

On the one hand, research and development of new methods are required to improve the diagnostic yield and accuracy, shorten the detection time, and to fully automate the complete procedure. On the other hand, critical clinical observation from multidisciplinary teams with specific knowledge of biofilm infections is also fundamental. As an example, just by observing whether a prosthesis failure occurs early (within the first 2 years after implantation), the probability that infection is the reason for the failure is around 70% compared with 16% probability of it being an aseptic loosening [13].

7 References

1. **Tande AJ, Patel R.** Prosthetic joint infection. *Clin Microbiol Rev.* 2014 Apr;27(2):302–345.
2. **Berbari E, Mabry T, Tsaras G, et al.** Inflammatory blood laboratory levels as markers of prosthetic joint infection: a systematic review and meta-analysis. *J Bone Joint Surg Am.* 2010 Sep 1;92(11):2102–2109.
3. **Bottner F, Wegner A, Winkelmann W, et al.** Interleukin-6, procalcitonin and TNF-alpha: markers of peri-prosthetic infection following total joint replacement. *J Bone Joint Surg Br.* 2007 Jan;89(1):94–99.
4. **Gollwitzer H, Dombrowski Y, Prodinger PM, et al.** Antimicrobial peptides and proinflammatory cytokines in periprosthetic joint infection. *J Bone Joint Surg Am.* 2013 Apr 3;95(7):644–651.
5. **Bracken CD, Berbari EF, Hanssen AD, et al.** Systemic inflammatory markers and aspiration cell count may not differentiate bacterial from fungal prosthetic infections. *Clin Orthop Relat Res.* 2014 Nov;472(11):3291–3294.
6. **Osmon DR, Berbari EF, Berendt AR, et al.** Executive summary: diagnosis and management of prosthetic joint infection: clinical practice guidelines by the Infectious Diseases Society of America. *Clin Infect Dis.* 2013 Jan;56(1):1–10.
7. **Della Valle C, Parvizi J, Bauer TW, et al.** American Academy of Orthopaedic Surgeons clinical practice guideline on: the diagnosis of periprosthetic joint infections of the hip and knee. *J Bone Joint Surg Am.* 2011 Jul 20;93(14):1355–1357.
8. **Moran E, Byren I, Atkins BL.** The diagnosis and management of prosthetic joint infections. *J Antimicrob Chemother.* 2010 Nov;65 Suppl 3:iii, 45–54.
9. **Zimmerli W, Trampuz A, Ochsner PE.** Prosthetic-joint infections. *N Engl J Med.* 2004 Oct 14;351(16):1645–1654.
10. **Glehr M, Friesenbichler J, Hofmann G, et al.** Novel biomarkers to detect infection in revision hip and knee arthroplasties. *Clin Orthop Relat Res.* 2013 Aug;471(8):2621–2628.
11. **Piper KE, Fernandez-Sampedro M, Steckelberg KE, et al.** C-reactive protein, erythrocyte sedimentation rate and orthopedic implant infection. *PLoS One.* 2010 Feb 22;5(2):e9358.
12. **Alijanipour P, Bakhshi H, Parvizi J.** Diagnosis of periprosthetic joint infection: the threshold for serological markers. *Clin Orthop Relat Res.* 2013 Oct;471(10):3186–3195.
13. **Portillo ME, Salvado M, Alier A, et al.** Prosthesis failure within 2 years of implantation is highly predictive of infection. *Clin Orthop Relat Res.* 2013 Nov;471(11):3672–3678.
14. **Jacovides CL, Parvizi J, Adeli B, et al.** Molecular markers for diagnosis of periprosthetic joint infection. *J Arthroplasty.* 2011 Sep;26(6 Suppl):99–103e1.
15. **Maharajan K, Patro DK, Menon J, et al.** Serum Procalcitonin is a sensitive and specific marker in the diagnosis of septic arthritis and acute osteomyelitis. *J Orthop Surg Res.* 2013 Jul 4;8:19.
16. **Shen CJ, Wu MS, Lin KH, et al.** The use of procalcitonin in the diagnosis of bone and joint infection: a systemic review and meta-analysis. *Eur J Clin Microbiol Infect Dis.* 2013 Jun;32(6):807–814.
17. **Chaganti RK, Purdue E, Sculco TP, et al.** Elevation of serum tumor necrosis factor alpha in patients with periprosthetic osteolysis: a case control study. *Clin Orthop Relat Res.* 2014 Feb;472(2):584–589.
18. **Konttinen YT, Xu JW, Waris E, et al.** Interleukin-6 in aseptic loosening of total hip replacement prostheses. *Clinical and experimental rheumatology* 2002 Jul-Aug;20(4):485–490.
19. **Villacis D, Merriman JA, Yalamanchili R, et al.** 3rd. Serum interleukin-6 as a marker of periprosthetic shoulder infection. *J Bone Joint Surg Am.* 2014 Jan 1;96(1):41–45.
20. **Wirtz DC, Heller KD, Miltner O, et al.** Interleukin-6: a potential inflammatory marker after total joint replacement. *Int Orthop.* 2000;24(4):194–196.
21. **Gedbjerg N, LaRosa R, Hunter JG, et al.** Anti-glucosaminidase IgG in sera as a biomarker of host immunity against Staphylococcus aureus in orthopaedic surgery patients. *J Bone Joint Surg Am.* 2013 Nov 20;95(22):e171.
22. **Scotece M, Conde J, Lopez V, et al.** Leptin in joint and bone diseases: new insights. *Curr Med Chem.* 2013;20(27):3416–3425.
23. **Drago L, Vassena C, Dozio E, et al.** Procalcitonin, C-reactive protein, interleukin-6, and soluble intercellular adhesion molecule-1 as markers of postoperative orthopaedic joint prosthesis infections. *Int J Immunopathol Pharmacol.* 2011 Apr-Jun;24(2):433–440.
24. **Société de Pathologie Infectieuse de Langue F, Collège des Universitaires de Maladies Infectieuses et T, Groupe de Pathologie Infectieuse P, et al.** Recommendations for bone and joint prosthetic device infections in clinical practice (prosthesis, implants, osteosynthesis). Société de Pathologie Infectieuse de Langue Française. *Médecine et maladies infectieuses.* 2010 Apr;40(4):185–211.
25. **Deirmengian C, Kardos K, Kilmartin P, et al.** The Alpha-defensin Test for Periprosthetic Joint Infection Outperforms the Leukocyte Esterase Test Strip. *Clin Orthop Relat Res.* 2015 Jan;473(1):198–203.
26. **Parvizi J.** New definition for periprosthetic joint infection. *Am J Orthop (Belle Mead NJ).* 2011 Dec;40(12):614–615.
27. **Trampuz A, Hanssen AD, Osmon DR, et al.** Synovial fluid leukocyte count and differential for the diagnosis of prosthetic knee infection. *Am J Med.* 2004 Oct 15;117(8):556–562.
28. **Ho G, Jr.** Bacterial arthritis. *Curr Opin Rheumatol.* 1991 Aug;3(4):603–609.
29. **Parvizi J, Jacovides C, Adeli B, et al.** Coventry Award: synovial C-reactive protein: a prospective evaluation of a molecular marker for periprosthetic knee joint infection. *Clin Orthop Relat Res.* 2012 Jan;470(1):54–60.
30. **Parvizi J, McKenzie JC, Cashman JP.** Diagnosis of periprosthetic joint infection using synovial C-reactive protein. *J Arthroplasty.* 2012 Sep;27(8 Suppl):12–16.
31. **Wiener E, Zanetti M, Hodler J, et al.** Lactate and T (2) measurements of synovial aspirates at 1.5 T: differentiation of septic from non-septic arthritis. *Skeletal Radiol.* 2008 Aug;37(8):743–748.
32. **Courtney P, Doherty M.** Joint aspiration and injection and synovial fluid analysis. *Best Pract Res Clin Rheumatol.* 2013 Apr;27(2):137–169.
33. **Schinsky MF, Della Valle CJ, Sporer SM, et al.** Perioperative testing for joint infection in patients undergoing revision total hip arthroplasty. *J Bone Joint Surg Am.* 2008 Sep;90(9):1869–1875.
34. **Borens O, Nussbaumer F, Baalbaki R, et al.** [Update on implant related infections in orthopaedic surgery. Diagnosis and treatment]. *Revue medicale suisse.* 2009 Dec 16;5(230):2563–2568. French.

35. **Trampuz A, Steinrucken J, Clauss M, et al.** [New methods for the diagnosis of implant-associated infections]. *Revue medicale suisse.* 2010 Apr 7;6(243):731–734. French.
36. **Legout L, Senneville E.** Periprosthetic joint infections: clinical and bench research. *ScientificWorldJournal.* 2013 Oct 27;2013:549091.
37. **Temmerman OP, Heyligers IC, Teule GJ, et al.** The value of contrast and subtraction arthrography in the assessment of aseptic loosening of total hip prostheses: a meta-analysis. *Eur J Radiol.* 2005 Oct;56(1):113–119.
38. **Parvizi J, Jacovides C, Antoci V, et al.** Diagnosis of periprosthetic joint infection: the utility of a simple yet unappreciated enzyme. *J Bone Joint Surg Am.* 2011 Dec 21;93(24):2242–2248.
39. **Wetters NG, Berend KR, Lombardi AV, et al.** Leukocyte esterase reagent strips for the rapid diagnosis of periprosthetic joint infection. *J Arthroplasty.* 2012 Sep;27(8 Suppl):8–11.
40. **Deirmengian C, Hallab N, Tarabishy A, et al.** Synovial fluid biomarkers for periprosthetic infection. *Clin Orthop Relat Res.* 2010 Aug;468(8):2017–2023.
41. **Nilsdotter-Augustinsson A, Briheim G, Herder A, et al.** Inflammatory response in 85 patients with loosened hip prostheses: a prospective study comparing inflammatory markers in patients with aseptic and septic prosthetic loosening. *Acta Orthop.* 2007 Oct;78(5):629–639.
42. **Saeed K, Dryden M, Sitjar A, et al.** Measuring synovial fluid procalcitonin levels in distinguishing cases of septic arthritis, including prosthetic joints, from other causes of arthritis and aseptic loosening. *Infection.* 2013 Aug;41(4):845–849.
43. **Barrack RL, Harris WH.** The value of aspiration of the hip joint before revision total hip arthroplasty. *J Bone Joint Surg Am.* 1993 Jan;75(1):66–76.
44. **Hughes JG, Vetter EA, Patel R, et al.** Culture with BACTEC Peds Plus/F bottle compared with conventional methods for detection of bacteria in synovial fluid. *J Clin Microbiol.* 2001 Dec;39(12):4468–4471.
45. **Ali F, Wilkinson JM, Cooper JR, et al.** Accuracy of joint aspiration for the preoperative diagnosis of infection in total hip arthroplasty. *J Arthroplasty.* 2006 Feb;21(2):221–226.
46. **Font-Vizcarra L, Garcia S, Martinez-Pastor JC, et al.** Blood culture flasks for culturing synovial fluid in prosthetic joint infections. *Clin Orthop Relat Res.* 2010 Aug;468(8):2238–2243.
47. **Cazanave C, Greenwood-Quaintance KE, Hanssen AD, et al.** Rapid molecular microbiologic diagnosis of prosthetic joint infection. *J Clin Microbiol.* 2013 Jul;51(7):2280–2287.
48. **Corvec S, Portillo ME, Pasticci BM, et al.** Epidemiology and new developments in the diagnosis of prosthetic joint infection. *Int J Artif Organs.* 2012 Oct;35(10):923–934.
49. **Shanmugasundaram S, Ricciardi BF, Briggs TW, et al.** Evaluation and Management of Periprosthetic Joint Infection-an International, Multicenter Study. *HSS J.* 2014 Feb;10(1):36–44.
50. **Mellado Santos JM.** Diagnostic imaging of pediatric hematogenous osteomyelitis: lessons learned from a multi-modality approach. *Eur Radiol.* 2006 Sept;16(9):2109–2119.
51. **Ardran GM.** Bone destruction not demonstrable by radiography. *Br J Radiol.* 1951 Feb;24(278):107–109.
52. **Ram PC, Martinez S, Korobkin M, et al.** CT detection of intraosseous gas: a new sign of osteomyelitis. *AJR Am J Roentgenol.* 1981 Oct;137(4):721–723.
53. **Chandnani VP, Beltran J, Morris SN, et al.** Acute experimental osteomyelitis and abscesses: detection with MR imaging versus CT. *Radiology.* 1990 Jan;174(1):233–236.
54. **Wing VW, Jeffrey MP, Federle MP.** Chronic osteomyelitis examined by CT. *Radiology.* 1985 Jan;154(1):171–174.
55. **Gold RH, Hawkins RA, Katz RD.** Bacterial osteomyelitis: findings on plain radiography, CT, MR, and scintigraphy. *JR Am J Roentgenol.* 1991 Aug;157(2):365–370,
56 **Boutin RD, Brossmann J, Sartoris DJ, et al.** Update on imaging of orthopedic infections. *Orthop Clin North Am.* 1998 Jan;29(1):41–66.
57 **Low KT, Peh WC.** Magnetic resonance imaging of diabetic foot complications. *Singapore Med J.* Jan;56;(1):23–34
58 **Gupta A, Subhas N, Primak AN, et al.** Metal artifact reduction: standard and advanced magnetic resonance and computed tomography techniques. *Radiol Clin North Am.* 2015 May;53(3):531–547.
59. **Chau CLF, Griffith JF.** Musculoskeletal infections: ultrasound appearances. *Clin Radiol.*2005 Feb;60(2):149–159,
60. **Cardinal E, Bureau NJ, Aubin B, et al.** Role of ultrasound in musculoskeletal infections. *Radiol Clin North Am.* 2001 Mar;39(2):191–201.
61. **Strobel K, Stumpe KD.** PET/CT in musculoskeletal infection. *Semin Musculoskelet Radiol.* 2007 Dec;11(4):353–364.
62. **Arteaga de Murphy C, Gemmel F, Balter J.** Clinical trial of specific imaging of infections. *Nucl Med Commun.* 2010 Aug;31(8):726–733,
63. **Schauwecker DS.** The scintigraphic diagnosis of osteomyelitis. *AJR Am J Roentgenol.* 1992 Jan;158(1):9–18.
64. **Song KM, Sloboda JF.** Acute hematogenous osteomyelitis in children. *J Am Acad Orthop Surg.* 2001 May-Jun;9(3):166–175.
65. **Kolindou A, Liu Y, Ozker K, et al.** In-111 WBC imaging of osteomyelitis in patients with underlying bone scan abnormalities. *Clin Nucl Med.*1996 Mar;21(3):183–191.
66. **Johnson JE, Kennedy EJ, Shereff MJ.** Prospective study of bone, indium-111-labeled white blood cell, and gallium-67 scanning for the evaluation of osteomyelitis in the diabetic foot. *Foot Ankle Int.* 1996 Jan;17(1):10–16.
67. **Rosenthall L, Kloiber R, Damtew B, et al.** Sequential use of radiophosphate and radiogallium imaging in the differential diagnosis of bone, joint and soft tissue infection: quantitative analysis. *Diagn Imaging.* 1982;51(5):249–258.
68. **Portillo ME, Salvado M, Alier A, et al.** Advantages of sonication fluid culture for the diagnosis of prosthetic joint infection. *J Infect.* 2014 Jul;69(1):35–41.
69. **Atkins BL, Athanasou N, Deeks JJ, et al.** Prospective evaluation of criteria for microbiological diagnosis of prosthetic-joint infection at revision arthroplasty. The OSIRIS Collaborative Study Group. *J Clin Microbiol.* 1998 Oct;36(10):2932–2939.
70. **Trampuz A, Piper KE, Jacobson MJ, et al.** Sonication of removed hip and knee prostheses for diagnosis of infection. *N Engl J Med.* 2007 Aug 16;357(7):654–663.
71. **Morgan PM, Sharkey P, Ghanem E, et al.** The value of intraoperative Gram stain in revision total knee arthroplasty. *J Bone Joint Surg Am.* 2009 Sep;91(9):2124–2129.
72. **Chimento GF, Finger S, Barrack RL.** Gram stain detection of infection during revision arthroplasty. *J Bone Joint Surg Br.* 1996 Sep;78(5):838–839.
73. **Johnson AJ, Zywiel MG, Stroh DA, et al.** Should gram stains have a role in diagnosing hip arthroplasty infections? *Clin Orthop Relat Res.* 2010 Sep;468(9):2387–2391.
74. **Spangehl MJ, Masterson E, Masri BA, et al.** The role of intraoperative gram stain in the diagnosis of infection during revision total hip arthroplasty. *J Arthroplasty.* 1999 Dec;14(8):952–956.

75. **Schafer P, Fink B, Sandow D, et al.** Prolonged bacterial culture to identify late periprosthetic joint infection: a promising strategy. *Clin Infect Dis.* 2008 Dec 1;47(11):1403–1409.
76. **Butler-Wu SM, Burns EM, Pottinger PS, et al.** Optimization of Periprosthetic Culture for Diagnosis of Propionibacterium acnes Prosthetic Joint Infection. *J Clin Microbiol.* 2011 Jul;49(7):2490–2495.
77. **Illiaquer M, Corvec S, Touchais S, et al.** Anaerobes isolated from bone and joint infections and their susceptibility to antibiotics. *J Infect.* 2012 Nov;65(5):473–475.
78. **Roux AL, Sivadon-Tardy V, Bauer T, et al.** Diagnosis of prosthetic joint infection by beadmill processing of a periprosthetic specimen. *Clin Microbiol Infect.* 2011 Mar;17(3):447–450.
79. **Bémer P, Plouzeau C, Tande D, et al.** Evaluation of 16S rDNA PCR Sensitivity and Specificity for Diagnosis of Prosthetic-Joint Infection: a prospective multicenter cross-sectional study. *J Clin Microbiol.* 2014 Oct;52(10):3583–3589.
80. **Velay A, Schramm F, Gaudias J, et al.** Culture with BACTEC Peds Plus bottle compared with conventional media for the detection of bacteria in tissue samples from orthopedic surgery. *Diagn Microbiol Infect Dis.* 2010 Sep;68(1):83–85.
81. **Spangehl MJ, Masri BA, O'Connell JX, et al.** Prospective analysis of preoperative and intraoperative investigations for the diagnosis of infection at the sites of two hundred and two revision total hip arthroplasties. *J Bone Joint Surg Am.* 1999 May;81(5):672–683.
82. **Schindler M, Christofilopoulos P, Wyssa B, et al.** Poor performance of microbiological sampling in the prediction of recurrent arthroplasty infection. *Int Orthop.* 2011 May;35(5):647–654.
83. **Tetreault MW, Wetters NG, Aggarwal VK, et al.** Should draining wounds and sinuses associated with hip and knee arthroplasties be cultured? *J Arthroplasty.* 2013 Sep;28(8 Suppl):133–136.
84. **Trampuz A, Piper KE, Hanssen AD, et al.** Sonication of explanted prosthetic components in bags for diagnosis of prosthetic joint infection is associated with risk of contamination. *J Clin Microbiol.* 2006 Feb;44(2):628–631.
85. **Toms AD, Davidson D, Masri BA, et al.** The management of peri-prosthetic infection in total joint arthroplasty. *J Bone Joint Surg Br.* 2006 Feb;88(2):149–155.
86. **Trampuz A, Zimmerli W.** Antimicrobial agents in orthopaedic surgery: Prophylaxis and treatment. *Drugs.* 2006;66(8):1089–1105.
87. **Ghanem E, Parvizi J, Clohisy J, et al.** Perioperative antibiotics should not be withheld in proven cases of periprosthetic infection. *Clin Orthop Relat Res.* 2007 Aug;461:44–47.
88. **Burnett RS, Aggarwal A, Givens SA, et al.** Prophylactic antibiotics do not affect cultures in the treatment of an infected TKA: a prospective trial. *Clin Orthop Relat Res.* 2010 Jan;468(1):127–134.
89. **Sendi P, Frei R, Maurer TB, et al.** Escherichia coli variants in periprosthetic joint infection: diagnostic challenges with sessile bacteria and sonication. *J Clin Microbiol.* 2010 May;48(5):1720–1725.
90. **Sendi P, Proctor RA.** Staphylococcus aureus as an intracellular pathogen: the role of small colony variants. *Trends Microbiol.* 2009 Feb;17(2):54–58.
91. **Esteban J, Alvarez-Alvarez B, Blanco A, et al.** Prolonged incubation time does not increase sensitivity for the diagnosis of implant-related infection using samples prepared by sonication of the implants. *Bone Joint J.* 2013 Jul;95-B(7):1001–1006.
92. **Cobo J, Del Pozo JL.** Prosthetic joint infection: diagnosis and management. *Expert Rev Anti Infect Ther.* 2011 Sep;9(9):787–802.
93. **Sierra JM, Garcia S, Martinez-Pastor JC, et al.** Relationship between the degree of osteolysis and cultures obtained by sonication of the prostheses in patients with aseptic loosening of a hip or knee arthroplasty. *Arch Orthop Trauma Surg.* 2011 Oct;131(10):1357–1361.
94. **Portillo ME, Salvado M, Trampuz A, et al.** Sonication versus vortexing of implants for diagnosis of prosthetic joint infection. *J Clin Microbiol.* 2013 Feb;51(2):591–594.
95. **Corvec S, Portillo ME, Pasticci BM, et al.** Epidemiology and new developments in the diagnosis of prosthetic joint infection. *Int J Artif Organs.* 2012 Oct;35(10):923–934.
96. **De Man FH, Graber P, Luem M, et al.** Broad-range PCR in selected episodes of prosthetic joint infection. *Infection.* 2009 Jun;37(3):292–294.
97. **Fenollar F, Levy PY, Raoult D.** Usefulness of broad-range PCR for the diagnosis of osteoarticular infections. *Current opinion in rheumatology.* 2008 Jul;20(4):463–470.
98. **Song DS, Kang BK, Lee SS, et al.** Use of an internal control in a quantitative RT-PCR assay for quantitation of porcine epidemic diarrhea virus shedding in pigs. *Journal of virological methods.* 2006 Apr;133(1):27–33.
99. **Levy PY, Fenollar F.** The role of molecular diagnostics in implant-associated bone and joint infection. *Clin Microbiol Infect.* 2012 Dec;18(12):1168–1175.
100. **Bergin PF, Doppelt JD, Hamilton WG, et al.** Detection of periprosthetic infections with use of ribosomal RNA-based polymerase chain reaction. *J Bone Joint Surg Am.* 2010 Mar;92(3):654–663.
101. **Gomez E, Cazanave C, Cunningham SA, et al.** Prosthetic joint infection diagnosis using broad-range PCR of biofilms dislodged from knee and hip arthroplasty surfaces using sonication. *J Clin Microbiol.* 2012 Nov;50(11):3501–3508.
102. **Achermann Y, Vogt M, Leunig M, et al.** Improved diagnosis of periprosthetic joint infection by multiplex PCR of sonication fluid from removed implants. *J Clin Microbiol.* 2010 Apr;48(4):1208–1214.
103. **Fenollar F, Roux V, Stein A, et al.** Analysis of 525 samples to determine the usefulness of PCR amplification and sequencing of the 16S rRNA gene for diagnosis of bone and joint infections. *J Clin Microbiol.* 2006 Mar;44(3):1018–1028.
104. **Gallo J, Kolar M, Dendis M, et al.** Culture and PCR analysis of joint fluid in the diagnosis of prosthetic joint infection. *New Microbiol.* 2008 Jan;31(1):97–104.
105. **Vandercam B, Jeumont S, Cornu O, et al.** Amplification-based DNA analysis in the diagnosis of prosthetic joint infection. *J Mol Diagn.* 2008 Nov;10(6):537–543.
106. **Esteban J, Alonso-Rodriguez N, Del-Prado G, et al.** PCR-hybridization after sonication improves diagnosis of implant-related infection. *Acta Orthop.* 2012 Jun;83(3):299–304.
107. **Portillo ME, Salvado M, Sorli L, et al.** Multiplex PCR of sonication fluid accurately differentiates between prosthetic joint infection and aseptic failure. *J Infect.* 2012 Dec;65(6):541–548
108. **Titecat M, Loiez C, Senneville E, et al.** Evaluation of rapid mecA gene detection versus standard culture in staphylococcal chronic prosthetic joint infections. *Diagn Microbiol Infect Dis.* 2012 Aug;73(4):318–321.

109. **Prod'hom G, Bizzini A, Durussel C, et al.** Matrix-assisted laser desorption ionization-time of flight mass spectrometry for direct bacterial identification from positive blood culture pellets. *J Clin Microbiol.* 2010 Apr;48(4):1481–1483.
110. **Ecker DJ, Sampath R, Massire C, et al.** Ibis T5000: a universal biosensor approach for microbiology. *Nat Rev Microbiol.* 2008 Jul;6(7):553–558.
111. **Costerton JW, Post JC, Ehrlich GD, et al.** New methods for the detection of orthopedic and other biofilm infections. *FEMS Immunol Med Microbiol.* 2011 Mar;61(2):133–140.
112. **Jacovides CL, Kreft R, Adeli B, et al.** Successful identification of pathogens by polymerase chain reaction (PCR)-based electron spray ionization time-of-flight mass spectrometry (ESI-TOF-MS) in culture-negative periprosthetic joint infection. *J Bone Joint Surg Am.* 2012 Dec 19;94(24):2247–2254.
113. **Greenwood-Quaintance KE, Uhl JR, Hanssen AD, et al.** Diagnosis of prosthetic joint infection by use of PCR-electrospray ionization mass spectrometry. *J Clin Microbiol.* 2014 Feb;52(2):642–649.
114. **Melendez DP, Uhl JR, Greenwood-Quaintance KE, et al.** Detection of prosthetic joint infection by use of PCR-electrospray ionization mass spectrometry applied to synovial fluid. *J Clin Microbiol.* 2014 Jun;52(6):2202–2205.
115. **Trampuz A, Osmon DR, Hanssen AD, et al.** Molecular and antibiofilm approaches to prosthetic joint infection. *Clin Orthop Relat Res.* 2003 Sep;(414):69–88.
116. **Trebse R.** The diagnostic protocol for evaluation of periprosthetic joint infection. *Hip Int.* 2012 Jul-Aug;22 Suppl 8:S25–35.
117. **Del Pozo JL, Patel R.** Clinical practice. Infection associated with prosthetic joints. *N Engl J Med.* 2009 Aug 20;361(8):787–794.
118. **Muller M, Morawietz L, Hasart O, et al.** Histopathologische Diagnose der periprothetischen Gelenkinfektion nach Hüftgelenkersatz. [Histopathological diagnosis of periprosthetic joint infection following total hip arthroplasty: use of a standardized classification system of the periprosthetic interface membrane]. *Der Orthopäde.* 2009 Nov;38(11):1087–1096. German.
119. **Morawietz L, Classen RA, Schroder JH, et al.** Proposal for a histopathological consensus classification of the periprosthetic interface membrane. *J Clin Pathol.* 2006 Jun;59(6):591–597.
120. **Nunez LV, Buttaro MA, Morandi A, et al.** Frozen sections of samples taken intraoperatively for diagnosis of infection in revision hip surgery. *Acta Orthop.* 2007 Apr;78(2):226–230.
121. **Bori G, Soriano A, Garcia S, et al.** Neutrophils in frozen section and type of microorganism isolated at the time of resection arthroplasty for the treatment of infection. *Arch Orthop Trauma Surg.* 2009 May;129(5):591–595.
122. **Grosso MJ, Frangiamore SJ, Ricchetti ET, et al.** Sensitivity of frozen section histology for identifying Propionibacterium acnes infections in revision shoulder arthroplasty. *J Bone Joint Surg Am.* 2014 Mar 19;96(6):442–447.
123. **Ahmadi S, Lawrence TM, Morrey BF, et al.** The value of intraoperative histology in predicting infection in patients undergoing revision elbow arthroplasty. *J Bone Joint Surg Am.* 2013 Nov 6;95(21):1976–1979.
124. **Tsaras G, Maduka-Ezeh A, Inwards CY, et al.** Utility of intraoperative frozen section histopathology in the diagnosis of periprosthetic joint infection: a systematic review and meta-analysis. *J Bone Joint Surg Am.* 2012 Sep 19;94(18):1700–1711.
125. **Corvec S, Portillo ME, Pasticci BM, et al.** Epidemiology and new developments in the diagnosis of prosthetic joint infections. *Int J Artif Organs.* 2012 Oct;35(10):923–934.
126. **Trampuz A, Steinhuber A, Wittwer M, et al.** Rapid diagnosis of experimental meningitis by bacterial heat production in cerebrospinal fluid. *BMC Infect Dis.* 2007 Oct 10;7:116.
127. **Trampuz A, Salzmann S, Antheaume J, et al.** Microcalorimetry: a novel method for detection of microbial contamination in platelet products. *Transfusion.* 2007 Sep;47(9):1643–1650.
128. **Borens O, Yusuf E, Steinrucken J, et al.** Accurate and early diagnosis of orthopedic device-related infection by microbial heat production and sonication. *J Orthop Res.* 2013 Nov;31(11):1700–1703.
129. **Yusuf E, Steinrucken J, Nordback S, et al.** Necrotizing fasciitis after breast augmentation: rapid microbiologic detection by using sonication of removed implants and microcalorimetry. *Am J Clin Pathol.* 2014 Aug;142(2):269–272.
130. **Trampuz A, Zimmerli W.** Diagnosis and treatment of implant-associated septic arthritis and osteomyelitis. *Curr Infect Dis Rep.* 2008 Sep;10(5):394–403.
131. **Nishitani K, Beck CA, Rosenberg AF, et al.** A Diagnostic Serum Antibody Test for Patients With Staphylococcus aureus Osteomyelitis. *Clin Orthop Relat Res.* 2015 Sep;473(9):2735–2749.
132. **Artini M, Romano C, Manzoli L, et al.** Staphylococcal IgM enzyme-linked immunosorbent assay for diagnosis of periprosthetic joint infections. *J Clin Microbiol.* 2011 Jan;49(1):423–425.
133. **Wang X, Sadovskaya I, Leterme D, et al.** A comparative study of antibodies against proteins extracted from staphylococcal biofilm for the diagnosis of orthopedic prosthesis-related infections in an animal model and in humans. *Diagn Microbiol Infect Dis.* 2013 Feb;75(2):124–129.
134. **Holinka J, Bauer L, Hirschl AM, et al.** Sonication cultures of explanted components as an add-on test to routinely conducted microbiological diagnostics improve pathogen detection. *J Orthop Res.* 2011 Apr;29(4):617–622.
135. **Piper KE, Jacobson MJ, Cofield RH, et al.** Microbiologic diagnosis of prosthetic shoulder infection by use of implant sonication. *J Clin Microbiol.* 2009 Jun;47(6):1878–1884.
136. **Esteban J, Gomez-Barrena E, Cordero J, et al.** Evaluation of quantitative analysis of cultures from sonicated retrieved orthopedic implants in diagnosis of orthopedic infection. *J Clin Microbiol.* 2008 Feb;46(2):488–492.
137. **Lutz MF, Berthelot P, Fresard A, et al.** Arthroplastic and osteosynthetic infections due to Propionibacterium acnes: a retrospective study of 52 cases, 1995–2002. *Eur J Clin Microbiol Infect Dis.* 2005 Nov;24(11):739–744.
138. **Vergidis P, Greenwood-Quaintance KE, Sanchez-Sotelo J, et al.** Implant sonication for the diagnosis of prosthetic elbow infection. *J Shoulder Elbow Surg.* 2011 Dec;20(8):1275–1281.
139. **Puig-Verdie L, Alentorn-Geli E, Gonzalez-Cuevas A, et al.** Implant sonication increases the diagnostic accuracy of infection in patients with delayed, but not early, orthopaedic implant failure. *Bone Joint J.* 2013 Feb;95-B(2):244–249.
140. **Nishitani K, Sutipornpalangkal W, de Mesy Bentley KL, et al.** Quantifying the natural history of biofilm formation in vivo during the establishment of chronic implant-associated Staphylococcus aureus osteomyelitis in mice to identify critical pathogen and host factors. *J Orthop Res.* 2015 Sep;33(9):1311–1319.

141. **Sorli L, Puig L, Torres-Claramunt R, et al.** The relationship between microbiology results in the second of a two-stage exchange procedure using cement spacers and the outcome after revision total joint replacement for infection: the use of sonication to aid bacteriological analysis. *J Bone Joint Surg Br.* 2012 Feb;94(2):249–253.
142. **Mariconda M, Ascione T, Balato G, et al.** Sonication of antibiotic-loaded cement spacers in a two-stage revision protocol for infected joint arthroplasty. *BMC Musculoskelet Disord.* 2013 Jun 24;14:193.
143. **Vasoo S, Mason EL, Gustafson DR, et al.** Desulfovibrio legallii Prosthetic Shoulder Joint Infection and Review of Antimicrobial Susceptibility and Clinical Characteristics of Desulfovibrio Infections. *J Clin Microbiol.* 2014 Aug;52(8):3105–3110.
144. **Farrell JJ, Larson JA, Akeson JW, et al.** Ureaplasma parvum prosthetic joint infection detected by PCR. *J Clin Microbiol.* 2014 Jun;52(6):2248–2250.
145. **Kloesel B, Beliveau M, Patel R, et al.** Bulleidia extructa periprosthetic hip joint infection, United States. *Emerg Infect Dis.* 2013 Jul;19(7):1170–1171.
146. **Tande AJ, Cunningham SA, Raoult D, et al.** A case of Q fever prosthetic joint infection and description of an assay for detection of Coxiella burnetii. *J Clin Microbiol.* 2013 Jan;51(1):66–69.
147. **Rohacek M, Weisser M, Kobza R, et al.** Bacterial colonization and infection of electrophysiological cardiac devices detected with sonication and swab culture. *Circulation.* 2010 Apr 20;121(15):1691–1697.
148. **Rieger UM, Pierer G, Luscher NJ, et al.** Sonication of removed breast implants for improved detection of subclinical infection. *Aesthetic Plast Surg.* 2009 May;33(3):404–408.

Section 2

Special situations

Section 2
Special situations

8 Open fractures

Charalampos G Zalavras

1 Basics

The defining characteristic of an open fracture is associated soft-tissue trauma that creates communication of the fracture site with the outside environment [1]. High-energy open fractures are more common in younger men and low-energy open fractures in older women [2]. Open diaphyseal fractures of the tibia, femur, and humerus are usually the result of high-energy trauma with road traffic injuries being the most common mechanism [2]. Open diaphyseal fractures of the tibia, femur, and humerus have resulted from road traffic injuries in 46%, 54%, and 50% of cases, respectively [2].

Open fractures carry an increased risk for complications, such as infection and nonunion, and require a principle-based approach to decrease the morbidity and improve the prognosis. The principles of open fracture management consist of careful assessment of the patient and the injury, early systemic antibiotic therapy that can be supplemented by local antibiotic delivery, thorough debridement, wound management with soft-tissue coverage, and stabilization of the fracture. Management of open fractures based on these principles will help prevent infection, achieve fracture healing, and restore function in these challenging injuries.

2 Assessment and classification

2.1 Patient and injury assessment

Open fractures may be associated with serious and potentially life-threatening abdominal, thoracic, head, or other injuries [2, 3]. The average injury severity score of patients with open diaphyseal fractures of the tibia, femur, and humerus was 13.5, 18.1, and 17.5, respectively [2]. Therefore, it is critical to perform a thorough assessment of every patient with an open fracture and to use appropriate resuscitation and manage other injuries as necessary according to advanced trauma life support protocols.

Evaluation of the injured extremity should include a careful neurovascular examination and assessment of the size, location, and contamination of the wound (**Fig 8-1a**). The wound is irrigated, gross contamination removed, and a sterile dressing applied. The fractured extremity should be grossly realigned and immobilized with a splint (**Fig 8-1b–c**). Intravenous antibiotic therapy should be started and tetanus prophylaxis should be given depending on the patient's immunization status.

The treating surgeon should be aware of the possibility of compartment syndrome despite the presence of the open wound fracture, especially in crush injuries [4] (**Fig 8-2**).

Fracture characteristics, such as articular involvement and comminution, should be evaluated by the appropriate imaging studies to plan fixation of the fracture.

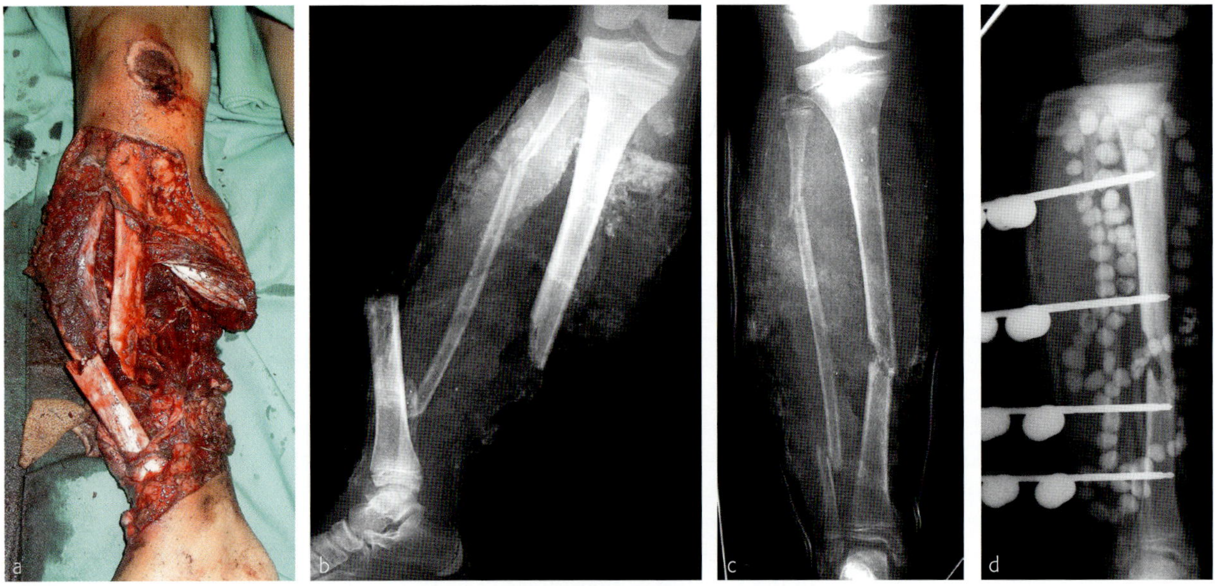

Fig 8-1a–d Open fracture of the tibia and fibula with severe soft-tissue injury and contamination.

- **a** Note the foreign particles and dirt embedded in the soft tissues.
- **b** There is severe deformity of the leg with excessive displacement and malrotation, as can be seen by evaluating the difference in the projections of the knee and ankle joints. Vascular compromise of the extremity may be the result of such fracture-site deformity and this x-ray should not have been taken before reduction and splinting of the injured leg.
- **c** Gross restoration of rotation and alignment of the extremity may restore perfusion and prevent further soft-tissue damage.
- **d** The fracture was stabilized intraoperatively with an external fixator. Note the antibiotic polymethylmethacrylate beads in place.

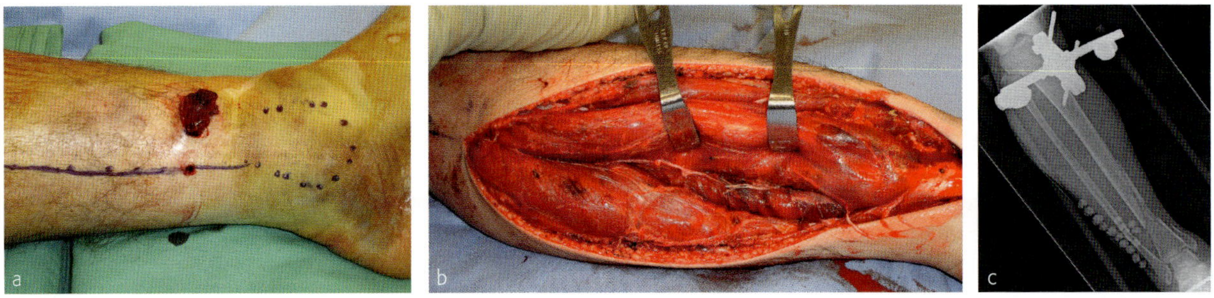

Fig 8-2a–c Patient with open distal tibial and fibular fractures developing compartment syndrome of the leg.

- **a** Traumatic wounds associated with the open fractures.
- **b** The smaller traumatic wound was incorporated into an incision that extended proximally and distally along the posterior border of the fibula to first decompress all four compartments of the leg and then perform debridement and irrigation of the open fractures.
- **c** An external fixator spanning the ankle joint was used as provisional fixation. When not being used for definitive fixation, external fixation is placed as a spanning construct leaving the zone of injury free of pins and easily accessible for imaging studies and future fixation. The surgeon should also be aware of future incision placement to avoid placing external fixation pins in these areas.

2.2 Classification of open fractures

The severity of the injury can vary considerably among patients. Classification systems of open fractures have been developed with the aim to describe the injury, guide treatment, determine prognosis, and compare treatment methods for research purposes.

The classification system of Gustilo and Anderson, subsequently modified by Gustilo, Mendoza, and Williams [5, 6], has been extensively used and comprises the following types:

- Type I: wound of 1 cm or less with minimal contamination or muscle crushing.
- Type II: wound more than 1 cm long with moderate soft-tissue damage and crushing. Bone coverage is adequate and comminution is minimal.
- Type IIIA: extensive soft-tissue damage, often due to a high-energy injury with a crushing component. Massively contaminated wounds and severely comminuted or segmental fractures are included in this subtype. Bone coverage is adequate.
- Type IIIB: extensive soft-tissue damage with periosteal stripping and bone exposure, usually with severe contamination and bone comminution. Flap coverage is required.
- Type IIIC: arterial injury requiring repair.

The risk of infection depends on the severity of the open fracture and ranges from 0–2% for type I open fractures, 2–10% for type II, and 10–50% for type III fractures [5, 7].

However, the reliability of this classification may be suboptimal. Brumback and Jones [8] evaluated the responses of orthopedic surgeons who were asked to classify open fractures of the tibia on the basis of videotaped case presentations, and found that the average agreement among observers was only 60% overall.

The Orthopaedic Trauma Association proposed a new classification system for determining the severity of open fractures, which is based on pathoanatomical characteristics of the injury and specifically evaluates skin, muscle, and arterial injury, bone loss, and contamination [9]. The average interobserver agreement was 86% overall but interobserver reliability on muscle injury and contamination was moderate [10].

Regardless of the system used, classification of the open fracture should not be done in the emergency department but instead in the operating room after wound exploration and debridement. Only then can the treating surgeon assess the extent and severity of the injury and the degree of contamination.

3 Antibiotics

3.1 Systemic antibiotic therapy

Most open fracture wounds are contaminated with microorganisms [5, 7, 11], therefore, antibiotics are not used for prophylaxis but for treatment of wound contamination. Antibiotic therapy reduces the risk of infection in patients with open fractures. Patzakis et al [11] established the important role of antibiotics in a prospective randomized study, which indicated a decreased infection rate when cefazolin was administered before debridement (2 of 84 fractures [2.3%]) compared with no antibiotics (11 of 79 fractures [13.9%]).

Antibiotic administration should be started as soon as possible on admission of the patient in the emergency department. Both animal and clinical studies [7, 12] have demonstrated the importance of early antibiotic therapy. Delay of more than 3 hours from injury to administration of antibiotics has been associated with an increased risk of infection [7].

The recommended duration of antibiotic therapy is 3 days [7, 13], although a study [14] comparing 1 day to 5 days of antibiotics reported similar infection rates and suggested that 1 day of antibiotics may be an option. An additional 3-day administration of antibiotics is recommended for subsequent surgical procedures, such as repeated debridement and wound coverage [7, 13, 15].

Open wound cultures are not useful in selecting the optimal antibiotic regimen. Culture results require a considerable delay and they often fail to identify the organism causing a subsequent infection [16, 17]. In most cases, infections are not caused by the organisms initially present in the wound but by nosocomial organisms, such as staphylococci and aerobic gram-negative bacilli. A randomized controlled trial (RCT) [18] reported that only 3 of 17 infections (18%) that developed in a series of 171 open fractures were caused by an organism identified by the initial cultures. Wound cultures obtained before wound debridement are not recommended [17]. After debridement, intraoperative cultures may help with antibiotic selection for subsequent procedures or for management of early infections.

A combination of gram-positive coverage (eg, a first-generation cephalosporin such as cefazolin) and gram-negative coverage (eg, an aminoglycoside such as gentamicin) is widely accepted for severe (type III) open fractures [7, 13, 15, 19, 20]. Systemic administration of aminoglycosides may not be necessary if aminoglycoside-impregnated beads are used for local antibiotic delivery.

Administration of a cephalosporin as a single agent in types I and II open fractures has been proposed by some authors, [13, 19, 20] whereas others [7, 15] have advocated combined gram-positive and gram-negative coverage for these less severe open fractures to provide coverage against contaminating gram-negative organisms. Patzakis and Wilkins reported that in open tibial fractures, combination therapy reduced the infection rate (5 of 109 [4.5%]) compared with cephalosporin only (25 of 192 [13%]) [7]. Fracture types I and II were not analyzed separately but the distribution of fracture types was comparable between the two groups. Moreover, a type IIIA open fracture with a wound of small size may be misclassified in the emergency department as type I or II open fracture and treated with a cephalosporin only (**Fig 8-3**).

Anaerobic coverage (eg, ampicillin or penicillin) should be added in injuries that may result in contamination with clostridial organisms (eg, farm injuries) and in vascular injuries that can create conditions of ischemia and low oxygen tension to prevent clostridial myonecrosis (ie, gas gangrene). It is critical to remember that antibiotic therapy is not a substitute for thorough surgical debridement.

The growing emergence of antimicrobial resistance in bacteria, and specifically the increase of methicillin-resistant *Staphylococcus aureus* (MRSA), has raised questions about the adequacy of current antibiotic protocols. An RCT compared administration of a combination of vancomycin and cefazolin to administration of only cefazolin in 101 patients who were followed up for a minimum of 30 days and for 10 months on average [21]. A significantly higher rate of MRSA infection was observed in patients with MRSA nasal colonization, but there was no difference in the infection rates between the group receiving vancomycin and cefazolin (19%) versus the group receiving only cefazolin (15%). There was one MRSA infection in each group [21]. The routine use of vancomycin in open fractures cannot be recommended based on available data and the potential for emergence of glycopeptide-resistant organisms is a serious concern.

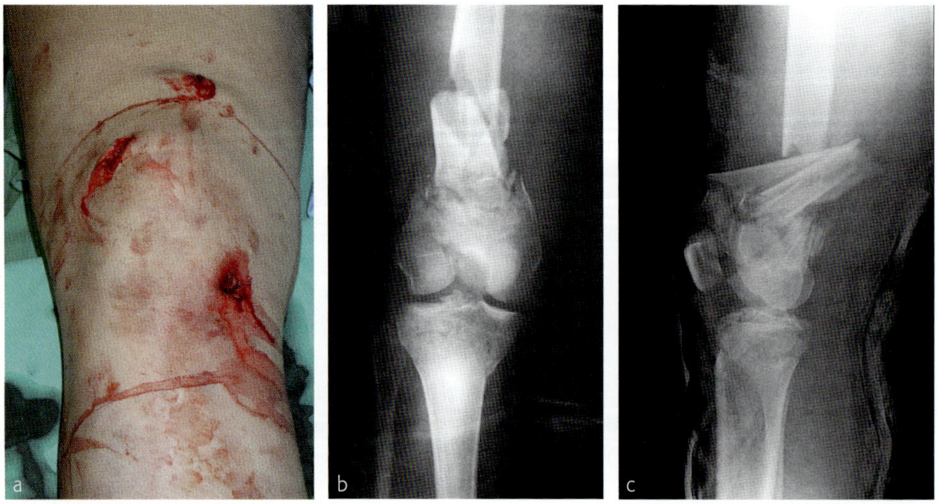

Fig 8-3a–c Open distal femoral fracture.
a The small size of the wounds around the knee area does not correspond to the severity of the injury.
b–c Extensive comminution is present in this open distal femoral fracture as can be seen in the AP (**b**) and lateral (**c**) views. This fracture may be erroneously classified as a type I or II instead of type IIIA open fracture.

3.2 Local antibiotic therapy

Local antibiotic therapy with antibiotic-impregnated delivery vehicles has been used in addition to systemic antibiotic therapy [22]. A commonly used delivery vehicle is polymethylmethacrylate (PMMA) cement, which can be molded to create beads of 5–10 mm diameter (**Fig 8-1d**) or spacer blocks of larger size. Bioabsorbable delivery vehicles, such as calcium sulfate, appear to be a promising alternative [23] (see chapter 6 Local delivery of antibiotics and antiseptics for further discussion).

Several antimicrobial agents have been successfully incorporated into PMMA cement for local delivery, including aminoglycosides, vancomycin, and cephalosporins [22]. An antibiotic appropriate for local delivery must be heat-stable, available in powder form, and active against the targeted microbial pathogens. In open fractures, aminoglycosides are common choices because of their broad spectrum of activity, heat stability, and low allergenicity.

Elution, which is the process of release of antibiotics from the delivery vehicle to the surrounding tissues, is determined by the difference in the concentration of antibiotics between the antibiotic delivery system and its environment. High concentration of antibiotics and increased porosity of the delivery vehicle facilitate elution [24, 25]. Elution depends on the type of antibiotic, and tobramycin has superior elution properties compared to vancomycin [26]. A fluid medium is necessary for elution and the rate of fluid turnover influences the local antibiotic concentration [27]. Elution of antibiotics from PMMA beads is characterized by an initial rapid phase and a secondary slow phase [28]. Following insertion of antibiotic-impregnated PMMA beads in the open fracture wound, the wound should be sealed by a semipermeable barrier, so that the eluted antibiotic remains at the involved area to achieve a high local concentration (**Fig 8-4**).

The antibiotic bead-pouch technique achieves a high local concentration of antibiotics without a high systemic concentration, thereby maximizing efficacy at the injury site and minimizing toxicity [29]. Sealing of the wound from the external environment by the semipermeable barrier prevents secondary contamination by nosocomial pathogens, establishes an aerobic wound environment, and promotes patient comfort by avoiding painful dressing changes.

The antibiotic bead-pouch technique has been shown to reduce the infection rate when used in addition to systemic antibiotics for management of severe open fractures [30, 31]. Ostermann et al [30] compared systemic antibiotics alone to combined treatment with both systemic antibiotics and the bead-pouch technique in a series of 1,085 open fractures. The infection rate was significantly reduced to 31 of 845 fractures (3.7%) in the antibiotic bead-pouch group compared to 29 of 240 fractures (12%) in open fractures treated only with systemic antibiotics. Analysis based on open fracture severity demonstrated that the reduction of infection was statistically significant only in type III fractures (6.5% versus 20.6%). Note that wound management differed between the two groups. In the systemic antibiotic group, 63% of wounds were left open initially, thereby predisposing the wound to secondary contamination. In the antibiotic bead pouch group, 95% of wounds were either closed primarily or sealed with the bead-pouch technique.

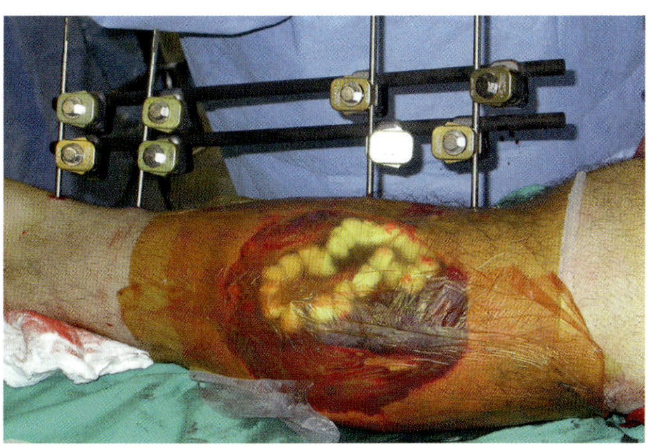

Fig 8-4 Antibiotic polymethylmethacrylate beads are in place in the area of the soft-tissue defect. Note the semipermeable membrane dressing, which seals the area to keep the fluid with eluted antibiotics in the wound, while at the same time maintaining an aerobic wound environment and preventing secondary contamination.

4 Debridement

Thorough surgical debridement is critical in the management of open fractures. The quality of surgical debridement is not only the most important factor in the treatment of osteomyelitis but also in the prevention of infection in open fractures [32, 33]. Devitalized tissue and foreign material promote the growth of microorganisms and development of biofilm and also constitute a barrier for the host's defense mechanisms.

4.1 Debridement principles

Debridement should be performed in the operating room. When the open fracture wound is insufficient for detailed evaluation of the injury, surgical extension of the wound is necessary (**Fig 8-2a-b**). Surgical extension should be done in a way that respects the vascularity of soft tissues and facilitates fracture fixation and any anticipated reconstructive procedures. If the location of a small traumatic wound is such that an incision incorporating the wound would not facilitate subsequent procedures, a surgical approach to the fracture can be done without incorporating the traumatic wound and the open fracture can be debrided through this approach.

Debridement should be performed in a systematic and atraumatic fashion while protecting adjacent neurovascular structures. Skin and subcutaneous tissue are sharply debrided back to bleeding edges. Muscle is sharply debrided until only viable tissue is present in the wound. Viable muscle is characterized by bleeding when cut and contractility upon touching the tissue with the cautery tip or squeezing it with forceps. Bone fragments should be left in place only if they have soft-tissue attachments, indicating vascularity of the fragments. Punctate bleeding from exposed bone surfaces helps determine viability of the bone. Free fragments are avascular and should be removed with the exception of articular fragments that are large enough to be useful in reconstruction of the involved joint. Large free diaphyseal fragments can be used as a guide to assist with reduction of the fracture and discarded afterward but should not be retained.

4.2 Irrigation

Irrigation of the open fracture wound following debridement may further mechanically remove small foreign bodies and reduce bacterial concentration. The author's preference is gravity irrigation (**Fig 8-5**). The type of solution and its delivery pressure remain controversial with most data derived from in vitro and animal studies.

Antiseptic solutions can be toxic to host cells and are not recommended [34]. Owens et al [35] used a goat model involving a complex musculoskeletal wound that was inoculated with *Pseudomonas aeruginosa* to compare irrigation with normal saline solution, bacitracin solution, castile soap, or benzalkonium chloride following wound debridement. Although normal saline was associated with the smallest reduction in bacterial counts immediately after irrigation (29% of pretreatment levels), it was also associated with the smallest rebound of bacterial counts at 48 hours (68% of pretreatment levels). In contrast, the castile soap group had the greatest reduction in bacterial counts immediately after irrigation (13% of pretreatment levels) and also the greatest rebound of bacterial counts at 48 hours (120% of pretreatment levels).

High-pressure pulsatile lavage has been associated with bacterial seeding into the intramedullary (IM) canal in an anatomical specimen study [36], with increased wound bacterial counts at 48 hours after irrigation [35] and with adverse effects on early new bone formation in a rabbit model [37].

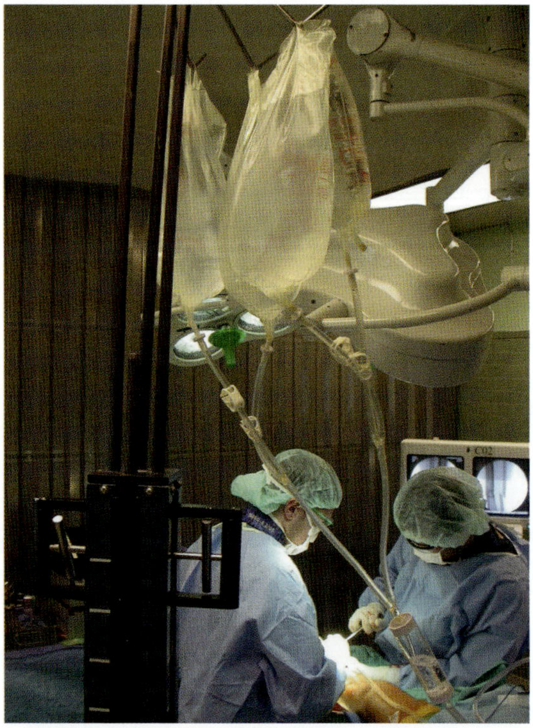

Fig 8-5 The author's preferred technique of gravity irrigation. Note that the saline fluid bags have been elevated as much as possible (approximately 3 m from the floor) using gravity to generate pressure.

Clinical data on irrigation of open fracture wounds are limited. Anglen [38] compared bacitracin solution to nonsterile castile soap solution for irrigation of open fractures in an RCT and found no difference in infection and nonunion rates, but an increased rate of wound-healing problems with bacitracin. Irrigation with normal saline was not evaluated in this study.

A pilot RCT [39] compared the effects of different irrigation methods (castile soap versus normal saline and high- versus low-pressure pulsatile lavage) on the reoperation rate and complication rate in patients with open fractures. Reoperation rates after a 1-year follow-up were similar in the castile soap group (13 of 56 [23%]) and the saline group (13 of 55 [24%]). Increased reoperation rate was seen in the high-pressure group (16 of 57 [28%]) compared to the low-pressure group (10 of 54 [19%]) but this was not significant. Note that the sample size was small and the protocol regarding antibiotics and wound management was not standardized among centers.

4.3 Timing of debridement

Urgent debridement of open fractures within 6 hours from injury has been considered important for prevention of infection; however, the literature has not supported this notion [7, 40–43].

Patzakis and Wilkins [7] reported in 1989 that the infection rate was similar in open fracture wounds debrided within 12 hours from injury (27 of 396 [6.8%]) and in those debrided after 12 hours from injury (50 of 708 [7.1%]) and concluded that elapsed time from injury to debridement is not a critical factor for development of infection in patients receiving antibiotic therapy.

Harley et al [40] demonstrated that time to surgical debridement either as a continuous or dichotomous (ie, before versus after 8 hours from injury) variable was not associated with increased infection or nonunion rates. Multivariate analysis showed that open fracture severity but not time to debridement was an independent predictor of infection and nonunion.

Skaggs et al [43] demonstrated that the rates of acute infection in children with open fractures were similar in the group that underwent surgical management within 6 hours (12 of 344 fractures [3%]) and in the group that underwent surgical management from 7 to 24 hours (4 of 202 fractures [2%]). No difference in infection rates was found after stratification of open fractures according to the Gustilo-Anderson classification. For type III open fractures, the infection rate was 6 of 61 in the early group (10%) compared to 2 of 36 in the delayed group (6%).

Pollak et al [41] found no relationship between time to surgical debridement and infection in 307 patients with severe open lower extremity fractures. The infection rate was 28%, 29%, and 26% in patients who underwent debridement earlier than 5 hours, 5–10 hours, and more than 10 hours from injury, respectively. Interestingly, the time between injury and admission to the definitive trauma treatment center was an independent predictor of the likelihood of infection.

Although bacterial populations in an untreated contaminated wound increase over time, it appears that early antibiotic administration and thorough surgical debridement can effectively reduce the contamination present. As a result, small delays in surgical management do not appear to translate in increased infection rates and may allow for stabilization and resuscitation of the patient, as well as for treatment of the patient by experienced surgical teams with all necessary equipment available.

4.4 Second-look debridement

A single thorough debridement executed by an experienced surgeon may be enough, especially in less severe open fractures, and this can be followed by primary closure, either complete or partial, of the open fracture wound (see topic 5 of this chapter).

On the other hand, a repeated debridement may be performed after 48 hours based on the degree of contamination and soft-tissue damage. In this case, delayed wound closure can be performed when the goal of a clean wound with viable, bleeding tissues has been achieved. In injuries requiring flap coverage, debridement should also be repeated at the time of the soft-tissue procedure.

5 Wound closure and soft-tissue coverage

5.1 Primary wound closure

Primary closure of open fracture wounds remains a controversial topic and the optimal time for wound closure is still debated [44]. Primary wound closure has traditionally not been advocated for open fractures because it has been associated with wound infections, including the catastrophic complication of gas gangrene (clostridial myonecrosis) that necessitates amputation of the involved extremity and may even lead to death of the patient [45, 46].

However, gas gangrene has mostly complicated military wounds with severe tissue injury, gross contamination, and inadequate antibiotic therapy or debridement. Clinical studies [7, 47–49] of civilian injuries comparing primary to delayed closure have not shown an increased infection rate following primary closure, and suggested that primary closure may prevent secondary contamination and reduce surgical morbidity, hospital stay, and cost [47, 48]. Patzakis and Wilkins [7] reported in 1989 that primary closure did not result in increased infection rate. Specifically, infection complicated 10.6% of wounds closed primarily compared to 13.4% of wounds closed with a delay [7]. DeLong et al [47] reported that primary closure was safe and was not associated with an increase in infection or nonunion, and a recent study by Jenkinson et al [48] showed a decreased infection rate with primary closure.

Primary closure of carefully selected open fracture wounds is a viable option under the following conditions:

1. There is no severe soft-tissue injury, vascular injury, or gross contamination, especially with soil or fecal matter.
2. Early administration of antibiotics has taken place.
3. A meticulous debridement has been executed by an experienced surgeon resulting in the presence of only healthy, bleeding tissue in the wound at the end of the procedure.
4. The wound edges can be approximated without tension. Partial wound closure is another option for less severe injuries [50].

The surgical extension of the wound created to assess the bone and soft tissues and to facilitate debridement can be closed primarily in types I and II open fractures, leaving only the injury wound open, to be closed in delayed fashion.

If there is any doubt about the viability of the tissues and/or the adequacy of the debridement, the wound should not be closed primarily and a second-look debridement should be undertaken with the plan to perform delayed wound closure or a soft-tissue coverage procedure, depending on the status of the soft-tissue envelope (**Fig 8-6**).

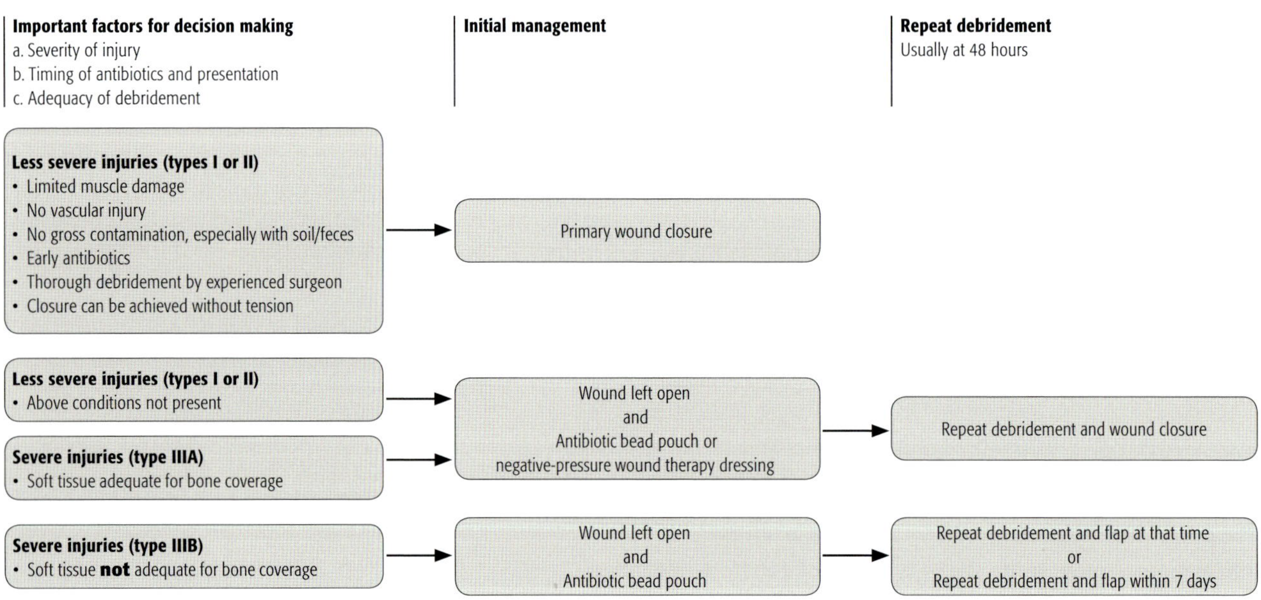

Fig 8-6 Algorithm for wound management in open fractures.

5.2 Delayed wound closure

Delayed wound closure prevents anaerobic conditions in the wound and the development of clostridial infections, permits drainage of the wound, and allows tissues of questionable viability to be discovered at the second-look debridement. On the other hand, a repeated surgical procedure is required, resulting in increased hospital stay and healthcare costs.

Delayed wound closure is recommended for more severe injuries with extensive soft-tissue damage and gross contamination in patients presenting with a considerable delay, in wounds with tissues of questionable viability at the end of the debridement, and in wounds that cannot be approximated without tension.

It should be emphasized that when a decision is made to close the open fracture wound with a delay, or when closure is not possible and a soft-tissue reconstructive procedure is needed, the wound should not be left exposed to the outside environment to prevent contamination with nosocomial pathogens. Instead the antibiotic bead-pouch technique [30] or negative-pressure wound therapy [51] should be used.

5.3 Soft-tissue coverage and reconstruction

In the presence of extensive soft-tissue injury, as in type IIIB open fractures, which precludes delayed wound closure and adequate bone coverage, soft-tissue reconstruction is required. Local or free muscle flaps can be transferred to achieve soft-tissue coverage of the open fracture. A vascular soft-tissue envelope promotes fracture healing, enhances antibiotic delivery, and achieves coverage of the wound that prevents secondary contamination as well as desiccation of exposed anatomical structures, such as bone, cartilage, and tendons. Soft-tissue reconstruction is usually achieved with local or free tissue transfers depending on the location and size of the soft-tissue defect [52–55]. Pollak et al [55] concluded that use of a free flap in limbs with a severe osseous injury was associated with fewer wound complications necessitating operative treatment compared to a rotational flap. A microvascular surgeon should participate early in management of an open fracture with extensive soft-tissue damage.

Soft-tissue reconstruction should be performed early, within the first 7 days. Delays beyond 7–10 days have been associated with increased rates of infection and flap complications [16, 56]. Godina [57] even argued in favor of flap coverage within 72 hours. Gopal et al [54] also utilized an early aggressive protocol in types IIIB and IIIC open fractures and observed deep infection in 4 of 63 fractures (6%) that were covered within 72 hours compared to 6 of 21 (29%) in the ones covered beyond 72 hours. It should be noted that in these studies the antibiotic bead pouch was not used, and therefore secondary contamination may have been an important confounding factor contributing to the infectious complications.

6 Fracture fixation

6.1 Fixation options

Stable fixation with restoration of length, alignment, and rotation of the fracture bone(s) is an important part of open fracture management. Stable fixation prevents further injury to the soft-tissue envelope by unstable fracture fragments, facilitates wound care, and permits early motion of adjacent joints and early patient mobilization and rehabilitation. Fracture stability also enhances the host response to contaminating organisms, despite the presence of implants [58].

Several options exist for fracture fixation. Fixation can be definitive or provisional, and methods include IM nailing, external fixation, and plate fixation. Selection among these options depends on careful evaluation of bone, soft tissue, and patient characteristics [15]. More than one method may be applicable to a specific injury and the surgeon's expertise and availability of implants should also be considered.

6.2 Intramedullary nailing

Intramedullary nailing is an effective and commonly used technique for fixation of diaphyseal fractures of the lower extremity (**Fig 8-7**) [59–61]. Statically interlocked IM nailing maintains length and alignment of the fractured bone, is biomechanically superior to other methods, and does not interfere with soft-tissue management. However, it disrupts the endosteal bone circulation to a variable degree, depending on reaming of the medullary canal.

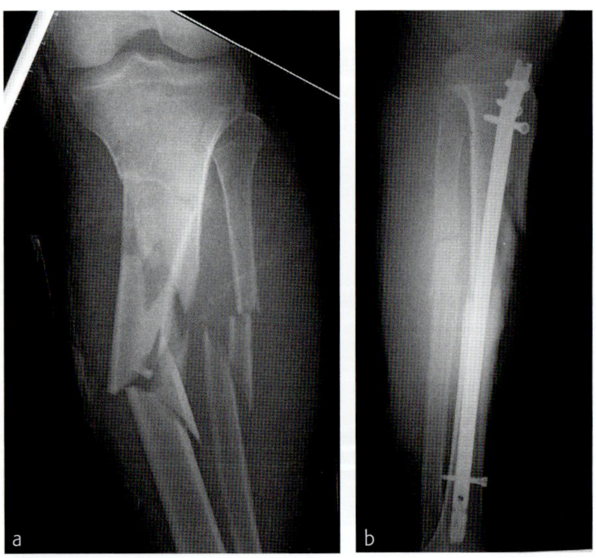

Fig 8-7a–b Open segmental fracture of the tibia and fibula (**a**) treated with an intramedullary nail (**b**).

Reamed IM nailing is commonly used for open diaphyseal fractures of the femur with good results. A study [61] on reamed IM nailing for these fractures reported no infections in 62 types I, II, and IIIA open fractures of the femur and 3 infections in 27 type IIIB open fractures (11%) [61].

Reamed and unreamed IM nailings have been used for open diaphyseal fractures of the tibia. Reamed nailing compromises the endosteal blood supply more than unreamed nailing but vascularity is gradually reconstituted [62, 63]. Reaming also facilitates insertion of larger diameter IM nails, thereby improving fracture-site stability.

Three randomized trials [64–66] comparing reamed to unreamed nailing for open tibial fractures did not demonstrate a significant difference in infection rates. Keating et al [64] reported that the infection rate was 1 of 40 (2.5%) in the unreamed nailing group compared to 2 of 45 (4.4%) in the reamed nailing group. Finkemeier et al [65] reported infection rates of 1 of 26 (3.8%) and 1 of 19 (5.3%) in the unreamed and reamed nailing group, respectively. Reamed nailing resulted in fewer screw failures in both studies. A multicenter RCT [66] comparing reamed to unreamed nailing in 400 open tibial fractures did not show any significant differences in the reoperation rate for infection (19 of 206 [9.2%]) in reamed nailing versus 16 of 194 (8.2%) in unreamed nailing) or in the overall reoperation rate. The optimal nailing technique for open fractures of the tibia remains uncertain.

6.3 External fixation

External fixation can be applied in a technically easy, safe, and expedient way, with minimal blood loss. For this reason it can be beneficial in damage-control situations, such as type IIIC open fractures to achieve prompt fracture stabilization, and in unstable polytrauma patients to minimize any additional inflammatory and physiological burden caused by surgery [67, 68].

External fixation preserves the vascularity of the fracture site and avoids implant insertion at the zone of injury. Therefore, it may be useful in wounds with severe soft-tissue damage and gross contamination, as in type IIIB open fractures (**Fig 8-1d**) [69–71]. External fixation can be used as the definitive fixation method for open diaphyseal fractures of the tibia with good results [69–71].

Two prospective randomized studies [59, 60], which compared external fixation to IM nailing as definitive fixation of open tibial fractures, found no differences in infection and nonunion rates [59, 60]. Instead, these complications were associated with increased severity of the open fracture [59]. However, external fixation requires patient compliance and is often complicated by pin-track infections and fracture malalignment if removed prematurely [59, 72].

Delayed conversion of external fixation to IM nailing has been associated with high infection rates of 44–50% [16, 73]. However, early conversion of the fixator to a nail within 2 weeks and in the absence of pin-track infection appears to be safe [74, 75].

External fixation can also be useful as provisional fixation in open periarticular fractures (**Fig 8-2c**) [76]. A joint-spanning external fixator can stabilize the fracture, restore length, alignment, and rotation of the involved bone and can be followed by definitive fixation at a second stage. Ring fixators may also be used for the definitive treatment of periarticular fractures with limited internal fixation as needed [77, 78].

6.4 Plate and screw fixation

Plate and screw fixation is useful in intraarticular and metaphyseal fractures because it allows anatomical reduction and restoration of joint congruency. It can be performed as definitive early fixation [79], or it can follow provisional stabilization of the fracture with a spanning external fixator [76]. Current locking plate designs and minimally invasive techniques have proved useful for the challenging injuries of open periarticular fractures (**Fig 8-8**) [80, 81]. Plate and screw fixation is recommended for open diaphyseal fractures of the forearm and humerus unless there is severe muscle damage and massive contamination [82, 83].

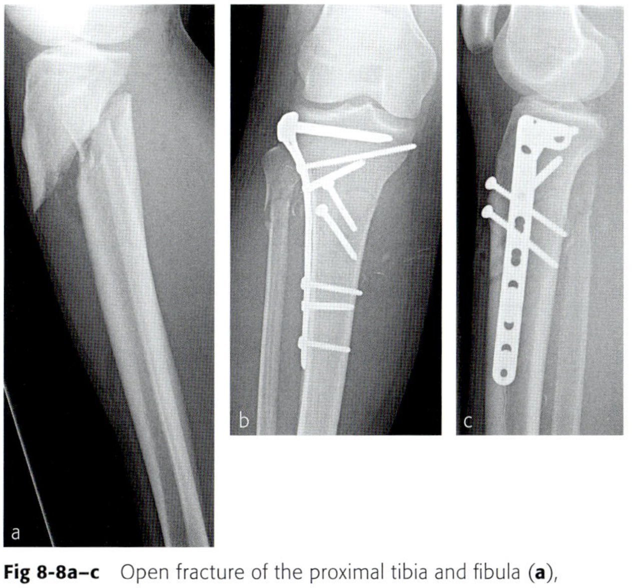

Fig 8-8a–c Open fracture of the proximal tibia and fibula (**a**), stabilized with a locking plate (**b–c**).

7 Mangled extremity

Salvage of a severely injured extremity (**Fig 8-9**) has been facilitated by surgical and medical advances but despite multiple reconstructive procedures, functional recovery of a severely injured extremity may be limited with associated morbidity, prolonged hospitalizations, psychological distress, and financial demands [84].

For this reason salvage of every mangled extremity, especially when a vascular injury is present, although technically possible, may be a disservice to the patient [85]. The alternative of below-knee amputation has even been considered as a superior alternative, leading to faster recovery and reduced long-term disability in comparison with successful limb salvage [84].

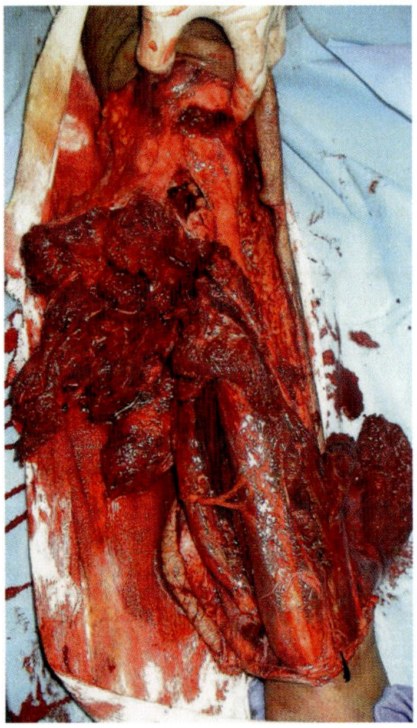

Fig 8-9 Mangled lower extremity with a type IIIC open fracture of the tibia and fibula with severe muscle damage and bone comminution.

A prospective observational multicenter study (Lower Extremity Assessment Project) evaluating limb-threatening lower extremity injuries in civilians provided useful information about the long-term functional outcome of these injuries [86–88]. Bosse et al [86] reported that patients who underwent amputation had functional outcomes that were similar to those of patients who underwent limb salvage at 2 years. The Sickness Impact Profile score was 12.6 in the amputation group versus 11.8 in the limb salvage group and the outcome remained similar between the two groups after adjusting for patient and injury characteristics. Return to work at 2 years was similar in the limb salvage group (49%) and the amputation groups (53%). However, limb salvage compared to amputation was associated with a significantly higher rate of repeated hospitalizations for complications (48% versus 34%, $P = .002$) and reoperations (19% versus 5%, $P < .001$). Functional outcome was adversely affected by several factors unrelated to the injury, such as low educational level, nonwhite race, poverty, lack of private health insurance, poor social support network, low self-efficacy, smoking, and involvement in litigation [86].

MacKenzie et al [88] demonstrated that disability following severe lower extremity trauma persisted at 7 years after the injury. Approximately half the patients who underwent either limb salvage or amputation had substantial disability at 7 years with no difference in functional outcomes between the two groups. Rehospitalization between 2 and 7 years from injury was required in 39% of patients who underwent limb salvage and in 33% of patients who underwent amputation [88].

The decision to amputate or proceed with limb salvage of a nonviable extremity with a type IIIC open fracture or a mangled extremity with a type IIIB fracture is often difficult and has important medical, psychological, and socioeconomic implications. The treating surgeon confronted with the dilemma of salvage versus amputation should evaluate and consider several patient and extremity factors. Patient factors include age, associated injuries, cardiopulmonary and hemodynamic status, preexisting medical problems, functional requirements, and socioeconomic support. Extremity factors include the previous functional status of the extremity and factors determined by the severity of injury, such as the extent of vascular injury, the time of warm ischemia, the degree of soft-tissue and bone damage, and anatomical disruption of the tibial nerve. Note that loss of plantar sensation upon presentation, which was considered an important adverse prognostic factor for limb salvage, is not associated with a worse functional outcome of limb salvage at 2 years compared to presence of a sensate foot [89]. In fact, more than half the patients presenting with an insensate foot regained sensation at 2 years [89].

Specialized scoring systems, such as the Mangled Extremity Severity Score (MESS), have been developed in an effort to offer guidelines for decision making in limb-threatening lower extremity injuries [90]. However, a prospective evaluation of the Mangled Extremity Severity Score (MESS) the Limb Salvage Index (LSI) the Predictive Salvage Index (PSI) as well as the Nerve Injury, Ischemia, Soft-Tissue Injury, Skeletal Injury, Shock, and Age of Patient Score (NISSSA) and the Hannover Fracture Scale-97 (HFS-97) did not support the utility of any of these scores for differentiating between extremities likely to be salvaged successfully and those requiring amputation [91]. Therefore, scores at or above the amputation threshold should not be relied upon to make a decision for amputation. On the other hand, low scores can predict the potential for limb salvage.

The final decision should be an individualized one, based on detailed evaluation of the patient and the extremity, sound judgment, and discussion with the patient and family if feasible [92].

8 Conclusion

Open fractures are challenging injuries, which are associated with a progressively increased risk for infection, nonunion, and even amputation, depending on their severity. Patients with open fractures should be evaluated for associated and potentially life-threatening injuries. The involved extremity should be evaluated for neurovascular injury and compartment syndrome, and the severity of contamination, soft-tissue damage, and bone injury should be determined, preferably intraoperatively. Systemic antibiotic therapy should be initiated upon patient presentation and local antibiotic delivery using antibiotic PMMA beads may be added in severe injuries. Thorough debridement with removal of all devitalized tissue and foreign bodies is a critical factor for prevention of infection. Primary wound closure is an option for less severe injuries if only healthy, viable tissue is present in the wound after a meticulous debridement performed by an experienced surgeon. Delayed closure with a second-look debridement after 48 hours is recommended for more severe injuries. At that time the wound can be closed if possible. In the case of extensive soft-tissue injury, a free or local flap may be required. Infections in open fractures usually result from secondary contamination with nosocomial organisms; therefore, the open fracture wound should not be left exposed but instead covered using the bead-pouch technique or negative-pressure wound therapy. Definitive or provisional stable fixation of the open fracture should be achieved. The timing and technique of fixation depend on bone, soft-tissue, and patient characteristics, and on the surgeon's expertise. Principle-based management of open fractures will help achieve the goals of infection prevention, fracture union, and restoration of function of the injured extremity.

9 References

1. **Zalavras CG, Patzakis MJ.** Open fractures: evaluation and management. *J Am Acad Orthop Surg.* 2003 May-Jun;11(3):212–219.
2. **Court-Brown CM, Bugler KE, Clement ND, et al.** The epidemiology of open fractures in adults. *A 15-year review. Injury.* 2012 Jun;43(6):891–897.
3. **Gustilo RB.** Management of open fractures. An analysis of 673 cases. *Minn Med.* 1971 Mar; 54(3):185–189.
4. **Blick SS, Brumback RJ, Poka A, et al.** Compartment syndrome in open tibial fractures. *J Bone Joint Surg Am.*1986 Dec;68(9):1348–1353.
5. **Gustilo RB, Anderson JT.** Prevention of infection in the treatment of one thousand and twenty-five open fractures of long bones: retrospective and prospective analyses. *J Bone Joint Surg Am.*1976 Jun;58(4):453–458.
6. **Gustilo RB, Mendoza RM, Williams DN.** Problems in the management of type III (severe) open fractures: a new classification of type III open fractures. *J Trauma.* 1984 Aug; 24(8):742–746.
7. **Patzakis MJ, Wilkins J.** Factors influencing infection rate in open fracture wounds. *Clin Orthop Relat Res.*1989 Jun;(243):36–40.
8. **Brumback RJ, Jones AL.** Interobserver agreement in the classification of open fractures of the tibia. The results of a survey of two hundred and forty-five orthopaedic surgeons. *J Bone Joint Surg Am.* 1994 Aug;76(8):1162–1166.
9. **Orthopaedic Trauma Association: Open Fracture Study Group.** A new classification scheme for open fractures. *Journal of orthopaedic trauma.* 2010 Aug;24(8):457–464.
10. **Agel J, Evans AR, Marsh JL, et al.** The OTA open fracture classification: a study of reliability and agreement. *Journal of orthopaedic trauma.* 2013 Jul; 27(7):379–384; discussion 384–375.
11. **Patzakis MJ, Harvey JP, Jr., Ivler D**. The role of antibiotics in the management of open fractures. *J Bone Joint Surg Am.* 1974 Apr;56(3):532–541.
12. **Penn-Barwell JG, Murray CK, Wenke JC.** Early antibiotics and debridement independently reduce infection in an open fracture model. *J Bone Joint Surg Br.* 2012 Jan;94(1):107–112.
13. **Templeman DC, Gulli B, Tsukayama DT, et al.** Update on the management of open fractures of the tibial shaft. *Clin Orthop Relat Res.* 1998 May;(350):18–25.
14. **Dellinger EP, Caplan ES, Weaver LD, et al.** Duration of preventive antibiotic administration for open extremity fractures. *Arch Surg.* 1988 Mar;123(3):333–339.
15. **Zalavras CG, Marcus RE, Levin LS, et al.** Management of open fractures and subsequent complications. *J Bone Joint Surg Am.* 2007 Apr;89(4):884–895.
16. **Fischer MD, Gustilo RB, Varecka TF.** The timing of flap coverage, bone-grafting, and intramedullary nailing in patients who have a fracture of the tibial shaft with extensive soft-tissue injury. *J Bone Joint Surg Am.*1991 Oct;73(9):1316–1322.
17. **Lee J.** Efficacy of cultures in the management of open fractures. *Clin Orthop Relat Res.* 1997 Jun;(339):71–75.
18. **Patzakis MJ, Bains RS, Lee J, et al.** Prospective, randomized, double-blind study comparing single-agent antibiotic therapy, ciprofloxacin, to combination antibiotic therapy in open fracture wounds. *J Orthop Trauma.* 2000 Nov:14(8):529–533.
19. **Hoff WS, Bonadies JA, Cachecho R, et al.** East Practice Management Guidelines Work Group: update to practice management guidelines for prophylactic antibiotic use in open fractures. *J Trauma.* 2011 Mar;70(3):751–754.
20. **Luchette FA, Bone LB, Born CT, et al.** EAST Practice Management Guidelines Workgroup: Practice management guidelines for prophylactic antibiotic use in open fractures. Eastern Association for the Surgery of Trauma. 2000. Available at http://www.east.org/tgp/openfrac.pdf. Accessed February, 2016.
21. **Saveli CC, Morgan SJ, Belknap RW, et al.** Prophylactic antibiotics in open fractures: a pilot randomized clinical safety study. *J Orthop Trauma.* 2013 Oct;27(10):552–557.
22. **Zalavras CG, Patzakis MJ, Holtom P.** Local antibiotic therapy in the treatment of open fractures and osteomyelitis. *Clin Orthop Relat Res.* 2004 Oct;(427):86–93.
23. **McKee MD, Wild LM, Schemitsch EH, et al.** The use of an antibiotic-impregnated, osteoconductive, bioabsorbable bone substitute in the treatment of infected long bone defects: early results of a prospective trial. *J Orthop Trauma.* 2002 Oct;16(9):622–627.
24. **Baker AS, Greenham LW.** Release of gentamicin from acrylic bone cement. Elution and diffusion studies. *J Bone Joint Surg Am.*1988 Dec;70(10):1551–1557.
25. **Beenken KE, Bradney L, Bellamy W, et al.** Use of xylitol to enhance the therapeutic efficacy of polymethylmethacrylate-based antibiotic therapy in treatment of chronic osteomyelitis. *Antimicrob Agents Chemother.* 2012 Nov;56(11):5839–5844.
26. **Greene N, Holtom PD, Warren CA, et al.** In vitro elution of tobramycin and vancomycin polymethylmethacrylate beads and spacers from Simplex and Palacos. *Am J Orthop (Belle Mead NJ).* 1998 Mar;27(3):201–205.
27. **Holtom PD, Patzakis MJ.** Newer methods of antimicrobial delivery for bone and joint infections. *Instr Course Lect.* 2003;52:745–749.
28. **Torholm C, Lidgren L, Lindberg L, et al.** Total hip joint arthroplasty with gentamicin-impregnated cement. A clinical study of gentamicin excretion kinetics. *Clin Orthop.* 1983 Dec;(181):99–106.
29. **Adams K, Couch L, Cierny G, et al.** In vitro and in vivo evaluation of antibiotic diffusion from antibiotic-impregnated polymethylmethacrylate beads. *Clinical orthopaedics and related research.*1992 May;(278):244–252.
30. **Ostermann PA, Seligson D, Henry SL.** Local antibiotic therapy for severe open fractures. A review of 1085 consecutive cases. *J Bone Joint Surg Br.* 1995 Jan;77(1):93–97.
31. **Keating JF, Blachut PA, O'Brien PJ, et al.** Reamed nailing of open tibial fractures: does the antibiotic bead pouch reduce the deep infection rate? *J Orthop Trauma.*1996; 10(5):298–303.
32. **Tetsworth K, Cierny G, 3rd.** Osteomyelitis debridement techniques. *Clin Orthop Relat Res.*1999 Mar;(360):87–96.
33. **Swiontkowski MF.** Criteria for bone debridement in massive lower limb trauma. *Clinical orthopaedics and related research.*1989 Jun;(243):41–47.
34. **Bhandari M, Adili A, Schemitsch EH.** The efficacy of low-pressure lavage with different irrigating solutions to remove adherent bacteria from bone. *J Bone Joint Surg Am.* 2001 Mar;83-A(3):412–419.
35. **Owens BD, White DW, Wenke JC.** Comparison of irrigation solutions and devices in a contaminated musculoskeletal wound survival model. *J Bone Joint Surg Am.* 2009 Jan;91(1):92–98.
36. **Bhandari M, Adili A, Lachowski RJ.** High pressure pulsatile lavage of contaminated human tibiae: an in vitro study. *J Orthop Trauma.* 1998 Sep-Oct;12(7):479–484.

37. **Dirschl DR, Duff GP, Dahners LE, et al.** High pressure pulsatile lavage irrigation of intraarticular fractures: effects on fracture healing. *J Orthop Trauma.* 1998 Sep-Oct;12(7):460–463.
38. **Anglen JO.** Comparison of soap and antibiotic solutions for irrigation of lower-limb open fracture wounds. A prospective, randomized study. *J Bone Joint Surg Am.* 2005 Jul;87(7):1415–1422.
39. **Petrisor B, Sun X, Bhandari M, et al.** Fluid lavage of open wounds (FLOW): a multicenter, blinded, factorial pilot trial comparing alternative irrigating solutions and pressures in patients with open fractures. *J Trauma.* 2011 Sep;71(3):596–606.
40. **Harley BJ, Beaupre LA, Jones CA, et al.** The effect of time to definitive treatment on the rate of nonunion and infection in open fractures. *J Orthop Trauma.* 2002 Aug;16(7):484–490.
41. **Pollak AN, Jones AL, Castillo RC, et al.** The relationship between time to surgical debridement and incidence of infection after open high-energy lower extremity trauma. *J Bone Joint Surg Am.* 2010 Jan;92(1):7–15.
42. **Schenker ML, Yannascoli S, Baldwin KD, et al.** Does timing to operative debridement affect infectious complications in open long-bone fractures? A systematic review. *J Bone Joint Surg Am.* 2012 Jun;94(12):1057–1064.
43. **Skaggs DL, Friend L, Alman B, et al.** The effect of surgical delay on acute infection following 554 open fractures in children. *J Bone Joint Surg Am.* 2005 Jan;87(1):8–12.
44. **Weitz-Marshall AD, Bosse MJ.** Timing of closure of open fractures. *J Am Acad Orthop Surg.* 2002 Nov;10(6):379–384.
45. **Patzakis MJ.** Clostridial myonecrosis. *Instr Course Lect.* 1990;39:491–493.
46. **Patzakis MJ, Dorr LD, Hammond W, et al.** The effect of antibiotics, primary and secondary closure on clostridial contaminated open fracture wounds in rats. *J Trauma.* 1978 Jan;18(1):34–37.
47. **DeLong WG, Jr., Born CT, Wei SY, et al.** Aggressive treatment of 119 open fracture wounds. *J Trauma.*1999 Jun;46(6):1049–1054.
48. **Jenkinson RJ, Kiss A, Johnson S, et al.** Delayed wound closure increases deep-infection rate associated with lower-grade open fractures: a propensity-matched cohort study. *J Bone Joint Surg Am.* 2014 Mar;96(5):380–386.
49. **Hohmann E, Tetsworth K, Radziejowski MJ, et al.** Comparison of delayed and primary wound closure in the treatment of open tibial fractures. *Arch Orthop Trauma Surg.* 2007; 127(2):131–136.
50. **Patzakis MJ, Wilkins J, Moore TM.** Considerations in reducing the infection rate in open tibial fractures. *Clin Orthop Relat Res.* 1983 Sep;(178):36–41.
51. **Stannard JP, Volgas DA, Stewart R, et al.** Negative pressure wound therapy after severe open fractures: a prospective randomized study. *J Orthop Trauma.* 2009 Sep;23(8):552–557.
52. **Shepherd LE, Costigan WM, Gardocki RJ, et al.** Local or free muscle flaps and unreamed interlocked nails for open tibial fractures. *Clin Orthop Relat Res.*1998 May;(350):90–96.
53. **Yaremchuk MJ.** Acute management of severe soft-tissue damage accompanying open fractures of the lower extremity. *Clin Plast Surg.* 1986 Oct;13(4):621–632.
54. **Gopal S, Majumder S, Batchelor AG, et al.** Fix and flap: the radical orthopaedic and plastic treatment of severe open fractures of the tibia. *J Bone Joint Surg Br.* 2000 Sep; 82(7):959–966.
55. **Pollak AN, McCarthy ML, Burgess AR.** Short-term wound complications after application of flaps for coverage of traumatic soft-tissue defects about the tibia. The Lower Extremity Assessment Project (LEAP) Study Group. *J Bone Joint Surg Am.* 2000 Dec; 82-A(12):1681–1691.
56. **Cierny G, 3rd, Byrd HS, Jones RE.** Primary versus delayed soft tissue coverage for severe open tibial fractures. A comparison of results. *Clin Orthop Relat Res.* 1983 Sep;(178):54–63.
57. **Godina M.** Early microsurgical reconstruction of complex trauma of the extremities. *Plast Reconstr Surg.*1986 Sep;78(3):285–292.
58. **Worlock P, Slack R, Harvey L, et al.** The prevention of infection in open fractures: an experimental study of the effect of fracture stability. *Injury.* 1994 Jan;25(1):31–38.
59. **Henley MB, Chapman JR, Agel J, et al.** Treatment of type II, IIIA, and IIIB open fractures of the tibial shaft: a prospective comparison of unreamed interlocking intramedullary nails and half-pin external fixators. *J Orthop Trauma.*1998 Jan;12(1):1–7.
60. **Tornetta P, 3rd, Bergman M, Watnik N, et al.** Treatment of grade-IIIb open tibial fractures. A prospective randomised comparison of external fixation and non-reamed locked nailing. *J Bone Joint Surg Br.* 1994 Jan;76(1):13–19.
61. **Brumback RJ, Ellison PS, Jr., Poka A, et al**. Intramedullary nailing of open fractures of the femoral shaft. *J Bone Joint Surg Am.*1989 Oct;71(9):1324–1331.
62. **Schemitsch EH, Kowalski MJ, Swiontkowski MF, et al.** Comparison of the effect of reamed and unreamed locked intramedullary nailing on blood flow in the callus and strength of union following fracture of the sheep tibia. *J Orthop Res.*1995 May;13(3):382–389.
63. **Schemitsch EH, Kowalski MJ, Swiontkowski MF, et al.** Cortical bone blood flow in reamed and unreamed locked intramedullary nailing: a fractured tibia model in sheep. *J Orthop Trauma.*1994 Oct;8(5):373–382.
64. **Keating JF, O'Brien PJ, Blachut PA, et al.** Locking intramedullary nailing with and without reaming for open fractures of the tibial shaft. A prospective, randomized study. *J Bone Joint Surg Am.*1997 Mar;79(3):334–341.
65. **Finkemeier CG, Schmidt AH, Kyle RF, et al.** A prospective, randomized study of intramedullary nails inserted with and without reaming for the treatment of open and closed fractures of the tibial shaft. *J Orthop Trauma.* 2000 Mar-Apr;14(3):187–193.
66. **Bhandari M, Guyatt G, Tornetta P, 3rd, et al.** Randomized trial of reamed and unreamed intramedullary nailing of tibial shaft fractures. *J Bone Joint Surg Am.* 2008 Dec;90(12):2567–2578.
67. **Roberts CS, Pape HC, Jones AL, et al.** Damage control orthopaedics: evolving concepts in the treatment of patients who have sustained orthopaedic trauma. *Instr Course Lect.* 2005;54: 447–462.
68. **Pape HC, Tornetta P, 3rd, Tarkin I, et al.** Timing of fracture fixation in multitrauma patients: the role of early total care and damage control surgery. *J Am Acad Orthop Surg.* 2009 Sep;17(9):541–549.
69. **Edwards CC, Simmons SC, Browner BD, et al.** Severe open tibial fractures. Results treating 202 injuries with external fixation. *Clin Orthop Relat Res.*1988 May;(230):98–115.
70. **Behrens F, Searls K.** External fixation of the tibia. Basic concepts and prospective evaluation. *J Bone Joint Surg Br.* 1986 Mar;68(2):246–254.
71. **Marsh JL, Nepola JV, Wuest TK, et al.** Unilateral external fixation until healing with the dynamic axial fixator for severe open tibial fractures. *J Orthop Trauma.*1991;5(3):341–348.
72. **Bhandari M, Guyatt GH, Swiontkowski MF, et al.** Treatment of open fractures of the shaft of the tibia. *J Bone Joint Surg Br.* 2001 Jan;83(1):62–68.
73. **McGraw JM, Lim EV.** Treatment of open tibial-shaft fractures. External fixation and secondary intramedullary nailing. *J Bone Joint Surg Am.* 1988 Jul;70(6):900–911.

74. **Blachut PA, Meek RN, O'Brien PJ.** External fixation and delayed intramedullary nailing of open fractures of the tibial shaft. A sequential protocol. *J Bone Joint Surg Am.* 1990 Jun;72(5):729–735.
75. **Scalea TM, Boswell SA, Scott JD, et al.** External fixation as a bridge to intramedullary nailing for patients with multiple injuries and with femur fractures: damage control orthopedics. *J Trauma.* 2000 Apr;48(4):613–621; discussion 621–613.
76. **Sirkin M, Sanders R, DiPasquale T, et al.** A staged protocol for soft tissue management in the treatment of complex pilon fractures. *J Orthop Trauma.* 1999 Feb;13(2):78–84.
77. **Tornetta P, 3rd, Weiner L, Bergman M, et al.** Pilon fractures: treatment with combined internal and external fixation. *J Orthop Trauma.* 1993;7(6):489–496.
78. **Watson JT.** High-energy fractures of the tibial plateau. *Orthop Clin North Am.* 1994 Oct;25(4):723–752.
79. **Benirschke SK, Agnew SG, Mayo KA, et al.** Immediate internal fixation of open, complex tibial plateau fractures: treatment by a standard protocol. *J Orthop Trauma.* 1992;6(1):78–86.
80. **Kregor PJ, Stannard JA, Zlowodzki M, et al.** Treatment of distal femur fractures using the less invasive stabilization system: surgical experience and early clinical results in 103 fractures. *J Orthop Trauma.* 2004 Sep;18(8):509–520.
81. **Stannard JP, Wilson TC, Volgas DA, et al.** The less invasive stabilization system in the treatment of complex fractures of the tibial plateau: short-term results. *J Orthop Trauma.* 2004 Sep;18(8):552–558.
82. **Moed BR, Kellam JF, Foster RJ, et al.** Immediate internal fixation of open fractures of the diaphysis of the forearm. *J Bone Joint Surg Am.* 1986 Sep;68(7):1008–1017.
83. **Vander Griend R, Tomasin J, Ward EF.** Open reduction and internal fixation of humeral shaft fractures. Results using AO plating techniques. *J Bone Joint Surg Am.* 1986 Mar;68(3):430–433.
84. **Georgiadis GM, Behrens FF, Joyce MJ, et al.** Open tibial fractures with severe soft-tissue loss. Limb salvage compared with below-the-knee amputation. *J Bone Joint Surg Am.*1993 Oct;75(10):1431–1441.
85. **Hansen ST, Jr.** The type-IIIC tibial fracture. Salvage or amputation. *J Bone Joint Surg Am.* 1987 Jul;69(6):799–800.
86. **Bosse MJ, MacKenzie EJ, Kellam JF, et al.** An analysis of outcomes of reconstruction or amputation after leg-threatening injuries. *The New England journal of medicine.* 2002 Dec; 347(24):1924–1931.
87. **MacKenzie EJ, Bosse MJ.** Factors influencing outcome following limb-threatening lower limb trauma: lessons learned from the Lower Extremity Assessment Project (LEAP). *J Am Acad Orthop Surg.* 2006;14(10 Spec No.):S205–210. Review.
88. **MacKenzie EJ, Bosse MJ, Pollak AN, et al.** Long-term persistence of disability following severe lower-limb trauma. Results of a seven-year follow-up. *J Bone Joint Surg Am.* 2005 Aug;87(8):1801–1809.
89. **Bosse MJ, McCarthy ML, Jones AL, et al.** The insensate foot following severe lower extremity trauma: an indication for amputation? *J Bone Joint Surg Am.* 2005 Dec;87(12):2601–2608.
90. **Johansen K, Daines M, Howey T, et al.** Objective criteria accurately predict amputation following lower extremity trauma. *J Trauma.* 1990 May;30(5):568–572; discussion 572–563.
91. **Bosse MJ, MacKenzie EJ, Kellam JF, et al.** A prospective evaluation of the clinical utility of the lower-extremity injury-severity scores. *The Journal of bone and joint surgery American volume.* 2001 Jan;83-A(1):3–14.
92. **Tornetta P, 3rd, Olson SA.** Amputation versus limb salvage. *Instr Course Lect.* 1997; 46:511–518.

9.1 Infection after fracture

Martin A McNally

1 Basics

Successful fracture care involves the prevention and treatment of complications which may arise during the fracturehealing period. Infection remains a serious problem after fracture, particularly with the increasing use of internal fixation. The attempted salvage of previously untreatable open limb injuries with bone loss, severe contamination, and major soft-tissue defects has provided a new group of patients with challenging infections and infected nonunions.

Our concepts of implant-related infection are changing with a better understanding of the complex interactions between microorganisms, implant surfaces, and host immunity. We are now familiar with the "biofilm approach" to the management of infection after prosthetic joint implantation [1–3]. In infection after fracture, treatment concepts are more varied and less well defined. Most studies report small cohorts with a single treatment modality. It is difficult to compare treatments and to define strategies for any specific patient group. However, the principles of eradication of infection after fracture have many similarities to the treatment of prosthetic joint infection. The decisions around retention or removal of an implant, the management of the soft tissues and the provision of local and systemic antimicrobial therapy are common to both clinical situations.

1.1 Etiology and incidence

It is rare for a nonoperatively treated closed fracture to become infected. Most infection after fracture occurs after an open injury or after internal fixation. Thus, infection after fracture is mainly exogenous with contamination occurring at the time of injury or during surgical intervention. This offers an important opportunity to prevent infection with appropriate early wound debridement, stabilization, and prophylactic antibiotics (see chapter 4 Prevention of intraoperative infection and chapter 8 Open fractures).

Occasionally, a fracture infection may develop long after fracture fixation and healing, as a result of hematogenous spread in a bacteremic patient. This should be suspected in those with a compromised immune system who present with a painful healed fracture that was previously pain free.

The incidence of infection after fracture is dependent on the severity of the bony lesion, the damage to the soft-tissue envelope, and the Gustilo-Anderson type [4]. In open fractures, infection occurs uncommonly in Gustilo-Anderson type I fractures at 0–2% but rises to 2–10% for type II, and to 10–50% for type III injuries [5]. Open fractures of the tibia are twice as likely to become infected as similar grade injuries to other bones [6].

Fractures of the pelvic ring can have high rates of deep infection, either as a result of open injuries with contamination or complicating the method of fixation. Posterior fixation of sacral and type C unstable fractures carry a 10% deep infection risk [7]. Overall, pelvic ring fractures have a 7% risk (2–11%) regardless of the method of treatment [8]. When a pelvic external fixator is used, the reported pin infection rates vary from 2.5% to 50% [8, 9]. Pin-site infection may have serious consequences with pin loosening and loss of fracture reduction.

Acetabular fractures are usually closed injuries but around 3–9% will suffer deep infection after treatment [10]. This rate may be higher in open injuries and in those with severe closed internal degloving of the soft tissues (ie, Morel-Lavallé lesion) [11]. The use of postoperative irradiation to reduce the incidence of heterotopic ossification may also increase the infection rate [12]. Deep infection after acetabular fracture will result in hip joint destruction in over half of cases with requirement for major staged reconstruction or amputation [10, 13].

Infection rates may also be high in fractures involving the foot. This high risk of infection may be related to reduced blood supply in diabetic patients and those with peripheral vascular disease, or to the prevalence of crush injuries to the soft tissues which often accompany foot fractures. Open injuries have the highest likelihood of developing an infection. In one series of 36 open calcaneal fractures treated with internal fixation, 60% of those with fracture comminution (type III fractures) were complicated by osteomyelitis [14]. Other studies have confirmed the high infection rates in open fractures. Even with early aggressive debridement, soft-tissue reconstruction and immediate antibiotics, an incidence of around 4–19% can be expected [15, 16]. The infection risk is most closely related to the degree of soft-tissue injury [16].

Local factors around the fracture are important but it has also been shown that the general health of the patient contributes to infection risk and outcome from treatment of established infection. The presence of one or two medical comorbidities increases the risk of infection in open fractures by almost three times while three or more comorbidities increase the risk by five to six times [17]. Tobacco smoking alone significantly increases infection rate and time to union in open tibial fractures [18].

1.2 Pathogenesis

Fractures are normally infected by bacteria living in highly organized colonies, attached to the surface of implants, fragments of dead bone, or poorly vascularized soft tissues. Bacteria in the planktonic state are quickly recognized by the host immune defences. In this state, they are metabolically active and can be eradicated by cellular or humoral host responses in the extracellular space. Most antibiotics which act on protein synthesis pathways or nuclear division are active against planktonic bacteria.

With exposure of bone in an open fracture or during operative fixation, the surface is initially contaminated by bacteria which rapidly adhere to the surface by a series of complex interactions, involving bacterial cell wall proteins known as adhesins. Within a short period, the bacteria secrete a polysaccharide extracellular matrix (glycocalyx) in which they can survive with reduced metabolic activity (stationary state) [19, 20]. This complex structure of bacterial colonies in polysaccharide is known as "biofilm" (see chapter 1 Implant-associated biofilm). Within biofilms, bacteria have increased organism to organism signaling (quorum sensing) which facilitates further development of the biofilm. They can also break free (emigration) and travel elsewhere or between segments of the biofilm, enhancing interactions and altering bacterial behavior [21].

The presence of foreign material in the tissues greatly increases the risk of clinical infection and reduces the inoculum required to create an infection [20]. There is also evidence that metal implants may cause alteration of the normal host immune cell response, with impaired granulocyte function on the surface of implants and inhibition of T-cell activation and plasma cell function [21].

This potent combination of isolation within the biofilm, very low metabolic activity, and impaired host immune response, allows bacteria to evade eradication and become much more resistant to antimicrobial therapy [20, 23]. It has also been shown that some organisms (particularly *Staphylococcus aureus*) can invade host cells and survive inside osteoblasts. This may be one cause of later recurrence of infection, long after treatment [24].

It is important to understand that most fracture implant infections occur with bacteria in biofilms [2, 20], so curative treatment of these must involve removal of the biofilm. The mechanisms described above mean that established fracture infections are very unlikely to be eradicated with antibiotics alone [25].

1.3 Histopathology

The histological features of infection after fracture are characterized by the presence of bone necrosis with surrounding inflammatory response. Bone death may be a result of the initial injury, the surgical approach to fixation, or thermal injury due to drilling and reaming with blunt or high-speed drills [26]. The infection can also kill bone by secreted toxins, thrombosis of nutrient vessels and by cortical bone stripping due to subperiosteal abscess formation.

Dead bone which remains in continuity with the living bone (such as an exposed tip of cortex at the end of a diaphyseal fracture fragment) can be revascularized by creeping substitution if it does not become infected. Once bacteria are adherent to the dead bone; the dead bone will either be separated from the living diaphysis, forming a sequestrum or will be resorbed by macrophage activity. A loose dead fracture fragment cannot be revascularized. It may be shed out of the limb through a sinus or may become encased in new bone formation (ie, involucrum) (**Fig 9.1-1**). Generally, this new bone is well vascularized and is resistant to colonization by bacteria. It will only form if there is living periosteum over the infected area.

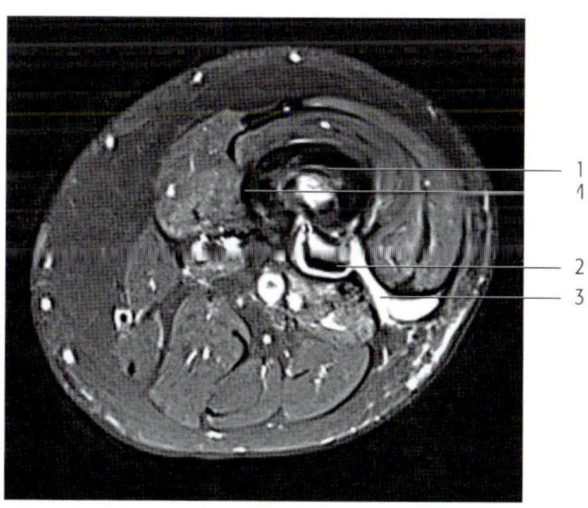

Fig 9.1-1 This magnetic resonance imaging scan shows all of the pathological features of osteomyelitis after intramedullary nailing of a femoral fracture. There is central dead bone lining the medullary canal (**1**), a separate cortical sequestrum (**2**), a sinus track extending to the skin surface (**3**), and periosteal new bone formation around the femur (**4**).

1.4 Classification of infection after fracture

Defining subgroups within a disease or condition is only useful if this adds to our understanding of the condition or helps to suggest methods of treatment for each subgroup.

The current classifications have been developed mostly around long bone osteomyelitis [27] and prosthetic joint infection [28]. These have significant omissions and limitations. For example, the most frequently used classification, Cierny-Mader [27], makes no reference to the soft tissues or to the microbiology of the infection. The only study attempting to classify the soft-tissue elements was published in 1977, before the main advances in plastic surgical cover of infected bone and soft-tissue defects [29]. A recent attempt to produce a more comprehensive classification of all bone and joint infections has collated seven features of the patients and the infection [30].

Classification based on the timing of the onset (presentation) of the infection is a useful concept. Infections after fracture can be divided into "early" (onset within 2 weeks of fracture), "delayed" (onset between 3–10 weeks after fracture), and "late" (onset more than 10 weeks after fracture) [25, 31] (**Table 9.1-1**). The rapid diagnosis of an early infection can be prevented by inappropriate empiric use of antibiotics in the first few weeks after fracture, delaying the onset of symptoms and signs.

The speed at which an infection presents after injury or fixation can be greatly affected by soft-tissue cover. Infection following fixation of superficial bones (eg, olecranon, lateral malleolus, patella) will often present rapidly with obvious skin breakdown or wound leakage in a well patient. Deep infection around an intramedullary nail or plate fixation of the proximal femur may present later after a period of increasing pain. The patient may exhibit systemic symptoms of fever or malaise but the surgical wound may appear well healed with few local signs of infection.

It is important to distinguish between an early acute infection and a later chronic infection. In acute infection, there may be limited amounts of dead bone and the initial fracture fixation may be stable. This situation can be treated promptly, without complex procedures, and in many cases will result in a good outcome with a healed fracture. In chronic infection, the presence of microorganisms for a prolonged period will be associated with established biofilm, dead tissue, and often fracture instability with fixation failure. This is a major complication which will require expert treatment in all cases to achieve union without persistent infection [25].

Initial presentation	Clinical features	Microbiology	Treatment principle
Early Up to 2 weeks after fracture or internal fixation	• Local pain, erythema, swelling, poor wound healing, systemic symptoms	• Virulent organisms • *S aureus* • Gram-negative bacilli • Group A streptococci	• Rapid diagnosis • Salvage of stable fixation before failure • Debridement with attention to soft tissues • Targeted antimicrobial therapy
Delayed 3–10 weeks after fracture or internal fixation	• Insidious onset of symptoms • Persistent pain • Impaired bone healing • Early loosening of implants	• Low-virulence organisms • Coagulase-negative staphylococci, skin flora	• Individual treatment needed • May involve exchange of fixation, major bony resection, soft-tissue reconstruction, and prolonged antibiotic treatment
Late More than 10 weeks after fracture or internal fixation	(**a**) Acute symptoms due to new hematogenous infection of an implant (rare) (**b**) Chronic symptoms with pain, instability, wound breakdown, and sinus formation	(**a**) *S aureus* and *Escheria coli* (**b**) Often polymicrobial. May be the result of poorly treated early or delayed infection producing resistant strains.	• Depends on degree of fracture healing

Table 9.1-1 Classification of infection after fracture, by timing of initial presentation.

1.4.1 Cierny-Mader classification

The Cierny-Mader classification of osteomyelitis [27] describes two essential components of bone infection which are relevant to infected fractures. First, the localization of the dead or infected bone, and second, the medical state of the patient. It is predominantly useful in chronic infections.

The contribution of the health of the patient cannot be overemphasized in the management of infected fractures. The Cierny-Mader classification divided patients into three groups depending on physiological health. Group A patients have no medical conditions which would impair the normal response to stress, trauma or infection, or wound healing. Group B patients have comorbidities which either affect the local conditions in the limb (preventing adequate wound healing) or affect the general health of the individual. Group C patients may be either too frail to undergo definitive treatment or may have few symptoms from the infection, thereby making extensive surgery unlikely to result in an improvement in quality of life.

In infected fractures, it is common to find young healthy individuals with severe open injuries (Group B with local compromise) or elderly patients with multiple comorbidities including peripheral vascular disease and diabetes mellitus (Group B with systemic and local compromise). In contrast to chronic hematogenous osteomyelitis, there are very few infected fractures which are asymptomatic and can be left untreated.

In a study of 1,651 patients with chronic infection treated with limb salvage protocols, Cierny and DiPasquale [33] showed that infection was eradicated in 96% of Group A hosts but only 73% of compromised Group B hosts. This highlights the need to fully assess the patient and to optimize general health, prior to beginning treatment. **Table 9.1-2** lists some of the conditions which can interfere with normal wound healing and the response to surgery.

The other element of the Cierny-Mader classification is the anatomical localization of the infection within the bone. They described four distinct patterns of bone involvement.

Local factors in the limb (B^L host)	Systemic factors (B^S host)
Arterial ischemia	Malnutrition
Venous insufficiency	Diabetes
Previous surgery	Smoking
Deep vein thrombosis	IV drug abuse
Lymphoedema	Bleeding diathesis
Radiation fibrosis	Hypoxia
Tissue scarring	Renal/liver failure
Retained foreign material/implants	Immunosuppression
Osteoporosis	Malignancy
Compartment syndrome	Sickle cell disease
Obesity	Drug inhibitors*
	Mental illness

Table 9.1-2 Conditions which impact the outcome of treatment of osteomyelitis by affecting wound healing.
Abbreviations: B^L, host with local comprise in the limb; B^S, host with systemic compromise; IV, intravenous.
*Eg, steroids, cytotoxic drugs, disease-modifying antirheumatic drugs, which may inhibit wound healing or produce immune compromise.

In type I, medullary osteomyelitis, the dead bone is confined to the medullary canal and endosteum (**Fig 9.1-2**, **Fig 9.1-3**). There may be significant areas of dead cancellous bone but the whole circumference of the cortex is alive with normal periosteal attachment. The surrounding soft tissues are intact and there is no sinus formation. There may be overlying soft-tissue erythema and edema. This type of infection is rare after trauma as it usually follows hematogenous spread of bacteria to the medullary canal.

In type II, superficial osteomyelitis, the dead bone is produced by a devascularization of the outer surface of the cortical bone. This can follow soft-tissue injury such as a pretibial degloving wound or burn or after bone exposure in the base of a pressure ulcer or area of venous stasis (**Fig 9.1-4**, **Fig 9.1-5**, **Fig 9.1-6**, **Fig 9.1-7**).

In type III, localized osteomyelitis, there is involvement of the cortex and underlying medullary bone. However, this occurs in a stable segment with a region of healthy, living bone bridging across the infected area. This is the most common form of infection in healed fractures with late presentation (**Fig 9.1-8**, **Fig 9.1-9**). The dead bone may be the result of fracture fragments which have lost blood supply during injury or internal fixation and have become buried in callus. It is tempting to assume that infection after intramedullary nailing will be a type I infection and infection after plating will be a type II infection but usually they are both type III.

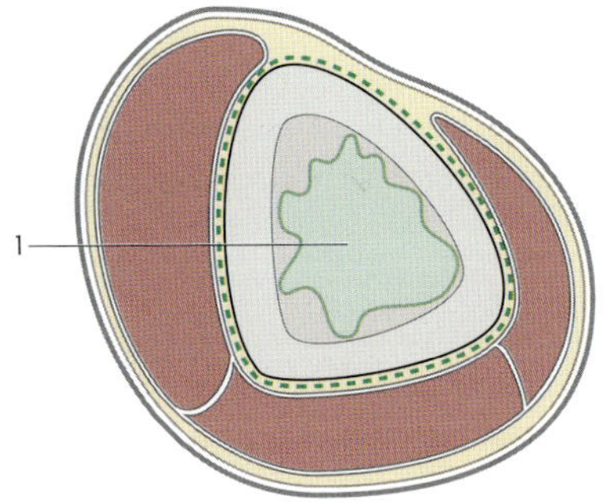

Fig 9.1-2 Cierny-Mader type I: medullary osteomyelitis. The infection (pale green) is confined to the medullary canal (**1**) with no dead cortical bone (grey) and intact periosteum around the bone (green dashed line).

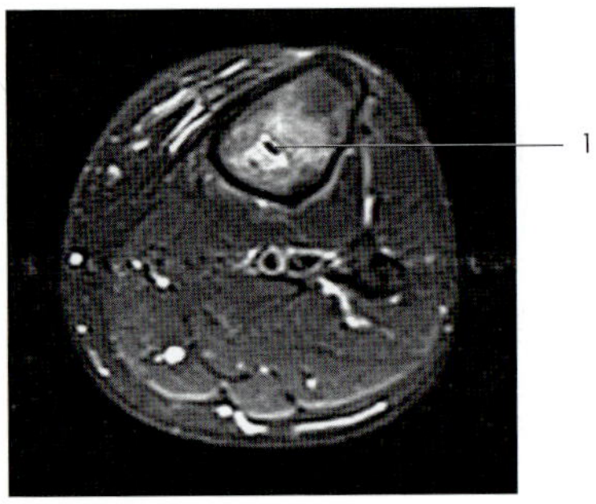

Fig 9.1-3 T1 magnetic resonance image of Cierny-Mader medullary osteomyelitis (type I) showing high signal from the medullary canal but normal cortex and no extension into the soft tissues. There is a central sequestrum (**1**).

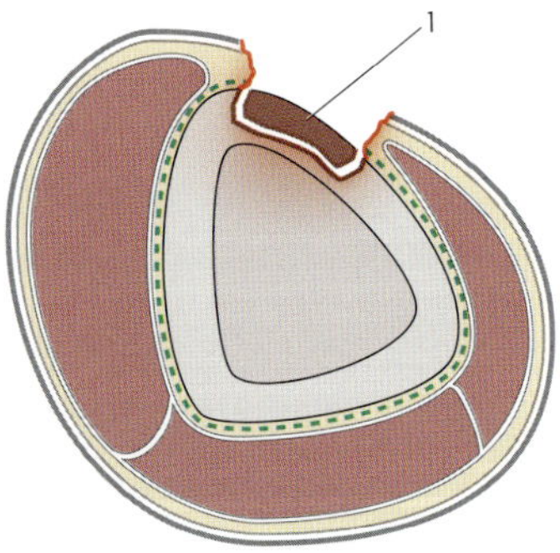

Fig 9.1-4 Cierny-Mader superficial osteomyelitis (type II). The dead bone (brown), (**1**) is confined to the cortex often with a major overlying soft-tissue defect.

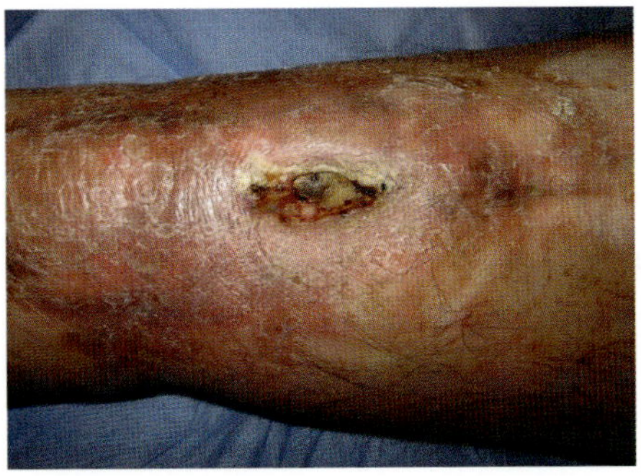

Fig 9.1-5 The sequestrum is easily seen in the middle of a large area of unstable skin from previous skin grafts.

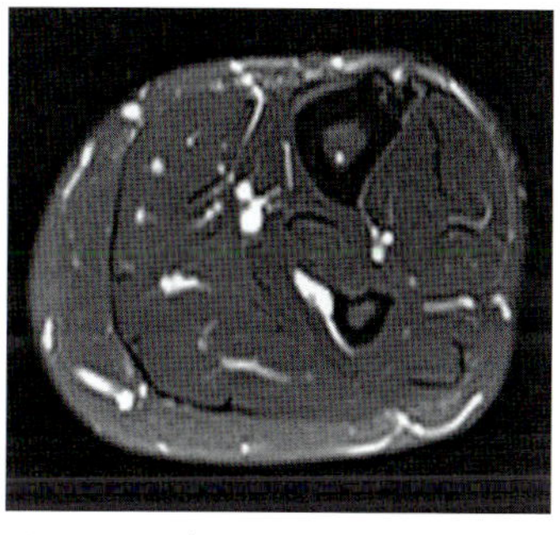

Fig 9.1-6 The magnetic resonance imaging shows the unaffected medullary canal with a normal nutrient artery, but magnetic resonance imaging is often unable to clearly demonstrate dead cortical bone in type II infections.

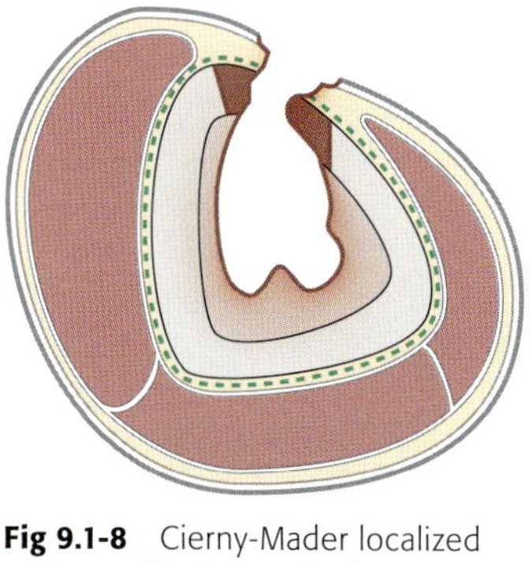

Fig 9.1-8 Cierny-Mader localized osteomyelitis (type III). There is involvement of the medullary and cortical bone, often with extension into the soft-tissues and sinus discharge from the skin.

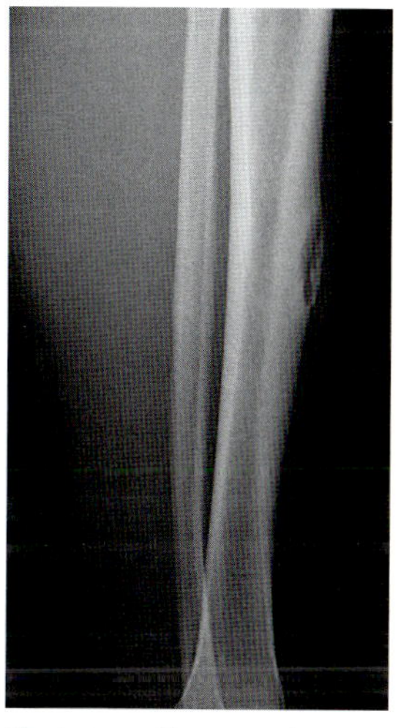

Fig 9.1-7 Cierny-Mader osteomyelitis (type II) with visible cortical sequestrum on the anterior surface of the tibia. Plain x-ray defines the sequestrum well.

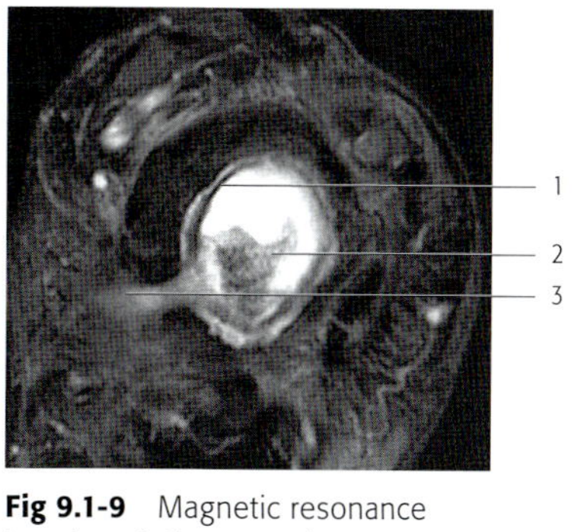

Fig 9.1-9 Magnetic resonance imaging of Cierny-Mader osteomyelitis (type III) of lower tibia after intramedullary nailing. There is obvious endosteal sequestration (**1**) and debris (a cancellous bone sequestrum) (**2**) within the medullary canal. There is a well-formed sinus through the cortex to the skin (**3**).

In type IV, diffuse osteomyelitis, there is segmental involvement with dead cortex and medulla across the entire cross section of the bone. There is often instability and subperiosteal abscess formation, stripping the outer surface of the cortex and producing further cortical bone death (**Fig 9.1-10**, **Fig 9.1-11**). All unhealed, infected fractures and infected nonunions are type IV. In early infections, the zone of bone death will be limited to fracture edges and to devascularized bone fragments but in late presenting cases and established infected nonunions, the infection may have spread throughout the medullary canal and adjacent cortex.

The Cierny-Mader-type infection can be inferred from the history and findings on imaging but should be confirmed during surgery. A type III localized infection may have very little healthy bridging bone. Adequate resection in these cases may produce a segmental defect, converting the case to a type IV.

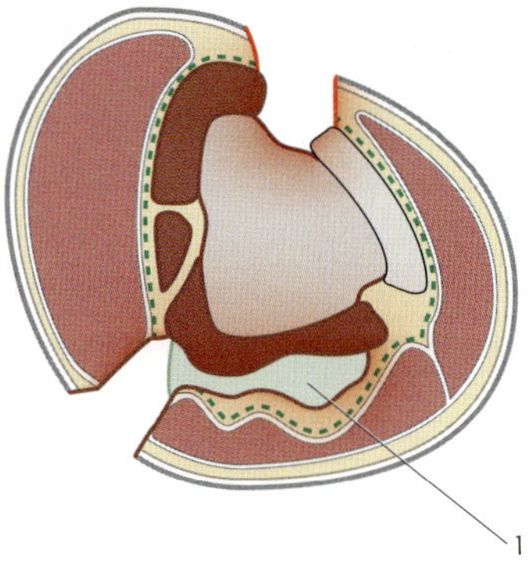

Fig 9.1-10 Cierny-Mader diffuse osteomyelitis (type IV). There is dead cortical and medullary bone (brown) extending across the whole bone diameter. Subperiosteal stripping by abscesses (**1**) cause further bone death and extension of the infection.

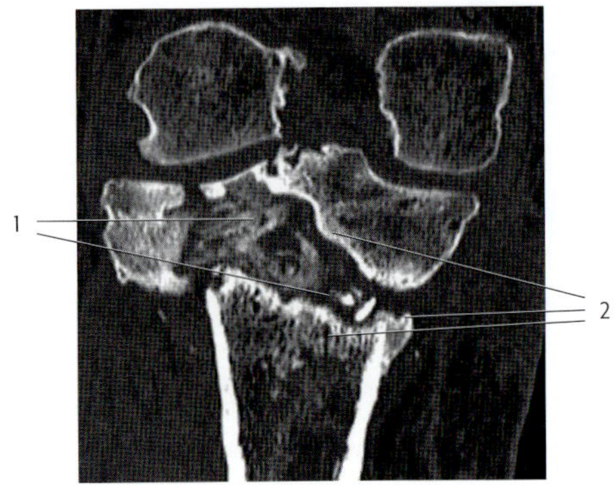

Fig 9.1-11 This computed tomographic scan of an infected Schatzker VI proximal tibial fracture shows the areas of sequestered dead bone (**1**) within new bone formation (**2**) in a Cierny-Mader type IV osteomyelitis.

1.5 Classification by method of fixation

The distribution of dead bone and hence infection in a fracture is determined by the fracture configuration, the method of fixation, and the soft-tissue disruption. In a typical Gustilo-Anderson type IIIB tibial fracture [4] (**Fig 9.1-12**), there will be devitalized ends of the bone from periosteal stripping. If there is fragmentation, some of the fragments may have lost all connection with the soft tissue and will be dead. Others may retain a small periosteal attachment and so will have some potential to resist infection and allow bone healing.

It has been noted that fixation with plates, intramedullary nails and external fixator pins produces distinct patterns of bone necrosis, which are predictable and are helpful in planning excision and reconstruction [26, 32].

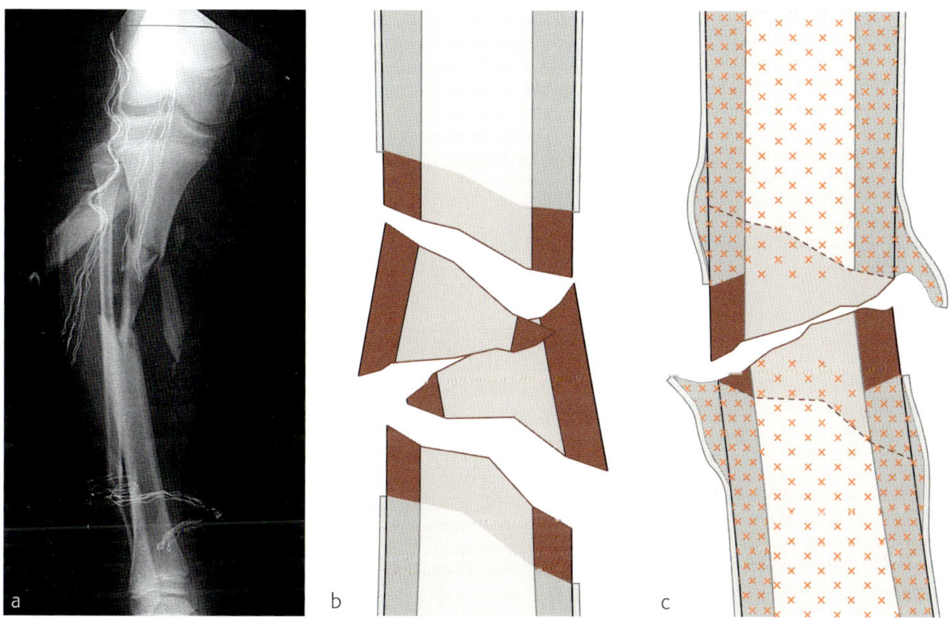

Fig 9.1-12a–c This open diaphyseal fracture has had a degree of periosteal stripping producing areas of poorly perfused or dead bone (central brown bone). Over several weeks, new bone develops in vital regions (crosses) but has not been able to fully revascularize the tips of the central fragments. These dead zones offer a surface for biofilm formation after bacterial colonization. If the patient presents late with an infected nonunion, the location of the dead bone can be predicted from the initial fracture pattern. It can be seen that over time, the main infected bone tends to become centralized within new bone formation [26].

1.5.1 Infection after plate osteosynthesis

A plate can only be placed on the surface of a bone by disrupting the soft-tissue envelope and periosteum covering the bone. Even percutaneous plating through small incisions will cause some periosteal stripping and devascularization of the underlying cortex. With good stability and in the absence of bacteria, small areas of dead cortical bone will be remodeled by creeping substitution. However, when bacteria contaminate the area, there is abundant surface available for colonization and biofilm formation. Infection will spread along implants and become established on dead fragments and on bone surfaces without periosteal cover.

If extensive periosteal stripping has been performed during fracture reduction and fixation, there may be widespread infection, passing around the whole bone with the potential for a segmental osteomyelitis (Cierny-Mader type IV) (**Fig 9.1-13**, **Fig 9.1-14**).

The addition of cerclage wires around plates (or nails) risks segmental cortical devascularization.

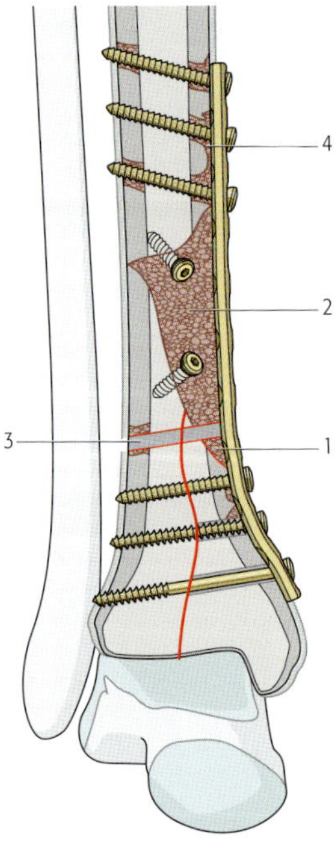

Fig 9.1-13 After plating, infection will develop on areas of dead bone under the plate (**1**), in nonvital fracture fragments (**2**), around empty screw holes (**3**), and in areas of thermal necrosis (**4**).

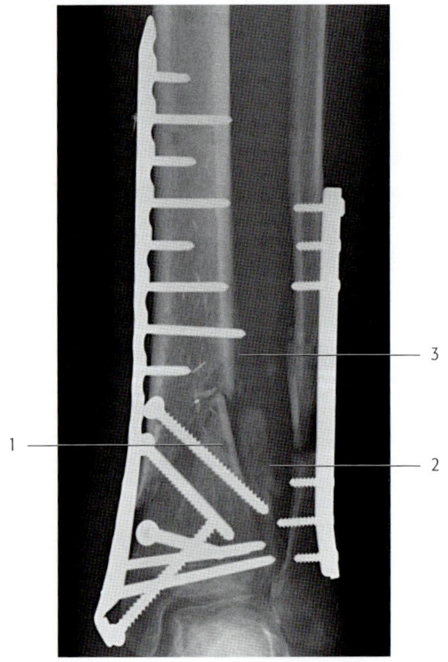

Fig 9.1-14 This poorly fixed tibial fracture demonstrates the devascularization seen after injury and fixation. The lateral side of the distal fragment has been stripped of periosteum (**1**) which has produced new bone away from the surface of the tibia (**2**). The distal tibial cortex shows no bone formation. Conversely, the proximal tibia has abundant periosteal bone formation on the lateral side (**3**).

1.5.2 Infection after intramedullary nailing

Closed reduction and intramedullary nailing limits the extraosseous soft-tissue injury around a fracture but causes new endosteal devascularization. Unreamed and reamed nails both produce endosteal bone death, but this will be increased by overreaming small medullary canals or reaming with blunt reamers, producing thermal necrosis of cortical bone.

Reaming also generates bone debris from the medullary cancellous bone, which is pushed out through the fracture site. Without infection, this may act like an autogenous bone graft and aid fracture healing. When an infection occurs, this collection of tiny dead bone fragments will act as multiple sequestra for bacterial adherence and can form a subperiosteal abscess around the fracture site (**Fig 9.1-15**).

Open reduction, prior to nailing, will have all of the disadvantages of exposure and periosteal stripping together with endosteal cortical necrosis. The presence of the "open" fracture with dead bone increases the risk of deep infection and nonunion.

When an intramedullary nail becomes infected, the bacteria will usually colonize all of the nail and locking screws, and any areas of dead cortical bone adjacent to the nail. Outside the bone, periosteal new bone formation may allow callus bridging and fracture healing, even in the presence of intramedullary nail osteomyelitis.

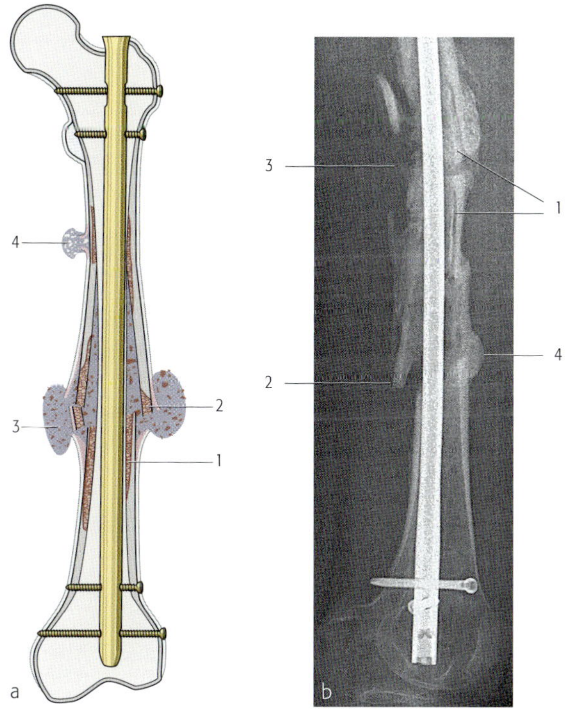

Fig 9.1-15a–b Dead bone is seen centrally around the nail (**1**) and at the fracture site (**2**). Reamings in the fracture hematoma can act as small sequestra in the presence of infection (**3**). Often, an infected fracture will continue to heal with periosteal new bone formed on the healthy exterior of the cortex (**4**).

1.5.3 Infection after external fixation

In general, a correctly applied external fixator allows fracture stabilization without any disturbance of the blood supply around the fracture (beyond that caused by the injury), but infection around external fixator pin sites is common. Extension of pin infection to the fracture site is infrequent if the fixator has been placed with pins outside the zone of injury.

Early infection can start from the time of fixator application due to thermal bone necrosis produced by drilling with blunt drills or high-speed drills. The correct drill size must be used for each pin diameter. During pin placement, an adequate skin incision must be made to avoid crushing the skin edge during drilling or pin passage. Such skin crushing is a potent cause of early pin-site infections (**Fig 9.1-16**).

Late pin infections are usually a result of pin loosening or soft-tissue infections around the pin, allowing ingress of bacteria. In tensioned fine-wire fixators (Ilizarov ring fixators), loss of wire tension during treatment can allow movement at the bone interface and pin osteomyelitis.

It can be seen that it is possible to define the pattern of infection around fractures and to classify groups of patients. Careful investigation of these issues will give the clinician a better understanding of each case before treatment is started. Failure to eradicate infection is often a reflection of a failure to appreciate the pathogenesis of infection in any given patient.

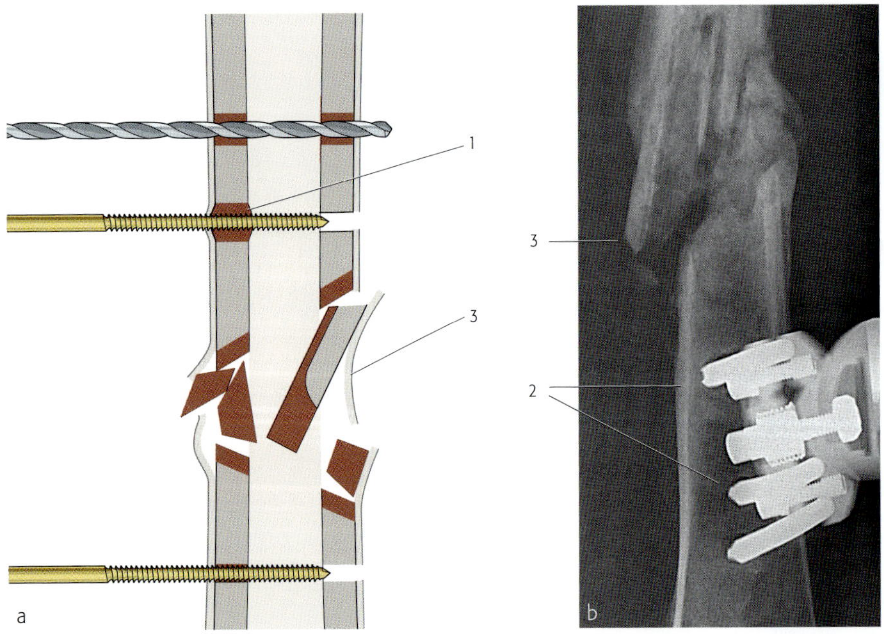

Fig 9.1-16a–b With external fixation, dead bone is seen around the pin sites (**1**) which may provoke pin loosening (**2**), and at the fracture site in nonvital fragments (**3**).

2 Diagnostics

There is no blood test or imaging procedure which will always distinguish an infected fracture from a normal healing fracture or aseptic nonunion. The definitive diagnosis of an infection is made on a group of features (clinical, hematological, microbiological, and imaging). However, the presence of a draining sinus from the fracture site or the laboratory culture of microorganisms from multiple, sterile, deep samples are pathognomonic of an infected fracture.

2.1 Clinical diagnosis

The presence of an infection after a fracture should be suspected when there is local pain, swelling, erythema, or tenderness around the fracture and impaired wound healing. In addition, patients may feel unwell with fever, malaise, anorexia, and tachycardia. There may be a history of recent illness or infection in another body site. Patients with polytrauma who have been treated in intensive care units may have significant respiratory and urinary tract infections which can predispose to early fracture infection.

It can be seen that in the early phase after an injury, the local clinical features of an infection in the limb may be very similar to those of a fracture hematoma or even a deep vein thrombosis. However, if there is increasing acute inflammation around the fracture, an infection should be suspected and early intervention undertaken.

The most important feature in infected fractures is the appearance of the wound. A healthy fracture wound should become dry within a few days and the surrounding redness and swelling of injury and surgery should be gradually improving over 7–10 days. Any deviation from this should raise concern about infection. Wound breakdown with discharge of fluid can represent the release of a fracture hematoma but these cases have a high risk of being infected or developing an infection in the open wound. In all cases, the wound should be addressed surgically (**Fig 9.1-17**).

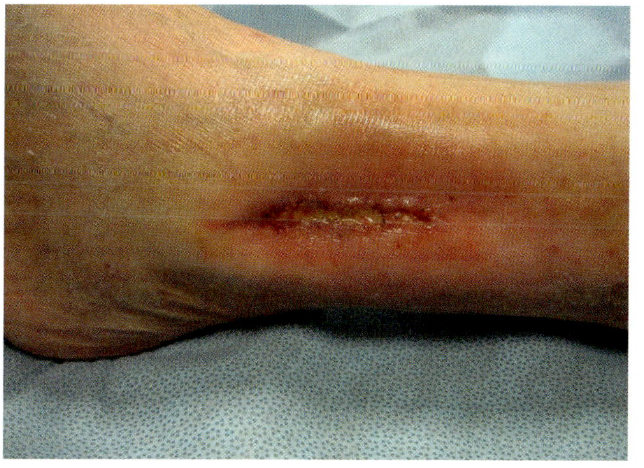

Fig 9.1-17 This patient had internal fixation of a fibular fracture. The wound remained red and swollen with minor leakage of fluid over a 4-week period. This was regularly dressed by a community nurse and was diagnosed as a "superficial wound infection". Oral flucloxacillin was given by the family doctor. At 6 weeks after injury, the wound opened and discharged copious pus. The patient was systemically unwell with pyrexia and malaise. The delay in treating this early fracture infection caused loosening of the fixation plate and prevented an early debridement and retention of the implant with good diagnostic sampling and appropriate antibiotic therapy.

2.2 Laboratory tests

In the first few days after fracture or fixation surgery, the C-reactive protein (CRP) level, white blood cell count, and erythrocyte sedimentation rate (ESR) will all be elevated. Within 1–2 weeks, the CRP should be returning to normal in most individuals so a persistent elevation with a high white blood cell count in a patient with clinical signs of infection can confirm the diagnosis of an early acute infection.

In later presenting cases, a previously normal blood screen may become abnormal but many patients do not develop a significant rise in inflammatory markers. Also, in patients with chronic discharge from an osteomyelitic segment, there may be very little systemic reaction and completely normal blood indices are present [20].

Routine blood culture is not normally diagnostic in infected fractures but when an unwell patient presents with high fever, blood cultures should be taken prior to giving parenteral antibiotics. This culture may be the only opportunity to obtain a microbiological diagnosis in the absence of antimicrobials [25].

2.3 Imaging studies

2.3.1 Plain x-rays

Serial plain radiology may be helpful in identifying areas of progressive bone lysis and loosening around fracture fixation devices (**Fig 9.1-18**). Rapid increase in bone lysis is usually due to infection. It is always important to compare later x-rays with the original fracture film and the immediate postoperative film. See chapter 7 Diagnostics for additional information.

After injury, disuse of the limb will produce increasing osteopenia until full weight bearing is restored. Osteopenia can only develop in bone which is well vascularized. Areas of cortex which remain with increased density (often wrongly described as sclerotic) despite surrounding osteopenia are usually avascular (**Fig 9.1-19**).

Plain x-rays cannot definitively diagnose or exclude infection as many of the signs are not specific to fracture infection.

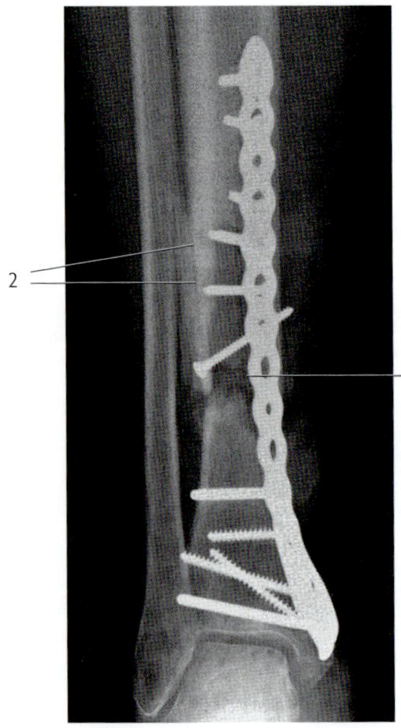

Fig 9.1-18 This infected open tibial fracture developed bone loss under the middle third of the plate and around the edges of the fracture (**1**). The lateral side of the fracture has living bone with good periosteal new bone formation above and below the fracture. The two screws above the fracture show major loosening (**2**) but the other screws have no obvious bone lysis around them. These changes progressed over 10 weeks from the initial injury.

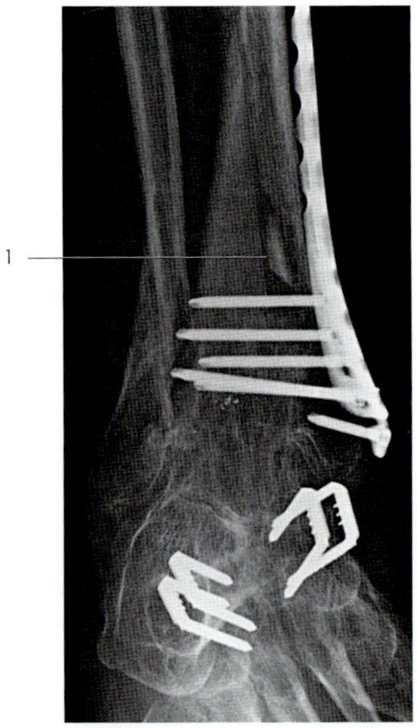

Fig 9.1-19 This open fracture occurred above a previous hindfoot fusion. An early infection developed and was treated by washout and antibiotic suppression. At 12 weeks, the fracture is healing and the surrounding bone is showing the usual osteopenia which occurs after injury. The central devascularized fragment remains without osteopenia (**1**), confirming that it is dead.

2.3.2 Ultrasonography

Ultrasonography is helpful in detecting joint effusions and fluid collections around implants. It may be used to obtain guided aspiration of collections in suspected early infections to distinguish hematoma from infection.

2.3.3 Computed tomography

Computed tomography (CT) is useful in defining the extent of bone necrosis and in planning excision surgery. It is particularly good for demonstrating small sequestra and areas of new bone formation on viable cortex (**Fig 9.1-11**, **Fig 9.1-20a**). It is less good at visualizing the soft tissues with fistulas. The presence of metal implants degrades the CT images but new metal artifact reduction software (MARS) can reduce this problem. With the advent of magnetic resonance imaging (MRI), the use of contrast with CT is rarely indicated.

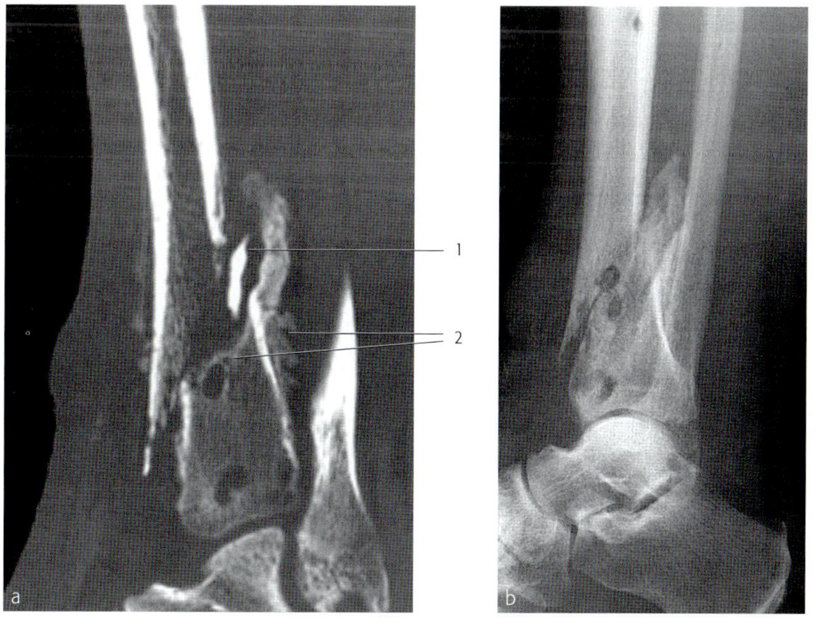

Fig 9.1-20a–b Computed tomography of this infected distal tibial fracture. It shows the large central sequestrum, which is not easily seen on the plain x-ray (**1**). It also shows the areas of healthy periosteum and endosteal new bone formation on the surface of the distal fragment (**2**).

2.3.4 Magnetic resonance imaging

In patients without metal implants, MRI is the imaging modality of choice for the diagnosis of bone infection. It gives excellent visualization of the soft tissues. It demonstrates sequestra (although not as well as CT), cloacae in the cortex, medullary abscesses, periosteal involucrum, and subperiosteal collections (**Fig 9.1-6**, **Fig 9.1-9**, **Fig 9.1-21**, **Fig 9.1-22**). It is not good at distinguishing dead cortex from living bone. Magnetic resonance imaging will also tend to overestimate the extent of bone infection due to edema in the medullary canal and soft tissues. Also, the MRI appearance of infected and uninfected nonunions can be very similar.

2.3.5 Nuclear imaging

A wide range of nuclear scans have been advocated for the diagnosis of bone infections [34], but generally they have little to add in the diagnosis of fracture-related infection. In the early stages after injury, isotope scans are nonspecific and in later cases, MRI with or without CT will give higher resolution imaging. The combination of a nuclear scan with a CT scan may allow improved resolution and better anatomical definition of infection (**Fig 9.1-22**).

In cases presenting with pain at a fracture many months or years after injury, a normal isotope bone scan may reassure the patient that infection is unlikely.

More recently, positron-emission tomography (PET) or PET with CT has been advocated in the diagnosis of infected implants [35]. The administration of radiolabelled glucose (^{18}FDG) with PET and CT can be useful in patients who have had numerous surgical procedures. Glucose is taken up very actively by phagocytes in the infected area and this can be identified by the PET and localized by CT. See chapter 7 Diagnostics for additional information.

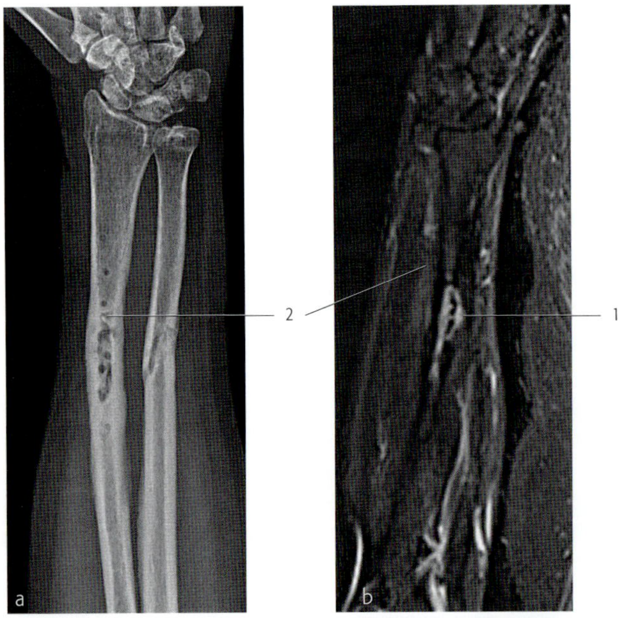

Fig 9.1-21a–b This radial fracture healed after internal fixation despite active infection. Removal of the plate without adequate bone excision allowed osteomyelitis to continue. The magnetic resonance imaging shows the sequestered cortical bone (**1**) and the extent of the medullary involvement. It clearly shows that the distal medulla is normal and that the infection has been limited to the fracture site by the formation of a healthy bar of endosteal new bone (medullary involucrum) (**2**).

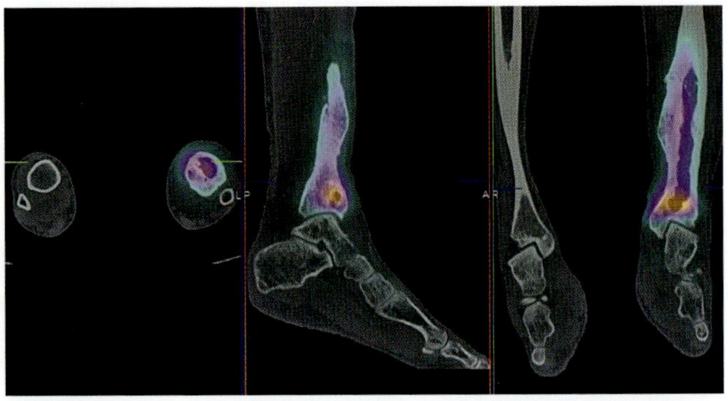

Fig 9.1-22 Single-photon emission computed tomography with superimposed x-ray computed tomography (SPECT/CT) scan of a chronically infected tibial fracture previously treated with an intramedullary nail, showing high uptake in the distal tibia with good localization around a medullary cavitary defect.

2.4 Microbiological diagnosis

Culture of pathogenic organisms from sterile samples taken from around the fracture remains the definitive diagnostic test. This is an essential step to confirm diagnosis and to guide appropriate antimicrobial therapy after surgery.

Superficial swabs should be avoided as they give unrepresentative and misleading microbiological results. Material for culture can be obtained from percutaneous biopsy but deep samples taken at surgery are recommended [25, 36]. Five or six clean, deep samples should be taken from around the infected zone. Each sample should be harvested with a separate instrument to avoid cross-contamination and samples (and instruments) should not touch the patient's skin. Samples for histological assessment should also be taken in parallel with the microbiological tissue [25].

If possible, all biopsies and deep samples should be taken when the patient has been taken off antibiotics for at least 2 weeks to improve the yield of cultured organisms.

Sonication of removed implants has been advocated to disrupt biofilm and improve diagnostic accuracy. This has been evaluated in prosthetic joint infection [37] but has not been shown to increase accuracy of diagnosis in early implant infections [38]. It is valuable in situations where there is little material for sampling. In infected fractures of phalanges or small bones, small tissue samples and removed screws or wires subjected to sonication may give reliable diagnosis.

3 Treatment of infected fractures

Effective treatment of all infected fractures is dependent on several important principles [39]:

- Preoperative:
  - Optimization of the general health of the patient
  - Full discussion of treatment options, potential complications, and realistic outcomes
  - Diagnostic tests for general health and condition of the limb
- Intraoperative:
  - Representative, uncontaminated deep sampling for microbiology and histology
  - Debridement and excision of dead and compromised tissue
  - Bone stabilization (retention or replacement of infected implants)
  - Delivery of antimicrobial therapy after sampling (local and systemic)
  - Management of dead spaces
  - Soft-tissue cover
- Postoperative:
  - Early functional rehabilitation
  - Continued, culture-specific antimicrobial therapy
  - Monitoring for early detection of complications
  - Staged secondary reconstruction for malunion, joint contracture, and nonunion

Delivery of these principles always requires the combined efforts and skills of orthopedic trauma surgeons, infectious disease physicians, radiologists, and plastic surgeons who are focused on the management of bone infections. There may also be patients who need vascular, urological, or other surgical specialties for specific injuries. While the treatment of an acute early infection should be possible in all trauma units, management of more complex infections, chronic infections, and infected nonunions should be done in specialist units with multidisciplinary teams [39, 40]. This approach has been shown to improve patient outcomes [41, 42].

Occasionally, emergency treatment may be needed in patients with severe early onset infection and systemic signs of sepsis (ie, pyrexia, hypotension, tachycardia). In this situation, there is little time to perform a full preoperative workup, but as a minimum, patients should be rehydrated and have blood cultures taken before administration of broad-spectrum intravenous antibiotics. Initial surgery is aimed at obtaining tissue for microbial culture and draining any collections of pus. This urgent intervention can be life or limb saving. It is not appropriate to embark on complex reconstruction in a systemically unwell patient. Wounds can be left open and dressed or managed with a temporary negative-pressure wound closure device for a very short period [43]. Definitive surgery, including wound closure, can then be performed when the patient's general condition improves.

3.1 Acute infection

It should be noted that early, acute infection after an open fracture or internal fixation is usually caused by a virulent organism (**Table 9.1-1**), which will produce rapid tissue destruction, bone loss, failure of fixation, and fracture nonunion. Urgent treatment is needed to salvage the fixation and prevent these sequelae.

There is no place for nonoperative treatment with antibiotics alone. It is widely accepted that fractures can heal in the presence of infection, providing they are stable, have good soft-tissue cover and have effective antimicrobial suppression. The aim of surgery is to reduce the bacterial load, ensure fracture stability, improve soft-tissue cover, and allow antibiotic suppressive therapy to union of the fracture.

All infected fractures presenting early should have a surgical exploration of the wound with collection of deep samples as described above. Abscesses are drained and all dead tissue should be removed, including nonviable fragments of bone. There should be no attempt to keep large dead bone fragments to preserve stability, as this will simply maintain bacterial biofilm and lead to an infected nonunion. If initial bony resection results in a segmental or major bone defect, this can be managed as for infected nonunion (see chapter 9.2 Infected nonunion). If smaller defects are created, these can be treated by secondary bone grafting after a period of antimicrobial therapy.

After resection, broad-spectrum intravenous antibiotics should be given, which will cover the range of causative organisms. In two independent series, the combination of a glycopeptide with an antipseudomonal agent (vancomycin and meropenem) was shown to be the most appropriate empiric regimen [36, 44]. This combination is given for a few days until microbial cultures allow selection of targeted therapy.

An early infection can often be treated with retention of the implant, but this should only be considered if the implant is stable and it is possible to achieve good soft-tissue cover over it [20, 45, 46]. The decision to keep an infected implant is difficult. Retained infected implants will be coated in biofilm, which will potentially allow persistence of organisms after debridement [47]. This problem may be only partly addressed by the use of biofilm-active antibiotics after surgery [48].

Removal of the implant will produce instability and alternative fixation will be required. In complex fracture patterns around joints, it may be very difficult to achieve stability without implant retention. In a series of 97 cases of deep infection following an ankle fracture, it has been shown that early implant removal prior to fracture union is a poor prognostic indicator with an increased risk of permanent complications [49].

Studies of treatment of early infected fractures with implant retention suggest that about 70% of cases will proceed to union [45, 46, 49], but there is often persistent infection after union (29–40%), requiring further surgery and later recurrence is common. In one study, only 49% of patients remained with an infection-free union at 6 months after treatment [46].

Several studies have shown that host comorbidities such as smoking, diabetes, and poor soft tissues after an open fracture are predictive of failure. In Cierny-Mader Group B hosts, infected implants should be removed if there is a reasonable alternative fixation possible.

Intramedullary nailing provides a load-sharing construct with relative fracture stability. With early infection, the stability is often compromised, particularly with unreamed, small diameter nails. There is also the problem of dead bone on the inner surface of the diaphysis (**Fig 9.1-15**) and the dead space inside a hollow nail, which can act as a reservoir for infection [50]. This combination makes it less likely that an infected fracture treated with nail retention will do well [51, 52]. It is therefore recommended that most infected nails should be removed. The canal should be reamed [53] and deep samples sent for culture. The use of the reamer irrigator aspirator (RIA) may be helpful in this situation [54]. The bone can be stabilized by insertion of a new nail, an antibiotic-loaded cement nail, or by application of an external fixator. An experimental study has indicated that there may be some advantage in using a solid titanium nail rather than a hollow steel nail to prevent infection recurrence [50]. Recently, antibiotic-coated nails have been reported in the treatment of infected nonunion of the femur and tibia [55] with a 60% success rate. Their efficacy in early infected fractures is not known.

After debridement, there may be bony defects in the cortex or within the medullary canal. Superficial defects can be filled with healthy soft tissue but deep cavities are more difficult. It is not recommended to use standard bone grafts in acute infection. Defects may be filled with antibiotic-eluting materials, which will reduce the bacterial load. Polymethylmethacrylate (PMMA) beads with gentamicin have been the best studied delivery system [25, 31, 33, 56], but there is now a range of bioabsorbable materials that can elute very high levels of antibiotic around the fracture site [57, 58]. See chapter 6 Local delivery of antibiotics and antiseptics for additional information. These materials include calcium sulphate and calcium sulphate/hydroxyapatite composites which dissolve over a variable period, negating the need for bead removal. However, none of these materials have sufficient mechanical strength to support an unhealed fracture and must be combined with fixation (**Fig 9.1-23**).

The outcome of treatment of an infected fracture is greatly affected by the condition of the soft tissues around the fracture. In the femur, proximal tibia, and humerus, it is usually possible to cover plates and infected fractures with adjacent soft tissues or transposed local muscle flaps. Infected fractures of the olecranon, distal fibula, and tibia are often associated with major open wounds after debridement and will need free microvascular tissue transfer to allow adequate cover for healing. The use of muscle flaps has been shown to improve vascularization around fractures, delivering oxygen, host immune cells, and antimicrobial agents. They are highly resistant to infection and aid elimination of bacteria [25].

In the past, it was common to have serial debridements with open wound treatment over several days or weeks. This approach results in delay of wound healing and does not improve outcome [20] and can lead to superinfection. Soft-tissue cover, including free muscle flap transfer, can safely be performed during the same operation as the initial debridement. If, for practical reasons, it cannot be achieved in this way, temporary occlusive dressings or a negative-pressure wound dressing can be used for a short period. However, negative-pressure wound therapy should not be used as the definitive management for the soft tissues in infected fractures. Negative-pressure wound sponges rapidly become colonized with bacteria and may induce secondary infection and promote antibiotic resistance [43]. In general, definitive wound closure should be achieved within 7 days of debridement or as soon as possible.

Effective management of suspected early infection will often allow retention of a stable implant and culture-guided antimicrobial therapy to fracture union. It is recommended that for a rapidly diagnosed and treated early infection, antibiotic therapy should be continued for 3 months [59] or until fracture union. Once union has occurred, the implant should be removed and any remaining dead bone excised. The resulting bone defect should be managed as for a chronic osteomyelitic cavity (see topic 3.2 of this chapter).

During antibiotic suppressive therapy, the patient must be carefully and regularly reviewed with x-rays and wound inspection. Wound breakdown, systemic upset (eg, pyrexia, tachycardia, anorexia), inability to tolerate antimicrobials, or deterioration on the x-ray, all suggest that suppressive therapy is not working and further intervention will be required. It is not appropriate to continue to watch a fracture with progressive bone loss, infected soft tissues, or a systemically ill patient (**Fig 9.1-24**).

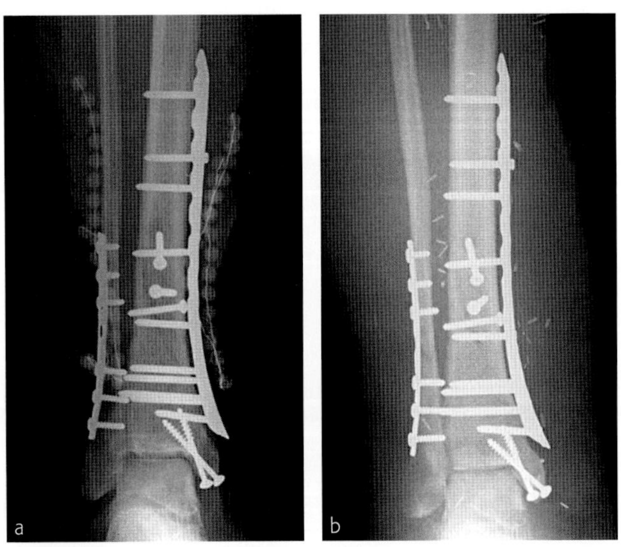

Fig 9.1-23a–b This tibial fracture developed an early infection. It was debrided and deep samples taken which grew *Staphylococcus aureus*. The surgeon retained the metalwork as he believed it was stable.

- **a** The wounds were filled with gentamicin-filled polymethylmethacrylate beads.
- **b** After 10 days the beads were removed and a free muscle flap was used to cover the defect. The patient continued on oral suppressive antibiotics.

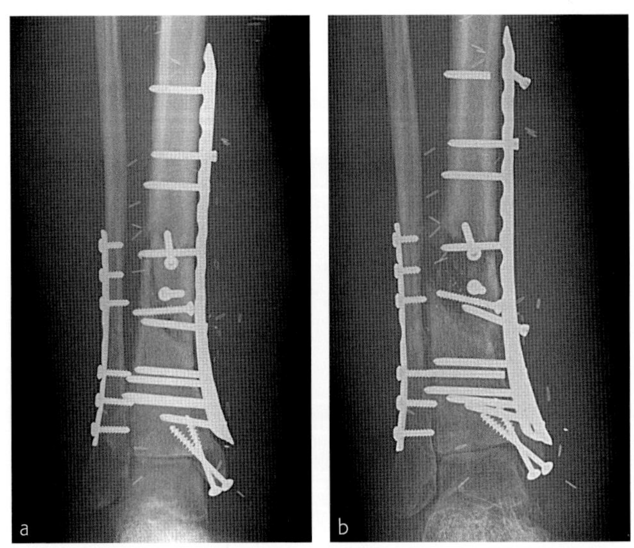

Fig 9.1-24a–b This fracture (as seen in **Fig 9.1-23**) was followed up over 5 months. The patient remained well and the wound was dry. The patient was seen on only two occasions with these x-rays at 2 (**a**) and 5 (**b**) months. The x-rays show progressive bone resorption, loosening of the fixation, and screw breakage, indicating a failure of early management and active infection of the fracture. This required segmental resection and Ilizarov bone transport to secure union.

3.2 Chronic infection

Chronic infection usually presents late in one of two ways. First, an early infection can be missed or treated poorly with antibiotics, allowing the infection to progress and eventually present with a much more developed picture. This will normally appear as a delayed presentation within 10–12 weeks of injury and with an unhealed fracture. Secondly, low-virulence organisms can cause subclinical infection with no early clinical signs. In such a situation, the patient will present with indolent pain or local swelling but rarely with fistulation or systemic ill health. Laboratory investigations are not usually helpful. Late infections may become clear when the fracture fails to unite and the fixation fails.

Diagnostic investigations should focus on establishing if the fracture is healed or not. Plain x-rays and CT scanning are the most useful in this. Occasionally, it is necessary to screen the fracture under image intensification with valgus and varus stress to confirm union.

3.2.1 Delayed presentation

In contrast to early infections, the longer duration of chronic infection allows late cases to develop extensive mature biofilm on implants and dead bone surfaces. Infection can spread into adjacent soft tissues with subperiosteal abscesses and sinus tracks. Intramedullary nails facilitate spread along the medullary canal to locking screw sites. In retrograde femoral nails or in antegrade tibial nails, the knee joint may develop septic arthritis. Metaphyseal plates can infect the adjacent joint. Any previous suboptimal antibiotic therapy may have also produced resistant bacterial strains. The success rate of treatment of late infections is dependent on the duration of the infection [23, 25].

Delay causes disuse osteopenia in the whole bone and localized bone lysis around the fracture and fixation device. This combination means that chronic infections will often have unstable fixation. In general, chronic infections with an unhealed fracture should be treated with removal of the original fixation implant. Replacement with new fixation will be needed if the fracture is not healed and, in most cases, this will involve conversion to an external fixator. While this may be inconvenient for the patient, it offers the best chance of infection-free union without revision surgery [40].

In delayed cases, there is often more extensive soft-tissue involvement and scarring with poor tissue perfusion. This is particularly problematic around the tibia after plating. Early assessment by a plastic surgeon is advised as many cases will need radical skin excision and free flap cover.

Bone excision should also be radical to remove any remnants of necrotic bone and biofilm and to reduce the bacterial load in the wound. This will likely produce significant bone defects which must be filled with living tissue (microvascular flaps) or antibiotic carriers (**Fig 9.1-25**).

The choice of replacement fixation may be difficult. In some infected fractures (eg, proximal humerus, proximal femur, pelvis) external fixation is not always possible and so new internal fixation may be needed. However, the use of internal fixation in active infection is associated with a higher infection recurrence rate and high reoperation rate [55, 40, 60].

Exchange nailing in chronic infections has been advocated but there is no consensus on its use [61]. In a carefully selected group of tibial infections, exchange nailing allowed less than half the fractures to heal without further intervention [62]. This concern has prompted some surgeons to perform staged nailing. In stage one, the infected nail is removed and the canal is reamed and sampled. A temporary antibiotic-loaded PMMA nail is inserted and after 3–4 weeks the PMMA nail is exchanged for an interlocking nail [61, 63].

3.2.2 Late presentation

After several months, an infected fracture will be either healed with an ongoing infection, or is unlikely to progress to healing without intervention, ie, infected nonunion. There is no urgency for treatment. It is more important to fully assess the patient and to correct any general medical conditions prior to surgery. Time is well spent on smoking cessation, improving nutrition, attention to diabetes care, rationalizing drug therapies, and improving vascular status [33, 39, 64]. If the patient is systemically well, antibiotic therapy should be stopped at least 2 weeks before surgery to improve the yield of bacteria in deep-tissue samples [25, 36].

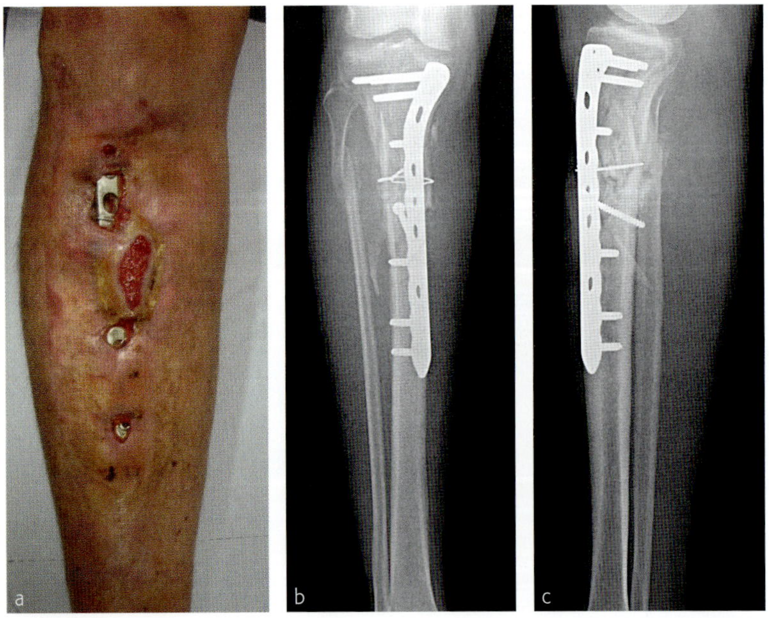

Fig 9.1-25a–c This open tibial fracture occurred after a motorcycle accident. The patient was referred to the Bone Infection Unit at the author's hospital 16 weeks after the injury with infection that had been present since the original injury.
a There was major skin breakdown with exposed metalwork.
b–c The fracture fixation was unstable, with loose fragments of dead bone and posterior involucrum/callus.

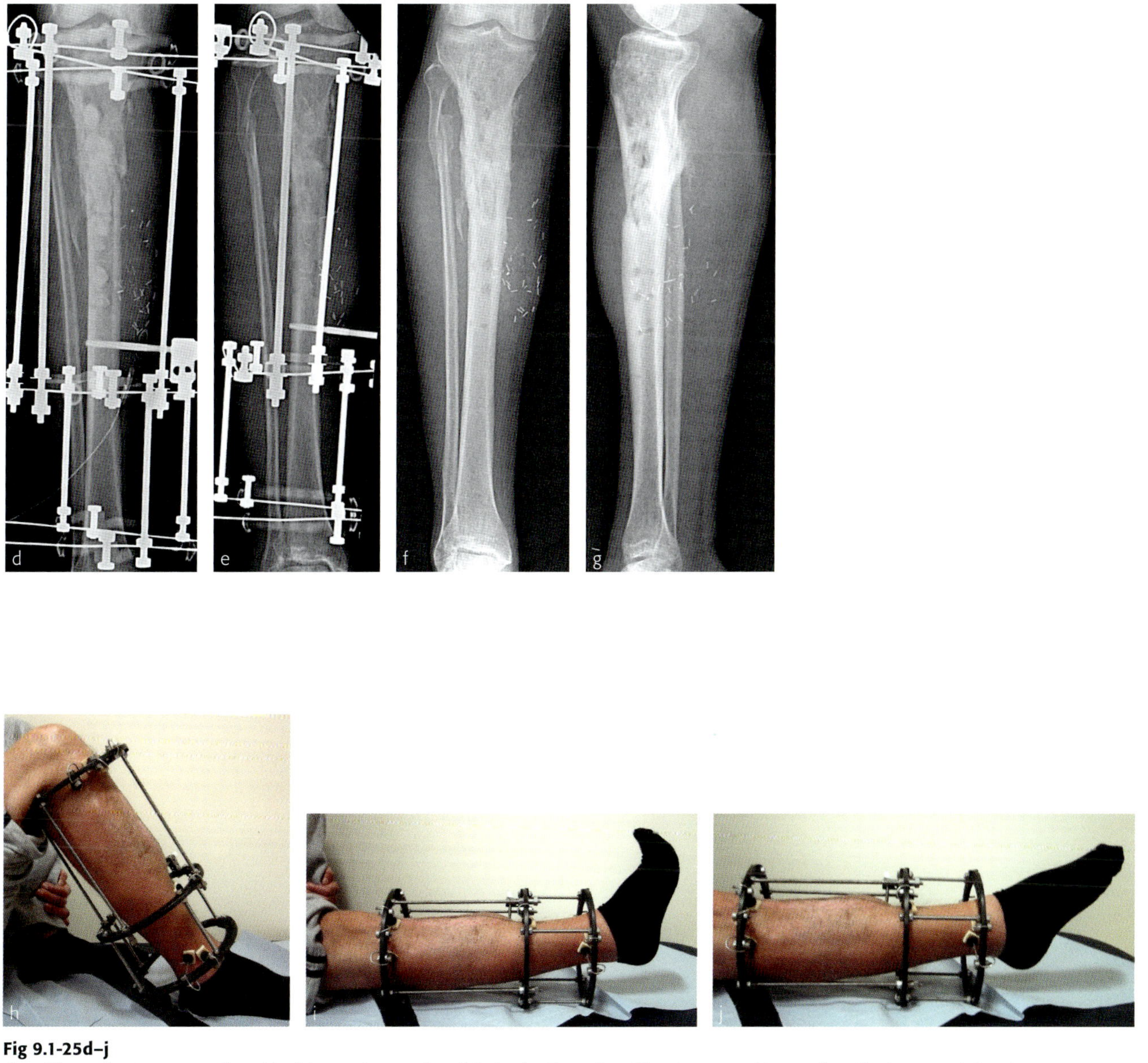

Fig 9.1-25d–j

d The patient was unwell and had been given oral antibiotics for 7 weeks without surgery. At operation, the loose metalwork was removed with several large fragments of necrotic cortical bone. The tibia was stabilized with an Ilizarov fixator and a free latissimus dorsi muscle flap transferred for skin cover. The large bone defect was filled with 20 mL of a calcium sulphate/hydroxyapatite bioabsorbable composite with gentamicin. Deep-tissue samples grew polymicrobial infection with *Staphylococcus aureus, Klebsiella* species and *Proteus* species.

e At 9 weeks, the biocomposite is remodelling and fracture healing is progressing.

f–g The fixator was removed at 13 weeks (29 weeks after injury) and the patient remained with an infection-free limb with bone union 9 months later.

h–j The patient regained excellent return of function in his frame.

Late presentation with a healed fracture

Infected fractures may present after bone healing with residual infection from an early infection. Occasionally, a well-healed, sterile fracture will become infected from a contiguous or remote focus by direct seeding or hematogenous spread. This is usually with a high-virulence organism and will present like acute osteomyelitis.

Patients usually complain of pain, swelling, and systemic symptoms prior to sinus discharge from the fracture or surgical scars. Rarely, a patient may present with a new pathological fracture through the area of infection after fixation removal.

Treatment employs the principles of management for chronic osteomyelitis of any etiology [20, 33, 39]. The implant should be removed and deep samples are taken for microbiology and histology. In these cases, there is always at least Cierny-Mader type III bone involvement with cortical and medullary infection. It is essential to perform an adequate bone resection after implant removal. Under plates, there is typically a layer of dead cortical bone and the screw holes will often contain dead or infected tissue (**Fig 9.1-26**).

After removal of an infected intramedullary nail, the canal should be reamed to at least 1–4 mm greater than the diameter of the nail being removed [61]. It has been suggested that the femur should be reamed to 17 mm (+/- 1.5 mm) and the tibia to 15 mm (+/- 1.5 mm) [53]. However, care should be taken with narrow bones to avoid penetration or fracture or bony necrosis due to thermal injury during reaming.

The canal must be carefully washed of debris. To facilitate this, a cortical window may be created distally. This can be created around the area of the locking screws.

Recurrence of infection after removal of an intramedullary nail is common. This is usually due to inadequate bone excision or failure to manage the medullary dead space. When infection has been present for a prolonged period around an intramedullary nail, it can produce dead bone outside the reach of a central reamer. There may be peripheral dead bone fragments at the fracture site, around locking screw holes, in cortical bone, and in the metaphyseal regions (**Fig 9.1-27**). These areas can only be resected by opening windows over the dead segments. Such areas can be identified by MRI or SPECT/CT after removal of the intramedullary nail.

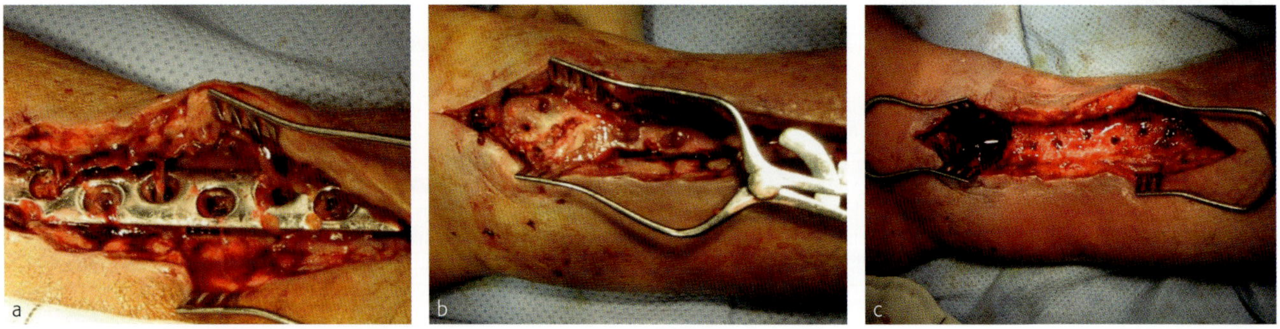

Fig 9.1-26a–c This originally closed tibial fracture was successfully treated with internal fixation. The patient presented late with pain, swelling and erythema.

- **a** The plate was removed and pus drained from the wound.
- **b** Under the plate there is a surface of dead bone and the edges of the fracture site are also dead (compare with **Fig 9.1-13** and **Fig 9.1-14**). The fracture has healed by surrounding callus.
- **c** After plate removal, the dead cortical bone must be removed and the screw holes overdrilled to prevent recurrence of the infection. The distal bone defect was managed with a bioabsorbable, gentamicin-loaded antibiotic carrier. After surgery, deep cultures grew coagulase-negative staphylococci, treated with a short course of oral antibiotics.

After implant removal and bone excision, the resulting bone defect must be managed. If there is a shallow defect on the surface of the bone, this can be filled with the surrounding living tissue. Deep, cavitary defects should not be left unfilled as this predisposes to recurrent infection and fracture [57, 65, 66]. Medullary defects can be filled with antibiotic-loaded PMMA beads or custom antibiotic-loaded PMMA rods [63] but both need to be removed within 4 weeks of implantation. The resulting defect may need second-stage bone grafting to avoid fracture [67].

Defect filling with absorbable calcium sulphate pellets has demonstrated good results in large series but does not promote reliable bone formation [57, 66]. Bioactive glass has been used in infected bone defects with encouraging early results [68]. The use of composite materials which deliver antibiotics and potentially promote bone ingrowth is an interesting recent development [69]. This is important as refracture after treatment of chronic infection has been reported between 3–8% [57].

External fixation pins may develop a characteristic chronic infection that can persist after pin removal. The plain x-ray will show a ring of dead bone, ie, ring sequestrum (**Fig 9.1-28**). This may be naturally expelled from the bone with resolution of the infection but more often needs to be removed and a short course of antibiotics given.

Late presentation with nonunion

Unhealed fractures presenting late after injury (> 3 months) with established infection remain one of the most difficult problems in orthopedic surgery. Close multidisciplinary teamwork is needed with a wide range of surgical skills and microbiological expertise to achieve good outcomes [25, 40, 41, 42]. See chapter 9.2 Infected nonunion.

4 Conclusion

Effective treatment of infected fractures requires an understanding of the etiology and pathogenesis of infection. Surgeons should be aware of the presence of biofilms and consider the anatomical distribution of dead bone around fractures and fixation devices. Treatment protocols must be delivered by multidisciplinary teams and must include the major principles described above. As a minimum, treatment must include optimization of the general health of patients, deep tissue sampling, adequate bony excision, stabilization, dead space management, soft-tissue cover and culture-specific antimicrobial therapy.

5 Acknowledgments

I am grateful to Geert Walenkamp, Peter Ochsner, and the late George Cierny III for developing many of the concepts described in this chapter and which have allowed successful treatment for many patients.

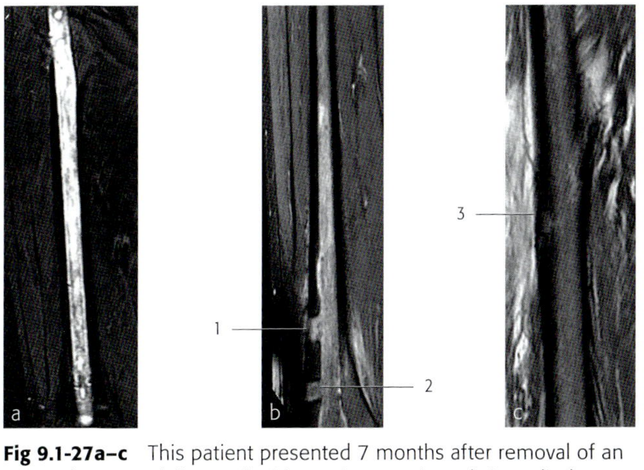

Fig 9.1-27a–c This patient presented 7 months after removal of an infected intramedullary nail with persistent pain and sinus discharge from the distal locking screw scars.
- **a** Magnetic resonance imaging demonstrates the central high signal in the medullary canal.
- **b** The presence of endosteal erosion (**1**) in the distal femur with dead bone around the locking screw holes (**2**).
- **c** An intracortical abscess at the old fracture site (**3**). These areas cannot be resected with medullary reaming alone.

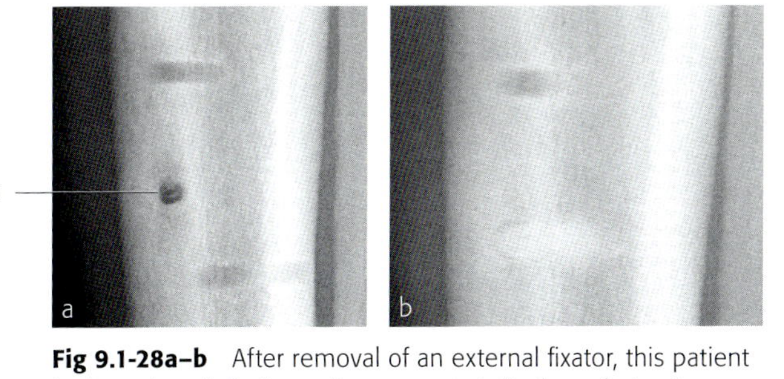

Fig 9.1-28a–b After removal of an external fixator, this patient had continued discharge from a central diaphyseal pin site over several weeks. All of the other pin sites healed without infection.
- **a** Plain x-ray shows a typical ring sequestrum in the midtibia with a central ring of dead bone and surrounding bone resorption (**1**).
- **b** The sequestrum was drilled out and the defect filled with an absorbable biocomposite with gentamicin to avoid fracture or recurrent infection.

6 References

1. **Zimmerli W, Trampuz A, Ochsner PE.** Prosthetic joint infections. *N Engl J Med.* 2004 Oct 14;351(16):1645–1654.
2. **Trampuz A, Osmon DR, Hanssen AD, et al.** Molecular and antibiofilm approaches to prosthetic joint infection. *Clin Orthop Relat Res.* 2003;414:69–88.
3. **Zimmerli W, Moser C.** Pathogenesis and treatment concepts of orthopaedic biofilm infections. *FEMS Immunol Med Microbiol.* 2012 Jul;65(2):158–168.
4. **Gustilo RB, Anderson JT.** Prevention of infection in the treatment of one thousand and twenty-five open fractures of long bones: retrospective and prospective analyses. *J Bone Joint Surg Am.* 1976 Jun; 58:453–458.
5. **Zalavras CG, Marcus RE, Levin SL, et al.** Management of open fractures and subsequent complications. *J Bone Joint Surg Am.* 2007 Apr;89(4):884–895.
6. **Patzakis MJ, Wilkins J.** Factors influencing infection rate in open fracture wounds. *Clin Orthop Relat Res.* 1989 Jun;(243):36–40.
7. **Suzuki T, Hak DJ, Ziran BH, et al.** Outcome and complications of posterior transiliac plating for vertically unstable sacral fractures. *Injury.* 2009 Apr;40(4):405–409.
8. **Papakostidis C, Kanakaris NK, Kontakis G, et al.** Pelvic ring disruptions: treatment modalities and analysis of outcomes. *Int Orthop.* 2009 Apr;33(2):329–338.
9. **Vaidya R, Kubiak EN, Bergin PF, et al.** Complications of anterior subcutaneous internal fixation for unstable pelvis fractures: a multicenter study. *Clin Orthop Relat Res.* 2012 Aug;470(8):2124–2131.
10. **Kim HT, Ahn JM, Hur JO, et al.** Reconstruction of acetabular posterior wall fractures. *Clin Orthop Surg.* 2011 Jun;3(2):114–120.
11. **Hak DJ, Olson SA, Matta JM.** Diagnosis and management of closed internal degloving injuries associated with pelvic and acetabular fractures: the Morel-Lavallée lesion. *J Trauma.* 1997 Jun;42(6):1046–1051.
12. **Haas ML, Kennedy AS, Copeland CC, et al.** Utility of radiation in the prevention of heterotopic ossification following repair of traumatic acetabular fracture. *Int J Radiat Oncol Biol Phys.* 1999 Sep 1;45(2):461–466.
13. **Matta J.** Fractures of the acetabulum: accuracy of reduction and clinical results in patients managed operatively within three weeks after the injury. *J Bone Joint Surg Am.* 1996 Nov;78(11):1632–1645.
14. **Siebert CH, Hansen M, Wolter D.** Follow-up evaluation of open intra-articular fractures of the calcaneus. *Arch Orthop Trauma Surg.* 1998;117(8):442–447.
15. **Berry GK, Stevens DG, Kreder HJ, et al.** Open fractures of the calcaneus: a review of treatment and outcome. *J Orthop Trauma.* 2004 Apr;18(4):202–206.
16. **Heier KA, Infante AF, Walling AK, et al.** Open fractures of the calcaneus: soft-tissue injury determines outcome. *J Bone Joint Surg Am.* 2003 Dec;85-A(12):2276–2282.
17. **Bowen TR, Widmaier JC.** Host classification predicts infection after open fractures. *Clin Orthop Relat Res.* 2005 Apr;(433):205–211.
18. **Castillo RC, Bosse MJ, MacKenzie EJ, et al.** Impact of smoking on fracture healing and risk of complications in limb-threatening open tibia fractures. *J Orthop Trauma.* 2005 Mar;19(3):151–157.
19. **Gristina AG, Costerton JW.** Bacterial adherence and the glycocalyx and their role in musculoskeletal infection. *Orthop Clin North Am.* 1984 Jul;15 (3):517–535.
20. **Trampuz A, Zimmerli W.** Diagnosis and treatment of infections associated with fracture-fixation devices. *Injury.* 2006 May;37 Suppl 2:S59–S66.
21. **Schmidt AH, Swiontkowski MF.** Pathophysiology of infections after internal fixation of fractures. *J Am Acad Orthop Surg.* 2000 Sep–Oct;8(5):285–291.
22. **Watnick P, Kolter R.** Biofilm, city of microbes. *J Bacteriol.* 2000 May;182(10):2675–2679.
23. **Stewart PS, Costerton JW.** Antibiotic resistance of bacteria in biofilms. *Lancet.* 2001 Jul 14;358(9276):135–138.
24. **Bosse MJ, Gruber HE, Ramp WK.** Internalization of bacteria by osteoblasts in a patient with recurrent, long-term osteomyelitis. A case report. *J Bone Joint Surg Am.* 2005 Jun;87(6):1343–1347.
25. **McNally MA, Sendi P.** Implant-Associated Osteomyelitis of Long Bones. In: Zimmerli W, ed. *Bone and Joint Infections: From Microbiology to Diagnostics and Treatment.* John Wiley & Sons, 2015:303–323.
26. **Ochsner PE, Hailemariam S.** Histology of osteosynthesis associated bone infection. *Injury.* 2006 May;37 Suppl 2:S49–S58.
27. **Cierny G, 3rd, Mader JT, Penninck JJ.** A clinical staging system for adult osteomyelitis. *Clin Orthop Relat Res.* 2003 Sep;(414):7–24.
28. **McPherson EJ, Woodson C, Holtom P, et al.** Periprosthetic total hip infection: outcomes using a staging system. *Clin Orthop Relat Res.* 2002 Oct;(403):8–15.
29. **Ger R.** Muscle transposition for treatment and prevention of chronic traumatic osteomyelitis of the tibia. *J Bone Joint Surg Am.* 1977 Sep;59(6):784–791.
30. **Romanò CL, Romanò D, Logoluso N, et al.** Bone and joint infections in adults: a comprehensive classification proposal. *Eur Orthop Traumatol.* 2011 May;1(6):207–217.
31. **Willenegger H, Roth B.** Behandlungstaktik und Spaetergebnisse bei Fruhinfarkt nach Osteosynthese. [Treatment tactics and late results in early infection following osteosynthesis]. *Unfallchirurgie.* 1986 Oct;12(5):241–246. German.
32. **Burri C.** *Post-traumatic osteomyelitis.* Bern Stuttgart Vienna: Hans Huber Publishers; 1975.
33. **Cierny G 3rd, DiPasquale D.** Treatment of chronic infection. *J Am Acad Orthop Surg.* 2006;14(10):S105–110.
34. **Ziran BH, Smith W, Rao N.** Orthopaedic infections and osteomyelitis. In Rockwood CA. Green RW, Buchholz JD, et al, eds. *Rockwood and Green's Fractures in Adults. Vol. 1,* Wolters Kluwer/Lippincott Williams and Wilkins, 7th ed, 2012 624–627.
35. **Schiesser M, Stumpe KD, Trentz O, et al.** Detection of metallic implant-associated infections with FDG PET in patients with trauma: correlation with microbiologic results. *Radiology.* 2003 Feb;226(2):391–398.
36. **Sheehy SH, Atkins BA, Bejon P, et al.** The microbiology of chronic osteomyelitis: prevalence of resistance to common empirical anti-microbial regimens. *J Infect.* 2010;60(5):338–343.
37. **Trampuz A, Piper KE, Jacobson MJ, et al.** Sonication of removed hip and knee prostheses for diagnosis of infection. *N Engl J Med.* 2007 Aug 16;357(7):654–663.
38. **Puig-Verdié L, Alentorn-Geli E, González-Cuevas A, et al.** Implant sonication increases the diagnostic accuracy of infection in patients with delayed, but not early, orthopaedic implant failure. *Bone Joint J.* 2013 Feb;95-B:244–249.
39. **McNally MA and Nagarajah K.** Osteomyelitis. *Orthop Trauma.* 2010;24(6):416–429.
40. **Bose D, Kugan R, Stubbs D, et al.** Management of infected nonunion of the long bones by a multidisciplinary team. *Bone Joint J.* 2015 Jun; 97-B:814–817.

41. **Ziran BH, Rao N, Hall RA.** A dedicated team approach enhances outcomes of osteomyelitis treatment. *Clin Orthop Relat Res.* 2003 Sep;(414):31–36.
42. **Salvana J, Rodner C, Browner BD, et al.** Chronic osteomyelitis: results obtained by an integrated team approach to management. *Conn Med.* 2005 Apr; 69(4):195–202.
43. **Diefenbeck M, Mennenga U, Gückel P, et al.** [Vacuum-assisted closure therapy for the treatment of acute postoperative osteomyelitis]. *Z Orthop Unfall.* 2011 Jun;149(3):336–341. German.
44. **Olesen UK, Juul R, Bonde CT, et al.** A review of forty-five open tibial fractures covered with free flaps. Analysis of complications, microbiology and prognostic factors. *Intern Orthop.* 2015 Jun;39(6):1159–1166.
45. **Berkes M, Obremskey WT, Scannell B, et al.** Maintenance of hardware after early postoperative infection following fracture internal fixation. *J Bone Joint Surg Am.* 2010 Apr;92(4):823–828.
46. **Rightmire E, Zurakowski D, Vrahas M.** Acute infections after fracture repair: management with hardware in place. *Clin Orthop Relat Res.* 2008 Feb;466(2):466–472.
47. **Nishitani K, Sutipornpalangkul W, de Mesy Bentley KL, et al.** Quantifying the natural history of biofilm formation in vivo during the establishment of chronic implant associated Staphylococcus aureus osteomyelitis in mice to identify critical pathogen and host factors. *J Orthop Res.* 2015 Sep;33(9):1311–1319.
48. **Zimmerli W, Widmer AF, Blatter M, et al.** Role of rifampin for treatment of orthopedic implant-related staphylococcal infections: a randomized controlled trial. Foreign-Body Infection (FBI) Study Group. *JAMA.* 1998 May 20;279(19):1537–1541.
49. **Ovaska MT, Mäkinen TJ, Madanat R, et al.** Predictors of poor outcomes following deep infection after internal fixation of ankle fractures. *Injury.* 2013 Jul;44(7): 1002–1006.
50. **Melcher GA, Hauke C, Metzdorf A, et al.** Infection after intramedullary nailing: an experimental investigation on rabbits. *Injury.* 1996; 27 Supp 3:SC23–26.
51. **Makridis KG, Tosounidis T, Giannoudis PV.** Management of infection after intramedullary nailing of long bone fractures: treatment protocols and outcomes. *Open Orthop J.* 2013 Jun;7:219–226.
52. **Al-Mayahi M, Betz M, Müller DA, et al.** Remission rate of implant-related infections following revision surgery after fractures. *Intern Orthop.* 2013 Nov;37(11):2253–2258.
53. **Ochsner PE, Gösele A, Buess P.** The value of intramedullary reaming in the treatment of chronic osteomyelitis of long bones. *Arch Orthop Trauma Surg.* 1990;109(6):341–347.
54. **Zalavras CG, Sirkin M.** Treatment of long bone intramedullary infection using the RIA for removal of infected tissue: indications, method and clinical results. *Injury.* 2010 Nov;41 Suppl 2:S43–47.
55. **Conway J, Mansour J, Kotze K, et al.** Antibiotic cement-coated rods: an effective treatment for infected long bones and prosthetic joint nonunions. *Bone Joint J.* 2014 Oct;96-B(10):1349–1354.
56. **Hanssen AD.** Local antibiotic delivery vehicles in the treatment of musculoskeletal infection. *Clin Orthop Relat Res.* 2005 Aug;(437):91–96.
57. **Ferguson JY, Dudareva M, Riley ND, et al.** The use of a biodegradable antibiotic-loaded calcium sulphate carrier containing tobramycin for the treatment of chronic osteomyelitis: a series of 195 cases. *Bone Joint J.* 2014 Jun;96-B(6):829–836.
58. **Zalavras CG, Patzakls MJ, Holtom P.** Local antibiotic therapy in the treatment of open fractures and osteomyelitis. *Clin Orthop Relat Res.* 2004 Oct;(427):86–93.
59. **Sendi P, Zimmerli W.** Antimicrobial treatment concepts for orthopaedic device-related infection. *Clin Microbiol Infect.* 2012 Dec;18(12):1176–1184.
60. **Prasarn ML, Ahn J, Achor T, et al.** Management of infected femoral nonunions with a single-staged protocol utilizing internal fixation. *Injury.* 2009 Nov;40(11):1220–1225.
61. **Brinker MR, O'Connor DP.** Exchange nailing of ununited fractures. *J Bone Joint Surg Am.* 2007 Jan; 89(1):177–188.
62. **Petrisor B, Anderson S, Court-Brown CM.** Infection after reamed intramedullary nailing of the tibia: a case series review. *J Orthop Trauma.* 2005 Aug;19(7):437–441.
63. **Madanagopal SG, Seligson D, Roberts CS.** The antibiotic cement nail for infection after tibial nailing. *Orthopedics.* 2004 Jul;27(7):709–712.
64. **Lazzarini L, Mader JT, Calhoun JH.** Osteomyelitis in long bones. *J Bone Joint Surg Am.* 2004 Oct;86-A(10):2305–2318.
65. **McKee MD, Li-Bland EA, Wild LM, et al.** A prospective, randomized clinical trial comparing an antibiotic-impregnated bioabsorbable bone substitute with standard antibiotic-impregnated cement beads in the treatment of chronic osteomyelitis and infected nonunion. *J Orthop Trauma.* 2010 Aug;24(8):483–490.
66. **Chang W, Colangeli M, Colangeli S, et al.** Adult osteomyelitis: debridement versus debridement plus Osteoset T pellets. *Acta Orthop Bel.* 2007 Apr;73(2):238–243.
67. **McNally MA, Small JO, Tofighi HG, et al.** Two stage management of chronic osteomyelitis of the long bones. The Belfast Technique. *J Bone Joint Surg Br.* 1993 May;75(3):375–380.
68. **Romanò CL, Logoluso N, Meani E, et al.** A comparative study of the use of bioactive glass S53P4 and antibiotic-loaded calcium sulphate bone substitutes in the treatment of chronic osteomyelitis. *Bone Joint J.* 2014 Jun;96-B:845–850.
69. **McNally MA, Ferguson JY, Lau A et al.** Single-stage treatment of chronic osteomyelitis with a new absorbable, gentamicin-loaded, calcium sulphate / hydroxyapatite biocomposite. A prospective series of 100 cases. *Bone Joint J.* 2016 98-B: 1289–1296.

9.2 Infected nonunion

Johan Lammens, Peter E Ochsner, Martin A McNally

1 Basics

An infected nonunion is defined as a fracture site where the presence of infection compromises healing of the fracture. Nonunion can be said to have occurred whenever no further progression of fracture healing can be observed and the fracture will not heal without intervention. In contrast to aseptic nonunions [1], these criteria for infected nonunion can be met much earlier. In the presence of gross instability, fulminant infection or major bone loss, it can be assumed that no healing will progress even shortly after injury.

There are multiple factors contributing to the development of an infected nonunion (**Table 9.2-1**). The most important are type III open fractures, extensive local soft-tissue damage, severe comminution of the bone, presence of devitalized bone, and initial surgical mismanagement (**Fig 9.2-1**) [2, 3].

The infection may be acute or chronic. As a rule, the infections are exogenous in origin. Hematogenous infection from a distant source is a rare cause of nonunion. Primary contamination of open wounds, insufficient debridement, destructive operative procedures, negative-pressure wound therapy for more than 7 days and too much delayed soft-tissue closure of the fracture sites are the most important factors to favor the development of infection and impaired bone healing.

Patient	Bone	Surgery
Obesity	Open fracture	Inadequate stabilization
Smoking	Fracture type	Excessive osteosynthesis
Drug abuse	Fracture site	Misalignment
Steroid use	Bone defect	Prolonged negative pressure wound therapy
Vascular insufficiency	Soft-tissue deficiency	Additional soft-tissue damage (approach, periosteal stripping)
Immunosuppression	Infection	
Metabolic disorders		
Endocrinological disorders		

Table 9.2-1 Overview of factors with a potential influence on the development and healing of infected nonunion.

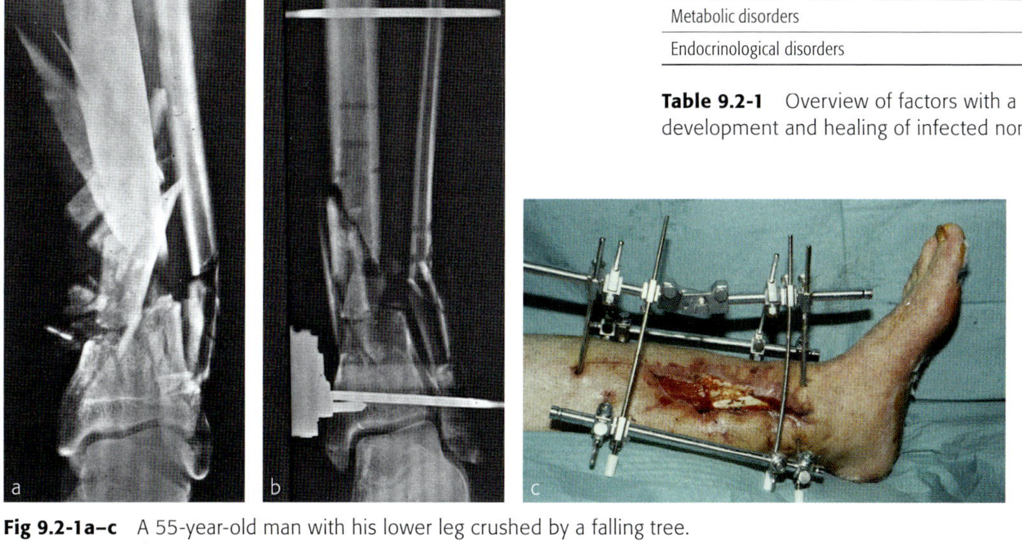

Fig 9.2-1a–c A 55-year-old man with his lower leg crushed by a falling tree.
a AP x-ray shows severe comminution.
b At admission after 3 months the x-ray shows almost no periosteal reaction suggesting that the bone is dead.
c On examination, there is a major soft-tissue defect with visible bone fragments. The fixation is unstable.

The classifications for nonunions without infection are of limited value in the evaluation of infected nonunions [4]. There may be signs of a hyper- or atrophic nonunion on x-ray, but the main indicators for the severity of an infected nonunion are the extent of bone necrosis, the presence of demarcated sequestra (**Fig 9.2-2**) and the virulence of the infection.

Periosteal new bone formation along the bone fragments is an important sign of vitality, whereas its absence after several months indicates that the bone is dead. It may present as a loose fragment surrounded by infected tissue (sequestrum) (**Fig 9.2-3**).

1.1 Classification

As in infected fractures (see topic 1.4 in chapter 9.1 Infection after fracture) it is helpful to subdivide infected nonunions to better understand the components of each case and to plan treatment. The classification of Weber and Cech [4], divides all nonunions (aseptic and septic) into two broad groups: viable and nonviable nonunions. Types A, B, and C are the "viable nonunions" with living bone present on both sides of the unhealed fracture. This is uncommon in established infected nonunions. Types D and E are "nonviable nonunions" with dead bone at one or both ends of the fracture site. Type E have separate dead fragments in the nonunion. Types F and G are also nonviable with bone

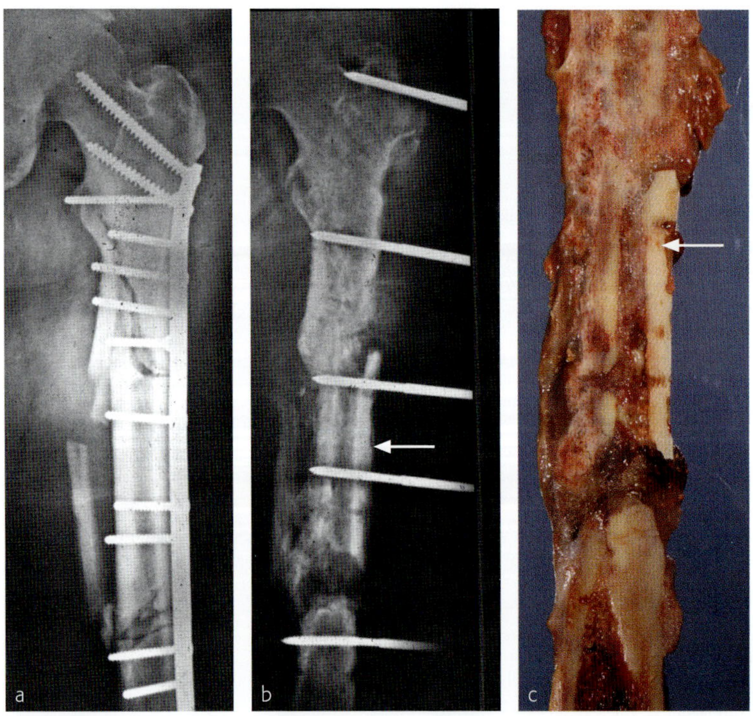

Fig 9.2-2a–c A 55-year-old man injured in a car accident.

a Open segmental femoral fracture, type 32-C2, with plate osteosynthesis changed to external fixation after 9 months because of severe posttraumatic osteomyelitis.

b–c The patient died after 1 year and the femur was examined at post mortem. Periosteal new bone formation is seen mainly on the medial side with partial remodeling of the central segment. There is demarcation of the lateral cortex with extensive granulation tissue and no signs of remodeling or periosteal new bone formation (arrows). Adequate debridement at this time would have required removal of, at least, the lateral part of the central segment (arrows) and all the granulation tissue.

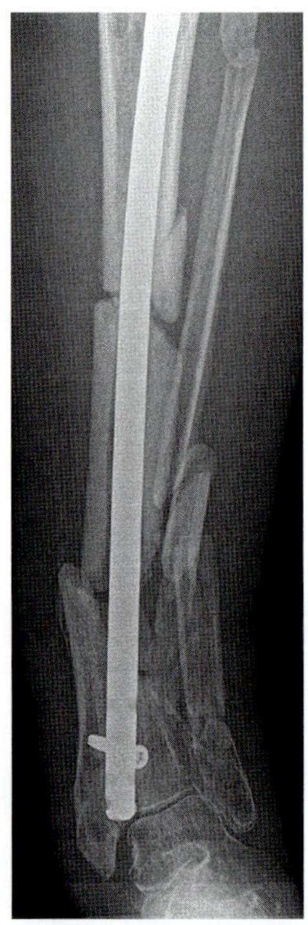

Fig 9.2-3 Infected nonunion of the tibia after intramedullary nailing. The distal fragment is viable with periosteal new bone formation on the medial side. The central and proximal fragments showed no periosteal reaction. The normal osteopenia of disuse is seen in the distal fragment but is absent from the central and proximal regions. There is also intraarticular malposition of the implant in the ankle joint and axial deviation.

gaps. **Fig 9.2-3** shows a typical Weber and Cech Type E infected nonunion with a central, nonviable, loose fragment. This classification is useful because it highlights the importance of identifying areas of dead bone which must be removed if infection is present.

There are many factors which contribute to the development of an infected nonunion and also to the difficulty or ease with which it can be treated. The Non-Union Scoring System (NUSS) proposed by Calori et al [5] (**Table 9.2-2**) includes the essential general and local risk factors contributing to the pathogenesis of a nonunion and allows calculation of a total numerical score for each case. Infection is seen as a single contributing factor in nonunion but is given increased weighting in the score. This NUSS may help in planning the therapy but also allows comparative analyses of infected nonunions [6]. A special "ladder strategy" is described consisting of an algorithm for the choice of treatment based on the severity as expressed by points from 0 to 50. It is suggested that the score be multiplied by two and that patients with a score from 0 to 25 can be treated with simple measures, patients in the 26–75 range will require more specialist treatments, and those over 75 points might be considered for amputation. However, this score and the treatment recommendations have not been well validated in infected cases and some issues are contentious. For example, why adequate stability and anatomical alignment have a negative impact on the total score is not discussed in the paper.

"The site of the infected non-union has a great impact on the choice of the treatment. Epiphyseal-metaphseal nonunions occur in cancellous bone with less tendency to sequestration. The contact surface of the two main fragments is relatively large. Diaphyseal non-unions tend to result in more extensive bone necrosis and sequestration after major trauma."

		Score	Max. score
Bone			
Quality	Good	0	
	Moderate, eg, mildly osteoporotic	1	
	Poor, eg, severe porosis or bone loss	2	
	Very poor (necrotic, appears avascular or septic)	3	3
Primary injury–open or closed fracture	Closed	0	
	Open 1° grade	1	
	Open 2–3° A grade	3	
	Open 3° B–C grade	5	5
Number of previous interventions on this bone to procure healing	None	1	
	< 2	2	
	< 4	3	
	> 4	4	4
Invasiveness of previous interventions	Minimally invasive: closed surgery, eg, screws, K-wires	0	
	Internal intramedullary (nailing)	1	
	Internal extramedullary	2	
	Any osteosynthesis which includes bone grafting	3	3
Adequacy of primary surgery	Inadequate stability	0	
	Adequate stability	1	1
Weber and Cech group	Hypertrophic	1	
	Oligotrophic	3	3
	Atrophic	5	5
Bone alignment	Nonanatomical	0	
	Anatomical	1	1
Bone defect–gap	0.5–1 cm	2	
	1–3 cm	3	
	> 3 cm	5	5
Soft tissues			
Status	Intact	0	
	Previous uneventful minor surgery, minor scarring	2	
	Previous treatment of soft-tissue defect, eg, skin loss, local flap cover, multiple incisions, compartment syndrome, old sinuses	3	
	Previous complex treatment of soft-tissue defect, eg, free flap	4	
	Poor vascularity: absence of distal pulses, poor capillary refill, venous insufficiency	5	
	Presence of actual skin lesion/defect, eg, ulcer, sinus, exposed bone or plate	6	6
Patient			
ASA grade	1 or 2	0	
	3 or 4	1	1
Diabetes	No	0	
	Yes: well controlled (HbA1c < 10)	1	
	Yes: poorly controlled (HbA1c > 10)	2	2
Blood tests	FBC: WCC > 12	1	
	ESR > 20	1	
	CRP > 20	1	3
Clinical infection status	Clean	0	
	Previously infected or suspicion of infection	1	
	Septic	4	4
Drugs	Steroids	1	
	NSAIDs	1	2
Smoking status	No	0	
	Yes	5	5

Table 9.2-2 Non-Union Scoring System (NUSS) according to Calori et al **[5]**.
Abbreviations: ASA, American Society of Anesthesiologists; FBC, full blood count; WCC, white cell count; ESR, erythrocyte sedimentation rate; CRP, C-reactive protein; NSAID, nonsteroidal antiinflammatory drug.

2 Clinical findings and imaging

The diagnosis of an infected nonunion is frequently obvious. An acute infection or a history of local drainage combined with the absence of fracture consolidation confirms the infected nonunion. However, some hypertrophic patterns may be very stiff with little fracture mobility. Clinical examination findings of infected nonunion include limping, use of crutches for the lower extremity due to pain, and impaired mobility of the neighboring joints. Occasionally there will be intermittent fistula formation with drainage, but also complete networks of different fistulae with interconnections may be found.

Laboratory tests rarely give useful information. The erythrocyte sedimentation rate, the C-reactive protein, and the white blood cell count are often normal or only moderately elevated.

Low-grade infections may be difficult to diagnose (see chapter 7 Diagnostics for further information). Without a draining fistula, the only sign may be a progressive osteolysis around the implants. The treating surgeon must be suspicious of any fracture which fails to heal despite adequate stabilization and closed soft tissues. If there was a previous history of an open fracture, a wound which was slow to heal, or other medical conditions (eg, diabetes, smoking, peripheral vascular disease), it should be suspected that low-grade infection is the cause of poor healing and appropriate investigations should be initiated.

Microbiological diagnosis should be established from deep tissue samples only (see chapter 9.1 Infection after fracture). Superficial wound or sinus swabs should not be used as they will culture skin commensals which are not representative of the true infecting pathogen.

2.1 Imaging procedures

The following imaging procedures are essential for the evaluation of a suspected infected nonunion (see chapter 7 Diagnostics for additional information):

- Standard x-rays are the most important basis for diagnosis. In addition to follow-up examinations, recent images in 4 views (AP, lateral, and internal and external oblique) are especially informative. The local condition of the nonunion is of particular interest, namely the extent of an existing bone defect, the periosteal reaction delivering information on the viability of the underlying bone, residual foreign bodies (eg, metal, cement beads), sequestra in the bone (**Fig 9.2-5a**, **9.2-12b**) and soft tissues, etc. Repeated x-rays are also suitable for monitoring the progress of healing.
- Computed tomography, possibly combined with a contrast sinogram is the most sensitive examination method to demonstrate sequestra, but extensive experience is needed to differentiate between minor bone irregularities following complicated bone healing and areas of infected bone necrosis and sequestrum formation. It is also helpful to identify nonintegrated bone substitutes.
- Three-phase and antigranulocyte scintigraphy may help to assess bone viability and to localize infection. A supplemental SPECT/CT provides better anatomical resolution. Nanocolloid can be an alternative [7].
- Magnetic resonance imaging clearly reveals zones of inflammation based on the edema provoked by the local infection but does not always reveal sequestra. It is best for soft-tissue extensions of pus around the bone and can delineate sinus tracts well. It plays a subordinate role in therapeutic decision making.
- Fistulography is particularly useful in the operating room. The fistula is injected with a mixture of methylene blue and x-ray contrast agent. This enables the fistulae to be traced with the image intensifier. During the operation the blue dye can be followed during dissection. The blue trace usually can be followed up to the bone but not inside the bone itself.
- Angiography is essential if there is any doubt about compromised circulation of the limb. After a prolonged period with chronic infection and nonunion, the blood vessels can be difficult to palpate. Angiography should be used to plan a vascularized free flap if the vessels cannot be identified on Doppler ultrasound.

2.2 Assessment of the functional status

Treatment of an infected nonunion may involve potentially very elaborate reconstructions, which may last from a few months to more than one year. Careful evaluation of the general conditions of the limb is mandatory before deciding on any treatment method. In deciding between a reconstruction attempt and amputation the following factors favor limb preservation:

- Foot: intact plantar sensation, no or correctable pes equinus, pain-free ankle joint either mobile or fixed at right angle
- Knee: no severe or painful osteoarthritis, no or correctable malposition (axis or rotation), active, pain-free mobility
- Upper limb nonunion with a well-functioning hand
- Patient who is able and determined to complete a reconstructive program

3 Treatment

Any treatment of an infected nonunion starts with an extensive debridement including harvesting of tissue samples for bacteriology and histology. The cure of infection is the basis for any definitive treatment of the nonunion. In metaphyseal nonunions compression alone is mostly sufficient to achieve bridging. In diaphyseal infected nonunions a hypertrophic nonunion site is rare. Frequently an extensive resection of dead bone is necessary to eliminate infection followed by a complex reconstruction of the bone. Extensive osteoplastic measures are then needed to achieve union with restoration of the normal length of the limb.

3.1 Approach, exploration and debridement

Approach: If possible, choose an approach along an old scar, allowing good access to the whole area to be debrided (**Fig 9.2-4a–b**). If you plan additional approaches think of eventual needs for a decortication and placement of a cancellous bone graft or of a plastic surgeon for connecting free flaps to the remaining vessels.

Exploration: Each operation on an infected nonunion must aim to clarify the condition of the bone and soft tissues. The extent of infection is determined; suitable sites for tissue sampling are identified. Tissue samples from the neighborhood of plates and nails are especially important (**Fig 9.2-4b**). The samples are cut in half sending one part for microbiological studies and the other part for histological examination. At least 3–6 samples should be taken with separate instruments for each sample to avoid cross-contamination. If metal implants or foreign material are present, they can be sent for sonication to culture organisms from biofilm on the material. Empiric antibiotic therapy should be given either immediately after sampling or 10 minutes prior to the release of a tourniquet.

Debridement: This step is mandatory in the treatment of every infected nonunion. The orthopedic implants and dead bone inhibiting bridging of the nonunion should be removed. A reduction of the number of bacteria favors the effectiveness of the immune system and antibiotics. To define the extent of fistulae and abscess cavities and the location of sequestra, a combined injection of a mixture of methylene blue and x-ray contrast agent can be helpful (**Fig 9.2-4b**). Extension of the abscess cavities is seen with the image intensifier and dissection is facilitated. Implants and all foreign bodies including previously inserted material such as gentamicin beads, remnants of bone substitutes or allografts are removed. Dead bone and sequestra, as well as infected membranes along the abscess cavities and fistulae are resected. The elimination of sequestra is relatively easy. They can be recognized preoperatively with standard x-rays or computed tomography and are surrounded by granulation tissue, scars, or pus. Sometimes they are buried in new bone formation in the medullary cavity or within peripheral callus.

It can be difficult to decide the correct extent of bone excision. A clear demarcation between viable and nonviable bone is not always obvious. It is a common error either not to remove all the dead bone or to be too aggressive in the resection of vital bone. In preoperative x-rays, necrotic bone may appear dense with clear cut margins (**Fig 9.2-1**, **Fig 9.2-2**). Bone under remodeling becomes metabolically active and appears osteopenic on x-ray and is covered with a new periosteal bone layer (**Fig 9.2-2**, **Fig 9.2-3**).

A simple and accurate way to demonstrate vitality is the intraoperative evaluation of the bleeding of the bone. Bleeding points can be observed after removal of the granulation tissue. A chisel can be used to remove a thin layer of bone to detect small punctate bleeding points, known as the "paprika sign" (**Fig 9.2-4c**) [8]. Using a chisel allows assessment of the bone quality. Dead bone is often brittle. Debridement can be done with a tourniquet inflated and point bleeding will be seen in vital bone without releasing it. At the end of the bone resection, the tourniquet is removed and the remaining bone observed for bleeding. Often, extensive medullary bleeding will obscure the vision but if any area does not bleed well, further resection is needed. After debridement, the surgical site should be copiously irrigated with a saline solution to reduce the bacterial load. The created defect can be left open or temporarily filled with a antibiotic loaded cement spacer.

Staged debridement: Usually, all removal of infected bone can be achieved in one stage and the operation can then proceed to reconstruction. In situations with extensive bone necrosis or with a systemically unwell patient, it may be better to wait for at least one week between the debridement and the bone and soft-tissue reconstruction. This opens the possibility for a second-look debridement before the reconstructive measures. At the same time one can begin with the definitive antibiotic therapy according to the susceptibility testing of the bacteria. Some surgeons advocate repeated surgical debridement in serious cases but this increases the risk of superinfection and is rarely needed if a careful debridement is performed at the first operation.

3.2 Stabilization

Achieving stability after bone resection is one of the most important components of treatment of an infected nonunion. Stability allows soft-tissue healing, bone bridging, and neoangiogenesis with delivery of antibiotics into the fracture site. Unstable bones will have a high risk of recurrent infection and persistent nonunion.

3.2.1 Temporary stabilization

As a rule, an infected nonunion becomes more unstable after debridement, such that stabilization is necessary. Generally, stabilization is performed with an external fixator. This allows bridging the site of infection without touching the infected focus and minimizing the chance of reinfection.

Occasionally, infected nonunions can be excised and left with a segmental defect. This may be appropriate in midfibular nonunions and infected nonunions of the midfoot, or middle metatarsals.

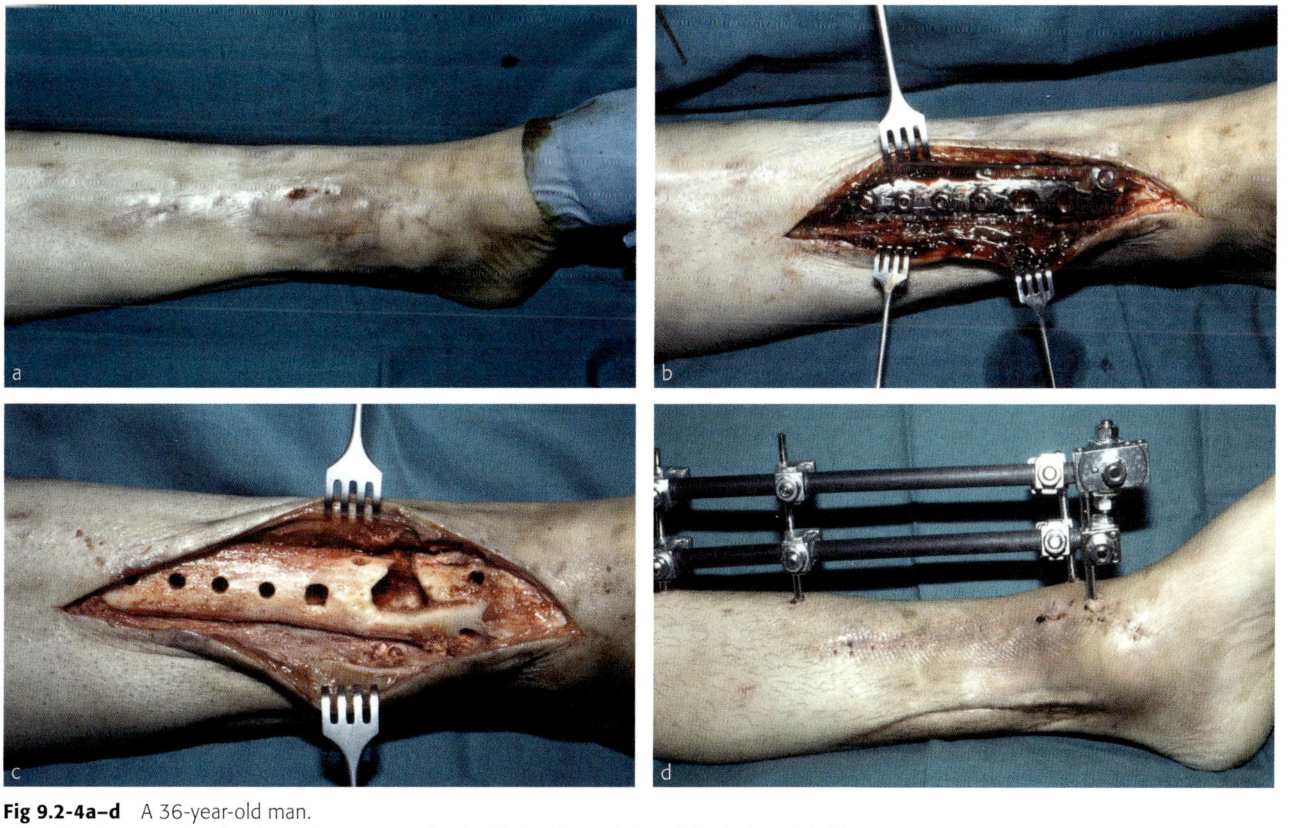

Fig 9.2-4a–d A 36-year-old man.

a Fistula 6 months after lower leg osteosynthesis, filled with methylene blue before debridement.

b The granulation tissue around the plate has been stained blue.

c After debridement.

d Wound healing after a local transposition flap, the denuded posterior area being covered with a mesh graft. The nonunion was stabilized with an external fixator.

3.2.2 Final stabilization

Once the local infection is eradicated, prolonged stabilization must be maintained until the nonunion site is bridged with callus. This can be a time-consuming affair, lasting many months.

3.2.3 External fixation

Definitive stabilization with an external fixation remains the treatment of choice in most centers. If there is to be plastic surgical reconstruction, the placement of the fixator should be discussed with the plastic surgeon prior to operation. A unilateral fixator (**Fig 9.2-4d**) is less bulky than a ring fixator and may give better access for plastic surgery. A ring fixator according to Ilizarov allows successive angular corrections during the application, eg, the correction of a pes equinus. It provides excellent angular and rotational stability and allows early weight bearing. The Ilizarov method of distraction osteogenesis is an essential technique in the management of infected nonunions.

3.2.4 Internal fixation

To combine early weight bearing with minimal inconvenience for the patient, surgeons have considered internal fixation after resection of infected nonunions. This can be performed acutely in the same operation as the debridement or as a second stage after a period of external fixation and antibiotic therapy.

Klemm tested the use of interlocking nails after a radical debridement, mainly local antibiotic treatment and external fixation [9]. He reported union in 89% of femoral infected nonunions but in only 62% of tibias. He concluded that the method was not as safe as external fixation [9]. Later papers compared Ilizarov fixation alone with a fixator exchanged to an interlocking nail as a secondary procedure. Both groups had comparable results but the patients with a change to an intramedullary (IM) nail experienced fewer restrictions [10]. Early conversion to IM nailing may be more cost-effective than completing the treatment with an external device, but risks for reinfection should not be underestimated [11]. A 27% risk for reintervention due to remaining problems of nonunion or recurrence of infection is reported. This may be considered as acceptable in view of the complex problem and the lesser morbidity compared to external fixation devices [12]. The presence of a nail after successful eradication and bone union will reduce the risk of refracture, but most centers would recommend nail removal to reduce infection recurrence risk. More recently, IM nails coated with antibiotic-loaded polymethylmethacrylate (PMMA) cement have been inserted after radical debridement and normalization of the serum parameters for infection (erythrocyte sedimentation rate, C-reactive protein, and white blood cell count) [13]. These may offer some advantages but there is still a substantial risk of recurrence of infection (25–40%) and the need for further surgery.

3.3 Osteoplastic measures

3.3.1 Decortication and cancellous autograft

Decortication

The best place to put autogenous bone graft is in a well-vascularized area. This is the case where there is visible new subperiosteal bone formation. Lifting this bone together with the periosteum and the adjacent muscles with a curved chisel creates a pocket around the nonunion lined on both sides by vital bone lamellae. This gap is filled with cancellous autograft [4] which undergoes quick remodeling in addition creating new bone.

Autogenous bone graft

Fresh autogenous cancellous bone graft brings living osteogenic osteoblasts and osteoinductive bone matrix to the nonunion site. It stimulates the environment to create new bone. A network of woven bone will develop within about 6 weeks linking the two sides of the nonunion. In the presence of adequate stability remodeling of this immature woven bone can begin. Cancellous autograft is the ideal material to add to nonunion sites with small bone defects if debridement of dead infected bone has been successful. Due to the limited quantity of cancellous bone available for reconstruction, segmental defects are limited to a length of about 3–4 cm. Beyond this limit other strategies should be considered. Cancellous autograft is still considered as the gold standard for promoting union and filling smaller defects [14].

Harvesting of cancellous autograft

Cancellous bone graft can mainly be extracted from the posterior and anterior iliac crests. For smaller quantities, the proximal tibia and femur, the distal tibia, and the distal radius can be considered. Milled cortical bone can be harvested in the medullary canal of the femur. Preferably the surgeon should extract the bone graft from the same side where there is the infected nonunion to repair:

- Posterior iliac crest, outer side: This is a good source for cancellous autograft. Place the patient in the lateral decubitus position and drape the receiving leg at the same time as the iliac crest. Use an incision along the iliac crest or an oblique one from cranial medial to distal lateral avoiding trauma to the cluneal nerves and the sciatic nerve. Prepare the outside of the ilium placed over the sacroiliac joint. A cortical window is opened from the iliac crest in distal direction for about 5 x 5 cm. The removed cortical section can be fragmented in small pieces. Underneath you can harvest a great quantity of cancellous bone using curettes, curved bone gouges, and chisels. Cut the bone pieces to the size of a pea and store them in a container covered with a moist gauze. Hemostasis is achieved by placing a collagen sponge. To avoid large blood loss, either do not drain the cavity or use a drain without vacuum. In some indications the patient can remain for the whole intervention in a prone position [15].
- Anterior iliac crest, inner side: The intervention is possible in supine position but the amount of grafts you are able to withdraw is more limited. When doing the approach, take care of the lateral femoral cutaneous nerve. As with the posterior approach, bone graft harvest may be followed by swelling, pain, hematoma, blood loss, and even infection [16].
- Femur: The reamer irrigator aspirator (RIA) method is a novel technique to obtain large amounts of autogenous graft and harvest bone from the inner cortex of the femur or tibia [17]. Large quantities of good quality bone graft may be obtained with proven cell viability equal to iliac crest graft [18]. As orthopedic and trauma surgeons are familiar with the reaming of fractured bones, it provides a familiar and simple technique. However, due to the different equipment and purpose of this reaming procedure attention should be paid to avoid unwanted complications, including fracture [19, 20]. The reamer irrigator aspirator is passed down the medullary canal only once in a pulsatile way, using a reamer of a size 1–4 mm larger than the narrowest portion of the medullary canal. The smallest available diameter is 12 mm, the largest 16.5 mm. A medullary canal with a diameter less than 10 mm or an excessively thin cortex should be considered unsuitable as donor sites. Eccentric reaming should be avoided as the sharp front and lateral cutting flute of the reamer could weaken or perforate the cortex leading to iatrogenic fractures. Because simultaneous irrigation and aspiration is performed during the reaming, high strain on the reamer should be avoided to prevent blockage of the suction device. Continuous aspiration can mask potential blood loss which should be anticipated. With a correct application the technique is safe with a reported morbidity less than 2% [21]. The technique is recommended for more extensive defects and often combined with a pretreatment of the defect with the Masquelet technique as described in topic 3.3.4 of this chapter [22].

Placement of the graft

- Approach: The recipient site is exposed. The fibrotic tissue between the main fragments is carefully resected but the periosteum is preserved as much as possible. The bone ends are exposed and additionally debrided if there are any nonviable areas.
- Where to arrange the graft (**Fig 9.2-5**): The graft should never be placed outside the periosteum where it cannot unite with the underlying bone. Therefore the best preparation for grafting is a decortication, allowing contact with healthy bone under periosteum. The graft should extend at least 2 cm beyond the limit of the defect or the nonunion. Most cancellous graft is packed under the decorticated lamellae. Fragments are also packed around the proximal and distal fragments and in between the bone ends in defect nonunions. After placement, the skin over the grafting site must be closed. If necessary, this may require a plastic surgical procedure with a local or free flap. Skin closure is easier in the lower leg if the graft is placed on the dorsolateral aspect of the tibia or between the tibia and the fibula where you may create a bony bridge.

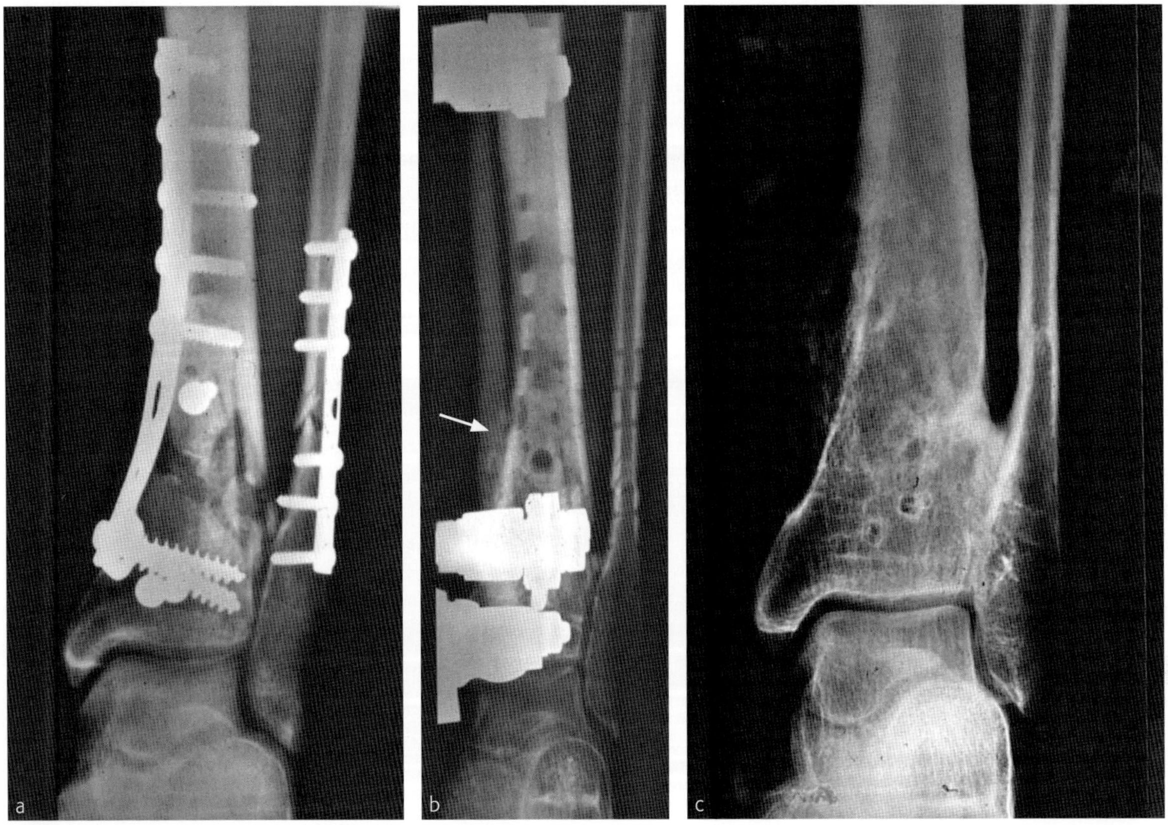

Fig 9.2-5a–c X-rays of the same patient as shown in **Fig 9.2-4**.
a Preoperative condition 5 months after osteosynthesis (see **Fig 9.2-4a**). There are visible sequestra in the nonunion area.
b Bridging autogenous cancellous bone graft (arrow), external fixation for 3 months.
c Ten years after revision: no recurrence, no osteoarthritis.

Papineau technique

Open cancellous bone grafting (Papineau technique), leaving the graft exposed beneath a nonadherent dressing, is an old technique for reconstructing nonunions with limited defects [23]. After debridement, the open wound is protected from superinfection by antiseptic bandages, eg, soaked with polyhexanide. As soon as the bone defect is covered with clean granulation tissue (**Fig 9.2-6a**), the cavity is filled with a surplus of cancellous autograft as a second step (**Fig 9.2-6b**). Wound care is continued with moist antiseptic dressings. Local superinfection is frequent. Superficial cancellous bone pieces will often fail to integrate and must be removed. As soon as the whole surface of the filled defect is covered with granulation tissue, a split-skin graft can be placed [24, 25]. As a modification, negative-pressure wound therapy has been used on top of the graft [26]. Papineau technique is simple and can be performed with limited resources, but it is time-consuming. Usually the remaining scar is unstable and has a tendency to open at intervals with recurrent infection (**Fig 9.2-6d**).

3.3.2 Allograft

Allograft is not a good option to overcome bone defects in the presence of active infection. After a short initial period of osteoinduction the allograft is subject to an immunological antibody reaction destroying the positive initial effect. Mixing allograft with cancellous autograft is contraindicated, often leading to the destruction of the positive effect of the autograft (**Fig 9.2-12c**, **Fig 9.2-13**).

3.3.3 Bone morphogenetic proteins and other substances to replace bone

The use of bone-inducing molecules has clinically been limited to bone morphogenetic protein (BMP)-2 and BMP-7. Both have been analyzed in multicenter studies; one for open fractures and one for nonunions.

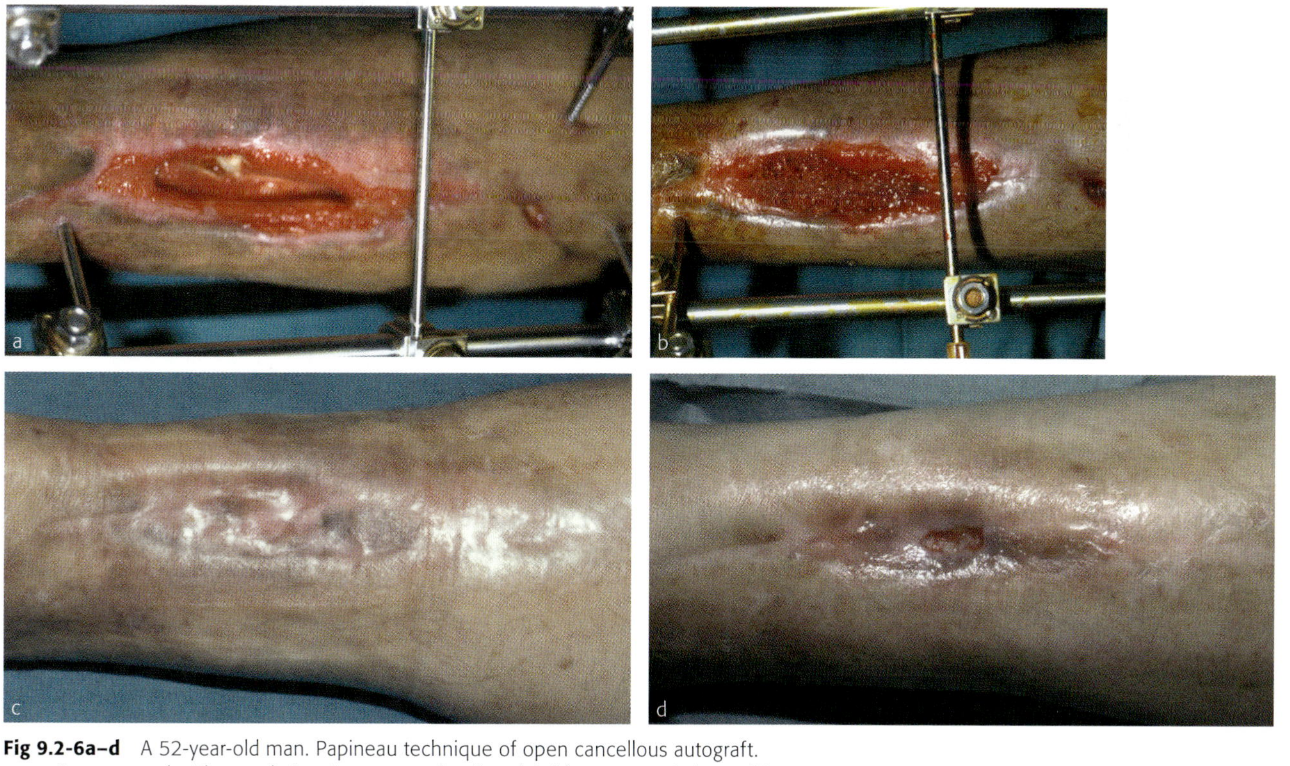

Fig 9.2-6a–d A 52-year-old man. Papineau technique of open cancellous autograft.
a Open wound with granulation tissue 3 weeks after debridement, ready for grafting.
b The defect is over-filled with morselized cancellous autograft.
c The wound is covered with scar tissue after 4½ months.
d Six years later, the patient had intermittent wound breakdown in the unstable scar.

The statistical analysis shows a slight to moderate beneficial effect of the application [27, 28]. Bone morphogenetic protein recruits and activates mesenchymal stem cells and directs them towards the osteogenic lineage [29] but its activity is very short-lived (up to 24 hours). The costs of BMP are high and this limits its use [30]. In the metaphyseal area and in normotrophic or hypertrophic diaphyseal nonunion there is no need for BMP. To be effective in atrophic diaphyseal nonunions and in defect pseudarthroses, BMP has to be combined with cancellous autograft or cultivated mesenchymal stem cells in combination with a scaffold such as tricalcium phosphate [31]. There are concerns that the use of BMP in supraphysiological doses as advocated by the manufacturer may provoke tumors [32].

The use of any BMP in infected nonunion has not been evaluated. It may be appropriate to consider BMP implantation in patients who have a poor biological response (eg, steroid use, previous radiotherapy to the limb, connective tissue disorder) for bone healing but this requires further study. Generally, it should be used only during a second-stage reconstruction after infection has been eradicated.

3.3.4 The induced membrane principle

In infected nonunions the surrounding soft tissues including periosteum have often been destroyed to a large extent. Masquelet described a method to create a new environment in the defect area favorable to bone reconstruction [33]. After thorough debridement, a PMMA spacer containing antibiotics effective against the pathogenic bacteria is prepared and inserted into the bone defect just before hardening, thereby slightly draping the cement around the bony edges (**Fig 9.2-7a–b**). The cement is carefully covered by closing the subcutaneous tissue followed by skin sutures. Over time, the PMMA block becomes covered by a fibrovascular membrane. After 4–8 weeks, the spacer is removed. The induced membrane around the cement can be seen to be vascularized with new blood vessel formation (**Fig 9.2-7c**). The presence of bone precursor cells and the production of bone-inducing growth factors have been demonstrated [34]. The space within this membrane is now packed with cancellous autograft. To guarantee stability, an external fixator is appropriate, although the use of nails has also been described [35]. The consolidation for defects of around 5 cm in length will last 1 year or more [36]. Loss of stability or general medical conditions can impair consolidation in many cases of large defects in the lower limb.

3.3.5 The Ilizarov method

Ilizarov developed a system for the stabilization of bone fragments, for correction of deformity, and bone defect filling, while allowing joint motion and rehabilitation. He described in detail the combination of callus distraction and segmental transportation [37]. The main advantage of this system is the regeneration of a segment of new autogenous bone "on the spot", ie, in the diseased limb itself without the need of a donor site [38]. The resulting regenerated bone has adequate diameter for the segment to be replaced and has mechanical strength superior to that resulting from cancellous autografts and free vascularized bone grafts. Of all the available methods, Ilizarov techniques remain the most reliable in achieving infection-free union (**Fig 9.2-8**).

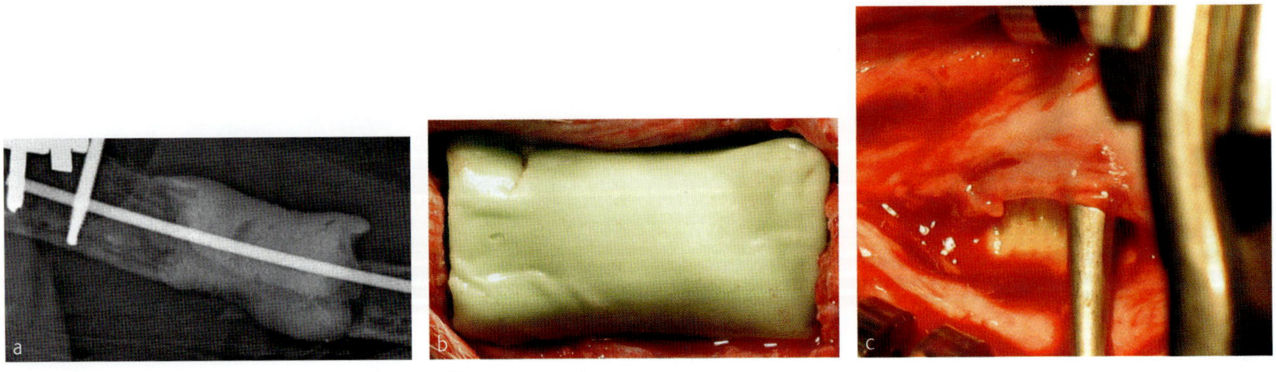

Fig 9.2-7a–c Induced membrane principle according to Masquelet.
a–b Placement of cement in the defect after debridement.
c Removal of the cement after 6 weeks shows that a thick membrane is formed.

Depending on the extent of shortening of the limb or length of bone defect, there are four different ways of treatment, as defined in the guidelines of the French Society of Orthopaedic Surgery and Traumatology (SOFCOT) [39]:

- Unifocal compression:
  Resection and compression alone. In case of minimal shortening after segmental resection, the site can be acutely compressed, accepting the shortening. The external fixator holds the reduction and allows further gradual compression, eg, 0.25 mm twice a day.
- Unifocal compression-distraction:
  Resection, acute shortening with compression, and secondary distraction (relengthening) at the site of the resected nonunion. The shortening should not exceed 3 cm. The resected nonunion is compressed during 2 or 3 weeks after which a distraction is initiated at 0.75 or 1 mm per day to restore the leg length.
- Bifocal compression-distraction:
  Resection, acute shortening with compression of the resection site, and secondary distraction through a corticotomy at a distant site. The shortening should not exceed 3–6 cm. The corticotomy is distracted 0.75 mm or 1 mm per day beginning after an interval of 7–10 days for secondary lengthening to restore normal leg length.
- Bifocal bone transport:
  Resection without shortening, distant corticotomy, and secondary segmental transportation until compression in the docking (resection) site. Useful for defects greater than 3 cm, up to 15 cm or more (**Fig 9.2-8**). The speed of the segmental transportation is 0.75 mm or 1 mm per day. If additional lengthening is needed in the tibia, a fibular osteotomy may be necessary.

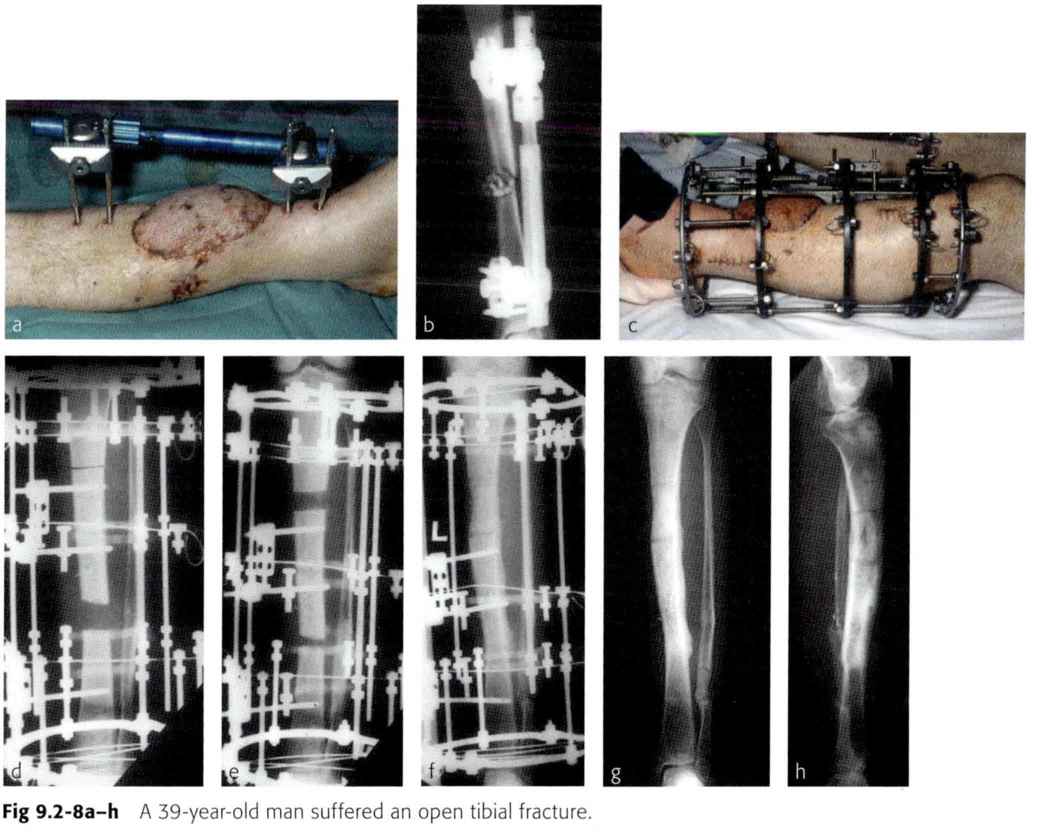

Fig 9.2-8a–h A 39-year-old man suffered an open tibial fracture.
a–b Patient was treated with external fixation and a free muscle flap and local polymethylmethacrylate antibiotic beads.
c Patient developed an early infection which was treated by a 5 cm segmental resection and Ilizarov bone transport.
d–e The limb was initially shortened by 2.5 cm to allow docking to occur more quickly.
f After docking, the lengthening was continued to full leg length.
g–h Final outcome at 14 months showed an infection-free limb with good alignment and good function. Bone transport proceeded under the muscle flap without difficulty.

The choice between solution 3 and 4 depends on several factors. Shortening in the lower leg of more than 3–4 cm is technically demanding and not without risk. There are problems with soft tissues including vascular risks. Careful observation of the blood supply to the hand or foot is needed during acute shortening of more than 3 cm. If ischemia is seen, the limb cannot be acutely shortened to bone contact and a bone transport will be needed.

Early bone contact in the segmental resection with acute compression will usually improve regenerate formation and maturation and allow shorter fixator times. However, in the lower leg a resection of the fibula will be necessary reducing the stability.

Surgical steps in distraction osteogenesis (Ilizarov method)

- Segmental resection: The debridement consists of a segmental resection of the site of nonunion (**Fig 9.2-8**). Because of the destabilization to be expected, the external fixation may be applied prior to the resection. Two parallel resection osteotomies are performed to secure a large contact area in the later docking site. Segmental resection transforms the infected nonunion into a defect nonunion. It is essential to perform an adequate segment removal to ensure that no residual dead bone is left at the margins of the defect. Conserving nonviable bone compromises the later healing of the docking site.
- Stabilization: A unilateral fixator (**Fig 9.2-10**) [40–42] or a circular frame (**Fig 9.2.8**, **Fig 9.2-9**, **Fig 9.2-11**) [43, 44] can be chosen. The use of IM devices is limited to cases with a proven small risk of recurrence of infection. The fixator should be built in a way that a bone fragment can be transported into the defect area continuously and compressed in the docking site without later change of the frame system (**Fig 9.2-8**, **Fig 9.2-10**).

The application of the external fixation systems is not particularly complicated if performed regularly. The progressive treatment, however, requires a meticulous follow-up and the ability to adjust the fixator whenever necessary. Pin-track infection, wire breakage, and loss of joint motion must all be addressed quickly to prevent permanent complications. It is the intensive aftercare in particular that makes an Ilizarov procedure more complicated than standard orthopedic procedures. Ilizarov treatment of infected nonunions should be performed in dedicated centers that have sufficient experience and logistical support.

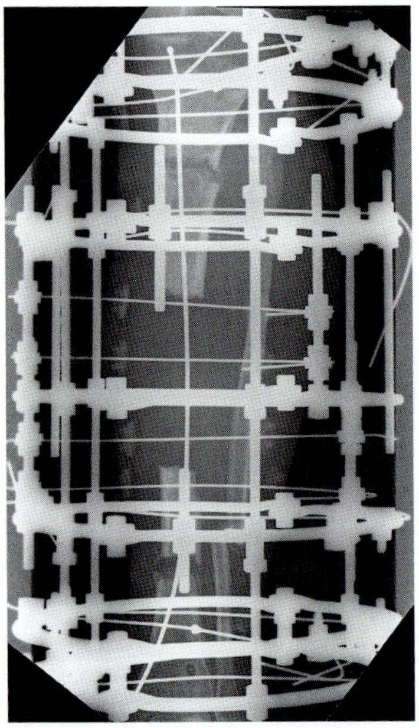

Fig 9.2-9 Example of an Ilizarov ring fixator applied for a trifocal bone transport to reconstruct a middiaphyseal tibial defect. In this case, there has been a central segmental resection with two corticotomies performed in the proximal and distal tibia. The two bone fragments are then transported towards each other over a thin intramedullary wire, to allow docking in the midtibia.

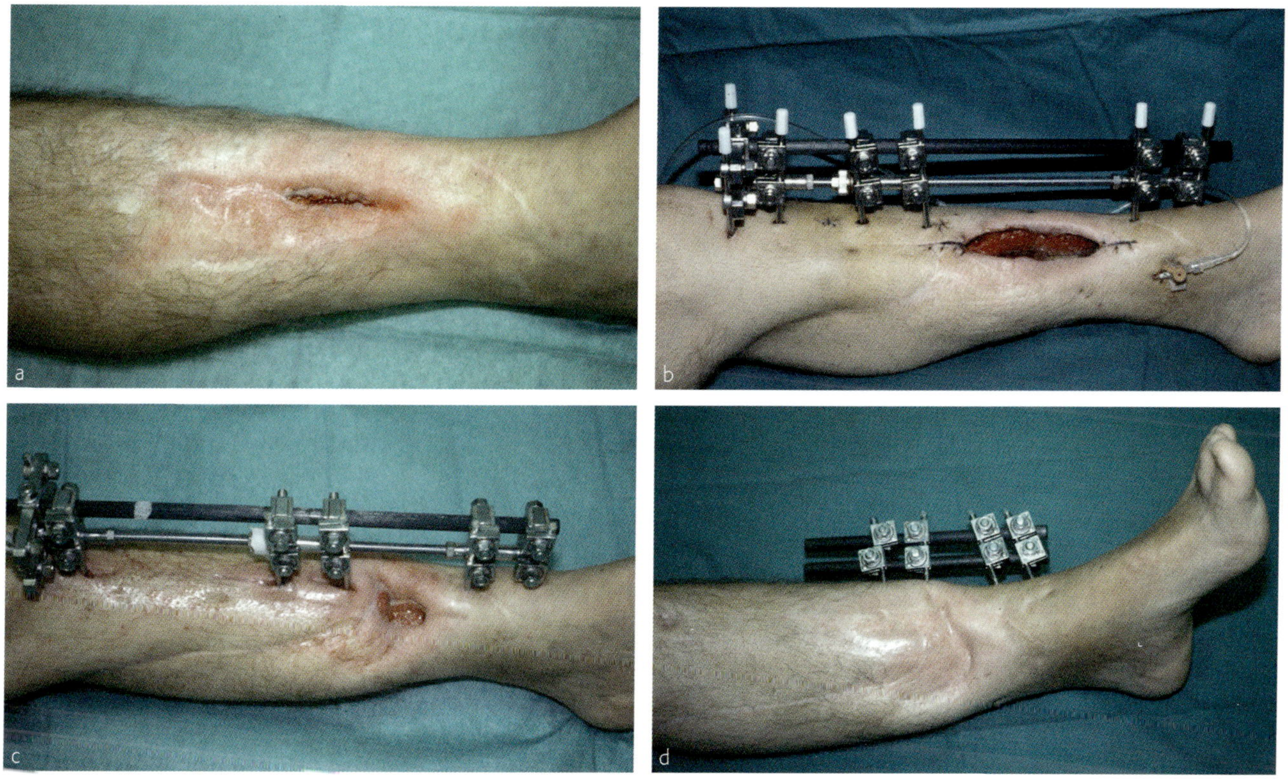

Fig 9.2-10a–d Infected nonunion of the tibia.
a–b Treatment with Ilizarov bone transport using a monolateral fixator after resection of an 8 cm bone segment.
c The skin defect has gradually closed as the central transport segment moves down the limb without the need of a skin graft.
d The fixator has been simplified towards the end of treatment for patient convenience.

- Soft-tissue handling: The soft tissues should be closed over the defect primarily if possible. Wound closure should not be forced after bone resection. Open areas are covered with bandages moistened with antiseptics such as polyhexanide. In parallel to bone transportation there is concomitant neo-histiogenesis of the adjacent soft tissue. The soft tissues are distracted together with the bone, which leads to a closure of the soft-tissue defect. This may avoid further reconstructive surgery or focus it at a precise localization at the end of the distraction (**Fig 9.2-10**). In special situations a separate progressive traction on the soft tissues can be installed with strong sutures on both edges of the wound and attached to the frame in a way that a gradual closure can be realized (**Fig 9.2-11**) [45]. In this way, significant open skin defects can be closed during the bone transport. However, this can increase the risk of secondary infection and failure of healing of the docking site. As an alternative, Ilizarov methods can be combined with free vascularized tissue transfer [46]. Care must be taken with frame design to accommodate the bulk of the flap during transport. When acute shortening is performed, a free muscle flap can be used to cover the docking site. Corticotomy distraction at a distant site will not affect the muscle flap.

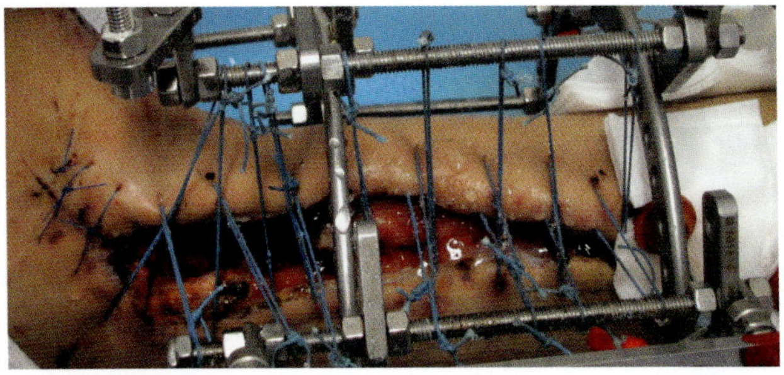

Fig 9.2-11 Gradual side-side closure of the skin is possible with the fixator and elastic bands.

- Corticotomy: In severe infection, particularly after IM nailing, the corticotomy for segmental distraction should be delayed by 1–2 weeks after the initial segmental resection. It is safer to choose the place for the corticotomy at a level with as large a diameter of the bone as possible. For a distal defect a proximal corticotomy is performed and vice versa. In case of a central defect both a proximal and distal osteotomy can double the speed of callus distraction but the shortening of the total healing period is less impressive (**Fig 9.2-9**). The corticotomy should be done in a minimally invasive way through a 1–2cm incision preserving the periosteum and reducing the damage to the medullary bone. The cortex can be weakened with drill holes and the corticotomy completed with a chisel. This is technically easier than the technique with a Gigli saw. Image intensifier use should confirm that the corticotomy is complete to avoid a failure of distraction or a premature fusion.
- Bone distraction: The fresh osteotomy is distracted during the operation by about 1 mm [37]. During the following 7–10 days (the latent period) callus is formed in the corticotomy gap. Then a daily distraction of 0.75–1 mm is made until the desired extension is performed. It is usual to divide the daily distraction into four episodes of 0.25 mm each time. Regular review with clinical and x-ray assessment is recommended every 2 weeks during distraction and every month during consolidation.
- Consolidation of the distraction site: The consolidation of the distraction site takes as a rough rule 5 (± 2) months in addition to the distraction period. This confirms that it is not worth retaining bone with doubtful vitality because the prolongation of the consolidation by resecting 1 cm more is around 10 days.
- Consolidation of the docking site: The external fixation can be continued till the complete healing of the docking site or may be reduced to a simpler system towards the end of healing (**Fig 9.2-10d**) [47]. Union with Ilizarov method alone and without additional osteoplastic measures is achieved in 50–80% of cases [43, 46]. Further treatment may be necessary such as decortication, cancellous autograft, addition of BMP, or secondary internal fixation [46, 48, 49]. The use of secondary internal fixation is associated with an increased infection recurrence rate [46].

3.3.6 Free vascularized bone transfer

The vascularized bone transfer is a distinct alternative to callus distraction. Vascularized bone can be transferred alone or as a composite graft combining bone, muscle and skin. There are some clear advantages of a free vascularized bone graft:

- The transplanted graft is vital and has an immediate biological healing potential on both of its ends.
- Debridement of the infected nonunion can leave irregular margins. Vascularized grafts can be adapted to fit the shape of the defect.
- Choosing a composite graft with bone and skin allows the immediate repair of a soft-tissue defect at the same time.
- The reconstruction can be functional after 3–4 months.
- In the upper limb, free fibular grafts are already similar in size to the host bones so little remodeling and hypertrophy is needed.

There are also some disadvantages:

- The thickness and the length of the bone grafts are limited.
- In the lower limb, free fibular grafts must undergo major hypertrophy. This may fail or require a very long period of time (> 2–3 years) resulting in stress fractures.
- Additional measures such as cancellous autografting may be needed to improve stability or secure union.
- To achieve bony integration, there is need for a better local stability than is needed for consolidation of callus distraction or a pure cancellous autograft. Nonunion at an integration site is common.

The following free vascularized bone grafts are useful:

- Fibula alone or as composite graft with muscle and skin: The fibula is long—up to about 20–25 cm can be harvested [50, 51]—but is thin. Without additional measures it is insufficient for the reconstruction of the tibia or the femur. Because of mechanical insufficiency fatigue fractures of the graft may happen [52]. Double grafting using the same fibula is possible. Problems of the donor site are not rare, particularly if a skin paddle is taken with the fibula.
- Scapula: The bone of the medial border is thin, but may have a remarkable extent up to 8 x 2 cm. A composite graft with muscle and skin is the rule. To reconstruct a full diameter of a tubular bone it needs additional osteoblastic measures, mainly cancellous autograft (**Fig 9.2-12**, **Fig 9.2-13**).
- Medial femoral condyle: This is a pure bone graft with a maximum extent of about 4 x 2 cm.
- Iliac crest as a composite graft with muscle up to the extent of 8 x 2 cm.
- Part of a rib with adjacent tissue up to about 6 cm of length. Not often considered outside the hand or foot due to poor bone quality and rib curvature.

Free vascular bone grafts require the skills of the orthopedic surgeon and a microvascular plastic surgeon. Careful preoperative planning is needed to define the resection, site of the vascular anastomosis and stabilization of the graft. The fixation of the graft in the nonunion site must be very stable. This can be achieved with an external fixator producing compression across the graft. If a rigid plate is used, this may stress shield the graft and prevent hypertrophy. Good stability is offered by an interlocking nail (**Fig 9.2-12**, **Fig 9.2-13**) but additional fixation may be needed for a better integration of the graft. Stabilization must allow immediate joint motion and early weight bearing. In the lower limb, immobilization may be needed for many months during graft remodeling.

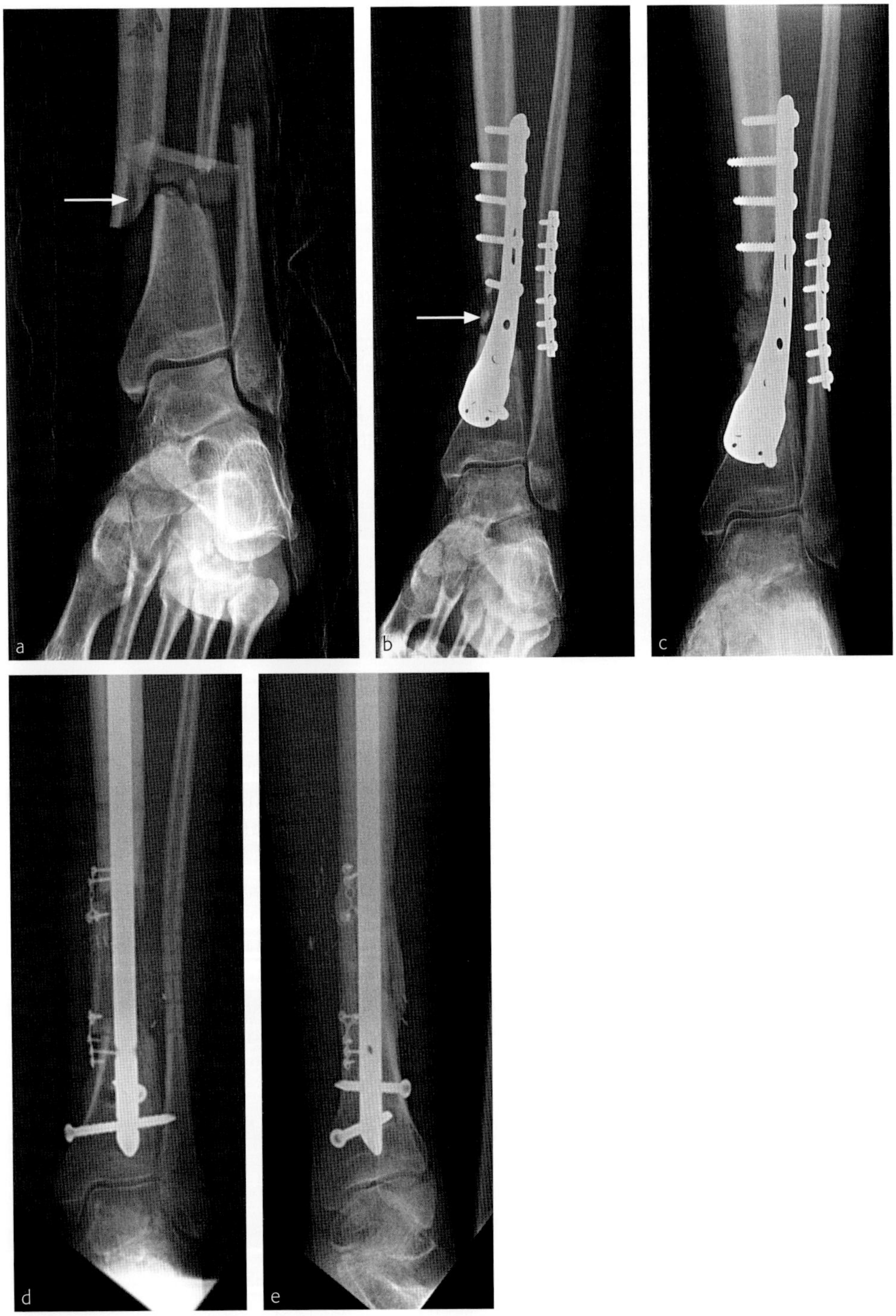

Fig 9.2-12a–e Severe open tibial fracture by a direct trauma in a 25-year-old man.

a Local comminution and displacement; plate osteosynthesis is decided.

b Within 6 months there was spontaneous resorption of the proximal tibial fragment (arrows) with resulting instability. Infection with enterococci and clostridia. Debridment and filling of the 5 cm defect with a mixture of morcelized auto- and allograft and pieces of collagen sponge containing gentamicin followed.

c Vanishing of the graft within 7 months (see **Fig 9.12-13**), no remaining infection.

d The infected defect was resected and filled with a vascularized composite bone, muscle and skin flap from the scapula with stable fixation using a nail and small plates and additional cancellous autograft.

e Full union with incorporation of the graft is seen at 9 months.

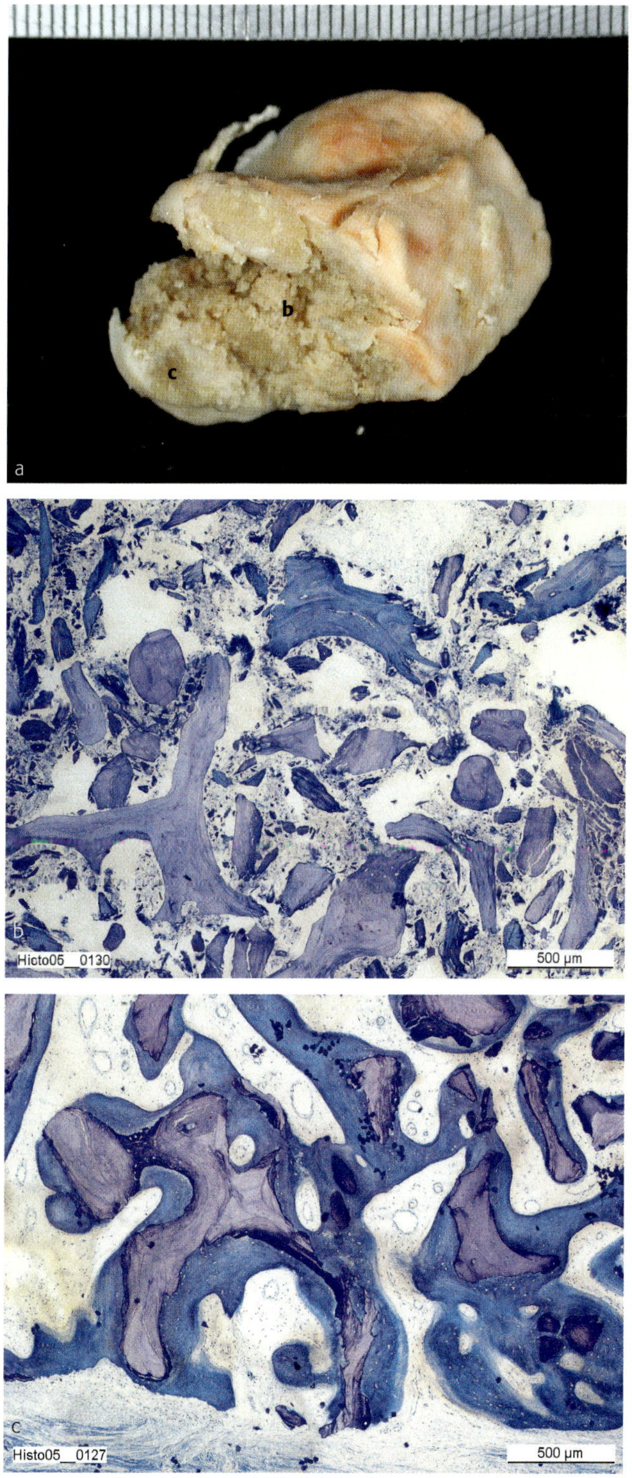

Fig 9.2-13a–c Same case as **Fig 9.2-12**. Failure of bridging of an infected nonunion with a composite graft containing morselized auto- and allograft and pieces of collagen sponge containing gentamicin.

- **a** Resected 4 cm long segment of failed reconstruction, mainly consisting of soft tissue containing brittle parts (b), only at one place having a bony resistance (c).
- **b** Histological analysis (undecalcified, Romanowsky stain) of the necrotic graft material without any new bone formation.
- **c** Single area of new bone formation (bright blue) around some cancellous autogaft pieces.

3.4 Closure of skin defects

The soft-tissue situation will determine whether wound closure will require reconstructive surgery using (free) tissue flaps or not. The treatment of infected nonunion is usually not urgent so a full assessment and discussion with a plastic surgeon can be arranged.

The most important means to cover defects are:

- Simple split-skin grafts on a well granulated bed
- Local rotation flaps (eg, gastrocnemius muscle flap)
- Free vascularized skin flaps (eg, lateral upper arm flap, which allows innervation), combined skin and muscle flaps (eg, latissimus dorsi flap) or muscle flaps (eg, gracilis flap)

There may be significant advantages in using free or local muscle flaps around infected nonunions. The flaps have been shown to resist infection, provide neo-vascularization of the bone from the muscle, deliver high levels of antibiotic to the site and recruit stem cells for tissue healing. In the lower leg, they also provide a good bulk of tissue over the subcutaneous anterior border of the tibia, reducing the risk of later injury causing bone exposure.

Negative-pressure wound therapy alone is not indicated in soft-tissue management of infected nonunions, unless it is used in combination with reconstructive surgery. Some techniques for the bony reconstruction can promote soft-tissue healing. This is the case for the Papineau technique, but the resulting scar tissue with or without split-skin graft results frequently in an unstable scar (**Fig 9.2-6**). The bone transport method in parallel can be accompanied with a 'de novo' soft-tissue regeneration (**Fig 9.5.10**, **Fig 9.2-11**).

4 Complications and outcomes

An infected nonunion is a complex problem requiring a long course of treatment, often with multiple surgeries. To some extent it has to be considered as a resection-reconstruction procedure with the final aim to eradicate the infection, to reconstruct the bone for full weight bearing and to regain a fully functional extremity. The important principles to avoid recurrence are the radical resection of the infected area, the adjuvant antibiotic therapy of an adequate length, dictated by careful tissue sampling and culture, followed by the early closure of any soft-tissue defect. Failure to address any of these issues will increase the chance of recurrent infection and persistent nonunion. In most series, up to 20% of cases will suffer one or both of these complications, requiring further intervention. However, after complete treatment, around 90% of cases can be successfully healed [43, 46, 53–55].

Restoration of full function is difficult in these cases as many patients have already developed joint contractures and chronic pain prior to the definitive treatment of their nonunion.

Delays in wound healing are frustrating for patients. Open wound techniques often require extensive nursing care and prolonged time in hospital, finally producing an unstable and vulnerable scar. As a result, combined reconstruction of the bone and soft tissues with free tissue transfer is now more common. This can safely be performed as a single procedure [46] or can be staged.

The production of advanced therapy medicinal products (ATMPs) containing expanded stem cells seeded on a absorbable scaffold and augmented with bone-inducing molecules are promising but not yet applicable in routine surgery. Therefore, the bone transport methods developed by GA Ilizarov remain the safest, least sophisticated, and most economical treatment method available for large bone defects resulting in functional bone replacement.

5 Conclusion

The currently available techniques are demanding, expensive and remain with some complications and problems. They require extensive surgical skill. In the future, we need methods which are more easily tolerated by patients and applicable in resource-poor parts of the world, where infected nonunion is common.

6 References

1. **Rosen H.** Treatment of nonunion: general principles. In: Chapman W, ed. *Operative Orthopaedics,* Philadelphia: Lippincott-Raven; 1988:489–509.
2. **Jain AK, Sinha S.** Infected nonunion of the long bones. *Clin Orthop Relat Res.* 2005 Feb;(431):57–65.
3. **Rodriguez-Merchan EC, Forriol F.** Nonunion: general principles and experimental data. *Clin Orthop Relat Res.* 2004 Feb;(419):4–12.
4. **Weber BG, Cech O.** *Pseudarthrosis: Pathology, biomechanics, therapy, results.* Berne, Switzerland: Hans Huber Medical Publisher; 1976.
5. **Calori GM, Phillips M, Jeetle S, et al.** Classification of non-union: need for a new scoring system? *Injury.* 2008 Sep;39 Suppl 2:S59–63.
6. **Calori GM, Colombo M, Mazza EL, et al.** Validation of the Non-Union Scoring System in 300 long bone non-unions. *Injury.* 2014 Dec;45 Suppl 6:S93–97.
7. **Propst-Proctor SL, Dillingham MF, McDougall IR, et al.** The white blood cell scan in orthopedics. *Clin Orthop Relat Res.* 1982 Aug;(168):157–165.
8. **Palmer MP, Altman DT, Altman GT, et al.** Can we trust intraoperative culture results in nonunions? *J Orthop Trauma.* 2014 Jul;28(7):384–390.
9. **Klemm KW.** Treatment of infected pseudarthrosis of the femur and tibia with an interlocking nail. *Clin Orthop Relat Res.* 1986 Nov;(212):174–181.
10. **Emara KM, Allam MF.** Ilizarov external fixation and then nailing in management of infected nonunions of the tibial shaft. *J Trauma.* 2008 Sep;65(3):685–691.
11. **Emara KM, Diab RA, Ghafar KA.** Cost of external fixation vs external fixation then nailing in bone infection. *World J Orthop.* 2015 Jan 18;6(1):145–149.
12. **Thonse R, Conway JD.** Antibiotic cement-coated nails for the treatment of infected nonunions and segmental bone defects. *J Bone Joint Surg Am.* 2008 Nov;90 Suppl 4:163–174.
13. **Conway J, Mansour J, Kotze K, et al.** Antibiotic cement-coated rods: an effective treatment for infected long bones and prosthetic joint nonunions. *Bone Joint J.* 2014 Oct;96-B(10):1349–1354.
14. **Meister K, Segal D, Whitelaw GP.** The role of bone grafting in the treatment of delayed unions and nonunions of the tibia. *Orthop Rev.* 1990 Mar;19(3):260–271.
15. **Gulan G, JotanoviĐ Z, Jurdana H, et al.** Treatment of infected tibial nonunion with bone defect using central bone grafting technique. *Coll Antropol.* 2012 Jun;36(2):617–621.
16. **Dimitriou R, Mataliotakis GI, Angoules AG, et al.** Complications following autologous bone graft harvesting from the iliac crest and using the RIA: a systematic review. *Injury.* 2011 Sep;42 Suppl 2:S3–15.
17. **Green J.** History and development of suction-irrigation-reaming. *Injury.* 2010 Nov;41 Suppl 2: S24–31.
18. **Belthur MV, Conway JD, Jindal G, et al.** Bone graft harvest using a new intramedullary system. *Clin Orthop Relat Res.* 2008 Dec;466(12):2973–2980.
19. **Giori NJ, Beaupre GS.** Femoral fracture after harvesting of autologous bone graft using a reamer/irrigator/aspirator. *J Orthop Trauma.* 2011 Feb;25(2):12–14.
20. **Pratt DJ, Papagiannopoulos G, Rees PH, et al.** The effects of medullary reaming on the torsional strength of the femur. *Injury.* 1987 May;18(3):177–179.
21. **Calori GM, Colombo M, Mazza EL, et al.** Incidence of donor site morbidity following harvesting from iliac crest or RIA graft. *Injury.* 2014 Dec;45 Suppl 6:S116–120
22. **Stafford PR, Norris BL.** Reamer-irrigator-aspirator bone graft and bi Masquelet technique for segmental bone defect nonunions: a review of 25 cases. *Injury.* 2010 Nov;41 Suppl 2: S72–77.
23. **Green SA, Dlabal TA.** The open bone graft for septic nonunion. *Clin Orthop Relat Res.* 1983 Nov;(180):117–124.
24. **Saleh M, Kreibich DN, Ribbans WJ.** Circular frames in the management of infected tibial non-union: a modification of the Papineau technique. *Injury.* 1996 Jan;27(1):31–33.
25. **Polyzois VD, Galanakos SP, Tsiampa VA, et al.** The use of Papineau technique for the treatment of diabetic and non-diabetic lower extremity pseudoarthrosis and chronic osteomyelitis. *Diabet Foot Ankle.* 2011;2.
26. **Archdeacon MT, Messerschmitt P.** Modern papineau technique with vacuum-assisted closure. *J Orthop Trauma.* 2006 Feb;20(2):134–137.
27. **Aro HT, Govender S, Patel AD, et al.** Recombinant human bone morphogenic protein-2: a randomized trial in open tibial fractures treated with reamed nail fixation. *J Bone Joint Surg Am.* 2001 May 4; 93(9):801–808.
28. **Friedlaender GE, Perry CR, Cole JD, et al.** Osteogenic protein-1 (bone morphogenetic protein-7) in the treatment of tibial nonunions. *J Bone Joint Surg Am.* 2001;83-A Suppl 1(Pt 2):S151–158.
29. **Bessa PC, Casal M, Reis RL.** Bone morphogenetic proteins in tissue engineering: the road from laboratory to clinic, part II (BMP delivery). *J Tissue Eng Regen Med.* 2008 Mar-Apr;2(2–3):81–96.
30. **Garrison KR, Donell S, Ryder J, et al.** Clinical effectiveness and cost-effectiveness of bone morphogenetic proteins in the non-healing of fractures and spinal fusion: a systematic review. *Health Technol Assess.* 2007 Aug;11(30):1–150, iii–iv.
31. **Calori GM, Colombo M, Ripamonti C, et al.** Polytherapy in bone regeneration: clinical applications and preliminary considerations. *Int J Immunopathol Pharmacol.* 2011 Jan-Mar;24(1 Suppl 2):85–90.
32. **Pountos I, Panteli M, Georgouli T, et al.** Neoplasia following use of BMPs: is there an increased risk? *Expert Opin Drug Saf.* 2014 Nov;13(11):1525–1534.
33. **Masquelet AC. Begue T.** The concept of induced membrane for reconstruction of long bone defects. *Orthop Clin North Am.* 2010 Jan;41(1):27–37; table of contents.
34. **Aho OM, Lehenkari P, Ristiniemi J, et al.** The mechanism of action of induced membranes in bone repair. *J Bone Joint Surg Am.* 2013 Apr 3;95(7):597–604.
35. **O'Malley NT, Kates SL.** Advances on the Masquelet technique using a cage and nail construct. *Arch Orthop Trauma Surg.* 2012 Feb; 132(2):245–248.
36. **Karger C, Kishi T, Schneider L, et al.** Treatment of posttraumatic bone defects by the induced membrane technique. *Orthop Traumatol Surg Res.* 2012 Feb;98(1):97–102.
37. **Ilizarov GA.** Clinical application of the tension-stress effect for limb lengthening. *Clin Orthop Relat Res.* 1990 Jan; (250):8–26.
38. **Fabry K, Lammens J, Delhey P, et al.** Ilizarov's method: a solution for infected bone loss. *Eur J Orthop Surg Traumatol.* 2006;16:103–109.
39. **Rigal S, Merloz P, Le Nen D, et al.** Bone transport techniques in posttraumatic bone defects. *Orthop Traumatol Surg Res.* 2012 Feb;98(1):103–108.
40. **Alonso JE, Regazzoni P.** The use of the Ilizarov concept with the AO/ASIF tubular fixateur in the treatment of segmental defects. *Orthop Clin North Am.* 1990 Oct;21(4):655–665.
41. **Harshwal RK, Sankhala SS, Jalan D.** Management of nonunion of lower-extremity long bones using mono-lateral external fixator--report of 37 cases. *Injury.* 2014 Mar;45(3):560–567.

42. **Arora S, Batra S, Gupta V, et al.** Distraction osteogenesis using a monolateral external fixator for infected non-union of the femur with bone loss. *J Orthop Surg (Hong Kong)*. 2012 Aug;20(2):185–190.
43. **Rozbruch SR, Pugsley JS, Fragomen AT, et al.** Repair of tibial nonunions and bone defects with the Taylor Spatial Frame. *J Orthop Trauma*. 2008 Feb;22(2):88–95.
44. **Megas P, Saridis A, Kouzelis A, et al.** The treatment of infected nonunion of the tibia following intramedullary nailing by the Ilizarov method. *Injury*. 2010 Mar;41(3):294–249.
45. **D'Hooghe P, Defoort K, Lammens J, et al.** Treatment of a large post-traumatic skin and bone defect using an Ilizarov frame. *Acta Orthop Belg*. 2006 Apr;72(2):214–218.
46. **Bose D, Kugan R, Stubbs D, et al.** Management of infected nonunion of the long bones by a multidisciplinary team. *Bone Joint J*. 2015 Jun;97-B(6):814–817.
47. **Laumen A, Lammens J, Vanlauwe J.** Reduction of treatment time in external ring fixation using the monofix device. *Acta Orthop Belg*. 2012 Aug;78(4):543–547.
48. **Lovisetti G, Sala F, Miller AN, et al.** Clinical reliability of closed techniques and comparison with open strategies to achieve union at the docking site. *Int Orthop*. 2012 Apr;36(4):817–825.
49. **Giotakis N, Narayan B, Nayagam S.** Distraction osteogenesis and nonunion of the docking site: is there an ideal treatment option? *Injury*. 2007 Mar;38 Suppl 1:S100–107.
50. **Kalra GS, Goel P, Singh PK.** Reconstruction of post-traumatic long bone defect with vascularised free fibula: A series of 28 cases. *Indian J Plast Surg*. 2013 Sep;46(3):543–548.
51. **Bumbasirevic M, Stevanovic M, Bumbasirevic V, et al.** Free vascularised fibular grafts in orthopaedics. *Int Orthop*. 2014 Jun;38(6):1277–1282.
52. **Falder S, Sinclair JS, Rogers CA, et al.** Long-term behaviour of the free vascularised fibula following reconstruction of large bony defects. *Br J Plast Surg*. 2003 Sep;56(6):571–584.
53. **Papakostidis C, Bhandari M, Giannoudis PV.** Distraction osteogenesis in the treatment of long bone defects of the lower limbs: effectiveness, complications and clinical results; a systematic review and meta-analysis. *Bone Joint J*. 2013 Dec; 95-B(12):1673–1680.
54. **Hollenbeck ST, Woo S, Ong S, et al.** The combined use of the Ilizarov method and microsurgical techniques for limb salvage. *Ann Plast Surg*. 2009 May; 62(5):486–491.
55. **Kugan R, Aslam N, Bose D, et al.** Outcome of arthrodesis of the hindfoot as a salvage procedure for complex ankle pathology using the Ilizarov technique. *Bone Joint J*. 2013 Mar; 95-B:371–377.

10 Infection after joint arthroplasty

Antonia F Chen, Carlo L Romanò, Lorenzo Drago, Javad Parvizi

1 Basics

Periprosthetic joint infection (PJI) after total joint arthroplasty (TJA) is a devastating complication. With the increase in the number of TJA cases performed annually, there will be a corresponding rise in the number of PJI with all of its associated morbidity, mortality, and costs to society. Thus, it is imperative to understand the etiology of PJI and effective strategies that exist to manage these. Thorough knowledge of the effective methods in prevention, diagnosis, and treatment of PJI is required. An infection around a prosthesis usually presents in an elusive manner and may evade detection unless a high index of suspicion is maintained. Thus, any patient with a painful prosthetic joint needs to be subjected to a thorough history taking, clinical examination, and laboratory and imaging investigation to confirm or refute the diagnosis of PJI. Once diagnosed, selection of the most appropriate surgical treatment combined with antibiotic therapy is critical for an optimal outcome.

1.1 Etiology

The etiology of infection after arthroplasty varies and includes endogenous and exogenous sources [1]. Contamination from within the joint at the time of index TJA may present as an infection that persists in the immediate postoperative period, or present later as an indolent infection. Late infections with acute presentations often result from hematogenous spread from other nidus of infection, such as oral or urinary sources. Infections can also spread from contiguous or direct sources, such as localized abscesses around the joint. Finally, infections may occur as a result of systemic sepsis or in the setting of a previously septic joint.

1.2 Localization

Commonly replaced joints are the knee, hip, shoulder, elbow, and ankle. All can become infected. Periprosthetic joint infection presents special diagnostic challenges when compared with other types of infections. It may be difficult to diagnose PJI, as isolation of bacteria from the joint may be difficult in approximately 30% of cases. Many cases present with a painful joint but no visible signs as would be found in cellulitis or other infections, ie, erythema, warmth, fluctuance, or tenderness. Thus, clinicians must rely on a high index of clinical suspicion based on history, presenting symptoms, imaging, and diagnostic workup to reach the diagnosis of an infection after arthroplasty. Aspiration of the joint and obtaining tissue samples for culture are the most important critical initial steps for diagnosis of PJI. If multiple joints have been replaced in a patient it is important to evaluate, examine, and possibly aspirate each one of them.

1.3 Incidence

The incidence of PJI may be underestimated, as approximately 30% of these cases are culture-negative and may not be reported as an infection. The prevalence of PJI is on the rise worldwide as more and more cases of arthroplasty are performed [2]. The incidence of PJI depends largely on what criteria are used to define this entity. The definition of PJI has changed over time. Traditionally, the definition of prosthetic joint infection was based on the criteria set forth by the Centers for Disease Control [3]. However, based on the more refined definition of PJI detailed below, the incidence of PJI in the United States from 2001–2009, using a national database, was found to be between 2–2.4%. Based on a projection study using the National Inpatient Sampling database, Kurtz et al [4] predicted that the total number of PJI cases would be on the rise on an almost exponential trajectory. A later study using the same database confirmed their initial projection predictions and stated that the number of PJI cases would rise to 65,555 per year by 2020 [5]. A similar trend, namely a substantial rise in the number of PJIs, has also been witnessed in European countries through registry data and data from individual hospitals [2, 6, 7].

1.4 Risk factors

There have been numerous studies attempting to evaluate the risk of a patient for PJI. Although patients with seemingly no risk factors for infection can develop PJI, the majority of patients that develop PJI have identifiable risk factors. The risk factors for PJI can be conveniently divided into host-related, surgical, and postoperative factors.

Infection around a prosthesis is likely to occur when infecting organisms find access to the implant. During an episode of bacteremia, the ability of a host to clear blood-borne pathogens depends on the patient's immune system. Thus, any immune-compromising conditions such as cancer, diabetes, human immunodeficiency virus, and inflammatory arthropathies would place the patient at a higher risk for PJI. Other modifiable risk factors, such as obesity which is defined as body mass index > 35 kg/m^2, excessive alcohol consumption, heavy smoking, and intravenous drug use, have also been associated with an increased risk for PJI [8–13]. Some nonmodifiable risk factors for PJI include older age [4, 14] and male sex [15, 16] (**Table 10-1**). Patients with other medical comorbidities such as cardiopulmonary comorbidities, depression, hemophilia, hepatitis C, malnutrition, hypertension, renal disease, liver disease, sickle cell hemoglobinopathies, and psoriasis also have a higher risk for infection [8, 11, 13, 17–23]. Finally, history of recent or remote infections such as previous infections in the same joint [24, 25], previous orthopedic infections [26], colonization with methicillin-resistant *Staphylococcus aureus* (MRSA) [13], and urinary tract infections [8, 27] may predispose patients to developing PJI.

To lower the risk of PJI, certain preoperative steps may be taken. Recent studies have identified some of these effective preventative methods. A recent International Consensus on PJI [28] evaluated all available literature pertinent to the mitigation of risks for PJI and identified the following as evidence-based strategies for prevention of surgical-site infections or PJI. The use of chlorhexidine skin wipes or soaps prior to elective TJA has been shown to be a very effective strategy for minimizing surgical-site infections including PJI and was strongly endorsed by the International Consensus Group (ICG) [29]. Optimization of medical conditions prior to arthroplasty, appropriate preparation of the skin with agents containing alcohol, and clipping of the hair around the incision site using clippers just prior to surgery were some of the other effective methods that are believed to be important for the prevention of PJI. Perhaps one of the most critical aspects of infection prevention, which incidentally has never been studied in a randomized and prospective manner, includes timely and dose-based administration of perioperative antibiotics. At this point, both the ICG and the Centers for Disease Control believe that first-generation cephalosporins or synthetic penicillins are still the best agents for this purpose. There are, however, occasions when an additional antibiotic needs to be used. For patients with penicillin allergies, vancomycin, carbapenems, teicoplanin, or clindamycin may be administered. Vancomycin may also be administered in patients who have a history of MRSA [30]. It is critical to note that vancomycin is not a preferred agent against methicillin-sensitive *S aureus* or other gram-

Modifiable risk factors for PJI		**Nonmodifiable risk factors for PJI**
Factor	**Modification**	**Factor**
Obesity	Lose weight to body mass index < 40 kg/m^2	Older age
Smoking	Decrease/cease smoking	Malignancy
Diabetes	Reduce HbA1c < 7–8	Rheumatoid arthritis
IV drug use	Stop drug use	Liver disease
Alcohol consumption > 4 units/day	Reduce/stop alcohol consumption	Renal failure
Immunosuppressive drugs	Stop certain medications prior to surgery	Sickle cell disease
Anemia	Iron supplementation, erythropoietin	Hepatitis C
Malnutrition (low albumin/protein/prealbumin/transferrin)	Improve diet with protein	HIV infection
Staphylococcus carrier	Decolonize patient	Male gender
		Psoriasis
		Cardiopulmonary disease
		Transplant patients

Table 10-1 Modifiable and nonmodifiable risk factors for developing a prosthetic joint infection.
Abbreviations: PJI, periprosthetic joint infection; IV, intravenous; HbA1c, glycosylated hemoglobin; HIV, human immunodeficiency virus.

positive agents, and hence its use should be combined with another agent with broader activity against other organisms.

There are a number of well-known surgical interventions that can be implemented to reduce the risk of PJI. Reduction of operative time, minimizing soft-tissue dissection, the use of regional anesthesia, reduction of blood loss with the use of agents such as tranexamic acid, the use of clean operating-room systems, and the use of occlusive dressings are examples of such methods [17, 31–34].

Perhaps one of the most important and yet understudied aspects of PJI prevention relates to the use of stringent postoperative protocols. Efforts to minimize hematoma formation, reduce wound drainage, and optimally manage medical conditions such as diabetes, arrhythmia, and cardiac conditions are important postoperative steps that can help reduce the incidence of PJI. In recent years, more efforts have been invested to reduce the need for allogeneic transfusion, which by virtue of immunomodulation, can increase the risk of surgical-site infection and PJI [35]. The administration of intraoperative tranexamic acid, the use of hypotensive regional anesthesia, and the use of less aggressive anticoagulants are all examples of such efforts to reduce blood loss and hematoma formation [36].

1.5 Classification

There are multiple classification systems for PJI, some using the time from index arthroplasty to diagnosis, duration of symptoms, host factors, and the type of microorganisms causing the infection. The most commonly used system is the Tsukayama classification, which provides a guideline for surgical intervention [37–39]. Based on that classification, an early infection is one that occurs within 1 month of the index procedure and may be treated with irrigation, debridement, exchange of mobile parts (if possible), and appropriate antibiotic therapy. Late chronic infections occur more than 1 month after the index procedure and should be treated by a one- or two-stage exchange arthroplasty procedure. Acute hematogenous infections may occur late in the setting of a well-functioning joint replacement. Such cases may be treated by irrigation, debridement, exchange of mobile parts with prosthesis retention, and administration of intravenous antibiotics.

The Zimmerli classification is a modification of the Tsukayama classification that stretches the time periods for each category. Acute infection is defined as one that occurs within 3 months of the index procedure, delayed infections occur between 3–24 months after the index procedure, and late infections occur more than 24 months after the index procedure [40]. This classification system proposes that acute infections are most likely due to seeding of organisms into the joint at the time of index arthroplasty, while late infections may be caused by hematogenous spread from another source of infection or by indolent organisms inoculated at the time of the initial surgery. The etiology of late infections is not well described in this system.

Finally, the McPherson classification evaluates multiple factors, including timing, host factors, and a local extremity grade. Infections occurring within 4 weeks of the surgical procedure are early postoperative infections. Late infections occur after 4 weeks and may have chronic symptoms [41]. Systemic host factors are graded into three categories similarly to those previously proposed in the Cierny-Mader classification [42]. Host type A is uncompromised, host type B has one to two compromising factors, and host type C has two or more compromising factors, such as chronic active infections at other locations or the presence of a neoplasm. The local extremity grade is a rating of the local wound infection site based on factors that may compromise healing, and is graded from 1 (no compromise) to 3 (two or more compromising factors). The presence of soft-tissue loss, multiple incisions, subcutaneous abscesses, fistulas, vascular insufficiency, and previous trauma and/or irradiation are all compromising factors that may affect a patient's ability to heal from a PJI. This classification system is the most comprehensive and clinically relevant of all classification systems. Based on this classification, a patient with early infection who has compromised soft tissues and/or a compromised host may not be a candidate for irrigation and debridement with retention of the prosthesis.

2 Symptoms

Patients who present with PJI may have overt or subtle symptoms of infection. Classically, an infected joint is expected to have redness, swelling, heat from the wound, pain, and loss of function. An example of infected total knee arthroplasty with erythema and edema is seen in **Fig 10-1**. However, many patients with PJI can present with subtle signs of infection and may exhibit none of the symptoms listed above. Pain is the most common presenting symptom of PJI [43]. Any patient presenting with painful prosthetic joint should be evaluated for PJI.

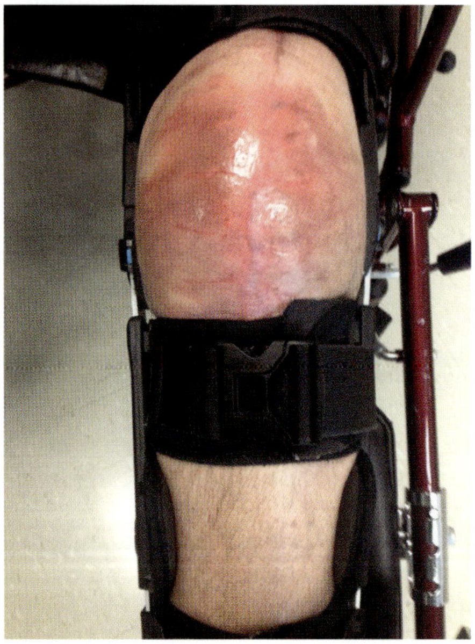

Fig 10-1 An example of infected total knee arthroplasty with erythema and edema.

3 Diagnostic workup

The diagnosis of PJI is challenging and requires a multifaceted approach. The workup of these patients involves taking a thorough history, performing detailed physical examination, and ordering the appropriate tests. The ICG on PJI proposed an algorithmic approach to the diagnosis of PJI that includes performing serological laboratory tests followed by aspiration of the joint (**Fig 10-2**). The aspirate should be analyzed for neutrophil count, polymorphonuclear (PMN) percentage, and should also be cultured. In recent years, the role of molecular biomarkers for diagnosis of PJI has been investigated with synovial α-defensin showing the greatest promise among all the markers with a sensitivity of 97% and specificity of 100% for the diagnosis of PJI [44].

3.1 Patient history

A patient's history should be the first step towards diagnosing an infected arthroplasty. Patients should be asked about recent infection exposure and procedures, as well as symptoms and their beginning.

Patients are at increased risk of PJI in the presence of an infection or inflammatory process in another part of the body, such as the genitourinary, respiratory, cardiac, gastrointestinal, skin, and bloodstream infections. The recent use of antibiotics is often indicative of a potential infectious agent that may seed the joint and result in an infected arthroplasty. Patients should be asked about the symptoms of urinary tract infection, such as urgency, dysuria, frequency, or urinary retention [45–47]. Patients should also be asked about respiratory symptoms, such as cough, dyspnea, and sputum production, which may implicate the upper respiratory tract as the source of possible PJI. Endocarditis can be a cardiac source of infection [48], while cholangitis and cholecystitis from the gastrointestinal tract can also seed a prosthetic joint [49, 50]. Finally, infections in other parts of the body, such as the oral cavity and the large intestine, may contain abscesses that lead to bacteremia and potential for seeding of prosthetic joints. Staphylococcal bacteremia has been reported to have a 30% risk of PJI [51].

Invasive procedures performed on the body may also release bacteria into the bloodstream and predispose patients with prosthetic joints to PJI. Invasive dental procedures, such as drainage of a periapical abscess, may result in the release of bacteria from the oral cavity such as *Treponema denticola, Actinomyces israelii, Actinomyces naeslundii,* and *Streptococcus viridans* and *Streptococcus oralis* [45, 47, 52, 53]. Gastrointestinal procedures such as colonoscopies and endoscopies may result in release of gram-negative organisms such as *Escherichia coli*

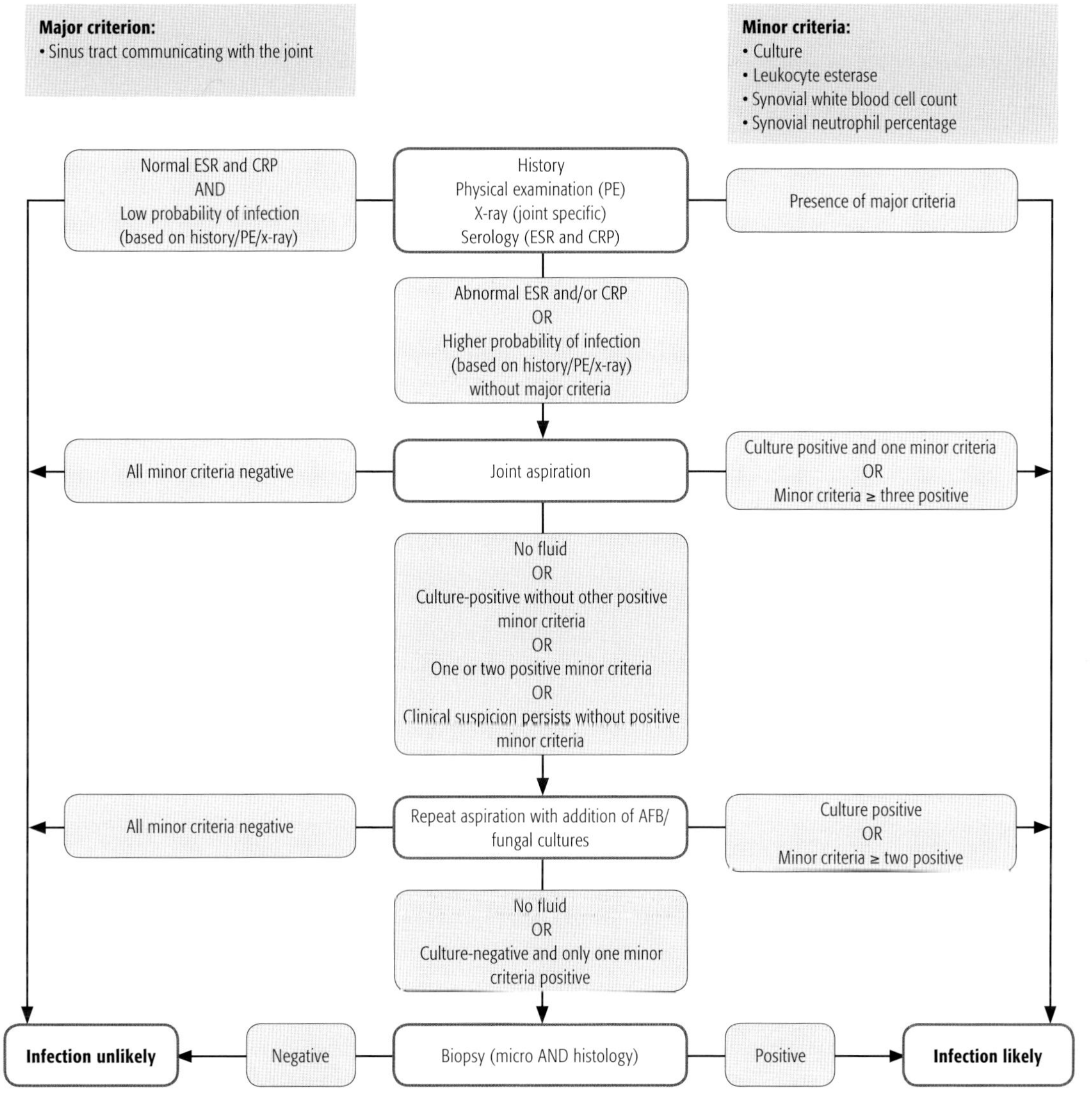

Fig 10-2 Algorithm for diagnosing periprosthetic joint infection.
Abbreviations: ESR, erythrocyte sedimentation rate; CRP, C-reactive protein; PE, physical examination; AFB, acid-fast *Bacillus*.
(Reprinted with permission from: **Parvizi J, Gehrke T.** *Proceedings of the International Consensus Meeting on Periprosthetic Joint Infection*. Towson: Data Trace Publishing Company; 2013:160.)

and *Klebsiella pneumoniae* [54]. Additionally, any recent surgical procedure where the skin has been compromised can increase the burden of commensal organisms, such as *S aureus* and *Staphylococcus epidermidis* [55]. Asking patients about recent procedural history may help targeted investigations for isolation of specific organisms emanating from these sources.

Detailed questioning should be conducted to inquire about the duration of symptoms, as this can dictate the potential treatment regimen for the patient. Symptoms that have an onset within 4 weeks after the index arthroplasty or have a duration of less than 4–6 weeks may be treated by less invasive surgical measures, such as irrigation and debridement combined, if possible, with exchange of mobile parts together with administration of antibiotics. Symptoms that occur much later after the index procedure and are greater than 4–6 weeks in duration may indicate chronic infection and require more aggressive surgical measures, such as one- or two-stage exchange arthroplasty.

3.2 Laboratory

The diagnosis of PJI can be difficult to establish in some cases. There are no specific tests that have been developed for this purpose. Traditionally, the workup of PJI starts with ordering screening serological tests, such as erythrocyte sedimentation rate (ESR) and C-reactive protein (CRP). Although traditionally ordered, serum white blood cell (WBC) count has been shown to have a very low sensitivity for diagnosis of PJI and has been abandoned by most as part of a routine workup [56]. The next step in diagnostic workup includes aspiration of the joint. The joint aspirate is sent for neutrophil count, PMN percentage, and culture. As already mentioned, in recent years, additional tests of the synovial fluid such as leukocyte esterase and molecular biomarkers have also been proposed that may provide additional data point for diagnosis of PJI [57]. Microbiological cultures can be obtained preoperatively from synovial fluid aspirates, or intraoperatively from synovial fluid or tissue samples.

As there is currently no absolute test for diagnosis of PJI, a working group from the Musculoskeletal Infection Society (MSIS) proposed a diagnostic criteria for PJI [58]. The MSIS criteria for PJI were recently slightly modified by the ICG [59]. The definition of PJI based on the ICG modification of the MSIS criteria is presented in **Table 10-2**. A PJI is believed to exist when either a single major criterion or three minor criteria are present.

Major criteria–one present for PJI	Minor criteria–three of five present for PJI
1. Two positive periprosthetic cultures with phenotypically identical organisms	1. Elevated serum CRP and ESR
2. A sinus tract communicating with the joint	2. Elevated synovial fluid WBC count or ++ change on leukocyte esterase test strip
	3. Elevated synovial fluid polymorphonuclear neutrophil percentage
	4. Positive histological analysis of periprosthetic tissue
	5. Single positive culture

Table 10-2 The International Consensus Group definition for periprosthetic joint infection.
Abbreviations: PJI, periprosthetic joint infection; CRP, C-reactive protein; ESR, erythrocyte sedimentation rate; WBC, white blood cell.

The minor criteria must be used in conjunction with other tests, as no single test paints a clear picture of PJI. For example, ESR and CRP are elevated when inflammation is present and are nonspecific for PJI. The threshold level for these tests is also dependent on the laboratory where the test is performed. Depending on the laboratory normal values, a normal ESR is less than 30 mm/h and a normal CRP is less than 1.0 mg/dL or 10 mg/L. When ordering CRP tests, one must order a quantitative CRP and not a high-sensitivity CRP or ultrasensitive CRP, unless a conversion factor is applied [60]. One must also take the timing of infection into account, as ESR and CRP are elevated in the early postoperative period. Erythrocyte sedimentation rate is elevated up to 6 weeks after surgery and CRP is elevated up to 2 weeks after surgery. Thus, these tests may have little utility in the early postoperative period for diagnosing PJI. But if used repeatedly they can provide important information on the kinetics of the CRP.

The criteria for elevated synovial WBC count and synovial PMN percentage can also be affected by the timing of infection and the joint being investigated. Numerous studies have been conducted with each proposing a different threshold for the level of synovial fluid WBC count and PMN percentage. The values have varied between 1,100–3,450 cells/µL for the synovial WBC count and 64–78% for PMN percentage for chronic infections [61–63]. On the other hand, for acute PJI (less than 6 weeks) the threshold for synovial WBC count and PMN percentage have been shown to be higher [64, 65]. The values for each of these tests depend on the time after the index TJA, and on the method used to measure these values. Traditionally, synovial WBC count and PMN percentage have been performed manually. In recent years, almost all laboratories around the world have converted to automated or semiautomated methods for measuring these values. Thus, it is unclear what influence automated measurement of WBC count and PMN percentage has on their value.

Additionally, serum WBC, synovial fluid WBC, PMN percentage, and culture can all be confounded by factors such as the administration of antibiotics. A recent study demonstrated that the administration of antibiotics can significantly reduce the detection of PJI based on positive synovial fluid and tissue cultures from 87% without antibiotics to 73% with antibiotics [66].

The literature highlights the challenges that exist with regard to interpretation of the results of tests that are ordered during workup of PJI. It is clear that the serological and synovial test results are influenced by numerous factors. However, in an attempt to standardize the diagnostic protocol for PJI, the MSIS and the ICG have proposed a threshold for each of these diagnostic parameters (**Table 10-3**).

Another criterion for diagnosing PJI is the histological analysis of synovial fluid or tissue culture. In many facilities, this is a commonly used test, but it may be unreliable. This test is dependent on a number of variables, including the location where the tissue sample was taken, how the test slide was prepared, and the pathologist review of the slides. Counting the number of neutrophils can be subjective and is based on training and experience. Additionally, different samples of tissue may have different neutrophil counts, necessitating a minimum of three biopsies [67]. Based on the American Academy of Orthopaedic Surgeons' criteria for the diagnosis of PJI, a positive test is one that detects ten or more neutrophils in at least five high-power fields using a microscope of at least 400 times magnification [68]. The American Academy of Orthopaedic Surgeons' guidelines suggest that frozen section may be used in patients suspected of having PJI in whom the diagnosis has not been confirmed.

Many orthopedic surgeons still believe that the presence of purulence is a major criterion for PJI, although patients are not often diagnosed with PJI based on purulence alone. This was placed in the minor criteria category for the MSIS definition and was removed from the ICG criteria for PJI, since the presence of purulence only has 82% sensitivity, 32% specificity, 91% positive predictive value, and 17% negative predictive value [69]. It is difficult to diagnose PJI based on a subjective criterion such as purulence, and it may be difficult to differentiate purulence resulting from infection versus inflammatory conditions such as the metal-on-metal failures.

When the diagnosis of infection by traditional methods proves ineffective, the use of serum and synovial biomarkers may aid the diagnosis of infection. Serum biomarkers that may be unique to PJI include interleukin (IL)-6, tumor necrosis factor (TNF)-α, procalcitonin, soluble intercellular adhesion molecule-1 (sICAM-1), short-chain exocellular lipoteichoic acid (sce-LTA), and monocyte chemoattractant protein (MCP)-1 [70–73]. These biomarkers may be more specific than ESR and CRP for diagnosing PJI. Some of the same molecules may be found in the synovial fluid of PJI cases, including IL-6 and TNF-α, while additional cytokines such as IL-1β, IL-8, IL-17, vascular endothelial growth factor (VEGF), and interferon (IFN)-δ may be elevated in the synovial fluid of PJI cases [74–76]. Recent attention has been placed on other synovial fluid markers, including α-defensin, leukocyte esterase, synovial CRP, cathelicidin LL-37, human β-defensin-2 (HBD-2), and HBD-3 [75, 77–79]. While serum may be easier to obtain than synovial fluid, synovial fluid markers may be more sensitive and specific for the diagnosis of PJI.

Laboratory test	Acute PJI (< 90 days)	Chronic PJI (> 90 days)
1. ESR	No threshold	30 mm/h
2. CRP	100 mg/L	10 mg/L
3. Synovial WBC count	10,000 cells/μL	3,000 cells/μL
4. Synovial polymorphonuclear %	90%	80%
5. Leukocyte esterase	+ or ++	+ or ++
6. Histological analysis of tissue	> 5 neutrophils/hpf in 5 hpf (x400 magnification)	> 5 neutrophils/hpf in 5 hpf (x400 magnification)

Table 10-3 Threshold of laboratory values for the minor diagnostic criteria from the International Consensus Group definition for periprosthetic joint infection.
Abbreviations: PJI, periprosthetic joint infection; ESR, erythrocyte sedimentation rate; CRP, C-reactive protein; WBC, white blood cell; hpf, high power field.

3.3 Imaging

Imaging modalities have limited use for diagnosing PJI (see chapter 7 Diagnostics). All TJA patients should have a plain x-ray of the suspected joint, as x-rays in a patient with PJI may be normal or demonstrate periosteal bone growth, transcortical sinus tracts, or loosening (**Fig 10-3**). Computed tomography (CT) and magnetic resonance imaging have limited use secondary to scatter from the implant, but may be used to evaluate the soft tissue with findings such as periprosthetic fluid collections and abscesses [80]. Nuclear imaging should not have a direct role in the diagnosis of PJI, but may be helpful for ruling out infection in a few cases. Positive emission tomography labeled with fluorodeoxyglucose can identify areas of increased biological activity, but is not limited to PJI [81, 82]. Patients with PJI may have increased uptake on triple-phase bone scans, but scans may also be positive if there is implant loosening or bone remodeling associated with normal bone ingrowth around the implant [83]. White blood cell indium scans or 99mTc-antigranulocyte single photon emission computed tomography (SPECT)/CT scans may be more specific for PJI, but will also show other areas of inflammation [84–86]. Bone scans, including WBC-labeled scans, should rarely be ordered during workup of a patient suspected of PJI as they carry low sensitivity.

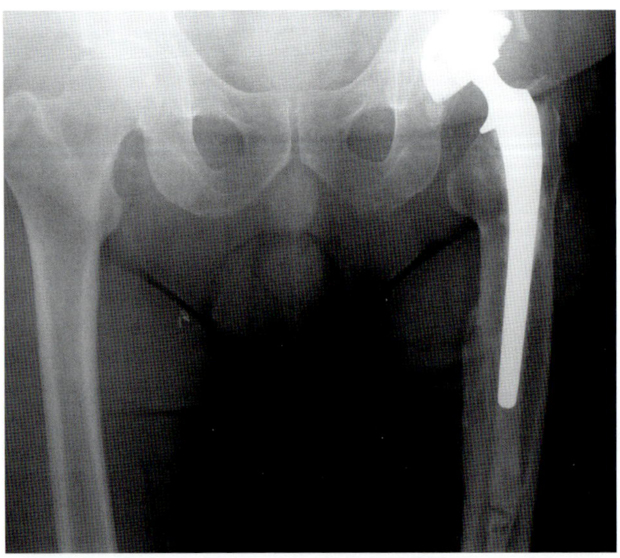

Fig 10-3 X-ray evidence of loosening secondary to periprosthetic joint infection.

4 Treatment options

Treatment of periprosthetic infection includes nonoperative and operative options.

Implant-related infections are characterized by the presence of biofilm(s)-embedded bacteria, hence the main goal of any treatment should be to completely remove all bacteria and biofilms adherent to the infected prosthesis and the surrounding tissues. Unfortunately, this may or may not be achieved by nonoperative means and may explain the relatively frequent infection recurrence after the least invasive therapeutic approaches.

On the other hand, surgical treatments are aimed at physical removal of biofilms and infected tissues and implants, but the best surgical modality for treating chronic periprosthetic joint infections remains controversial, with a lack of controlled, randomized, comparative studies.

Surgical procedures range from simple debridement with implant retention or change of modular implant parts to staged joint reimplantation, arthrodesis, or amputation. Once again, available data show that success is directly related to the surgeon's ability to completely remove all infected materials, and less invasive surgical treatments such as debridement and retention have approximately half the rate of success, compared to those involving implant removal. Complete removal of an infected implant, accurate debridement, and joint reconstruction can be extremely challenging, with high risk of complications, need for specifically trained teams, and high associated costs. Moreover, there is some evidence that a less invasive approach may work relatively well in otherwise healthy patients and fail in more immunocompromised hosts.

In some cases, in which all other treatments failed or were refused by the patients, salvage procedures like resection arthroplasty, arthrodesis, or amputation may be the only possible option.

In spite of growing research and scientific evidence in this field and the many efforts to produce a universal algorithm to drive the most appropriate treatment in any given patient, treatment choice still largely relies on each team's experience and on an open discussion with the patient about possible risk and benefits of different options according to his or her specific condition and needs.

4.1 Nonsurgical treatment

Given the biofilm-related nature of PJIs, medical treatments are often of limited value and unable to achieve prolonged infection control when used alone [87]. The rate of failure is markedly higher when the PJI fulfills the criteria of chronic infection, even when patients did undergo open debridement without implant removal [88, 89].

With the lack of effective antibiofilm agents for systemic administration [90], nonoperative treatment mainly relies on symptomatic treatments (eg, antiinflammatory drugs, analgesics, orthopedic brace) and on suppressive antibiotic therapy. Suppressive antibiotic therapy is defined as the prolonged use of oral antibiotics for the prevention of relapsing symptoms and functional failure in those patients with implant retention.

Nonsurgical treatment is generally reserved for patients with a nonpainful septic prosthesis caused by microorganisms that are sensitive to oral antibiotics. In particular, suppressive antibiotic treatment may be indicated for patients in whom one or more of the following are present [28, 59]:

- Refusal of surgical treatment
- Cannot be surgically treated because of a high surgical risk due to comorbidities
- Have an infection that has not been eradicated after previous surgical treatment(s), according to clinical, laboratory, or imaging data
- Not painful and well-osseointegrated infected implants, in which an increased disability and/or large bone defect secondary to removal of the prosthesis may be foreseen

There is no clear evidence that one antibiotic regimen is more effective than another [28, 59] and many recommendations are largely based on empirie decisions. Identification of the microorganism and selection of the antibiotic therapy based on the susceptibility pattern of the isolated pathogen, preferably obtained from deep samples by joint aspiration or surgical debridement, is generally recommended. Taking into account the low probability of infection eradication and limited scientific data available, antibiotic treatment can be divided in two steps:

1. Induction to remission
2. Chronic suppression

The first step is usually achieved by using a bactericidal oral or intravenous combination of antibiotics, including rifampin, that should never be used alone for the high risk of inducing bacterial resistance, in cases of gram-positive infection, or fluoroquinolone in cases of gram-negative infection, whenever possible. The first phase of antibiotic treatment should be maintained until clinical signs of infection disappear and systemic inflammatory parameters, eg, CRP or ESR, improve for 6–12 weeks. After this period, chronic oral antibiotic suppression should be initiated using monotherapy or an association of antibiotics with a good safety profile and high oral bioavailability.

The optimal antibiotic treatment duration has not been established, but it may last several months and often depends on clinical conditions and on its tolerability by the patient. Ideally, effective suppressive therapy should be administered for the rest of the patient's life, but this is rarely observed. According to the literature, the average length of oral antibiotic suppression is approximately 2 years, ranging from 4 to 100 months in patients with chronic PJI with a reported success rate higher than 60% after prolonged follow-up periods [91–94]. Other authors did not observe similar results and reported a high rate of adverse events associated with chronic antibiotic therapy [95].

There is no clinical experience about the consequences of stopping suppressive antibiotic treatments and the risk of relapse or infection dissemination and secondary sepsis. Experience from chronic osteomyelitis suggests that these infections generally remain localized [96].

4.2 Debridement and retention

Debridement and implant retention, also known as irrigation and debridement, aims at preserving the already implanted prosthesis, treating the patient with surgical cleaning of the prosthesis, with or without changing modular parts of the implant, and debridement of the surrounding tissues followed by antibiotic treatment.

There is a general consensus for the potentially positive aspects of an irrigation and debridement procedure [90, 97] compared with exchange surgeries: reduced risk of complications and blood loss, bone stock and function preservation and reduced costs. Still, the success rates of this debridement procedure are low and variable in the literature, ranging from 15% to 75%, with an average eradication rate of 44.9% at a mean 52 months follow-up in a recent systematic review, including periprosthetic knee and hip infections [98].

Indications for performing an irrigation and debridement are not well defined and range from the presence of a working joint with a well-fixed implant to the duration of symptoms [99].

If irrigation and debridement is performed, it is imperative to ensure that the prostheses are well-fixed, not painful and well-positioned and there is a good soft-tissue envelope to cover the prosthesis.

Moreover, the literature suggests that irrigation and debridement should be preferred over surgical removal of the existing implant when symptoms are sufficiently "recent". Symptoms' duration may range from early, postsurgical, infections from 3 to 12 weeks from index procedure, and from 3 to 4 weeks for late hematogenous infections [97, 100–104].

A higher success rate for this procedure has been reported in healthier patients and in infections with low-virulence organisms [89, 105–110].

Absolute contraindication for irrigation and debridement include the inability to close a wound or the presence of a loose prosthesis. Relative contraindications are the presence of a sinus tract, an infection with highly virulent organisms such as MRSA [109, 111] or polymicrobial infections [112], often as a result of the presence of a sinus, and in patients with extensive comorbidities, in particular those with immunocompromised status [107, 113]. Marculescu et al [92] found that the presence of a sinus tract leads to an odds ratio of 2.84 for failure of irrigation and debridement.

Concerning surgical technique, there is a consensus [28, 59] that irrigation and debridement should be performed meticulously and according to the following steps:

1. Preoperative optimization of the patient; irrigation and debridement should not be regarded as an emergency procedure. The patient, without generalized sepsis, should be optimized prior to the procedure.
2. Good visualization and thorough debridement by open access. Surgical access should preferably be obtained through an already existing scar. Endoscopic or arthroscopic access has no role in irrigation and debridement of an infected prosthetic joint, since several studies demonstrate that the outcome of irrigation and debridement is markedly worse when debridement is performed using arthroscopy [101, 106, 114].
3. Removal and exchange of all modular parts of the infected implant whenever possible. Although there is no clear evidence in the literature regarding the role of exchanging modular components [97] and the fact that this practice results in added expenses, prolongs the surgery, and could potentially increase morbidity, it has also been pointed out that it can reduce bacterial burden by removing microorganisms adherent on the removed components and it allows access to parts of the joint that otherwise could not be reached, thus improving the debridement procedure.
4. Obtain multiple tissue-culture samples, preferably not swabs [115], and send the removed implant components for microbiological analysis and biofilm-disrupting sonication [116, 117] or chemical processing [118]; four to six tissue samples should be taken from areas that macroscopically appear most clinically infected. These should include the superficial, deep, and periprosthetic layers and the interfaces between modular components. The samples should be submitted for aerobic and anaerobic culture. Antibiotic prophylaxis at the time of induction does not alter the results of the microbiological cultures obtained during the surgery and should not be withheld [119].
5. Copious joint irrigation with approximately 6–9 L of saline. There is no evidence that using antiseptic solutions provides any benefit over saline. The use of high-pressure pulsatile lavage has recently been shown to be ineffective in dislodging biofilms [120] and some reports suggested that it may even spread infection deeper [121, 122].
6. Remove the prosthesis if loosened. Even if preoperative assessments did show that the implant is well fixed, the prosthesis should be tested intraoperatively for its stability and osseointegration. In the case the implant should be found loosened intraoperatively, it should be removed, shifting to a resection arthroplasty or to a one- or two-stage procedure. This eventuality should be discussed in advance with the patient and the decision anticipated as part of the informed consent.

Repeated irrigation and debridement offers limited improvement in the eradication rate at final follow-up [123] and is not recommended [90] unless within a specific protocol and with adequate patient information [120]. An increase in the failure rate of implant revision surgery, in the case of infection relapse after previous unsuccessful irrigation and debridement procedures, has been shown [124, 125].

Irrigation and debridement is usually followed by a variable period of antibiotic treatment, ranging from 4 to 12 weeks. Antibiotic treatment should be administered systemically and targeted to the isolated pathogen(s) whenever possible. There is insufficient evidence to support administration of continuous intraarticular antibiotics for the treatment of PJI and this is not currently recommended [90, 28].

Similarly, there is no conclusive evidence that the use of any local antibiotic-impregnated resorbable material significantly improves the outcome of surgical intervention for irrigation and debridement, although their use does not appear to be contraindicated [126, 127].

4.3 One- and two-stage exchanges

Exchange arthroplasty surgery for infection, one- or two-stage surgery, is a challenging procedure and should be reserved for experienced centers and surgeons. The morbidity and mortality associated with such surgery should not to be ignored. Teamwork is paramount to the success of the surgery. A multidisciplinary approach with microbiologists, infectious diseases physicians, critical-care anesthesiologist, plastic surgeons, and orthopedic surgeons with a particular interest in infection is essential [39].

Currently, two-stage exchange arthroplasty surgery is the most popular surgical regime for the management of PJI in North America and in several other countries worldwide; however, to date no randomized controlled trial provided absolute indications or contraindications for one- or two-stage exchange arthroplasty and comparative large prospective studies are lacking [39, 100, 128].

Patient selection bias, variability in surgical techniques, including time periods prior to reimplantation or the use of cemented or cementless implants, wide differences in the reported rates of infection eradication and in morbidity and mortality make direct comparisons between one- and two-stage procedures particularly difficult [129, 130].

A recent systematic review examined two-stage knee exchange in 38 studies and 1,421 patients to provide, on average, a better outcome compared to one-stage, as reported in six papers and 204 patients, ie, 89.8% infection eradication rate at a mean 44.7 months follow-up versus 81.9% at 40.7 months [131]. Similar findings were reported for the hip, with an average infection eradication rate of 81.7% after a single-stage (20 papers and 1,221 patients, at 58.4 months mean follow-up) and 91.1% after two-stage (63 papers, 3,360 patients, 67.3 months follow-up) [132]. Considering a single-stage cementless exchange (n = 81, only three studies available), the average infection eradication rate was 91.4% at a mean follow-up of 81 months. On the other side, satisfactory results have been recently reported in selected patients treated with "partial" two-stage revision surgery, in which only one component of a hip prosthesis had been exchanged in a two-stage procedure [133].

Concerning the shoulder prosthesis, a recent systematic review revealed no clear difference in infection control comparing one- or two-stage revision surgery, with an average better functional results in patients treated with a one-stage procedure [134].

Although definitive indications and contraindications to one- or two-stage exchange are lacking, there is some consensus [28, 90] that one-stage exchange can be a reasonable option for the treatment of PJI in circumstances where effective antibiotics are available but not in patients with systemic manifestations of infection, ie, sepsis, in whom resection arthroplasty and reduction of bioburden may be necessary. Relative contraindications to performing a one-stage exchange may include lack of identification of an organism preoperatively or the presence of multi-resistant bacteria, the presence of a sinus tract or severe soft-tissue involvement that may lead to the need for flap coverage [28, 135].

The immunocompromised patient or the presence of medical comorbidities, including obesity, metastatic disease, advanced cardiac disease, and renal and/or liver dysfunction (**Fig 10-4**), have been shown to impact on the infection eradication success rates and certainly influence morbidity and mortality. The presence of comorbidities may reduce the success rate of one-stage revision, thus representing a relative contraindication to this surgical option [137].

Conditions in which one-stage is considered to be contraindicated can be managed through a two-stage approach. These include:

- Patients with systemic manifestations of infection (ie, sepsis)
- Infection appears obvious but no organism has been identified preoperatively or preoperative cultures identified are difficult-to-treat and antibiotic-resistant organisms
- Presence of a sinus tract or inadequate and nonviable soft-tissue coverage

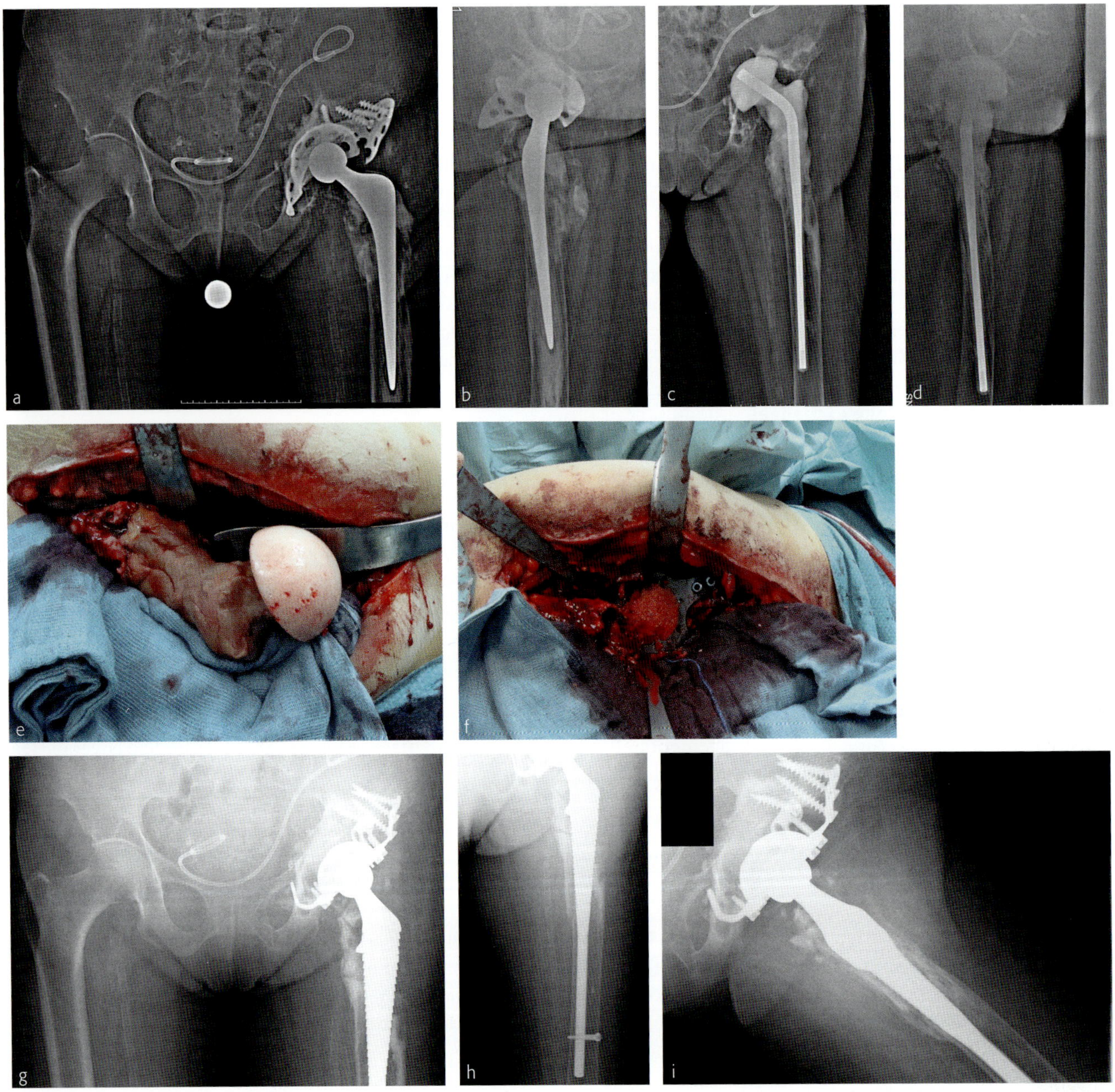

Fig 10-4a–i A 50-year-old woman with renal transplant. After six previous hip surgeries, she came with a chronic periprosthetic hip infection with draining sinus and severe bone loss. Cultures grew out multiresistant *Escherechia coli* and *Pseudomonas aeruginosa*.

a–b Preoperative x-rays.
c–d After septic prosthesis and cement removal and preformed hip spacer implant.
e At the time of spacer removal. Note the large bone defect of the proximal third of the femur.
f Intraoperative acetabulum reconstruction with morcellized bone grafts and uncemented prosthesis.
g–i Postoperative x-rays 2 years after reimplantation. Note bone remodeling both at the femoral and acetabular sites.

Concerning two-stage exchange, there is no definitive evidence in the literature as to the spacer choice or optimal time interval between the two stages: reports vary from 2 weeks to several months [39, 127, 128, 132]. Videos demonstrating techniques on proper spacer fabrication for hip (**Video 10-1**, **Video 10-2**), knee (**Video 10-3**), and shoulder (**Video 10-4**) can be viewed. Intravenous antibiotic therapy lasting 4–6 weeks with subsequent cessation of antibiotics for 2–8 weeks prior to reimplantation is most commonly employed.

There is also no definitive evidence concerning economic impact of one- versus two-stage revision; differences in cost between one-stage and two-stage exchange arthroplasty are not straightforward to analyze. Costs may vary due to factors associated with hospital facilities, patients, surgeons, and the infecting organism. However, it may generally be accepted that patient morbidity, operative time, operating room use, hospital and surgeon fees, and duration of antibiotic administration are less when undergoing one procedure versus a minimum of two major procedures. A cost analysis by Klouche et al [137] revealed that two-stage revision of septic total hip arthroplasty cost 1.7 times more than a one-stage revision. If the results of one-stage and two-stage exchange arthroplasty are comparable, one-stage may be preferred due to the advantages of decreased patient morbidity, lower cost, improved mechanical stability of the affected limb, and shorter period of disability [138].

4.4 Salvage procedures and amputation

Salvage procedures for periprosthetic infections include resection arthroplasty or permanent spacer and arthrodesis. Resection hip arthroplasty can be very successful in the control of infection and allow for assisted ambulation, although functional outcome is often rather poor [139].

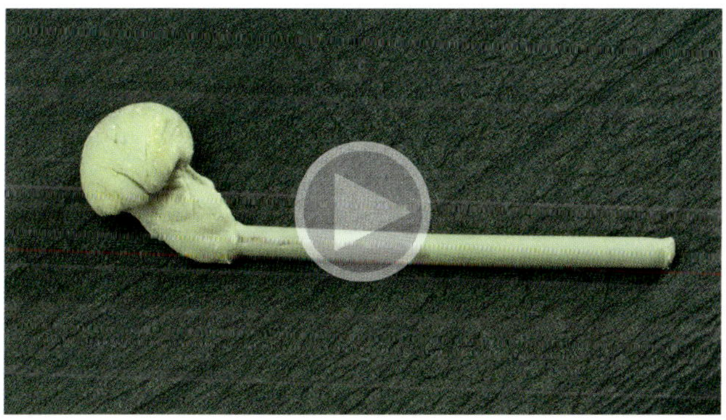

Video 10-1 The making a hip spacer video demonstrates a method for creating an articulating antibiotic hip spacer to replace an infected hip replacement.

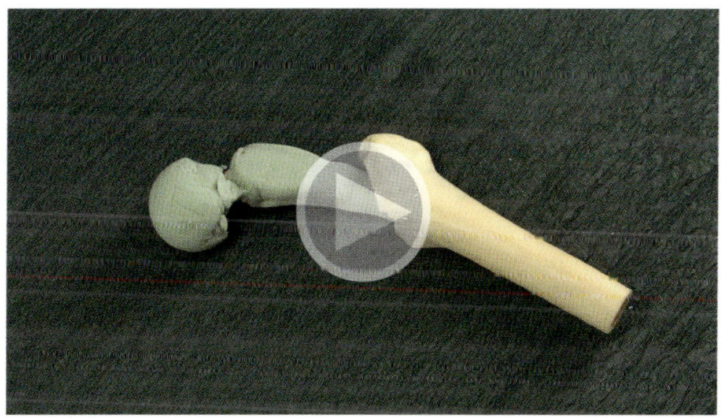

Video 10-2 The coating a femoral stem video demonstrates a method for creating an articulating antibiotic hip spacer to replace an infected hip replacement.

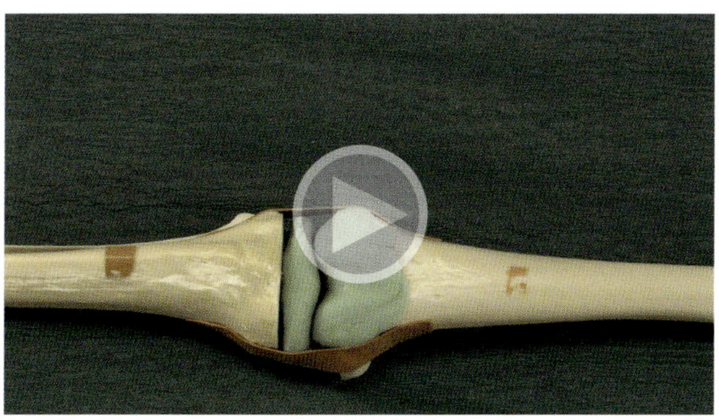

Video 10-3 The making an articulating knee spacer video demonstrates a way to create an antibiotic cement spacer to manage an infected total knee replacement. Although there are a number of ways to create such a spacer, this particular method is a reasonable option to do so.

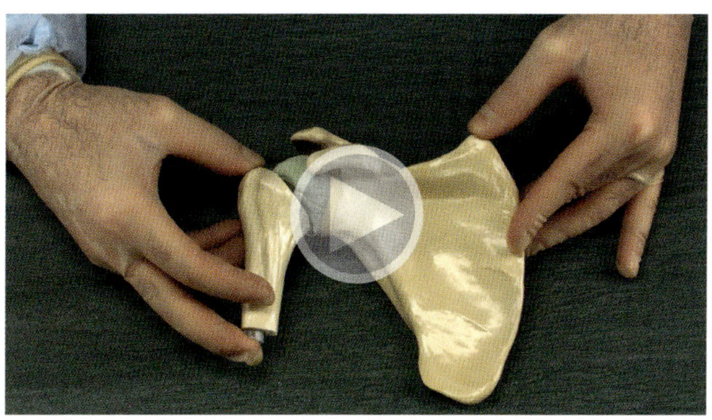

Video 10-4 The making a shoulder spacer video demonstrates creation of an antibiotic articulating spacer for managing an infected shoulder replacement.

Similarly, resection arthroplasty or the "permanent" use of an articulating spacer have been described as possible options to manage periprosthetic shoulder infection with high success rate on infection control, but with relatively poor functional results [133].

Knee arthrodesis or a fixed knee prosthesis may be appropriate options for patients who have had failed multiple attempts at reconstruction and stand an unacceptably high risk of recurrent infection with repeat arthroplasty procedures and/or have a deficient extensor mechanism or inadequate soft-tissue coverage, extensive bone loss, and a painful and/or unstable joint [126, 135, 140–144].

Severely immunocompromised hosts, alcohol, or intravenous drug abusers, and/or the presence of polymicrobial infections or those due to highly resistant organisms for which there is no effective antimicrobial therapy may also benefit from knee arthrodesis [145, 146].

Relative contraindications might apply to nonambulatory patients or those with extensive medical comorbidity that precludes multiple surgeries. In fact, knee arthrodesis may be performed as one- or two-stage, the decision depending on the individual circumstances and the host factors. One-stage arthrodesis, using an external fixation device, is most successful when conducted in cases of PJI caused by low-virulence organisms and minimal soft-tissue compromise [147]. Eradication of infection prior to arthrodesis allows an expanded armamentarium for fixation, such as the use of intramedullary and plating devices, with a reported success rate in infection control exceeding 90% [135, 148, 149].

The choice between arthrodesis and amputation needs to take into account the clinical situation of the individual and patient preference.

Amputation for treatment of PJI affecting the knee or the hip may be appropriate in selected cases involving a non-ambulatory patient, necrotizing fasciitis resistant to aggressive debridement, extremely severe bone loss, or complex periprosthetic infected fractures, inadequate soft-tissue coverage, multiple failed attempts at staged exchange and resection arthroplasty or severe peripheral vascular disease, neurovascular injury, and pain [132, 136, 150, 151]. Except in emergency cases, referral to a center with specialist experience in the management of PJI is advised before amputation is carried out, due to high mortality rates [146, 152, 153].

4.5 Treatment algorithm

Several classifications of PJIs have been proposed in the last few decades, aimed at driving treatment choice [38, 42, 154–156]; however, no single algorithm is universally recognized and accepted in the clinical use [28, 90].

Treatment algorithms, based on various periprosthetic infection classifications, are mainly focused on the time of onset of the infection; this probably relies on the implicit assumption that the shorter the time from onset of an infection, the less the spreading of bacterial colonization and hence the higher the chance to save an implant by a less invasive surgical approach, like debridement and retention.

To the authors' knowledge, the algorithm that has been extensively tested and validated clinically, by the same authors that have developed the protocol, is the one proposed by Zimmerli et al [89, 157, 158]. This algorithm, with only slight modifications, has been recently included in the Infectious Diseases Society of America guidelines [160]; it relies on the time from onset of infection and on some other variables, to progressively drive decisions from the least invasive debridement and retention (**Table 10-4**) to prosthesis exchange (**Table 10-5**, **Table 10-6**), or to other options (**Table 10-7**).

Presentation		Observation		Action
Duration of symptoms < 3 weeks OR Joint age < 30 days	Yes	Well-fixed prosthesis Absence of sinus tract Susceptible to oral antimicrobial agents	No	Removal of prosthesis
			Yes	Debridement and retention
	No			Removal of prosthesis

Table 10-4 Treatment algorithm to decide debridement and retention, rewritten and according to Infectious Diseases Society of America guidelines [154].

Presentation	Action
• THA • Good soft tissue • Identity of the organisms determined preoperatively • Good bone stock • Susceptible to oral agents with high oral bioavailability • Use of antibiotics-impregnated bone cement for fixation • No bone grafting required	One-stage exchange

Table 10-5 Treatment algorithm to decide one-stage exchange, rewritten and according to Infectious Diseases Society of America guidelines [154].
Abbreviation: THA, total hip arthroplasty.

Among several limitations that can be found in this or other treatment algorithms, the questionable role of time from infection onset is worth noting. Although the assumption that an implant-related infection is a time-dependent process looks intuitive, as it is often the case for parenchymal organs, currently available data on biofilm formation contradict the simple equation "early infection = less invasive approach and better prognosis", suggesting that time may not be the (only) reliable parameter to predict the success of implant retention. In fact, there is increasing evidence that mature biofilm(s) are formed within a few hours or days after bacterial adhesion. This finding may explain why implant retention often fails, even if performed within days or weeks after surgery and it raises important questions such as whether the time limits of 3 weeks, 30 days, or 90 days are based on a scientifically sound rationale or only on an insufficient understanding of the biofilm-related infections.

In this regard it should also be noted that currently available classifications and treatment algorithms of periprosthetic infection do not consider another variable that may be at least as important as time to drive the choice and the success of a given surgical treatment: the localization of bacteria around the implant. The site of bacterial colonization may in fact be such that it is not technically possible to remove the colonizing microorganisms even if debridement is performed at a very early stage of infection onset. In fact, even a few bacteria adhering to the implant-bone interface may not be reached by surgical debridement with implant retention, thus maintaining the infection, which may eventually recur after weeks or months after surgical debridement. Current classifications and treatment algorithms probably omit localization of biofilm and bacteria as a key factor to the success of surgery simply because we do not have appropriate techniques to demonstrate them prior to or during surgery.

Moreover, there is growing evidence that our technical ability to dislodge established biofilms from a surface is particularly limited, as, for example, simple scraping or curettage may only be partially effective as revealed by electron-scan images, while pulse lavage has been recently reported to be ineffective [160], thus further limiting the efficacy of any less invasive approach.

Presentation		Action
• Poor soft tissue OR • Difficult to treat microorganisms, AND • No prior two-stage exchange for infection or prior two-stage exchange and reason for failure, AND • Delayed reimplantation technically feasible, AND • Anticipated good functional outcome	Yes	Two-stage exchange
	No	See **Table 10-7**

Table 10-6 Treatment algorithm to decide two-stage exchange, rewritten and according to Infectious Diseases Society of America guidelines [154].

Presentation		Observation		Action
• Necrotizing fasciitis OR • Severe bone loss OR • Inability or failure of soft-tissue coverage OR • Prior failed attempt of resection arthroplasty or arthrodesis to control infection OR • No medical therapy available OR • Functional benefit to amputation over resection arthroplasty or arthrodesis	No	Patient comorbidities OR Patients preferences preclude additional surgery	No	Resection arthroplasty OR Arthrodesis
			Yes	Medical therapy only
	Yes			Consider amputation Referral to specialty hospital

Table 10-7 Treatment algorithm to decide other options, rewritten and according to Infectious Diseases Society of America guidelines [154].

Another important variable that most of the current algorithms do not consider is the host's type. The study of Simpson et al [161, 162] found that a less invasive approach to bone infection may work in Cierny-Mader type A, immunocompetent hosts, but not in type B or C patients. Also, currently available classifications of host's type look largely based on empiric observation and not on scientific data, with substantial differences between scoring systems [38, 152, 153]. Little is truly known about the host's immune system at the present time.

Based on these considerations, the authors find it more appropriate to provide a profile of possible candidates to the various treatment strategies based on current knowledge and with the relative chance of infection eradication rate (**Table 10-8**, **Table 10-9**, **Table 10-10**).

This schema, although necessarily incomplete and subject to further update as new data will become available, may serve as a basis to discuss risk and benefits of different treatment options in any given patient.

Presentation	Type of treatment	Average infection eradication rate
Patients who refuse surgical treatment OR Patients who cannot be surgically treated because of a high surgical risk due to comorbidities AND Patients who have an infection that has not been eradicated according to clinical, laboratory, or imaging data AND Patients who have an infection caused by pathogens sensitive to oral antibiotics AND Not painful and well-osteointegrated infected implants OR In which an increased disability and/or large bone defect secondary to removal of the prosthesis may be foreseen	Less invasive treatment (ie, prolonged suppressive antibiotic treatment)	Variable, but up to 60% in some reports
Short symptoms' duration (< 4–12 weeks from index procedure or < 4 weeks from first diagnosis for late hematogenous infections) OR Patients who refuse surgical removal of the existing implant OR Patients who cannot be treated with implant removal because of a high surgical risk due to comorbidities AND Not painful and well-osteointegrated infected implants, with good soft-tissue envelope to cover the prosthesis AND/OR In which an increased disability and/or large bone defect secondary to removal of the prosthesis may be foreseen AND/OR Type A hosts AND/OR Low-virulence organisms AND/OR No sinus tracts	Debridement and implant retention (irrigation and debridement)	15–75% (both for hip or knee) On average approximately 45% at 50 months follow-up

Table 10-8 Proposed patient's profile for implant retention in periprosthetic hip or knee infections.

Presentation	Type of treatment	Average infection eradication rate
Longer symptom duration (> 4–12 weeks from index procedure or > 4 weeks from first diagnosis for late hematogenous infections OR Periprosthetic chronic joint infection OR Painful or loosened infected implants, with good soft-tissue envelope to cover the prosthesis AND/OR Type A hosts AND/OR Low-virulence organisms AND/OR No sinus tracts	One-stage exchange	57–100% (hip) and from 73–100% (knee) On average approximately 80% at 60 months follow-up
Longer symptoms' duration (> 4–12 weeks from index procedure or > 4 weeks from first diagnosis for late hematogenous infections OR Periprosthetic chronic joint infection OR Painful or loosened infected implants, with good soft-tissue envelope to cover the prosthesis AND/OR All microorganism types or unidentified pathogen AND/OR Presence of a sinus tract or inadequate and nonviable soft-tissue coverage AND/OR Generalized sepsis	Two-stage exchange	74–100% (both for hip or knee) On average approximately 90% at 60 months follow-up

Table 10-9 Proposed patient's profile for hip or knee exchange procedures.

Presentation	Type of treatment	Average infection eradication rate
Periprosthetic chronic joint infection AND/OR Failed multiple attempts at reconstruction AND/OR A painful and/or unstable joint AND/OR Unacceptably high risk of recurrent infection AND/OR With a deficient extensor mechanism AND/OR Inadequate soft-tissue coverage AND/OR Extensive bone loss AND/OR Severely immunocompromised hosts, alcohol, or drug abusers AND/OR Polymicrobial infections or due to highly-resistant organisms for which there is no effective antimicrobial therapy	Arthrodesis or fixed joint prosthesis (knee)	> 90%
Periprosthetic chronic joint infection AND/OR Failed multiple attempts at reconstruction AND/OR A painful and/or unstable joint AND/OR Unacceptably high risk of recurrent infection AND/OR Inadequate soft-tissue coverage AND/OR Extensive bone loss AND/OR Severely immunocompromised hosts, alcohol, or drug abusers AND/OR Polymicrobial infections or due to highly resistant organisms for which there is no effective antimicrobial therapy	Resection arthroplasty (hip)	> 90%
Failure, refusal, or contraindications to other salvage procedures OR Necrotizing fasciitis resistant to aggressive debridement AND/OR Severe bone loss that precludes arthrodesis (knee) AND/OR Inadequate soft-tissue coverage AND/OR Periprosthetic fracture AND/OR Peripheral vascular disease and neurovascular injury or neuropathy	Amputation	

Table 10-10 Proposed patient's profile for hip or knee salvage procedures or amputation.

5 Conclusion

Periprosthetic infection is a challenging condition, which requires prompt recognition, accurate diagnostic evaluation, and adequate treatment.

Given the central role played by biofilms, both the microbiological and surgical approaches should be specifically directed to identify biofilm-embedded bacteria, prevent bacterial adherence on implant surface, and dislodge bacteria and biofilms, when implant surface become colonized by microorganisms.

Unfortunately our knowledge of the pathogenesis of the infection is limited and hence most current diagnostic and treatment approaches remain inadequate or only partially effective.

Moreover, we still have a lack of understanding of the host's role and very few ways to improve the ability of a compromised host to resist biofilm-related infections.

In spite of these limitations, recent new technologies, more standardized treatment protocols, and dedicated centers and teams have raised the overall infection eradication rate after PJI to approximately 80–90%, with acceptable function restoration in most of the cases. Based on current research, it may be anticipated that our ability to improve early diagnosis, prevent, and treat implant-related infection will improve in the future, when specifically designed diagnostic tools (**Fig 10-5**), antibacterial implant coatings (**Fig 10-6**), and antibiofilm agents become available.

A universal algorithm to select the appropriate clinical decision for a given patient is not yet available. The treatment choice should still rely on each team's experience, open-minded approach, and frank discussion with the patient about possible risks and benefits of different options, according to specific conditions and needs.

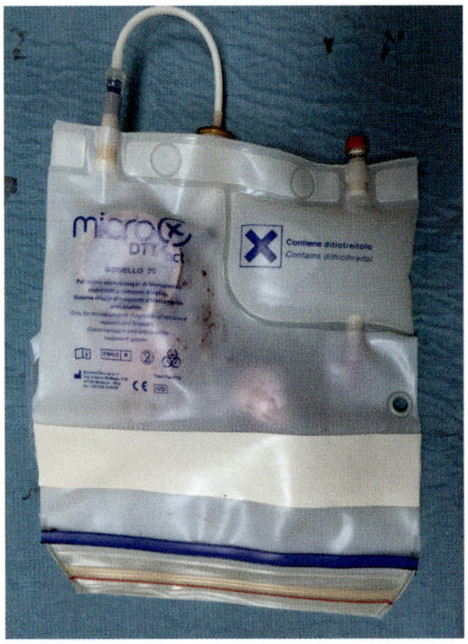

Fig 10-5 Microbiological diagnosis can be improved by closed systems that allow collection, transportation, and processing of retrieved implants and tissues. The MicroDTTect system frees biofilm-embedded bacteria eventually present on a sample by using dithiothreitol, a chemical compound able to destroy bacterial biofilms, without affecting pathogen vitality **[118]**.

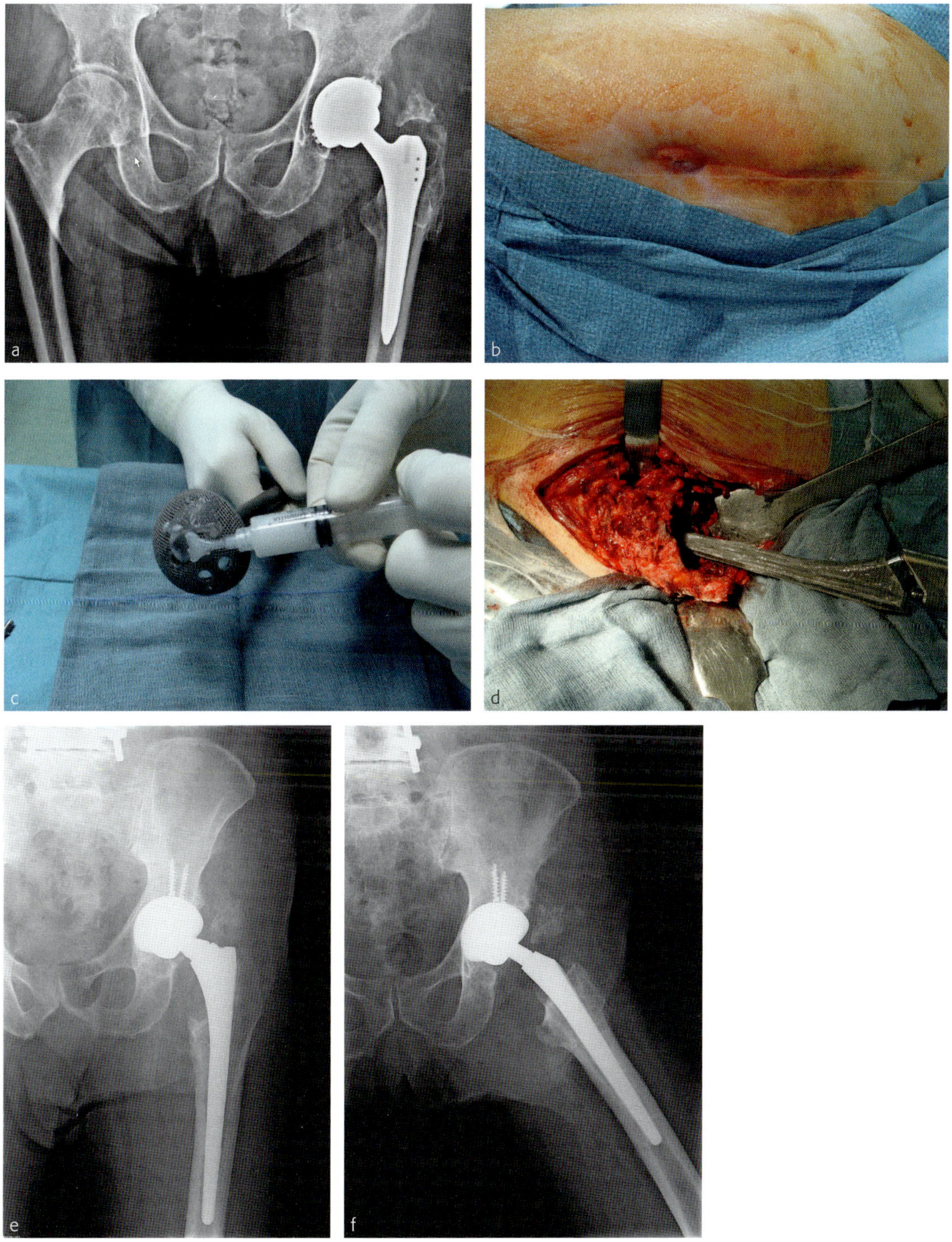

Fig 10-6a–f An 87-year-old cardiopathic man. Chronic periprosthetic hip infection with draining sinus. Cultures grew out multiresistant *Staphylococcus epidermidis.*

a Preoperative x-ray.
b Clinical aspect at the time of surgery.
c–d Coating of the cementless implant with a fast-resorbable vancomycin-loaded hydrogel and one-stage exchange.
e–f X-ray taken 2 years after implantation. The patient is free of symptoms.

6 References

1. **Schmalzried TP, Amstutz HC, Au MK, et al.** Etiology of deep sepsis in total hip arthroplasty. The significance of hematogenous and recurrent infections. *Clin Orthop Relat Res.* 1992 Jul(280):200–207.
2. **Dale H, Fenstad AM, Hallan G, et al.** Increasing risk of prosthetic joint infection after total hip arthroplasty. *Acta Orthop.* 2012 Oct;83(5):449–458.
3. **Mangram AJ, Horan TC, Pearson ML, et al.** Guideline for Prevention of Surgical Site Infection, 1999. Centers for Disease Control and Prevention (CDC) Hospital Infection Control Practices Advisory Committee. *Am J Infect Control.* 1999 Apr;27(2):97–132; quiz 133–134; discussion 96.
4. **Kurtz SM, Lau E, Schmier J, et al.** Infection burden for hip and knee arthroplasty in the United States. *J Arthroplasty.* 2008 Oct;23(7):984–991.
5. **Kurtz SM, Lau E, Watson H, et al.** Economic burden of periprosthetic joint infection in the United States. *J Arthroplasty.* 2012 Sep;27(8 Suppl):61–65 e1.
6. **Phillips JE, Crane TP, Noy M, et al.** The incidence of deep prosthetic infections in a specialist orthopaedic hospital: a 15-year prospective survey. *J Bone Joint Surg Br.* 2006 Jul;88(7):943–948.
7. **Dale H, Hallan G, Hallan G, et al.** Increasing risk of revision due to deep infection after hip arthroplasty. *Acta Orthop.* 2009 Dec;80(6):639–645.
8. **Bozic KJ, Ong K, Lau E, et al.** Estimating risk in Medicare patients with THA: an electronic risk calculator for periprosthetic joint infection and mortality. *Clin Orthop Relat Res.* 2013 Feb;471(2):574–583.
9. **Lehman CR, Ries MD, Paiement GD, et al.** Infection after total joint arthroplasty in patients with human immunodeficiency virus or intravenous drug use. *J Arthroplasty.* 2001 Apr;16(3):330–335.
10. **Namba RS, Paxton L, Fithian DC, et al.** Obesity and perioperative morbidity in total hip and total knee arthroplasty patients. *J Arthroplasty.* 2005 Oct;20(7 Suppl 3):46–50.
11. **Peersman G, Laskin R, Davis J, et al.** Infection in total knee replacement: a retrospective review of 6489 total knee replacements. *Clin Orthop Relat Res.* 2001 Nov(392):15–23.
12. **Moucha CS, Clyburn TA, Evans RP, et al.** Modifiable risk factors for surgical site infection. *Instr Course Lect.* 2011;60:557–564.
13. **Everhart JS, Altneu E, Calhoun JH.** Medical comorbidities are independent preoperative risk factors for surgical infection after total joint arthroplasty. *Clin Orthop Relat Res.* 2013 Oct;471(10):3112–3119.
14. **Soohoo NF, Farng E, Lieberman JR, et al.** Factors that predict short-term complication rates after total hip arthroplasty. *Clin Orthop Relat Res.* 2010 Sep;468(9):2363–2371.
15. **Jamsen E, Huhtala H, Puolakka T, et al.** Risk factors for infection after knee arthroplasty. A register-based analysis of 43,149 cases. *J Bone Joint Surg Am.* 2009 Jan;91(1):38–47.
16. **Dale H, Skramm I, Lower HL, et al.** Infection after primary hip arthroplasty: a comparison of 3 Norwegian health registers. *Acta Orthop.* 2011 Dec;82(6):646–654.
17. **Namba RS, Inacio MC, Paxton EW.** Risk factors associated with deep surgical site infections after primary total knee arthroplasty: an analysis of 56,216 knees. *J Bone Joint Surg Am.* 2013 May 1;95(9):775–782.
18. **Parvizi J, Sullivan TA, Pagnano MW, et al.** Total joint arthroplasty in human immunodeficiency virus-positive patients: an alarming rate of early failure. *J Arthroplasty.* 2003 Apr;18(3):259–264.
19. **Pour AE, Matar WY, Jafari SM, et al.** Total joint arthroplasty in patients with hepatitis C. *J Bone Joint Surg Am.* 2011 Aug 3;93(15):1448–1454.
20. **Yi PH, Frank RM, Vann E, et al.** Is potential malnutrition associated with septic failure and acute infection after revision total joint arthroplasty? *Clin Orthop Relat Res.* 2015 Jan;473(1):175–182.
21. **Sunday JM, Guille JT, Torg JS.** Complications of joint arthroplasty in patients with end-stage renal disease on hemodialysis. *Clin Orthop Relat Res.* 2002 Apr(397):350–355.
22. **Silva M, Luck JV, Jr.** Long-term results of primary total knee replacement in patients with hemophilia. *J Bone Joint Surg Am.* 2005 Jan;87(1):85–91.
23. **Chiang CC, Chen PQ, Shen MC, et al.** Total knee arthroplasty for severe haemophilic arthropathy: long-term experience in Taiwan. *Haemophilia.* 2008 Jul;14(4):828–834.
24. **Cherney DL, Amstutz HC.** Total hip replacement in the previously septic hip. *J Bone Joint Surg Am.* 1983 Dec;65(9):1256–1265.
25. **Jupiter JB, Karchmer AW, Lowell JD, et al.** Total hip arthroplasty in the treatment of adult hips with current or quiescent sepsis. *J Bone Joint Surg Am.* 1981 Feb;63(2):194–200.
26. **Pruzansky JS, Bronson MJ, Grelsamer RP, et al.** Prevalence of modifiable surgical site infection risk factors in hip and knee joint arthroplasty patients at an urban academic hospital. *J Arthroplasty.* 2014 Feb;29(2):272–276.
27. **Pulido L, Ghanem E, Joshi A, et al.** Periprosthetic joint infection: the incidence, timing, and predisposing factors. *Clin Orthop Relat Res.* 2008 Jul;466(7):1710–1715.
28. **Parvizi J, Gehrke T, Chen AF.** Proceedings of the International Consensus on Periprosthetic Joint Infection. *Bone Joint J.* 2013 Nov;95-B(11):1450–1452.
29. **Tokarski AT, Blaha D, Mont MA, et al.** Perioperative skin preparation. *J Arthroplasty.* 2014 Feb;29(2 Suppl):26–28.
30. **Hansen E, Belden K, Silibovsky R, et al.** Perioperative antibiotics. *J Arthroplasty.* 2014 Feb;29(2 Suppl):29–48.
31. **Fairclough JA, Johnson D, Mackie I.** The prevention of wound contamination by skin organisms by the pre-operative application of an iodophor impregnated plastic adhesive drape. *J Int Med Res.* 1986;14(2):105–109.
32. **Salvati EA, Robinson RP, Zeno SM, et al.** Infection rates after 3175 total hip and total knee replacements performed with and without a horizontal unidirectional filtered air-flow system. *J Bone Joint Surg Am.* 1982 Apr;64(4):525–535.
33. **Taylor GJ, Bannister GC.** Infection and interposition between ultraclean air source and wound. *J Bone Joint Surg Br.* 1993 May;75(3):503–504.
34. **Clarke JV, Deakin AH, Dillon JM, et al.** A prospective clinical audit of a new dressing design for lower limb arthroplasty wounds. *J Wound Care.* 2009 Jan;18(1):5–8, 10–11.
35. **Friedman R, Homering M, Holberg G, et al.** Allogeneic blood transfusions and postoperative infections after total hip or knee arthroplasty. *J Bone Joint Surg Am.* 2014 Feb 19;96(4):272–278.
36. **Huang R, Buckley P, Parvizi J, et al.**, eds. Aspirin as Prophylaxis against Venous Thromboembolism Results in Lower Incidence of Periprosthetic Joint Infection. Lecture presented at: American Association of Hip and Knee Surgeons; November 8, 2014; Dallas.

37. **Segawa H, Tsukayama DT, Kyle RF, et al.** Infection after total knee arthroplasty. A retrospective study of the treatment of eighty-one infections. *J Bone Joint Surg Am.* 1999 Oct;81(10):1434–1445.
38. **Tsukayama DT, Estrada R, Gustilo RB.** Infection after total hip arthroplasty. A study of the treatment of one hundred and six infections. *J Bone Joint Surg Am.* 1996 Apr;78(4):512–523.
39. **Osmon DR, Berbari EF, Berendt AR, et al.** Diagnosis and management of prosthetic joint infection: clinical practice guidelines by the Infectious Diseases Society of America. *Clin Infect Dis.* 2013 Jan;56(1):e1–e25.
40. **Zimmerli W, Trampuz A, Ochsner PE.** Prosthetic-joint infections. *N Engl J Med.* 2004 Oct 14;351(16):1645–1654.
41. **McPherson EJ, Woodson C, Holtom P, et al.** Periprosthetic total hip infection: outcomes using a staging system. *Clin Orthop Relat Res.* 2002 Oct(403):8–15.
42. **Cierny G, 3rd, Mader JT, Penninck JJ.** A clinical staging system for adult osteomyelitis. *Clin Orthop Relat Res.* 2003 Sep(414):7–24.
43. **Bozic KJ, Rubash HE.** The painful total hip replacement. *Clin Orthop Relat Res.* 2004 Mar(420):18–25.
44. **Deirmengian C, Kardos K, Kilmartin P, et al.** Combined Measurement of Synovial Fluid alpha-Defensin and C-Reactive Protein Levels: Highly Accurate for Diagnosing Periprosthetic Joint Infection. *J Bone Joint Surg Am.* 2014 Sep 3;96(17):1439–1445.
45. **David TS, Vrahas MS.** Perioperative lower urinary tract infections and deep sepsis in patients undergoing total joint arthroplasty. *J Am Acad Orthop Surg.* 2000 Jan-Feb;8(1):66–74.
46. **Waterhouse N, Beaumont AR, Murray K, et al.** Urinary retention after total hip replacement. A prospective study. *J Bone Joint Surg Br.* 1987 Jan;69(1):64–66.
47. **Walton JK, Robinson RG.** An analysis of a male population having total hip replacement with regard to urological assessment and post-operative urinary retention. *Br J Urol.* 1982 Oct;54(5):519–521.
48. **Meehan AM, Osmon DR, Duffy MC, et al.** Outcome of penicillin-susceptible streptococcal prosthetic joint infection treated with debridement and retention of the prosthesis. *Clin Infect Dis.* 2003 Apr 1;36(7):845–849.
49. **Cordero-Ampuero J, de Dios M.** What are the risk factors for infection in hemiarthroplasties and total hip arthroplasties? *Clin Orthop Relat Res.* 2010 Dec;468(12):3268–3277.
50. **Fabry K, Verheyden F, Nelen G.** Infection of a total knee prosthesis by Candida glabrata: a case report. *Acta Orthop Belg.* 2005 Feb;71(1):119–121.
51. **Sendi P, Banderet F, Graber P, et al.** Periprosthetic joint infection following Staphylococcus aureus bacteremia. *J Infect.* 2011 Jul;63(1):17–22.
52. **Strazzeri JC, Anzel S.** Infected total hip arthroplasty due to Actinomyces israelii after dental extraction. A case report. *Clin Orthop Relat Res.* 1986 Sep(210):128–131.
53. **Wust J, Steiger U, Vuong H, et al.** Infection of a hip prosthesis by Actinomyces naeslundii. *J Clin Microbiol.* 2000 Feb;38(2):929–930.
54. **Steffen EK, Berg RD, Deitch EA.** Comparison of translocation rates of various indigenous bacteria from the gastrointestinal tract to the mesenteric lymph node. *J Infect Dis.* 1988 May;157(5):1032–1038.
55. **Anderson DJ, Arduino JM, Reed SD, et al.** Variation in the type and frequency of postoperative invasive Staphylococcus aureus infections according to type of surgical procedure. *Infect Control Hosp Epidemiol.* 2010 Jul;31(7):701–709
56. **Toossi N, Adeli B, Rasouli MR, et al.** Serum white blood cell count and differential do not have a role in the diagnosis of periprosthetic joint infection. *J Arthroplasty.* 2012 Sep;27(8 Suppl):51–54 e1.
57. **Deirmengian C, Kardos K, Kilmartin P, et al.** The Alpha-defensin Test for Periprosthetic Joint Infection Outperforms the Leukocyte Esterase Test Strip. *Clin Orthop Relat Res.* 2015 Jan;473(1):198–203.
58. **Parvizi J, Zmistowski B, Berbari EF, et al.** New definition for periprosthetic joint infection: from the Workgroup of the Musculoskeletal Infection Society. *Clin Orthop Relat Res.* 2011 Nov;469(11):2992–2994.
59. **Parvizi J, Gehrke T, International Consensus Group on Periprosthetic Joint Infection.** Definition of periprosthetic joint infection. *J Arthroplasty.* 2014 Jul;29(7):1331.
60. **Milone MT, Kamath AF, Israelite CL.** Converting between high- and low-sensitivity C-reactive protein in the assessment of periprosthetic joint infection. *J Arthroplasty.* 2014 Apr;29(4):685–689.
61. **Cipriano CA, Brown NM, Michael AM, et al.** Serum and synovial fluid analysis for diagnosing chronic periprosthetic infection in patients with inflammatory arthritis. *J Bone Joint Surg Am.* 2012 Apr 4;94(7):594–600.
62. **Ghanem E, Parvizi J, Burnett RS, et al.** Cell count and differential of aspirated fluid in the diagnosis of infection at the site of total knee arthroplasty. *J Bone Joint Surg Am.* 2008 Aug;90(8):1637–1643.
63. **Dinneen A, Guyot A, Clements J, et al.** Synovial fluid white cell and differential count in the diagnosis or exclusion of prosthetic joint infection. *Bone Joint J.* 2013 Apr;95-B(4):554–557.
64. **Bedair H, Ting N, Jacovides C, et al.** The Mark Coventry Award: diagnosis of early postoperative TKA infection using synovial fluid analysis. *Clin Orthop Relat Res.* 2011 Jan;469(1):34–40.
65. **Yi PH, Cross MB, Moric M, et al.** The 2013 Frank Stinchfield Award: Diagnosis of infection in the early postoperative period after total hip arthroplasty. *Clin Orthop Relat Res.* 2014 Feb;472(2):424–429.
66. **Shahi A, Deirmengian C, Chen AF, et al., eds.** Premature Antibiotic Treatment Can Potentially Compromise The Diagnosis of PJI. Lecture presented at: Musculoskeletal Infection Society; August 8–9, 2014;Charleston.
67. **Pace TB, Jeray KJ, Latham JT, Jr.** Synovial tissue examination by frozen section as an indicator of infection in hip and knee arthroplasty in community hospitals. *J Arthroplasty.* 1997 Jan;12(1):64–69.
68. **Parvizi J, Della Valle CJ.** AAOS Clinical Practice Guideline: diagnosis and treatment of periprosthetic joint infections of the hip and knee. *J Am Acad Orthop Surg.* 2010 Dec;18(12):771–772.
69. **Adeli B, Said J, Parvizi J, eds.** Detection of Intraoperative Purulence is not Reliable for Diagnosis of Periprosthetic Joint Infection. Lecture presented at: Musculoskeletal Infection Society; August 5–6, 2011;Rochester.
70. **Bottner F, Wegner A, Winkelmann W, et al.** Interleukin-6, procalcitonin and TNF-alpha: markers of peri-prosthetic infection following total joint replacement. *J Bone Joint Surg Br.* 2007 Jan;89(1):94–99.
71. **Glehr M, Friesenbichler J, Hofmann G, et al.** Novel biomarkers to detect infection in revision hip and knee arthroplasties. *Clin Orthop Relat Res.* 2013 Aug;471(8):2621–2628.
72. **Worthington T, Dunlop D, Casey A, et al.** Serum procalcitonin, interleukin-6, soluble intercellular adhesin molecule-1 and IgG to short-chain exocellular lipoteichoic acid as predictors of infection in total joint prosthesis revision. *Br J Biomed Sci.* 2010;67(2):71–76.

73. **Drago L, Vassena C, Dozio E, et al.** Procalcitonin, C-reactive protein, interleukin-6, and soluble intercellular adhesion molecule-1 as markers of postoperative orthopaedic joint prosthesis infections. *Int J Immunopathol Pharmacol.* 2011 Apr-Jun;24(2):433–440.
74. **Deirmengian C, Hallab N, Tarabishy A, et al.** Synovial fluid biomarkers for periprosthetic infection. *Clin Orthop Relat Res.* 2010 Aug;468(8):2017–2023.
75. **Gollwitzer H, Dombrowski Y, Prodinger PM, et al.** Antimicrobial peptides and proinflammatory cytokines in periprosthetic joint infection. *J Bone Joint Surg Am.* 2013 Apr 3;95(7):644–651.
76. **Jacovides CL, Parvizi J, Adeli B, et al.** Molecular markers for diagnosis of periprosthetic joint infection. *J Arthroplasty.* 2011 Sep;26(6 Suppl):99–103 e1.
77. **Parvizi J, McKenzie JC, Cashman JP.** Diagnosis of periprosthetic joint infection using synovial C-reactive protein. *J Arthroplasty.* 2012 Sep;27(8 Suppl):12–16.
78. **Deirmengian C, Kardos K, Kilmartin P, et al.** Diagnosing periprosthetic joint infection: has the era of the biomarker arrived? *Clin Orthop Relat Res.* 2014 Nov;472(11):3254–3262.
79. **Parvizi J, Jacovides C, Antoci V, et al.** Diagnosis of periprosthetic joint infection: the utility of a simple yet unappreciated enzyme. *J Bone Joint Surg Am.* 2011 Dec 21;93(24):2242–2248.
80. **Cyteval C, Hamm V, Sarrabere MP, et al.** Painful infection at the site of hip prosthesis: CT imaging. *Radiology.* 2002 Aug;224(2):477–483.
81. **Chryssikos T, Parvizi J, Ghanem E, et al.** FDG-PET imaging can diagnose periprosthetic infection of the hip. *Clin Orthop Relat Res.* 2008 Jun;466(6):1338–1342.
82. **Delank KS, Schmidt M, Michael JW, et al.** The implications of 18F-FDG PET for the diagnosis of endoprosthetic loosening and infection in hip and knee arthroplasty: results from a prospective, blinded study. *BMC Musculoskelet Disord.* 2006 Mar 3;7:20.
83. **Nagoya S, Kaya M, Sasaki M, et al.** Diagnosis of peri-prosthetic infection at the hip using triple-phase bone scintigraphy. *J Bone Joint Surg Br.* 2008 Feb;90(2):140–144.
84. **Glithero PR, Grigoris P, Harding LK, et al.** White cell scans and infected joint replacements. Failure to detect chronic infection. *J Bone Joint Surg Br.* 1993 May;75(3):371–374.
85. **Graute V, Feist M, Lehner S, et al.** Detection of low-grade prosthetic joint infections using 99mTc-antigranulocyte SPECT/CT: initial clinical results. *Eur J Nucl Med Mol Imaging.* 2010 Aug;37(9):1751–1759.
86. **Magnuson JE, Brown ML, Hauser MF, et al.** In-111-labeled leukocyte scintigraphy in suspected orthopedic prosthesis infection: comparison with other imaging modalities. *Radiology.* 1988 Jul;168(1):235–239.
87. **Jacqueline C, Caillon J.** Impact of bacterial biofilm on the treatment of prosthetic joint infections. *J Antimicrob Chemother.* 2014 Sep;69 Suppl 1:i37–40.
88. **Koyonos L, Zmistowski B, Della Valle CJ, et al.** Infection control rate of irrigation and debridement for periprosthetic joint infection. *Clin Orthop Relat Res.* 2011Nov;469(11):3043–3048.
89. **Giulieri SG, Graber P, Ochsner PE, et al.** Management of infection associated with total hip arthroplasty according to a treatment algorithm. *Infection.* 2004 Aug;32(4):222–228.
90. **Romanò CL, Toscano M, Romanò D, et al.** Antibiofilm agents and implant-related infections in orthopaedics: where are we? *J Chemother.* 2013 Apr;25(2):67–80.
91. **Rao N, Crossett LS, Sinha RK, et al.** Long-term suppression of infection in total joint arthroplasty. *Clin Orthop Relat Res.* 2003 Sep;(414):55–60.
92. **Marculescu CE, Berbari EF, Hanssen AD, et al.** Outcome of prosthetic joint infections treated with debridement and retention of components. *Clin Infect Dis.* 2006 Feb;42(4):471–478.
93. **Lentino JR.** Prosthetic joint infections: bane of orthopedists, challenge for infectious disease specialists. *Clin Infect Dis.* 2003 May;36(9):1157–1161.
94. **Segreti J, Nelson JA, Trenholme GM.** Prolonged suppressive antibiotic therapy for infected orthopedic prostheses. *Clin Infect Dis.* 1998 Oct;27(4):711–713.
95. **Gallo J, Smizanský M, Radová L, et al.** Porovnání léčebných postupů používaných v terapii infekce kloubních náhrad kyčle a kolena. [Comparison of therapeutic strategies for hip and knee prosthetic joint infection]. *Acta Chir Orthop Traumatol Cech.* 2009 Aug;76(4):302–309. Czech.
96. **Esposito S, Leone S, Bassetti M, et al.** Italian guidelines for the diagnosis and infectious disease management of osteomyelitis and prosthetic joint infections in adults. *Infection.* 2009 Dec;37(6):478–496.
97. **Trampuz A, Zimmerli W.** Prosthetic joint infections: update in diagnosis and treatment. *Swiss Med Wkly.* 2005 Apr;135(17–18):243–251.
98. **Romanò CL, Logoluso N, Drago L, et al.** Role for Irrigation and Debridement in Periprosthetic Infections. *J Knee Surg.* 2014 Aug;27(4):267–272.
99. **Moran E, Masters S, Berendt AR, et al.** Guiding empirical antibiotic therapy in orthopaedics: the microbiology of prosthetic joint infection managed by debridement, irrigation and prosthesis retention. *J Infect.* 2007 Jul;55(1):1–7.
100. **Marculescu CE, Berbari EF, Hanssen AD, et al.** Outcome of prosthetic joint infections treated with debridement and retention of components. *Clin Infect Dis.* 2006 Feb;42(4):471–478.
101. **Zimmerli W, Ochsner PE**. Management of infection associated with prosthetic joints. *Infection.* 2003 Mar;31(2):99–108.
102. **Laffer RR, Graber P, Ochsner PE, Zimmerli W.** Outcome of prosthetic knee-associated infection: evaluation of 40 consecutive episodes at a single centre. *Clin Microbiol Infect.* 2006 May;12(5):433–439.
103. **Azzam KA, Seeley M, Ghanem E, et al.** Irrigation and debridement in the management of prosthetic joint infection: traditional indications revisited. *J Arthroplasty.* 2010 Oct;25(7):1022–1027.
104. **Martínez-Pastor JC, Muñoz-Mahamud E, Vilchez F, et al.** Outcome of acute prosthetic joint infections due to gram-negative bacilli treated with open debridement and retention of the prosthesis. *Antimicrob Agents Chemother.* 2009 Nov;53(11):4772–4777.
105. **Odum SM, Fehring TK, Lombardi AV, et al.** Irrigation and debridement for periprosthetic infections: does the organism matter? *J Arthroplasty.* 2011 Sep;26(6 Suppl):114–118.
106. **Aboltins CA, Page MA, Buising KL, et al.** Treatment of staphylococcal prosthetic joint infections with debridement, prosthesis retention and oral rifampicin and fusidic acid. *Clin Microbiol Infect.* 2007 Jun;13(6):586–591.
107. **Byren I, Bejon P, Atkins BL, et al.** One hundred and twelve infected arthroplasties treated with 'DAIR' (debridement, antibiotics and implant retention): antibiotic duration and outcome. *J Antimicrob Chemother.* 2009 Jun;63(6):1264–1271.

108. **Lora-Tamayo J, Murillo O, Iribarren JA, et al.** A large multicenter study of methicillin-susceptible and methicillin-resistant Staphylococcus aureus prosthetic joint infections managed with implant retention. *Clin Infect Dis.* 2013 Jan;56(2):182–194.
109. **Vilchez F, Martinez-Pastor JC, Garcia-Ramiro S, et al.** Outcome and predictors of treatment failure in early post-surgical prosthetic joint infections due to Staphylococcus aureus treated with debridement. *Clin Microbiol Infect.* 2011 Mar;17(3):439–444.
110. **Zmistowski B, Fedorka CJ, Sheehan E, et al.** Prosthetic joint infection caused by gram-negative organisms. *J Arthroplasty.* 2011 Sep;26(6 Suppl):104–108.
111. **Buller LT, Sabry FY, Easton RW, et al.** The preoperative prediction of success following irrigation and debridement with polyethylene exchange for hip and knee prosthetic joint infections. *J Arthroplasty.* 2012 Jun;27(6):857–864.e1–4.
112. **Westberg M, Grogaard B, Snorrason F.** Early prosthetic joint infections treated with debridement and implant retention: 38 primary hip arthroplasties prospectively recorded and followed for median 4 years. *Acta Orthop.* 2012 Jun;83(3):227–232.
113. **Peel TN, Cheng AC, Choong PF, et al.** Early onset prosthetic hip and knee joint infection: treatment and outcomes in Victoria, Australia. *J Hosp Infect.* 2012 Dec;82(4):248–253.
114. **Waldman BJ, Hostin E, Mont MA, et al.** Infected total knee arthroplasty treated by arthroscopic irrigation and debridement. *J Arthroplasty.* 2000 Jun;15(4):430–436.
115. **Aggarwal VK, Higuera C, Deirmengian G, et al.** Swab cultures are not as effective as tissue cultures for diagnosis of periprosthetic joint infection. *Clin Orthop Relat Res.* 2013 Oct; 471(10): 3196–3203.
116. **Trampuz A, Piper KE, Hanssen AD, et al.** Sonication of explanted prosthetic components in bags for diagnosis of prosthetic joint infection is associated with risk of contamination. *J Clin Microbiol.* 2006 Feb;44(2):628–631.
117. **Trampuz A, Piper KE, Jacobson MJ, et al.** Sonication of removed hip and knee prostheses for diagnosis of infection. *N Engl J Med.* 2007 Aug;357(7):654–663.
118. **Drago L, Signori V, De Vecchi E, et al.** Use of dithiothreitol to improve the diagnosis of prosthetic joint infections. *J Orthop Res.* 2013 Nov;31(11):1694–1699.
119. **Ghanem E, Parvizi J, Clohisy J, et al.** Perioperative antibiotics should not be withheld in proven cases of periprosthetic infection. *Clin Orthop Relat Res.* 2007 Aug;461:44–47.
120. **Mont MA, Waldman B, Banerjee C, et al.** Multiple irrigation, debridement, and retention of components in infected total knee arthroplasty. *J Arthroplasty.* 1997 Jun;12(4):426–433.
121. **Kalteis T, Lehn N, Schroder HJ, et al.** Contaminant seeding in bone by different irrigation methods: an experimental study. *J Orthop Trauma.* 2005 Oct;19(9):591–596.
122. **Muñoz-Mahamud E, García S, Bori G, et al.** Comparison of a low-pressure and a high-pressure pulsatile lavage during débridement for orthopaedic implant infection. *Arch Orthop Trauma Surg.* 2011 Sep;131(9):1233–1238.
123. **Romanò CL, Manzi G, Logoluso N, et al.** Value of debridement and irrigation for the treatment of peri-prosthetic infections. A systematic review. *Hip Int.* 2012 Jul-Aug;22 Suppl 8:S19–24.
124. **Sherrell JC, Fehring TK, Odum S, et al.** The Chitranjan Ranawat Award: fate of two-stage reimplantation after failed irrigation and débridement for periprosthetic knee infection. *Clin Orthop Relat Res.* 2011Jan;469(1):18–25.
125. **Hartman MB, Fehring TK, Jordan L, et al.** Periprosthetic knee sepsis. The role of irrigation and debridement. *Clin Orthop Relat Res.* 1991 Dec;(273):113–118.
126. **Tintle SM, Forsberg JA, Potter BK, et al.** Prosthesis retention, serial debridement, and antibiotic bead use for the treatment of infection following total joint arthroplasty. *Orthopedics.* 2009 Feb;32(2):87.
127. **Kuiper JW, Brohet RM, Wassink S, et al.** Implantation of resorbable gentamicin sponges in addition to irrigation and debridement in 34 patients with infection complicating total hip arthroplasty. *Hip Int.* 2013 Mar-Apr;23(2):173–180.
128. **Jackson WO, Schmalzried TP.** Limited role of direct exchange arthroplasty in the treatment of infected total hip replacements. *Clin Orthop Relat Res.* 2000 Dec;(381):101–105.
129. **Jamsen E, Stogiannidis J, Malmivaara A, et al.** Outcome of prosthesis exchange for infected knee arthroplasty: the effect of treatment approach. A systematic review of the literature. *Acta Orthopaedica.* 2009 Feb;80(1):67–77.
130. **Lange J, Troelsen A, Thomsen RW, et al.** Chronic infections in hip arthroplasties: comparing risk of reinfection following one-stage and two-stage revision: a systematic review and meta-analysis. *Clin Epidemiol.* 2012;4:57–73.
131. **Romanò CL, Gala L, Logoluso N, et al.** Two-stage revision of septic knee prosthesis with articulating knee spacers yields better infection eradication rate than one-stage or two-stage revision with static spacers. *Knee Surg Sports Traumatol Arthrosc.* 2012 Dec;20(12):2445–2453.
132. **Romanò D, Drago L, Romanò CL, et al.** Does two-stage revision of septic hip prosthesis provides better infection eradication rate than one-stage? Paper presented at: 14th EFORT Congress; 2013; Istanbul.
133. **Lombardi AV Jr, Berend KR, Adams JB.** Partial two-stage exchange of the infected total hip replacement using disposable spacer moulds. *Bone Joint J.* 2014 Nov;96-B(11 Supple A):66–69.
134. **George DA, Volpin A, Scarponi S.** Does exchange arthroplasty of an infected shoulder prosthesis provide better eradication rate and better functional outcome, compared to a permanent spacer or resection arthroplasty? a systematic review. *BMC Musculoskelet Disord.* 2016 Feb 1;17(1):52.
135. **Rasouli MR, Tripathi MS, Kenyon R, et al.** Low rate of infection control in enterococcal periprosthetic joint infections. *Clin Orthop Relat Res.* 2012 Oct;470(10):2708–2716.
136. **Wolf M, Clar H, Friesenbichler J.** Prosthetic joint infection following total hip replacement: results of one-stage versus two-stage exchange. *Int Orthop.* 2014 Jul;38(7):1363–1368.
137. **Klouche S, Sariali E, Mamoudy P.** Total hip arthroplasty revision due to infection: a cost analysis approach. *Orthop Traumatol Surg Res.* 2010 Apr;96(2):124–132.
138. **De Man FH, Sendi P, Zimmerli W, et al.** Infectiological, functional, and radiographic outcome after revision for prosthetic hip infection according to a strict algorithm. *Acta Orthop.* 2011 Feb;82(1):27–34.
139. **Cabrita HB, Croci AT, Camargo OP, et al.** Prospective study of the treatment of infected hip arthroplasties with or without the use of an antibiotic-loaded cement spacer. *Clinics (Sao Paulo).* 2007 Apr;62(2):99–108.
140. **Parvizi J, Azzam K, Ghanem E, et al.** Periprosthetic infection due to resistant staphylococci: serious problems on the horizon. *Clin Orthop Relat Res.* 2009 Jul;467(7):1732–1739.

141. **Azzam K, McHale K, Austin M, et al.** Outcome of a second two-stage reimplantation for periprosthetic knee infection. *Clin Orthop Relat Res.* 2009 Jul;467(7):1706–1714.
142. **Bejon P, Berendt A, Atkins BL, et al.** Two-stage revision for prosthetic joint infection: predictors of outcome and the role of reimplantation microbiology. *J Antimicrob Chemother.* 2010 Mar;65(3):569–575.
143. **Rand JA, Bryan RS, Chao EY.** Failed total knee arthroplasty treated by arthrodesis of the knee using the Ace-Fischer apparatus. *J Bone Joint Surg Am.* 1987 Jan;69(1):39–45.
144. **Scarponi S, Drago L, Romanò D, et al.** Cementless modular intramedullary nail without bone-on-bone fusion as a salvage procedure in chronically infected total knee prosthesis: long-term results. *Int Orthop.* 2014 Feb;38(2):413–418.
145. **Damron TA, McBeath AA.** Arthrodesis following failed total knee arthroplasty: comprehensive review and meta-analysis of recent literature. *Orthopedics.* 1995 Apr;18(4):361–368
146. **Knutson K, Hovelius L, Lindstrand A, et al.** Arthrodesis after failed knee arthroplasty. A nationwide multicenter investigation of 91 cases. *Clin Orthop Relat Res.* 1984 Dec;(191):202–211.
147. **Rand JA, Bryan RS, Chao EY.** Failed total knee arthroplasty treated by arthrodesis of the knee using the Ace-Fischer apparatus. *J Bone Joint Surg Am.* 1987 Jan;69(1):39–45.
148. **Ellingsen DE, Rand JA.** Intramedullary arthrodesis of the knee after failed total knee arthroplasty. *J Bone Joint Surg Am.* 1994 Jun;76(6):870–877.
149. **Scarponi S, Drago L, Romanò D, et al.** Cementless modular intramedullary nail without bone-on-bone fusion as a salvage procedure in chronically infected total knee prosthesis: long-term results. *Int Orthop.* 2014 Feb;38(2):413–418. .
150. **Isiklar ZU, Landon GC, Tullos HS.** Amputation after failed total knee arthroplasty. *Clin Orthop Relat Res.* 1994 Feb;(299):173–178.
151. **Sierra RJ, Trousdale RT, Pagnano MW.** Above-the-knee amputation after a total knee replacement: prevalence, etiology, and functional outcome. *J Bone Joint Surg Am.* 2003 Jun;85-A(6):1000–1004.
152. **Fedorka CJ, Chen AF, McGarry WM, et al.** Functional ability after above-the-knee amputation for infected total knee arthroplasty. *Clin Orthop Relat Res.* 2011 Apr;469(4):1024–1032.
153. **Zalavras CG, Rigopoulos N, Ahlmann E, et al.** Hip disarticulation for severe lower extremity infections. *Clin Orthop Relat Res.* 2009 Jul;467(7):1721–1726.
154. **Zimmerli W.** Prosthetic device infection. In: Root RK, Waldvogel FA, Corey L, Stamm WE, eds. *Clinical infectious diseases: a practical approach.* Oxford: Oxford University Press; 1999:801–808.
155. **Cierny G 3rd, DiPasquale D.** Periprosthetic total joint infections. Staging, treatment, and outcomes. *Clin Orthop Relat Res.* 2002 Oct;(403):23–28.
156. **Romanò CL, Romanò D, Logoluso N, et al.** Bone and joint infections in adults: a comprehensive classification proposal. *Eur Orthop Traumatol.* 2011 May;1(6):207–217.
157. **De Man FH, Sendi P, Zimmerli W, et al.** Infectiological, functional, and radiographic outcome after revision for prosthetic hip infection according to a strict algorithm. *Acta Orthop.* 2011 Feb;82(1):27–34.
158. **Laffer RR, Graber P, Ochsner PE, et al.** Outcome of prosthetic knee-associated infection: evaluation of 40 consecutive episodes at a single centre. *Clin Microbiol Infect.* 2006 May;12(5):433–439.
159. **Osmon DR, Berbari EF, Berendt AR, et al.** Diagnosis and management of prosthetic joint infection: clinical practice guidelines by the Infectious Diseases Society of America. *Clin Infect Dis.* 2013 Jan;56(1):e1–e25.
160. **Urish KL, Demuth PW, Craft DW, et al.** Pulse lavage is inadequate at removal of biofilm from the surface of total knee arthroplasty materials. *J Arthroplasty.* 2014 Jun;29(6):1128–1132.
161. **Ramaesh R, Gaston MS, Simpson AH.** Chronic osteomyelitis of the pelvis. *Acta Orthop Belg.* 2013 Jun;79(3):280–286.
162. **Simpson AH, Deakin M, Latham JM.** Chronic osteomyelitis. The effect of the extent of surgical resection on infection-free survival. *J Bone Joint Surg Br.* 2001 Apr;83(3):403–407.

11.1 Septic arthritis

Anna Conen, Olivier Borens

1 Basics

Acute septic arthritis refers to bacterial, or rarely, fungal infections of a joint. It is a medical and surgical emergency because of the rapid destruction of the joint (**Fig 11.1-1**). Immediate therapeutic intervention is necessary to decrease the associated morbidity and mortality. A delay between symptom onset and initiation of adequate therapy is the major determinant of poor outcome.

1.1 Etiology

In native joints, septic arthritis is commonly caused by hematogenous seeding of microorganisms from a distant infection focus [1–4]. Because the synovial membrane is highly vascularized and contains no limiting basement membrane, microorganisms can quickly pass from the blood into the joint space resulting in an acute onset of purulent joint inflammation. Patients at high risk for hematogenous seeding are intravenous (IV) drug users, patients with indwelling vascular catheters, patients with infective endocarditis, immunocompromised hosts, and elderly people [5, 6]. Other pathomechanisms in the emergence of septic arthritis are direct inoculation of microorganisms into the joint as a result of intraarticular injections, surgical interventions, open joint injury, or trauma [7, 8]. Rarely, microorganisms enter the joint space by spread from a contiguous focus, such as cellulitis, bursitis, or osteomyelitis.

Microorganisms in the joint space trigger an acute synovial inflammatory response. Within a few hours, activated inflammatory cells fill the closed synovial space. The inflammatory cells release enzymes and cytokines and the microorganisms produce in addition toxins that can kill eukaryotic cells. The consequences are chemical toxic damage of the cartilage and underlying subchondral bone but also pressure damage due to the increased joint pressure due to the large accumulated inflammatory effusion [3, 9].

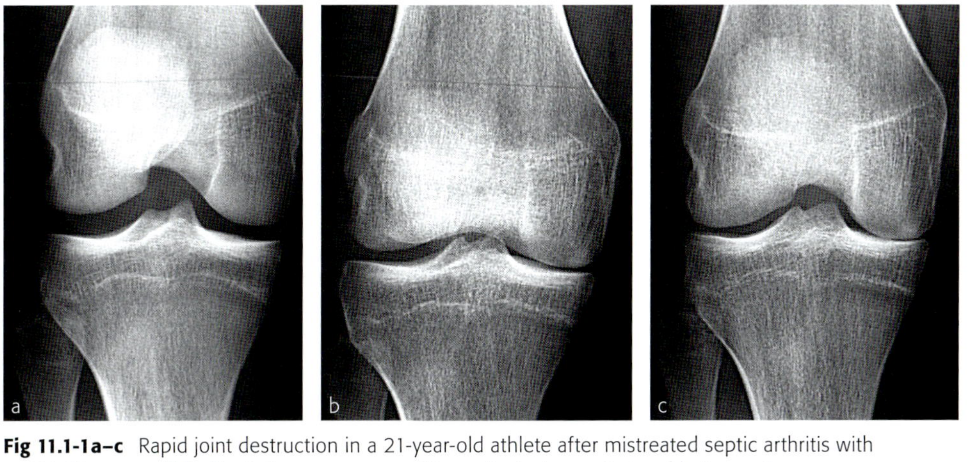

Fig 11.1-1a–c Rapid joint destruction in a 21-year-old athlete after mistreated septic arthritis with methicillin-susceptible *Staphylococcus aureus* (3 months between first and last x-rays).

1.2 Incidence

Septic arthritis is diagnosed in 2 to 10 persons per 100,000 people per year and in 5 to 10 patients per 10,000 patients hospitalized in an acute care facility per year. The incidence is considerably higher in patients suffering from rheumatoid arthritis, ie, 28 to 38 patients per 100,000 patients with rheumatoid arthritis per year. The incidence is increasing in recent years not only because of the aging population and the increasing use of immunosuppressive treatments and indwelling vascular catheters, but also because of the growing numbers of joint interventions [3]. Overall, the risk of postinterventional septic arthritis is small. For joint infiltrations it relates to 1 case per 22,000 interventions/infiltrations and for arthroscopy to 1 case per 250–1,000 interventions, respectively [4, 10].

1.3 Risk factors

Most patients who develop septic arthritis have at least one risk factor. Each factor has a modest impact on the risk of septic arthritis, but in combination they can substantially increase the risk [5, 11]. The most important risk factor is preexisting arthropathy, such as degenerative and chronic inflammatory joint diseases [4, 8]. Older age (> 80 years), comorbidities including diabetes mellitus, cutaneous ulcers, alcoholism, and immunosuppression are also associated with an increased risk for septic arthritis [12]. Diseases with an increased risk for bacteremia, such as IV drug use and infective endocarditis, are other important risk factors, as is the skin colonization with *Staphylococcus aureus*. Furthermore, the presence of distant infection foci with the possibility of secondary bacteremia increases the risk for septic arthritis, including skin, urogenital, gastrointestinal, and pulmonary infections. Overall, the risk for septic arthritis after a joint intervention is low as mentioned above, ie, < 0.01% after synovial fluid aspiration and 0.01–0.4% after arthroscopy. Intraarticular steroid injections further increase the risk, especially if associated with arthroscopy, where the risk is 27.4 times higher than without the administration of steroids [13, 14].

1.4 Location of involved joints

In 90% of patients with septic arthritis only one joint is involved (monoarthritis), and 10% suffer from multiple joint involvement (oligoarthritis). Oligoarthritis is mainly found in patients with underlying rheumatoid arthritis [15]. Predominantly weight-bearing joints are affected, such as knee joints in 45–55% and hip joints in 15–25%, followed by shoulder, wrist, ankle, and elbow joints (together in 5–10%) [4, 16]. Rarely sacroiliac or sternoclavicular joints and the symphysis pubis are infected and infection is more prevalent in IV drug users (sacroiliac or sternoclavicular joints and symphysis) and after gynecological and urological interventions (sacroiliac joint and symphysis) [17, 18]. In children the hip joint is most commonly affected in 60%, followed by the knee joint in 35%.

1.5 Which microbes cause septic arthritis?

Overall, *S aureus* is the predominant causative microorganism in 40–60%, followed by streptococci in 20–30% [1, 2, 9, 19, 20]. Methicillin-resistant *S aureus* has to be considered in countries with a high prevalence of methicillin-resistance [21]. Gram-negative bacilli are found in 4–20%, especially in IV drug users, immunocompromised hosts, elderly patients, or after trauma [9]. Culture-negative septic arthritis cases are described in 10–20% as a consequence of antimicrobial pretreatment or fastidious to grow microorganisms. Polymicrobial infections are rare (maximum of 8%) and often associated with penetrating trauma.

Depending on the clinical context and the presence of risk factors, one can anticipate the causative microorganism in septic arthritis. Therefore, the medical history is an essential element in narrowing the microbiological differential diagnosis (**Table 11.1-1**). In patients without any risk factor for septic arthritis, or in patients with diabetes mellitus or rheumatoid arthritis *S aureus* is the predominant cause. In IV drug users *S aureus* is the most common microorganism as well, but also *Pseudomonas aeruginosa* (because of tap water use to wash syringe), group A streptococci (because of a concomitant septic phlebitis) and *Candida* species (spp.) (because of contaminated lemon juice used for drug solution) have to be considered. Cat or dog bites usually result in infections with *Pasteurella multocida* and *Capnocytophaga canimorsus*, rat bites in infections with *Streptobacillus moniliformis* and human bites in infections with microorganisms of the oral cavity such as the HACEK group (*Haemophilus* spp., *Aggregatibacter actinomycetemcomitans, Cardiobacterium hominis, Eikenella corrodens*, and *Kingella kingae*) or anaerobes. After joint infiltration or surgical intervention, microorganisms of the skin flora, including *S aureus* and coagulase-negative staphylococci, should be considered. In children younger than 2 years of age predominantly *Kingella kingae* is found. If there is a sexual risk behavior, gonococci have to be considered, especially if there is a concomitant macular exanthema and polyarticular involvement [22]. After gynecological interventions (eg, curettage or childbirth) and mainly in patients with impaired humoral immune function *Mycoplasma hominis* can be found. *Brucella* spp. should be considered in patients who visited the Mediterranean areas or in case of the consumption of unpasteurized milk products. Special culture media and serology are required for diagnosis. If the patient history indicates oligoarthritis in combination with gastrointestinal symptoms and mesenteric lymphadenopathy, one should also be aware of *Tropheryma whipplei*. *Borrelia* spp. (ie, Lyme arthritis) should be considered in case of an oligoarticular involvement and after a stay in an endemic area, even if no tick bite was recognized.

Microorganism	Clinical clues/risk factors
Staphylococcus aureus	Healthy adults, presence of risk factors (eg, diabetes mellitus, skin breakdown, cutaneous infection), previously damaged joint (eg, rheumatoid arthritis, IV drug users, infective endocarditis)
Coagulase-negative staphylococci	After invasive articular manipulation (ie, synovial fluid aspiration, joint infiltration, arthroscopy)
Streptococcus spp.	Healthy adults, splenic dysfunction, cutaneous infection, infective endocarditis
Neisseria gonorrhoeae	Sexually active patients, promiscuity, complement deficiency, associated tenosynovitis, and vesicular pustules
Enterobacteriaceae	Elderly patients, immunocompromised hosts, urogenital or gastrointestinal infection
Pseudomonas aeruginosa	IV drug users, immunocompromised hosts
Mycoplasma hominis	Immunocompromised hosts, urogenital manipulations
Candida spp.	IV drug users, immunocompromised hosts

Table 11.1-1 Microorganisms causing septic arthritis according to patient's risk factors.
Abbreviation: IV, intravenous.

2 Symptoms

Most patients (ie, 78–85%) present with an acute onset of joint swelling and pain. The pain is present at rest, aggravated with weight bearing, and the joint motion is limited. Joint erythema and excess heat are present in most cases. Fever is only found in about 50% of patients, possibly because analgesic and antiinflammatory medications are used [11]. About half of the patients have a distant infection focus and may report dysuria, urinary frequency, flank pain, nausea, vomiting, diarrhea, or a productive cough.

3 Diagnostic procedures

3.1 Clinical examination

The affected joint is painful on palpation and movement. Erythema, excess heat, and a palpable effusion are present. In hip arthritis the latter signs can be absent and pain during movement and axial compression is the only clue for infection. Generally, a monoarthritis is present, in case of oligoarthritis one should bear in mind gonococccal arthritis, especially if a coexisting exanthema is found. The skin should always be examined for underlying skin diseases, either as the primary infection focus (eg, abscesses, cellulitis) or as a predisposing factor for the colonization with *S aureus* (eg, eczema, psoriasis). Furthermore, the patient should be examined for other primary infection foci, including urogenital, gastrointestinal, or pulmonary infections.

The differential diagnosis of septic arthritis manifesting as acute monoarthritis includes predominantly crystal-induced arthritis such as gout (urate crystals) and pseudogout (calcium-pyrophosphate crystals) (**Table 11.1-2**) [11, 23]. The differentiation between septic and crystal-induced arthritis is most challenging and often impossible both clinically and based on the synovial white blood cell (WBC) count. Other differential diagnoses include inflammatory osteoarthritis, inflammatory joint diseases (eg, rheumatoid arthritis, psoriatic arthritis, sarcoidosis, Still's disease) or reactive arthritis after gastrointestinal (eg, *Campylobacter* spp.) or urogenital infections (eg, *Chlamydia* spp.) among others [24, 25]. Furthermore, trauma, hemarthrosis, fracture, meniscus tears, or osteonecrosis (after trauma or in steroid-treated patients) should be considered. Extraarticular diseases can also simulate septic arthritis, such as tenosynovitis, skin infections (eg, cellulitis or erysipelas), bursitis, or erythema nodosum.

3.2 Laboratory tests

If septic arthritis is suspected, blood inflammatory parameters should be examined, including differential WBC count and C-reactive protein (CRP). The sensitivity of a WBC count > 10,000 cells/µL is 90% and a CRP > 100 mg/L is 77%, but both parameters are nonspecific [11]. As the predominant pathomechanism in septic arthritis is hematogenous seeding, two pairs of blood culture should be drawn for microbiological analysis; they are positive in about 50% of patients. Furthermore, urine and sputum cultures should be obtained if urogenital or respiratory tract are suspected to be the primary infection focus.

3.3 Imaging

Imaging is rarely necessary in the acute management of septic arthritis. Conventional x-ray detects preexisting joint diseases (ie, osteoarthritis, rheumatoid arthritis, osteomyelitis, or chondrocalcinosis). Ultrasound can be useful to guide joint aspiration. Bone scintigraphy is usually positive after 10 days, is not specific but may be helpful in the diagnosis of sacroiliac joint infection. Computed tomography is sensitive for the detection of bone erosions, joint effusion and soft-tissue infections. Magnetic resonance imaging is even more sensitive; however, it is only required for the diagnosis of sternoclavicular or sacroiliac arthritis, symphysitis, or post-operative arthritis following cruciate ligament reconstruction [26, 27].

Differential diagnosis	Specific diagnosis
Septic arthritis	Bacterial, fungal, viral, mycobacterial arthritis
Crystal-induced arthritis	Gout, pseudogout
Activated osteoarthritis	Degenerative joint disease
Reactive arthritis	Underlying urogenital (ie, *Chlamydia* spp. *N gonorrhoeae*) or gastrointestinal infections (ie, *Campylobacter* spp., *Salmonella* spp., *Shigella* spp., *Yersinia* spp.)
Systemic rheumatic diseases	Rheumatoid arthritis, psoriatic arthritis, sarcoidosis, systemic lupus erythematosus
Trauma	Hemarthrosis, fracture, osteonecrosis, meniscal tear
Tumor	Osteosarcoma, chondrosarcoma, metastatic disease
Extraarticular disease	Tenosynovitis, bursitis, cellulitis, erysipelas, erythema nodosum, Baker's cyst

Table 11.1-2 Differential diagnosis of acute monoarthritis.

3.4 Synovial fluid analysis

The examination of the synovial fluid is the most important diagnostic tool in every patient with suspected septic arthritis. Arthrocentesis should be performed before any antimicrobial treatment is initiated [11, 28]. The synovial fluid should be analyzed for the following parameters (ordered by significance):

1. Differential WBC count (use EDTA tubes to avoid coagulation)
2. Gram stain and microbiological culture (inoculate preferentially pediatric blood culture bottles to increase culture sensitivity)
3. Presence of crystals (use native tubes) (**Table 11.1-3**)

In septic arthritis, the synovial fluid macroscopically is turbid or purulent in 80–90% of patients. The differential WBC count helps to narrow the differential diagnosis: a WBC count of > 50,000 cells/µL has a sensitivity of 62% and a specificity of 92% for septic arthritis; but mainly in earlier stages of infection and in immunocompromised patients lower WBC counts can be expected, therefore a limit of > 20'000 cells/µL should be considered to be highly suspicious for septic arthritis. If the proportion of the polymorphonuclear leukocytes is > 90%, then sensitivity is 73% and specificity 79% [11]. Other inflammatory joint diseases, eg, rheumatoid arthritis or crystal-induced arthritis, can present with WBC counts of 2,000–50,000 cells/µL as well and especially crystal-induced arthritis mimics septic arthritis. The Gram stain is positive in only 50% but microbiological culture in up to 90% of patients with septic arthritis [11]. The microbiological diagnostic yield can be increased if the synovial fluid is inoculated into pediatric blood culture bottles [29]. If culture results are negative because patients were pretreated with antimicrobials or because of fastidious to grow or atypical microorganisms, bacterial DNA can be identified by polymerase chain reaction [30]. Crystals, ie, urate and calcium-pyrophosphate crystals, can be detected by polarized light microscopy of the synovial fluid. Note that the presence of crystals does not rule out septic arthritis, as coexistence of crystals and infection has been described [31, 32].

Clinical entity/Parameter	Normal	Degenerative joint disease	Inflammatory joint disease	Crystal-induced arthritis	Septic arthritis
Clarity	Transparent	Transparent	Translucent-turbid	Turbid	Turbid
Leukocyte count, cells/µL	< 200	200–2,000	2,000–20,000	> 20,000	> 20,000
Polymorphonuclear leukocytes, [%]	< 25	25–75	70–90	> 90	> 90
Culture	Negative	Negative	Negative	Negative	Positive

Table 11.1-3 Differential diagnosis of arthritis based on synovial fluid analysis.

4 Treatment principles

The key to successful management of septic arthritis is early recognition of the diagnosis, the rapid initiation of appropriate antimicrobial therapy, and joint drainage. Antimicrobial treatment alone is insufficient to cure septic arthritis [33]. If septic arthritis is suspected, the patient should be managed as such until the diagnosis is definitively excluded (**Fig 11.1-2**). The main treatment goal is the restoration of a painless full joint function by the eradication of infection with antimicrobial agents and by joint decompression with the removal of inflammatory effusion [3, 9, 34, 35].

Before any antimicrobial treatment is started in a clinically stable patient, microbiological analysis of blood and synovial fluid is essential to identify the causative microorganism. For the mechanical and surgical treatment of septic arthritis, different strategies can be followed:

- Repetitive needle aspirations until there is a significant reduction of inflammation (ie, decreasing WBC counts) and negative microbiological culture results
- Arthroscopy
- Arthrotomy(**Table 11.1-4**)

There are only a few studies comparing different surgical treatment strategies [36, 42]. Therefore, the selection of the drainage procedure is dependent on the affected joint (large versus small joints), the soft-tissue condition (presence of abscesses or fistula), the patient's comorbidities, the time lag between the onset of symptoms and the initiation of treatment (chronic inflammation with compartmentalization), and the Gächter stage (**Table 11.1-5**) [43–46].

The use of irrigation-suction drainage systems increases the risk of secondary infections and should be avoided. Joint irrigation with antiseptics is contraindicated because most antiseptics (chlorhexidine and polyhexanide) lead to chondrolysis and destruction of the joint [47]. The administration of intraarticular antimicrobial treatment is also contraindicated because a chemical synovitis can be induced [2]. Moreover, systemic antimicrobial therapy achieves excellent drug levels in the infected joint, as the inflamed synovia is well perfused [48].

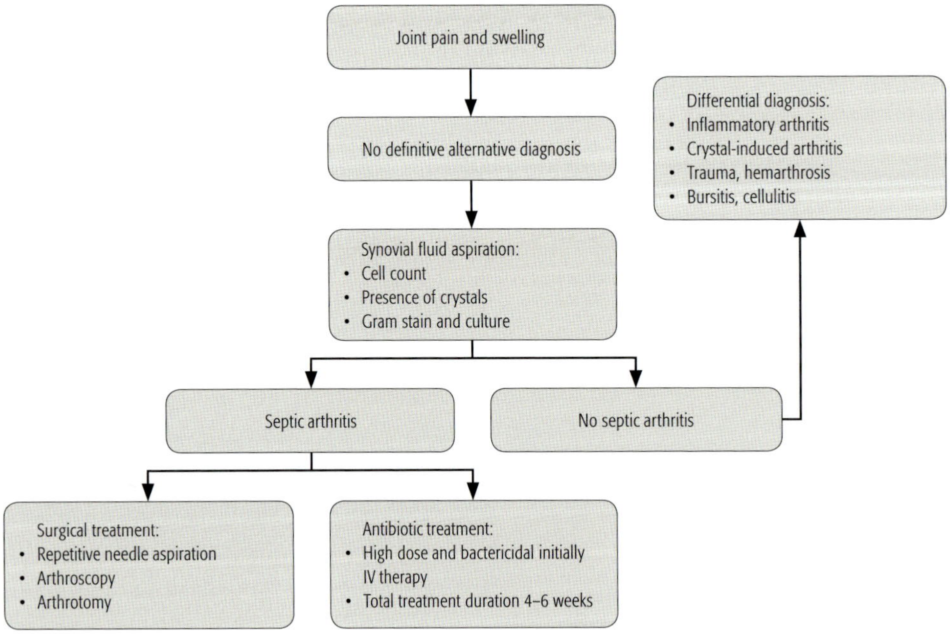

Fig 11.1-2 Management algorithm for septic arthritis.
Abbreviation: IV, intravenous.

4.1 Joint aspiration

Small peripheral joints (eg, finger and toe joints, wrist) can be treated with repetitive needle aspirations, if all necrotic and purulent material can be removed [38, 39]. Otherwise, arthroscopic or open surgical drainage must be performed, especially if compartmentalized fluid collections are present. In case of repetitive needle aspirations, daily aspirations are necessary until treatment response is documented not only clinically but also microbiologically (ie, culture results turn negative) and by decreasing WBC counts in synovial fluid analysis.

The diagnostic arthrocentesis can already alleviate pain symptoms in most patients and is therefore not only a diagnostic but also a first therapeutic intervention. It removes the inflamed synovial fluid with harmful enzymes and toxins that are damaging the cartilage. However, one aspiration is rarely enough and is mainly in large and weight-bearing joints (ie, knee, hip, shoulder, elbow, and ankle) only a provisional treatment and should be followed by rapid and aggressive surgical joint lavage via arthroscopy to avoid persisting joint damage.

Repetitive needle aspirations*	Arthroscopy	Arthrotomy†
Small joints (eg, finger or toe joints and wrist)	Large, weight-bearing joints (eg, knee, hip, shoulder, elbow, and ankle)	Periarticular infection (eg, abscess and fistula)
Patients with persistent or recurrent (reactive) synovial effusion after repetitive arthroscopic lavages‡	Joints difficult to puncture and drain by needle aspiration (eg, hip and shoulder)	Osteomyelitis, presence of bone sequestra
Patients with high perioperative mortality	Treatment failure of repetitive needle aspirations (eg, compartmentalized joint effusion, adhesions)	Need for emergency decompression
	Gächter stages 1, 2, and 3	Gächter stage 4
		Prosthetic joint

Table 11.1-4 Interventional and surgical treatment: when to use repetitive needle aspirations, arthroscopy, and arthrotomy?

* Daily repetition until white blood cell count in synovial fluid is decreasing and culture results turn negative; ineffective in compartmentalized joint effusions; no joint irrigation possible.

† Higher intraoperative and postoperative morbidity than arthroscopy in nonprosthetic joints.

‡ Prior documentation of microbiological response (negative culture results).

Stage	Criteria
1	Synovitis, cloudy fluid, possible petechiae, no radiological changes
2	Highly inflammatory synovitis, clumps of fibrin, pus, no radiological changes
3	Thickening of the synovial membrane (possibly several centimeters), adhesions with pouch formation, no radiological changes visible
4	Pannus formation, proliferation of aggressive synovitis on and later beneath the cartilage (ie, subchondral erosions), radiological changes visible

Table 11.1-5 Staging of septic arthritis as defined by Gächter.

4.2 Arthroscopy

In large weight-bearing joints (eg, hip, knee, shoulder, elbow, and ankle) repetitive needle aspirations are not enough to rapidly clean the joint and eliminate inflammatory effusion. Therefore, in these joints, if a Gächter stage 1, 2, or 3 is present (**Table 11.1-5**) and in patients with encapsulated inflammatory fluid collections, arthroscopic joint lavage as soon as possible with high-volume fluid irrigation (about 9 L of either Ringer's solution or NaCl 0.9% solution) is the therapeutic method of choice [45, 46, 49–51]. Compared to needle aspiration, arthroscopy allows the visualization of the joint, the removal of collections and adhesions, leading to a rapid decompression and mechanical cleaning of the joint. More severe infections, patients with a history of inflammatory arthropathy and infections caused by *S aureus* often require repeated arthroscopic interventions [51, 52]. The general approach is to repeat arthroscopy every 2–3 days if necessary, dependent on the initial intraoperative presentation and the clinical response to surgical and antimicrobial treatment (**Fig 11.1-3**). If a recurrent synovial effusion after multiple arthroscopies is present, interim needle aspirations can be performed if adequate response to antimicrobial therapy has been proven before (synovial cultures turn negative). A final arthroscopy might be useful to document the end of treatment results. The outcome is dependent on the initial stage of infection. Cure rates of > 80% have been documented.

4.3 Arthrotomy and possible treatment failures

Open surgical intervention, ie, arthrotomy, is necessary if the infection is not controlled by repetitive arthroscopy, in Gächter stage 4 disease (**Table 11.1-5**), if there is underlying osteomyelitis or the presence of bone sequestra or in patients with a contiguous spread of the infection into the surrounding soft tissue with abscess formation [45]. Furthermore, open surgical debridement is mandatory in patients with implants or prosthetic joints [53]. In earlier studies, arthrotomy was associated with a worse functional outcome and a prolonged hospitalization when compared with arthroscopy [40, 41]. Compared with repetitive needle aspirations, arthrotomy was associated with a lower mortality rate and a trend for a shorter hospitalization [38, 39, 42]. However, in all these older, retrospective and single-institution studies, the patient numbers were small and a selection and treatment assignment bias cannot be excluded. The selection of the treatment modality, ie, needle aspiration versus arthrotomy or arthroscopy, might depend on the medical department initially involved, ie, surgical or medical, and on the general health state of the patient: patients with many comorbidities and therefore a higher surgical intervention risk might be excluded from more invasive procedures and vice versa. Recently, two small studies compared arthrotomy and arthroscopy in the treatment of septic arthritis and confirmed the earlier findings [36, 37]. Both studies found high cure rates for both treatment modalities (80–100%), but a higher risk for a relapse of infection and a worse functional outcome in patients treated with arthrotomy.

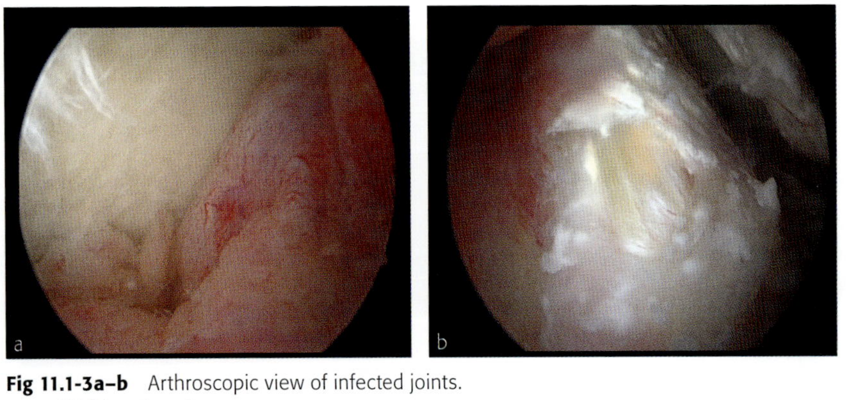

Fig 11.1-3a–b Arthroscopic view of infected joints.
a Gächter stage 1.
b Gächter stage 2.

4.4 Synovectomy

For Gächter stages 1 and 2 (**Table 11.1-5**), synovectomy should not be carried out as this reduces the diffusion of antimicrobial agents into the joint, which is facilitated by the strong perfusion in the inflamed synovial membrane. For Gächter stage 3, arthroscopic shaving may also be considered, while an arthrotomy is preferable if the synovial membrane is thick. For Gächter stage 4, an open synovectomy is recommended [45, 49, 51].

4.5 Antimicrobial treatment

In addition to the surgical and mechanical treatment, the administration of high-dose and bactericidal systemic antimicrobial therapy is mandatory in the management of septic arthritis. Neither treatment strategy alone is sufficient [33]. The isolation of the causative microorganism is essential for a targeted antimicrobial therapy with a long treatment duration. There are no randomized controlled studies evaluating the efficacy of different antimicrobial treatments.

Following arthrocentesis, empiric antimicrobial therapy is administered intravenously and guided by the presence of risk factors for septic arthritis (**Table 11.1-1**) and the results of the synovial Gram stain. In case no microorganisms can be detected in the Gram stain, the most common microorganisms causing septic arthritis should be covered, ie, staphylococci and streptococci. Intravenous amoxicillin/clavulanate 2.2 g every 8 hours or in penicillin-allergic patients IV cefazolin 2 g every 8 hours or IV cefuroxime 1.5 g every 8 hours are recommended. In countries with a high prevalence of methicillin-resistant *S aureus* empiric treatment should contain IV vancomycin 15 mg/kg body weight every 12 hours (vancomycin trough levels should be held at 15–20 mg/L). If gram-positive cocci are detected in the Gram stain (suggestive for staphylococci or streptococci) the same treatment regimen as for patients with a negative Gram stain result is recommended. If the Gram stain shows gram-negative cocci (suggestive for gonococci or meningococci) IV ceftriaxone 2 g per day is suggested, and if gram-negative bacilli are present IV ceftriaxone 2 g per day or IV cefepime 2 g every 8 hours if *P aeruginosa* is suspected. As soon as synovial culture results and susceptibility testings are available, targeted treatment is initiated [3, 54]. The targeted antimicrobial treatment is summarized in **Table 11.1-6**.

When changing IV to oral antimicrobial therapy, the following points have to be respected. Only antimicrobial agents with a good bioavailability and bone penetration should be used; otherwise insufficient drug levels in the bone are achieved with a consecutive treatment failure. Therefore, the authors do not recommend using oral amoxicillin/clavulanate or oral cephalosporins for staphylococcal septic arthritis [55]. Furthermore, if an infective endocarditis is present, the use of an oral therapy is contraindicated. Infective endocarditis usually is treated with a high-dose IV therapy for 4–6 weeks (2 weeks in streptococcal infective endocarditis if combination therapy is used). The authors also advise against bacteriostatic treatment regimens in septic arthritis, including clindamycin for staphylococci or streptococci and linezolid for staphylococci, streptococci, or enterococci. Be aware that oral treatment combinations with rifampin should not be used in patients with staphylococcal septic arthritis if they are scheduled for a prosthetic joint implantation in the near future (within a year). The reason is that rifampin-resistant skin flora emerges which—in case of a later postoperative prosthetic joint infection—increases the probability of an infection with a difficult-to-treat microorganism (ie, rifampin-resistant staphylococci) [53].

The duration of antimicrobial therapy is between 2–4 weeks for septic arthritis caused by streptococci and *Haemophilus* spp. and between 4–6 weeks for septic arthritis caused by *S aureus* and gram-negative bacilli [3, 56, 57]. Intravenous treatment duration usually is 1–2 weeks, dependent on the causing microorganism and its susceptibility pattern, the clinical response to treatment, and the presence of a concomitant osteomyelitis (Gächter stage 4). An earlier switch to the oral therapy is possible if the microorganisms are susceptible to bactericidal oral treatment regimens with a good bioavailability and bone penetration, such as rifampin-containing regimens for staphylococci and fluoroquinolones for enterobacteriaceae.

Microorganism	Antimicrobial agent	Daily dose	Application
Staphylococci: *S aureus* and coagulase-negative staphylococci			
Methicillin-susceptible staphylococci	Flucloxacillin[*,†]	4 x 2 g	IV
	Levofloxacin **AND**	2 x 500 mg	Oral
	Rifampin[‡]	2 x 450 mg	Oral
	OR		
	Trimethoprim/sulfamethoxazol **AND**	3 x 160/800 mg	Oral
	Rifampin[‡]	2 x 450 mg	Oral
	OR		
	Fusidic acid **AND**	3 x 500 mg	Oral
	Rifampin[‡]	2 x 450 mg	Oral
	OR		
	Doxycycline **AND**	2 x 100 mg	Oral
	Rifampin[‡]	2 x 450 mg	Oral
Methicillin-resistant staphylococci	Vancomycin[#], OR	2 x 15 mg/kg body weight	IV
	Teicoplanin, OR	1 x 400 mg[§]	IV
	Daptomycin	1 x 8 mg/kg body weight	IV
	Levofloxacin **AND**	2 x 500 mg	Oral
	Rifampin[‡]	2 x 450 mg	Oral
	OR		
	Trimethoprim/sulfamethoxazol **AND**	3 x 160/800 mg	Oral
	Rifampin[‡]	2 x 450 mg	Oral
	OR		
	Fusidic acid **AND**	3 x 500 mg	Oral
	Rifampin[‡]	2 x 450 mg	Oral
	OR		
	Doxycycline **AND**	2 x 100 mg	Oral
	Rifampin[‡]	2 x 450 mg	Oral
Streptococcus spp.	Penicillin G[†]	4 x 5 Mio Units	IV
	Ceftriaxon	1 x 2 g	IV
	Amoxicillin	3 x 750 mg	Oral
Enterococcus spp.	Amoxicillin[†]	4 x 2 g	IV
	With or without aminoglycoside[‖], OR		IV
	Daptomycin	1 x 10 mg/kg body weight	IV
	Amoxicillin	3 x 750 mg	Oral
Enterobacteriaceae, gonococci, meningococci (quinolone susceptible)	Ceftriaxon	1 x 2 g	IV
	Ciprofloxacin	2 x 750 mg	Oral
Nonfermenters[¶] (eg, *P aeruginosa*)	Cefepime, OR	3 x 2 g	IV
	Ceftazidime, OR	3 x 2 g	IV
	Piperacillin/tazobactam, OR	3 x 4.5 g	IV
	Meropenem	3 x 2 g	IV
	AND consider all with aminoglycoside[**]		
	Ciprofloxacin	2 x 750 mg	Oral
Candida spp.	Fluconazole	1 x 400 mg[††]	Oral
	Caspofungin	1 x 70 mg	IV
	Anidulafungin	1 x 100 mg[‡‡]	IV

Table 11.1-6 Targeted antimicrobial treatment in septic arthritis.
Note: The results of antimicrobial susceptibility testing are required for targeted treatment. Intravenous treatment duration is 1–2 weeks, and total treatment duration is 2–6 weeks, dependent on the microorganism, the clinical response to treatment, and the presence of a concomitant osteomyelitis.

The indicated dosages are for adult patients with normal body mass index, and normal renal and liver function. Abbreviation: IV, intravenous.

* In patients with a delayed-type hypersensitivity to penicillin, IV cefazolin 3 x 2 g or IV cefuroxime 3 x 1.5 g per day can be used.

† In patients with an immediate-type hypersensitivity to penicillin, IV vancomycin 2 x 15 mg/kg body weight per day (vancomycin trough level 15–20 mg/L) or IV daptomycin 1 x 8 mg/kg body weight (and 1 x 10 mg/kg body weight in enterococcal infections) per day should be used.

‡ Rifampin combinations should not be used if a prosthetic joint implantation is planned within the upcoming year. Oral treatment combinations should not be used if an underlying infective endocarditis is present.

§ After a single IV loading dose of 1 x 800 mg.

‖ Intravenous gentamicin 1 x 3 mg/kg body weight.

¶ Two weeks IV treatment recommended.

\# Vancomycin trough level 15–20 mg/L.

** Intravenous gentamicin 1 x 3 (-5) mg/kg body weight or IV tobramycin 1 x 3 (-5) mg/kg body weight.

†† After a single oral loading dose of 1 x 800 mg.

‡‡ After a single IV loading dose of 1 x 200 mg.

4.6 Physiotherapy

Physiotherapy of the infected joint is important and necessary to ensure that the cartilage is supplied with nutrients through diffusion [37, 54]. An infected joint should never be immobilized with external fixation or in a splint. Passive range-of-motion and isometric exercises to build up strength accelerate rehabilitation and reduce the risk of subsequent joint stiffness, furthermore they prevent muscular atrophy. For the knee and hip, a passive motion brace is useful. In the acute phase until drains have been removed the joint should not bear any weight, ie, bed rest or relief through two crutches is recommended, as is the placement in a functionally favorable position to avoid contractures (not fully extended).

4.7 Prognosis

The prognosis of septic arthritis has not improved in recent years despite better antimicrobial drugs and surgical intervention strategies. The functional prognosis is directly related to the presence of preexisting joint disease, the virulence of the causing microorganism, and the therapeutic delay between onset of symptoms and start of adequate therapy [2, 45, 56, 50, 59]. Despite adequate therapy, 25–50% of patients with septic arthritis experience permanent joint damage with impaired joint function. The mortality rate is dependent on age, the presence of comorbidities, and immunosuppression and ranges between 5–15% [56, 58]. In patients with a polyarticular infection, mortality rate is higher and may reach 30% [15].

5 Conclusion

A high index of suspicion for septic arthritis especially if risk factors are present allows a rapid initiation of therapy and a reduction of complications. Early signs of infection should prompt synovial fluid aspiration, which is the most important diagnostic workup (**Fig 11.1-2**). The key to successful management of septic arthritis is the rapid initiation of appropriate antimicrobial therapy, and joint drainage. Antimicrobial treatment alone is insufficient to cure septic arthritis. Joint drainage can be achieved by arthroscopy, repetitive needle aspirations or arthrotomy dependent on the involved joint, the extent and Gächter stage of the infection. High-dose and bactericidal systemic antimicrobial therapy is administered initially intravenously. Thereafter, oral treatments with a high bioavailability and bone penetration are necessary. Although treatment is highly efficient, permanent joint damage is the most important complication if adequate therapy is delayed.

6 References

1. **Morgan DS, Fisher D, Merianos A, et al.** An 18 year clinical review of septic arthritis from tropical Australia. *Epidemiol Infect.* 1996 Dec;117(3):423–428.
2. **Goldenberg DL, Reed JI.** Bacterial arthritis. *N Engl J Med.* 1985 Mar 21;312(12):764–771.
3. **Mathews CJ, Weston VC, Jones A, et al.** Bacterial septic arthritis in adults. *Lancet.* 2010 Mar 6;375(9717):846–855.
4. **Kaandorp CJ, Dinant HJ, van de Laar MA, et al.** Incidence and sources of native and prosthetic joint infection: a community based prospective survey. *Ann Rheum Dis.* 1997 Aug;56(8):470–475.
5. **Gavet F, Tournadre A, Soubrier M, et al.** Septic arthritis in patients aged 80 and older: a comparison with younger adults. *J Am Geriatr Soc.* 2005 Jul;53(7):1210–1213.
6. **Sapico FL, Liquete JA, Sarma RJ.** Bone and joint infections in patients with infective endocarditis: review of a 4-year experience. *Clin Infect Dis.* 1996 May;22(5):783–787.
7. **Babcock HM, Matava MJ, Fraser V.** Postarthroscopy surgical site infections: review of the literature. *Clin Infect Dis.* 2002 Jan 1;34(1):65–71.
8. **Kaandorp CJ, Van Schaardenburg D, Krijnen P, et al.** Risk factors for septic arthritis in patients with joint disease. A prospective study. *Arthritis Rheum.* 1995 Dec;38(12):1819–1825.
9. **Goldenberg DL.** Septic arthritis. *Lancet.* 1998 Jan 17;351(9097):197–202.
10. **Geirsson AJ, Statkevicius S, Vikingsson A.** Septic arthritis in Iceland 1990-2002: increasing incidence due to iatrogenic infections. *Ann Rheum Dis.* 2008 May;67(5):638–643.
11. **Margaretten ME, Kohlwes J, Moore D, et al.** Does this adult patient have septic arthritis? *JAMA.* 2007 Apr 4;297(13):1478–1488.
12. **Mader JT, Shirtliff ME, Bergquist S, et al.** Bone and joint infections in the elderly: practical treatment guidelines. *Drugs Aging.* 2000 Jan;16(1):67–80.
13. **Armstrong RW, Bolding F, Joseph R.** Septic arthritis following arthroscopy: clinical syndromes and analysis of risk factors. *Arthroscopy.* 1992;8(2):213–223.
14. **Cole BJ, Schumacher HR, Jr.** Injectable corticosteroids in modern practice. *J Am Acad Orthop Surg.* 2005 Jan-Feb;13(1):37–46.
15. **Dubost JJ, Fis I, Denis P, et al.** Polyarticular septic arthritis. *Medicine (Baltimore).* 1993 Sep;72(5):296–310.
16. **Gupta MN, Sturrock RD, Field M.** A prospective 2-year study of 75 patients with adult-onset septic arthritis. *Rheumatology (Oxford).* 2001 Jan;40(1):24–30.
17. **Ross JJ, Hu LT.** Septic arthritis of the pubic symphysis: review of 100 cases. *Medicine (Baltimore).* 2003 Sep;82(5):340–345.
18. **Ross JJ, Shamsuddin H.** Sternoclavicular septic arthritis: review of 180 cases. *Medicine (Baltimore).* 2004 May;83(3):139–48.
19. **Mathews CJ, Coakley G.** Septic arthritis: current diagnostic and therapeutic algorithm. *Curr Opin Rheumatol.* 2008 Jul;20(4):457–462.
20. **Dubost JJ, Soubrier M, De Champs C, et al.** No changes in the distribution of organisms responsible for septic arthritis over a 20 year period. *Ann Rheum Dis.* 2002 Mar;61(3):267–269.
21. **Frazee BW, Fee C, Lambert L.**How common is MRSA in adult septic arthritis? *Ann Emerg Med.* 2009 Nov;54(5):695–700.
22. **Wise CM, Morris CR, Wasilauskas BL, et al.** Gonococcal arthritis in an era of increasing penicillin resistance. Presentations and outcomes in 41 recent cases (1985-1991). *Arch Intern Med.* 1994 Dec 12-26;154(23):2690–2695.
23. **Baker DG, Schumacher HR, Jr.** Acute monoarthritis. *N Engl J Med.* 1993 Sep 30;329(14):1013–1020.
24. **Mathur T, Manadan AM, Hota B, et al.** Pseudo-septic hip arthritis as the presenting symptom of ankylosing spondylitis: a case series and review of the literature. *Clin Exp Rheumatol.* 2010 May-Jun;28(3):416–418.
25. **Singleton JD, West SG, Nordstrom DM.** "Pseudoseptic" arthritis complicating rheumatoid arthritis: a report of six cases. *J Rheumatol.* 1991 Sep;18(9):1319–1322.
26. **Learch TJ, Farooki S.** Magnetic resonance imaging of septic arthritis. *Clin Imaging.* 2000 Jul-Aug;24(4):236–242.
27. **Turpin S, Lambert R.** Role of scintigraphy in musculoskeletal and spinal infections. *Radiol Clin North Am.* 2001 Mar;39(2):169–189.
28. **Carpenter CR, Schuur JD, Everett WW, et al.** Evidence-based diagnostics: adult septic arthritis. *Acad Emerg Med.* 2011 Aug;18(8):781–796.
29. **Hughes JG, Vetter EA, Patel R, et al.** Culture with BACTEC Peds Plus/F bottle compared with conventional methods for detection of bacteria in synovial fluid. *J Clin Microbiol.* 2001 Dec;39(12):4468–4471.
30. **Louie JS, Liebling MR.** The polymerase chain reaction in infectious and post-infectious arthritis. A review. *Rheum Dis Clin North Am.* 1998 May;24(2):227–236.
31. **Soderquist B, Jones I, Fredlund H, et al.** Bacterial or crystal-associated arthritis? Discriminating ability of serum inflammatory markers. *Scand J Infect Dis.* 1998;30(6):591–596.
32. **Gordon TP, Reid C, Rozenbilds MA, et al.** Crystal shedding in septic arthritis: case reports and in vivo evidence in an animal model. *Aust N Z J Med.* 1986 Jun;16(3):336–340.
33. **Riegels-Nielsen P, Frimodt-Moller N, Sorensen M, et al.** Antibiotic treatment insufficient for established septic arthritis. Staphylococcus aureus experiments in rabbits. *Acta Orthop Scand.* 1989 Feb;60(1):113–115.
34. **Smith RL, Merchant TC, Schurman DJ.** In vitro cartilage degradation by Escherichia coli and Staphylococcus aureus. *Arthritis Rheum.* 1982 Apr;25(4):441–446.
35. **Balabaud L, Gaudias J, Boeri C, et al.** Results of treatment of septic knee arthritis: a retrospective series of 40 cases. *Knee Surg Sports Traumatol Arthrosc.* 2007 Apr;15(4):387–392.
36 **Böhler C, Dragana M, Puchner S, et al.** Treatment of septic arthritis of the knee: a comparison between arthroscopy and arthrotomy. *Knee Surg Sports Traumatol Arthrosc.* 2015 May 28.
37. **Peres LR, Marchitto RO, Pereira GS, et al.** Arthrotomy versus arthroscopy in the treatment of septic arthritis of the knee in adults: a randomized clinical trial. *Knee Surg Sports Traumatol Arthrosc.* 2015 Dec 24.
38. **Goldenberg DL, Brandt KD, Cohen AS, et al.** Treatment of septic arthritis: comparison of needle aspiration and surgery as initial modes of joint drainage. *Arthritis Rheum.* 1975 Jan-Feb;18(1):83–90.
39. **Broy SB, Schmid FR.** A comparison of medical drainage (needle aspiration) and surgical drainage (arthrotomy or arthroscopy) in the initial treatment of infected joints. *Clin Rheum Dis.* 1986 Aug;12(2):501–522.
40. **Sammer DM, Shin AY.** Comparison of arthroscopic and open treatment of septic arthritis of the wrist. *J Bone Joint Surg Am.* 2009 Jun;91(6):1387–1393.
41. **Wirtz DC, Marth M, Miltner O, et al.** Septic arthritis of the knee in adults: treatment by arthroscopy or arthrotomy. *Int Orthop.* 2001;25(4):239–241.

42. **Ravindran V, Logan I, Bourke BE.** Medical vs surgical treatment for the native joint in septic arthritis: a 6-year, single UK academic centre experience. *Rheumatology (Oxford).* 2009 Oct;48(10):1320–1322.
43. **Butt U, Amissah-Arthur M, Khattak F, et al.** What are we doing about septic arthritis? A survey of UK-based rheumatologists and orthopedic surgeons. *Clin Rheumatol.* 2011 May;30(5):707–710.
44. **Donatto KC.** Orthopedic management of pyogenic arthritis. *Compr Ther.* 1999 Aug-Oct;25(8-10):411–417.
45. **Vispo Seara JL, Barthel T, Schmitz H, et al.** Arthroscopic treatment of septic joints: prognostic factors. *Arch Orthop Trauma Surg.* 2002 May;122(4):204–211.
46. **Gächter A.** [The Infected Joint]. *Inform Arzt.* 1985;6:35-43. German.
47. **van Huyssteen AL, Bracey DJ.** Chlorhexidine and chondrolysis in the knee. *J Bone Joint Surg Br.* 1999 Nov;81(6):995–996.
48. **Frimodt-Moller N, Riegels-Nielsen P.** Antibiotic penetration into the infected knee. A rabbit experiment. *Acta Orthop Scand. [Comparative Study].* 1987 Jun;58(3):256–259.
49. **Parisien JS, Shaffer B.** Arthroscopic management of pyarthrosis. *Clin Orthop Relat Res.* 1992 Feb(275):243–247.
50. **Bussiere F, Beaufils P.** [Role of arthroscopy in the treatment of pyogenic arthritis of the knee in adults. Report of 16 cases]. *Rev Chir Orthop Reparatrice Appar Mot.* 1999 Dec;85(8):803–810. French.
51. **Stutz G, Kuster MS, Kleinstuck F, et al.** Arthroscopic management of septic arthritis: stages of infection and results. *Knee Surg Sports Traumatol Arthrosc.* 2000;8(5):270–274.
52. **Hunter JG, Gross JM, Dahl JD, et al.** Risk factors for failure of a single surgical debridement in adults with acute septic arthritis. *J Bone Joint Surg Am.* 2015 Apr 1;97(7):558–564.
53. **Trampuz A, Zimmerli W.** Diagnosis and treatment of implant-associated septic arthritis and osteomyelitis. *Curr Infect Dis Rep.* 2008 Sep;10(5):394–403.
54. **Shirtliff ME, Mader JT.** Acute septic arthritis. *Clin Microbiol Rev.* 2002 Oct;15(4):527–544.
55. **Landersdorfer CB, Bulitta JB, Kinzig M, et al.** Penetration of antibacterials into bone: pharmacokinetic, pharmacodynamic and bioanalytical considerations. *Clin Pharmacokinet.* 2009;48(2):89–124.
56. **Ross JJ, Saltzman CL, Carling P, et al.** Pneumococcal septic arthritis: review of 190 cases. *Clin Infect Dis.* 2003 Feb 1;36(3):319–327.
57. **Weston V, Coakley G, British Society for Rheumatology Standards G, et al.** Guideline for the management of the hot swollen joint in adults with a particular focus on septic arthritis. *J Antimicrob Chemother.* 2006 Sep;58(3):492–493.
58. **Kaandorp CJ, Krijnen P, Moens HJ, et al.** The outcome of bacterial arthritis: a prospective community-based study. *Arthritis Rheum.* 1997 May;40(5):884–892.
59. **Weston VC, Jones AC, Bradbury N, et al.** Clinical features and outcome of septic arthritis in a single UK Health District 1982-1991. *Ann Rheum Dis.* 1999 Apr;58(4):214–219.

11.2 Septic arthritis after anterior cruciate ligament surgery

Parag Sancheti, AJ Electricwala, Ashok Shyam, Kailash Patil

1 Basics

Infection after anterior cruciate ligament (ACL) reconstruction is an uncommon but potentially serious complication, which can cause significant morbidity, and complications including arthrofibrosis and articular cartilage loss [1]. Infection can result in permanent impairment of knee function that does not meet the high-demand performance expectations of the patients undergoing this surgery. Early diagnosis and treatment are the key factors in avoiding these consequences and reducing the length of hospitalization [1].

There are many algorithms suggested for treatment, but there is no consensus about the best treatment modality [2–5]. Many authors advocate either open or arthroscopic debridement together with intravenous antibiotic therapy, but there is considerable controversy about graft retention [2, 6, 7]. There is little evidence in the literature on functional outcomes of these patients, especially with long-term follow-up [1, 2, 7].

1.1 Epidemiology

Infection after arthroscopic ACL reconstruction (ACLR) is a rare complication with a reported incidence of 0.3–0.48% [2–4, 8–12] and a prevalence ranging from 0.14 to 1.7% [3, 4, 7, 10, 13–16]. The incidence of infection after ACLR does not vary by age, sex, or region [17].

The reported rates of infection after ACLR have been consistent over the past two decades in the literature [17].

1.2 Causative microorganisms

- *Staphylococcus* species, specifically the subspecies of *Staphylococcus aureus*, including methicillin-resistant *S aureus* (31%) and coagulase-negative *Staphylococcus epidermidis* (44%), are the bacteria responsible for the majority of reported infections. *Staphylococcus* forms biofilms that protect it from antimicrobials, opsonization, and phagocytosis making eradication difficult [18].
- *Propionibacterium saprophyticus* is a rare causative organism [18]
- Wind and colleagues in 2001 reported one case of *Candida albicans* infection following routine arthroscopy of the knee, which eventually resulted in a knee fusion [19].

1.3 Recognition of infection and confirmation of the diagnosis

Diagnosis of septic arthritis is based on patient history, physical examination, laboratory parameters suggestive of an infectious process, and a culture of joint aspirate [15].

1.3.1 Time to presentation

The average time to presentation of infection is 9.5 days (median: 8 days) after reconstruction. However, clinical features may develop as early as 4 days and as late as 20 days after surgery [20].

1.3.2 Clinical parameters

Typical parameters are [20]:

- Fever with a temperature ranging from 37.6° C to 39.6° C, general malaise
- Progressive increase in knee pain and swelling
- Large postoperative hematoma
- Increasing infection parameters in the blood (C-reactive protein (CRP), leukocytes, erythrocyte sedimentation rate (ESR))
- Other less frequent symptoms such as local incisional drainage, local warmth, and erythema
- On physical examination, painful restriction in knee range of movement, swelling, redness, and discharge from the wound may be found (**Fig 11.2-1**)
- Purulent discharge from the wound, hyperemic wound edges with local rise in temperature may be present (**Fig 11.2-2**)

Indolent presentation of septic arthritis after anterior cruciate ligament reconstruction

Indolent presentation of the disease was emphasized by Schollin-Borg et al [20]. They highlight that well-known symptoms of infection may be missing, and the situation can be easily interpreted as normal postoperative findings [20]. However, postoperative pain out of proportion to the surgical pain, long-lasting pain, and the absence of improvement in symptoms should raise the level of suspicion for septic arthritis [15].

The incision for the tibial tunnel is the most common site for deep-wound infection because of its superficial anatomical location [15].

1.3.3 Laboratory parameters

The parameters include:

- Both CRP and ESR may be helpful in discriminating a normal joint from a septic joint and in evaluating the response of infection to treatment. C-reactive protein is a more sensitive and reliable indicator of postoperative infection. The threshold values of 41 mg/L for CRP and 32 mm/h for ESR have the most optimal sensitivity (63%) and specificity (82%) [21]. The peak CRP level occurs earlier than the peak ESR level after treatment of postoperative infection and returns to normal more quickly [13]. Explanation: CRP is a rapid-response indicator that allows prompt treatment. Erythrocyte sedimentation rate reflects changes in the fibrinogen level, which increases after 24–48 hours of infection, whereas the CRP level increases within 6–8 hours of an inflammatory process. C-reactive protein reaches its peak value within the first 3 days and then shows a faster return to a normal value, which further proves that CRP is a more sensitive and reliable indicator of postoperative infection [13].
- Total leukocyte count > 10,000/cu mm is suggestive of infection [13].

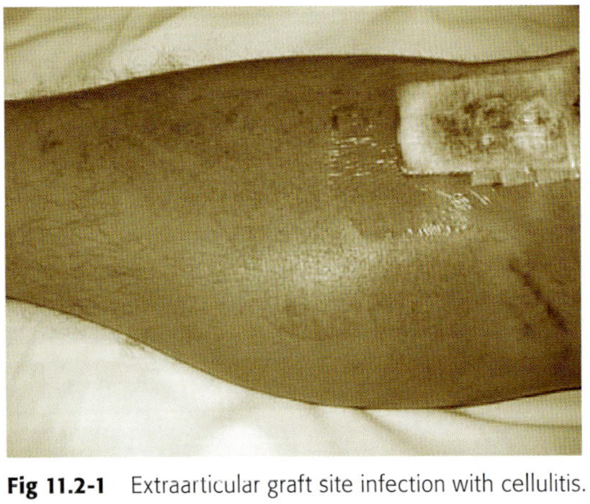

Fig 11.2-1 Extraarticular graft site infection with cellulitis.

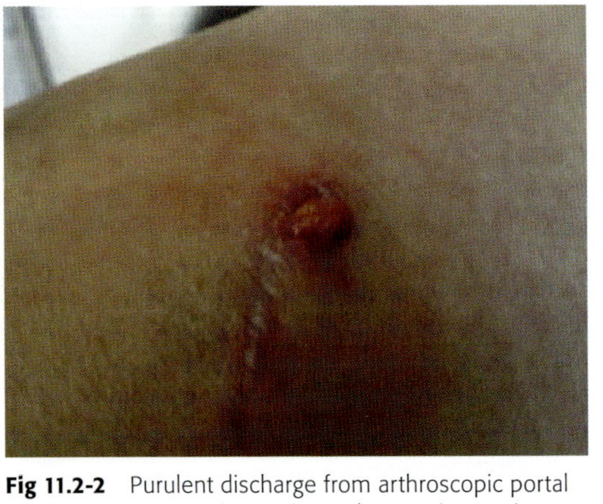

Fig 11.2-2 Purulent discharge from arthroscopic portal in a case of septic arthritis after arthroscopic anterior cruciate ligament reconstruction.

1.3.4 Synovial fluid aspiration

Joint aspiration should be performed as soon as the diagnosis of infection is suspected. The joint fluid obtained must be analyzed (white blood cell count, differential, crystals, and biochemistry) and cultured for aerobic and anaerobic organisms with antibiotic sensitivity [15]:

- Elevated leukocyte count of aspirated knee-joint fluid (average of 49.4 ×109/L, normal: 4–11) with > 92% polymorphonuclear cells is strongly indicative of septic arthritis [20].
- Culture for aerobic and anaerobic organisms and antibiotic sensitivity must be taken.

1.3.5 Radiological parameters

- Radiological evaluation must include anteroposterior, lateral, and Merchant patellar views [2]. X-rays may reveal loosening of implant hardware (**Fig 11.2-3**).
- Magnetic resonance imaging scan: suggestive imaging signs of infection are appearances of synovitis, bone erosions, periarticular edema, and fluid collections or abscesses [22–24].

2 Indications for surgical management

Clinical parameters suggestive of infection after ACLR:

- Fever ranging from 37.6° C to 39.6° C, feeling of general malaise
- Progressively increasing knee pain and swelling
- Increasing infection parameters
- Large postoperative hematoma
- Other less frequent symptoms such as local incisional drainage, local warmth, and erythema
- On physical examination, painful restriction in knee range of movement, swelling, redness, and discharging wound
- Purulent discharge from the wound, hyperemic wound edges with local increase in temperature

Once the diagnosis of septic arthritis is confirmed by the synovial aspirate as well as laboratory data, surgical debridement must be carried out [15].

3 Preoperative planning and surgical approach

Early diagnosis and treatment have been found to be the most critical factors in the healing process and avoidance of complications.

3.1 Steps of arthroscopic lavage

The list of steps to be taken includes [15]

1. Standard anteromedial and anterolateral portals can be used. A superolateral portal may be added for better inflow
2. Extensive washout of the joint with 10–15 L of normal saline solution
3. Debridement of inflamed or devitalized tissue
4. Removal of fibrin clots and old coagulated blood
5. Synovectomy—if significant synovitis is found
6. Gentle removal of the fibrin layer that covers the graft surface
7. Macroscopic evaluation of the graft for integrity
8. Synovial fluid and debrided tissue must be sent for new culture and antibiotic sensitivity

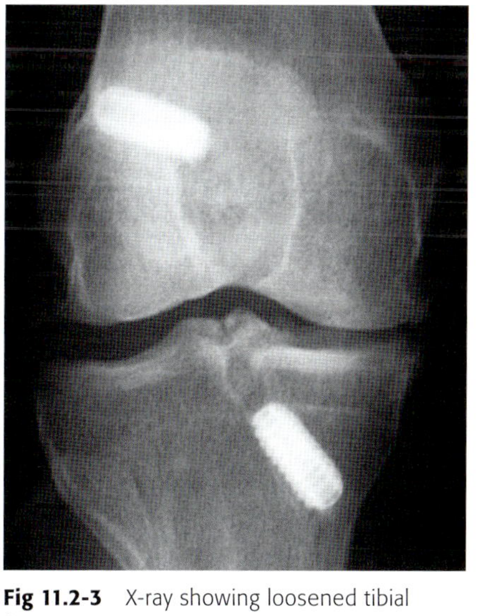

Fig 11.2-3 X-ray showing loosened tibial fixation screw.

4 Management and surgical debridement

Despite low incidence of infection after ACLR, it is important to recognize infection and treat it without delay to prevent the devastating consequences such as articular cartilage damage and arthrofibrosis. However, optimal clinical guidelines have not been established; there is no consensus about the best treatment modality. Burk and colleagues have published on this subject and found that opinions differed for graft preservation, type and duration of antibiotics, and time of revision [16]. Many authors recommend either an open or arthroscopic debridement together with intravenous antibiotic therapy, but there is considerable controversy regarding graft preservation [2–5]. Most authors agree that preserving the graft and repeating arthroscopic lavage as many times as necessary would be the best policy [2, 6]. However, some still believe that graft removal is an essential part of the healing process [7].

4.1 Antibiotic therapy

The aim of preoperative intravenous antibiotics is to achieve adequate plasma and tissue levels of antibiotics to reduce the risk of bacterial exposure. However, it is difficult or impossible to achieve antibiotic tissue levels above the minimum inhibitory concentration in the reconstructed ACL [18, 25–30]. In patients with a suspicion of septic arthritis, an empiric intravenous trial with a combination of broad-spectrum antibiotic such as ceftazidime (2 g per 8 hours) and vancomycin (1 g per 12 hours) must be started [18, 25–30]. The antibiotic therapy must be later changed according to the sensitivity of the microorganism cultured from the aspirate. Parenteral antibiotics can be replaced with oral antibiotics after 2–3 weeks. Antibiotics must be administered for a minimum of 6 weeks, and they must not be withdrawn until complete normalization of the clinical and laboratory parameters. The authors recommend parenteral antibiotics to be given until the clinical and laboratory parameters improve (CRP < 20, negative-joint aspirate), or for a minimum of 2 weeks. Oral antibiotics would be given thereafter until normalization of clinical and laboratory parameters (CRP < 10), or for a minimum of 4 weeks. The authors recommend a minimum total duration of administration of antibiotics of 6 weeks.

4.2 Surgical irrigation and debridement

Early diagnosis and treatment have been found to be the most critical factors in the healing process and avoiding complications. Typical arthroscopic findings are demonstrated in **Fig 11.2-4** and **Fig 11.2-5**.

Since the pioneering work of Ballard, the treatment for septic arthritis has been based on a combination of open debridement and joint irrigation [15, 31]. Riel and colleagues reported on one of the first series of patients with septic arthritis treated arthroscopically instead of with open lavage after ACLR that had successful outcomes [32]. Since then, this technique has been adopted worldwide by the orthopedic community [15, 32]. Once the diagnosis of septic arthritis is confirmed by the synovial aspirate and Gram stain as well as laboratory data, an arthroscopic procedure must be carried out [15]. After the initial debridement, clinical and laboratory parameters are rechecked. If not improved after 48–72 hours, arthroscopic irrigation and debridement is repeated. Arthroscopic debridement may be repeated until the clinical and laboratory parameters normalize. In the authors' opinion, several arthroscopic debridements are usually necessary.

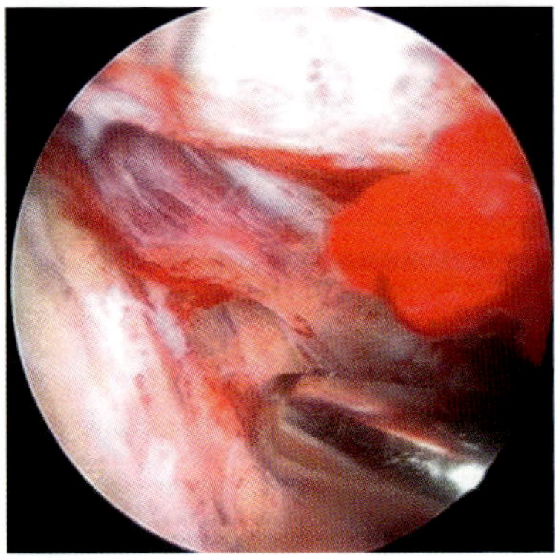

Fig 11.2-4 An infection-related fibrin layer of the reconstructed anterior cruciate ligament.

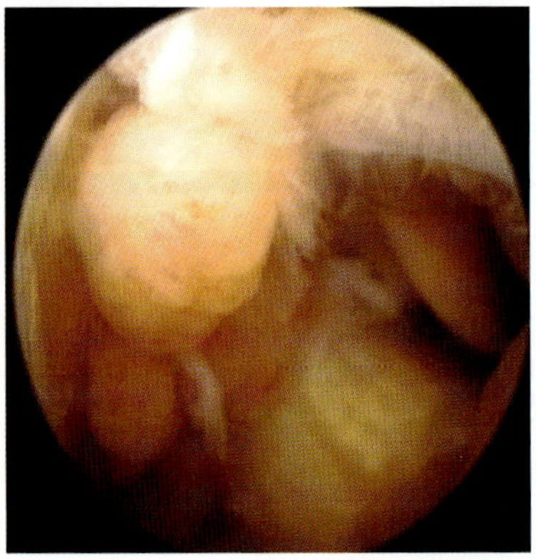

Fig 11.2-5 A bacteria-induced slime layer over the previously reconstructed anterior cruciate ligament with extensive synovitis.

5 Graft preservation versus graft removal and two-staged revision

An algorithmic approach is presented in **Fig 11.2-6**.

- Culture-specific intravenous antibiotics and arthroscopic joint irrigation with graft retention are recommended as initial treatment.
- Recommended indications for graft excision and hardware removal are infections caused by resistant organisms and graft infection [7].
- In such cases two-staged revision is recommended:
  - Stage 1: radical debridement, graft, and hardware removal.
  - Stage 2: revision ACLR after all clinical and laboratory parameters have returned to normal.
- Indications for two-staged revision at the authors' institution are:
  - If the recognition of infection after ACLR has been delayed by more than 2 weeks after the onset of clinical symptoms.
  - When the graft looks infected and the articular cartilage appears to be at risk of damage at the time of the first arthroscopic debridement.
  - When there is no progressive improvement in clinical and laboratory parameters after four consecutive arthroscopic debridements where graft has been preserved.
  - Persistent positive-culture joint fluid after three consecutive arthroscopic debridements.

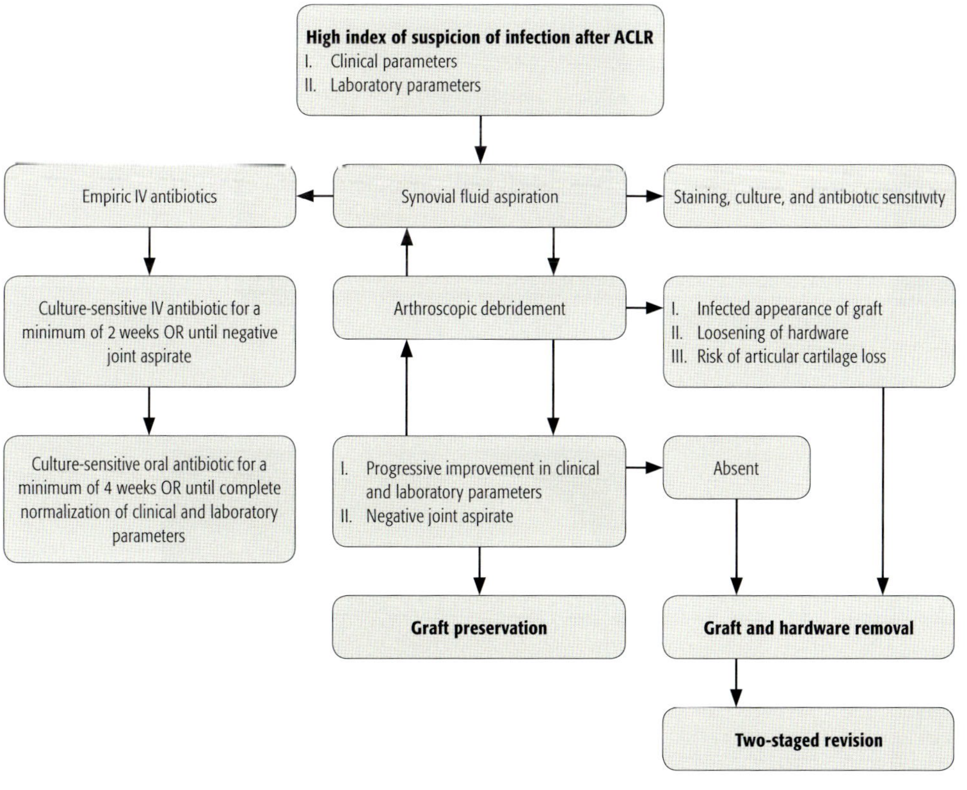

Fig 11.2-6 Algorithm for the management of infection after arthroscopic anterior cruciate ligament reconstruction. Abbreviations: ACLR, anterior cruciate ligament reconstruction; IV, intravenous.

6 Postoperative management and rehabilitation

Once the clinical symptoms have normalized, a physiotherapy program is initiated. The rehabilitation protocol is not significantly different from cases without infection [15]. At the authors' center, this rehabilitation program is followed:

- Continuous passive motion of the knee joint is begun at the earliest possible time to prevent knee stiffness.
- One week after surgery, a graded knee-strengthening program, including quadriceps and hamstrings strengthening through progressive isometric, isotonic, and isokinetic exercises, is started.
- Range of motion is progressively increased until at least 120° of flexion is achieved.
- Weight bearing is allowed at 4 weeks until the patient is ambulatory with crutches.

7 Complications

7.1 Arthrofibrosis

One of the most common complications of infections after ACLR is arthrofibrosis, which involves the development of fibrous scar tissue within and around the synovium in at least one compartment of the joint (**Fig 11.2-7**, **Fig 11.2-8**). This may also develop diffusely [22]. This condition is treated with arthroscopic or open lysis of adhesions.

7.2 Articular cartilage damage

Articular cartilage damage and early onset osteoarthritis is a devastating complication of infection in a joint (**Fig 11.2-9**, **Fig 11.2-10**). Hence, a high index of suspicion, early diagnosis, and treatment of infection after ACLR are key to preventing this complication.

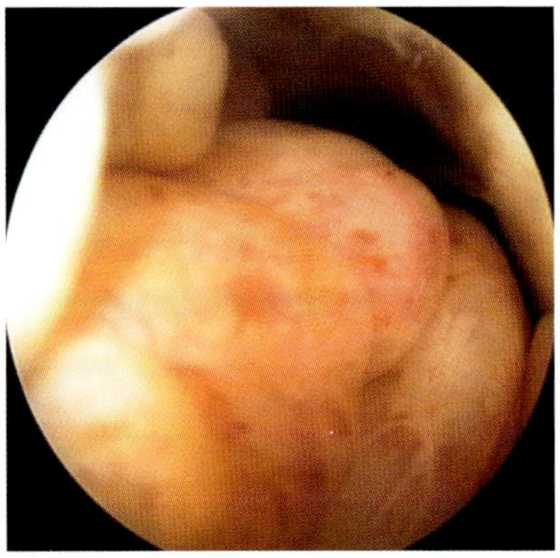

Fig 11.2-7 Extensive synovitis 3 weeks after anterior cruciate ligament reconstruction.

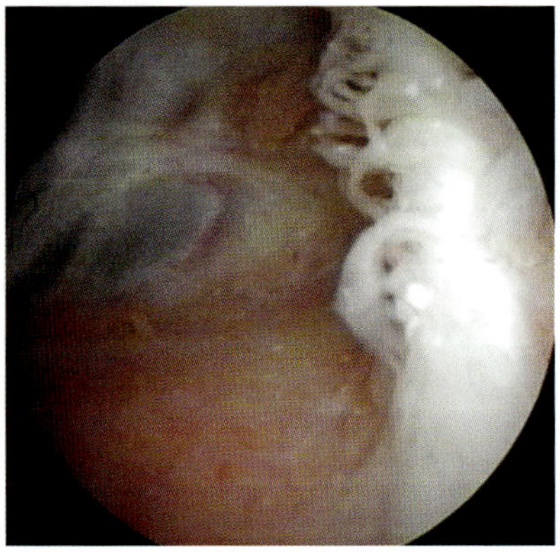

Fig 11.2-8 Infectious granulation tissue and adhesions in a case of stiff knee postinfection after anterior cruciate ligament reconstruction.

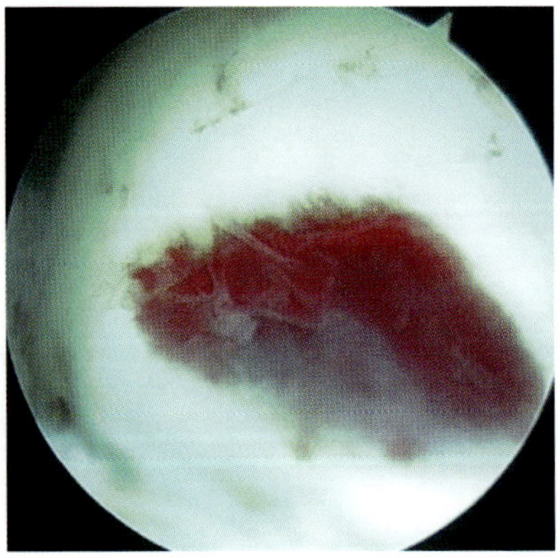

Fig 11.2-9 A crater formation with "cat-bite appearance" of the medial femoral condyle in a case of septic arthritis after anterior cruciate ligament reconstruction.

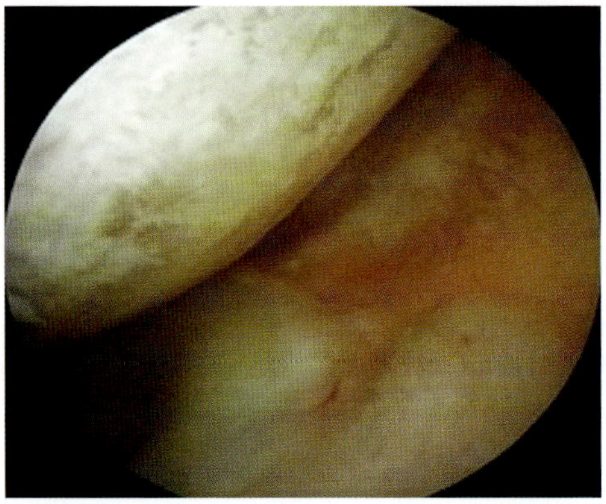

Fig 11.2-10 Articular cartilage loss in a case of indolent presentation of septic arthritis secondary to anterior cruciate ligament reconstruction.

8 Prevention methods

- Proper sterilization of surgical equipment: inappropriate sterilization technique of the hamstring graft harvester may be associated with the increased infection rate. Disassembling instruments with this type of configuration (ie, tube within a tube) is appropriate [33].
- Prevention of autograft contamination: a high rate (12%) of autograft contamination can be expected during autograft preparation for ACLR [34, 35].
- Routine surveillance for surgical-site infections: Periodic visible surveillance may help keep surgical-site infection rates down by encouraging adherence to infection control guidelines [17].
- Avoid intraarticular corticosteroid injections [17].
- Avoid preoperative razor shaving: if hair removal must be performed, it should be done immediately before the operation and with electric clippers [17].
- Avoid flash sterilization: flash sterilization is not recommended for routine sterilization because it meets only minimum sterilization standards for time and temperature. This is a particular concern with instruments such as arthroscopes, which have a long narrow lumen difficult to disinfect adequately without standard practices. Flash-sterilized instruments are also easily contaminated during transport back to the operative field because they are not enclosed in a sterile container [17].

9 Outcome

- Septic arthritis after ACLR often does not result in inferior objective knee function compared with uncomplicated ACLR [36].
- Subjectively, infection patients are as satisfied as noninfection patients, but rehabilitation takes longer and fewer patients return to play sports [36].

10 Conclusion

- *Staphylococcus*, specifically the subspecies of *S aureus*, including methicillin-resistant *S aureus* (31%) and coagulase-negative *S epidermidis* (44%), are the bacteria responsible for the majority of reported infections.
- Infection after ACLR may be intraarticular or extraarticular. Intraarticular infection presents with features of septic arthritis. Extraarticular infection presents with local wound complications.
- The average time to presentation of infection is 9.5 days.
- Indolent presentation of septic arthritis may be present where well-known symptoms of infection may be missing. Postoperative pain out of proportion to the surgical pain and the absence of improvement in symptoms should be suggestive for septic arthritis.
- C-reactive protein is a fairly sensitive and reliable indicator of postoperative infection.
- Surgical irrigation and debridement combined with parenteral antibiotics form the mainstay of treatment.
- A high index of suspicion, early diagnosis, and treatment of infection after ACLR are the keys to preventing complications of septic arthritis like arthrofibrosis and articular cartilage damage.
- Early appropriate surgery is essential.
- "Prevention is better than cure". Proper sterilization of surgical equipment, prevention of autograft contamination, and ideal operating room environment are key to prevention.

11 References

1. **Calvo R, Figueroa D, Anastasiadis Z, et al.** Septic arthritis in ACL reconstruction surgery with hamstring autografts. Eleven years of experience. *Knee.* 2014 Jun;21(3):717–720.
2. **Binnet MS, Başarir K.** Risk and outcome of infection after different arthroscopic anterior cruciate ligament reconstruction techniques. *Arthroscopy.* 2007 Aug;23(8):862–868.
3. **McAllister DR, Parker RD, Cooper AE, et al.** Outcomes of postoperative septic arthritis after anterior cruciate ligament reconstruction. *Am J Sports Med.* 1999 Sept-Oct;27(5):562–570.
4. **Indelli PF, Dillingham M, Fanton G, et al.** Septic arthritis in postoperative anterior cruciate ligament reconstruction. *Clin Orthop Relat Res.* 2002 May;(398):182–188.
5. **Matava MJ, Evans TA, Wright RW, et al.** Septic arthritis of the knee following anterior cruciate ligament reconstruction: results of a survey of sports medicine fellowship directors. *Arthroscopy.* 1998 Oct;14(7):717–725.
6. **D'Angelo GL, Ogilvie-Harris DJ.** Septic arthritis following arthroscopy with cost/benefit analysis of antibiotic prophylaxis. *Arthroscopy.* 1988;4(1):10–14.
7. **Viola R, Marzano N, Vianello R.** An unusual epidemic of Staphylococcus-negative infections involving anterior cruciate ligament reconstruction with salvage of the graft and function. *Arthroscopy.* 2000 Mar;16(2):173–177.
8. **Maletis GB, Inacio MC, Reynolds S, et al.** Incidence of postoperative anterior cruciate ligament reconstruction infections: graft choice makes a difference. *Am J Sports Med.* 2013 Aug;41(8):1780–1785.
9. **Barker JU, Drakos MC, Maak TG, et al.** Effect of graft selection on the incidence of postoperative infection in anterior cruciate ligament reconstruction. *Am J Sports Med.* 2010 Feb;38(2):281–286.
10. **Judd D, Bottoni C, Kim D, et al.** Infections following arthroscopic anterior cruciate ligament reconstruction. *Arthroscopy.* 2006 Apr;22(4):375–384.
11. **Katz LM, Battaglia TC, Patino P, et al.** A retrospective comparison of the incidence of bacterial infection following anterior cruciate ligament reconstruction with autograft versus allograft. *Arthroscopy.* 2008 Dec;24(12):1330–1335.
12. **Sonnery-Cottet B, Archbold P, Zayni R, et al.** Prevalence of septic arthritis after anterior cruciate ligament reconstruction among professional athletes. *Am J Sports Med.* 2011 Nov;39(11):2371–2376.
13. **Wang C, Ao Y, Fan X, et al.** C-reactive protein and erythrocyte sedimentation rate changes after arthroscopic anterior cruciate ligament reconstruction: Guideline to diagnose and monitor postoperative infection. *Arthroscopy.* 2014;30:1110–1115.
14. **Williams RJ 3rd, Laurencin CT, Warren RF, et al.** Septic arthritis after arthroscopic anterior cruciate ligament reconstruction. Diagnosis and management. *Am J Sports Med.* 1997 Mar-Apr;25(2):261–267.
15. **Torres-Claramunt R, Pelfort X, Erquicia J, et al.** Knee joint infection after ACL reconstruction: prevalence, management and functional outcomes. *Knee Surg Sports Traumatol Arthrosc.* 2013 Dec;21(12):2844–2849.
16. **Burks RT, Friederichs MG, Fink B, et al.** Treatment of postoperative anterior cruciate ligament infections with graft removal and early reimplantation. *Am J Sports Med.* 2003 May-Jun;31(3):414–418.
17. **Babcock HM, Carroll C, Matava M, et al.** Surgical site infections after arthroscopy: Outbreak investigation and case control study. *Arthroscopy.* 2003 Feb;19(2):172–181.
18. **Vertullo CJ, Quick M, Jones A, et al.** A surgical technique using presoaked vancomycin hamstring grafts to decrease the risk of infection after anterior cruciate ligament reconstruction. *Arthroscopy.* 2012 Mar;28(3):337–342.
19. **Wind WM, McGrath BE, Mindell ER.** Infection following knee arthroscopy. *Arthroscopy.* 2001 Oct;17(8):878–883.
20. **Schollin-Borg M, Michaëlsson K, Rahme H.** Presentation, outcome, and cause of septic arthritis after anterior cruciate ligament reconstruction: a case control study. *Arthroscopy.* 2003; Nov 19(9):941–947.
21. **Hussain TM, Kim DH.** C-reactive Protein and Erythrocyte Sedimentation Rate in Orthopaedics. *University of Pennsylvania Orthopedic Journal.* 2002 Spring;15:13–16.
22. **Kulczycka P, Larbi A, Malghem J, et al.** Imaging ACL reconstructions and their complications. *Diagnostic Interv Imaging.* 2015 Jan;96(1):11–19.
23. **Bencardino JT, Beltran J, Feldman MI, et al.** MR imaging of complications of anterior cruciate ligament graft reconstruction. *Radiographics.* 2009 Nov;29(7):2115–2126.
24. **Papakonstantinou O, Chung CB, Chanchairujira K, et al.** Complications of anterior cruciate ligament reconstruction: MR imaging. *Eur Radiol.* 2003 May;13(5):1106–1117.
25. **Lew DP, Waldvogel FA. Osteomyelitis.** *Lancet.* 2004 Jul 24-30;364(9431):369–379.
26. **Antoci V Jr, Adams CS, Hickok NJ, et al.** Antibiotics for local delivery systems cause skeletal cell toxicity in vitro. *Clin Orthop Relat Res.* 2007 Sep;462:200–206.
27. **Lawson KJ, Marks KE, Brems J, et al.** Vancomycin vs tobramycin elution from polymethylmethacrylate: an in vitro study. *Orthopedics.* 1990 May;13(5):521–524.
28. **Lin SS, Ueng SW, Lee SS, et al.** In vitro elution of antibiotic from antibiotic-impregnated biodegradable calcium alginate wound dressing. *J Trauma.* 1999 Jul;47(1):136–141.
29. **Whiteside LA, Peppers M, Nayfeh TA, et al.** Methicillin-resistant Staphylococcus aureus in TKA treated with revision and direct intra-articular antibiotic infusion. *Clin Orthop Relat Res.* 2011 Jan;469(1):26–33.
30. **Grayson JE, Grant GD, Dukie S, et al.** The in vitro elution characteristics of vancomycin from tendons. *Clin Orthop Relat Res.* 2011 Oct;469(10):2948–2952.
31. **Ballard A, Burkhalter WE, Mayfield GW, et al.** The functional treatment of pyogenic arthritis of the adult knee. *J Bone Joint Surg Am.* 1975 Dec;57(8):1119–1123.
32. **Riel KA, Primbs J, Bernett P.** [Arthroscopic distension irrigation in acute postoperative infection of the knee joint–long-term follow-up]. *Chirurg.* 1994 Nov;65(11):1023–1027. German.
33. **Tuman J, Diduch DR, Baumfeld JA, et al.** Joint infection unique to hamstring tendon harvestor used during anterior cruciate ligament reconstruction surgery. *Arthroscopy.* 2008 May;24(5):618–620.
34. **Wu GK, Ng GY, Mak AF.** Effects of knee bracing on the sensorimotor function of subjects with anterior cruciate ligament reconstruction. *Am J Sports Med.* 2001 Sep-Oct;29(5):641–645.
35. **Hantes ME, Basdekis GK, Varitimidis SE, et al.** Autograft contamination during preparation for anterior cruciate ligament reconstruction. *J Bone Joint Surg Am.* 2008 Apr;90(4):760–764.
36. **Boström Windhamre H, Mikkelsen C, Forssblad M, et al.** Postoperative septic arthritis after anterior cruciate ligament reconstruction: does it affect the outcome? A retrospective controlled study. *Arthroscopy.* 2014 Sep;30(9):1100–1109.

12 Spondylodiscitis

Paul W Millhouse, Caleb Behrend, Alexander R Vaccaro

1 Basics

Historically, infections of the vertebral column were devastating diseases. Spinal epidural abscesses were once rare but almost universally fatal disorders [1, 2]. With the advent of antibiotics, advanced imaging, and improvements in surgical methods, morbidity and mortality have been dramatically reduced. Now, a timely diagnosis and appropriate directed antimicrobial therapy, and when necessary, the use of surgery are the essential elements of successful management of these conditions. This chapter reviews strategies used for the correct identification of patients at increased risk for infection, typical presentations, principles of diagnosis, and the approach to treatment of spondylodiscitis [3].

1.1 Definition

Spondylodiscitis is infection or inflammation of the disc space, adjacent endplate, and possibly the vertebral body. The infection may involve one or more of these spinal structures and adjacent spinal segments as well as contiguous anatomical regions. In its most severe form, spondylodiscitis can lead to sepsis, spinal cord injury (SCI) from associated abscess, spinal instability, and even death.

1.2 Pathogenesis

Mechanisms by which microorganisms infect the vertebral body or the disc space include hematogenous or contiguous spread and direct inoculation of the disc space. The latter can be traumatic or iatrogenic associated with diagnostic or therapeutic interventions, such as spinal injection, discography, and surgery. The incidence of iatrogenic spondylodiscitis is increasing due to the increased use of invasive treatments.

Hematogenous spread of infection is more common when associated with another active infection, transient bacteremia, or injection as with intravenous (IV) drug use. The most frequent sources of hematogenous vertebral osteomyelitis are urinary tract infections or the transient bacteremia associated with genitourinary procedures, followed by soft-tissue and respiratory infections [3]. One commonly accepted mechanism for hematogenous spread involves a bacterial infection of the low flow regions of the vertebra with subsequent involvement of the endplate with eventual destruction of the intervertebral disc. The anatomy of the disc, endplate, and metaphysis vary with age, leading to different patterns of infection in children and adults.

1.3 Epidemiology

The distribution of pyogenic spinal infections is bimodal, occurring both in younger patients, often related to IV drug abuse, and in those 50–70 years old. Approximately half of those with osteomyelitis are older than 50 years and an even greater predominance of patients are male. Historically, mortality from spinal infections was high (up to 71%) [3]. With the advent of improved diagnostic imaging, antibiotic therapy, and surgical intervention, the morbidity and mortality has decreased. However, when the patient is septic or when an epidural abscess is present, relatively high mortality has still been reported (12–34%) in some series [4–7]. When an epidural abscess coexists there is also an associated high rate of paralysis (22–34%) that is irreversible in most cases if more than 24 hours have passed from the time of onset [6–8]. If identified early, the treatment and course can be more benign with most cases responding to antibiotic therapy alone. However, the condition is often misdiagnosed (up to 50% of cases) or undermanaged which contributes to the magnitude of resulting disability and mortality [9].

The incidence of pyogenic spinal infections in recent studies has been higher than in the past. This is thought to be due to an aging population, greater prevalence of various co-morbid conditions including alcoholism, IV drug use, and immunosuppression, as well as increased use of spinal interventions. Improved diagnostic ability may also play a role with more frequent use of magnetic resonance imaging (MRI) in the last three decades [2, 7, 10, 11].

Risk factors for established infection include the various forms of immunosuppression, such as diabetes mellitus, immunosuppressive medications, and genetic or acquired immunodeficiency. In addition, pregnancy, trauma, IV drug use, end-stage renal disease, alcohol abuse, malignancy, and known septicemia are all contributing conditions. Lastly, recent spinal injections or surgery are known risk factors [2, 7, 10, 12].

2 Symptoms and clinical suspicion

The course for infection can be prolonged by misdiagnosis. Most patients will have symptoms for several weeks or more before identification. Nearly all patients will present with back pain (87%), and many will have fever (52–70%). Most cases will not have an associated epidural abscess. When abscess or deformity is present, up to 70% of patients will have some neurological finding ranging from radiculopathy with corresponding pain and weakness, to more significant SCI [9].

The differential diagnosis for back pain without fever includes many common conditions that overburden emergency department staff and spine specialists alike. The list includes:

- Osteodiscitis
- Compression fractures
- Degenerative disc disease
- Facet arthropathy
- Spondylosis or spondylolisthesis
- Osteoporosis
- Psoriatic arthritis and other spondyloarthropathies
- Psychiatric disorders or addiction problems with malingering

In part, this difficulty contributes to the problem of misdiagnosis. Patients who have a history of substance abuse or psychiatric issues with a focus on spinal complaints have a higher association with IV drug use, alcoholism, poorly managed diabetes, and other risk factors for spinal epidural abscess. These patients are also more likely to have visited the emergency department in the past, increasing the likelihood of missing the diagnosis of an existing discitis. When fever or neurological deficits are present, the differential diagnostic possibilities are dramatically fewer.

3 Spinal diagnostic workup

Spondylodiscitis is often diagnosed in a delayed fashion due to its nonspecific presenting symptoms. This poses a clinical challenge because early diagnosis and medical treatment with culture-directed antibiotic therapy can reduce the risk for associated paravertebral abscess, epidural abscess, spinal deformity, and systemic involvement. Early diagnosis also decreases the need for surgical intervention.

Plain x-rays are often common early in an infection. Within 2–4 weeks x-rays may show disc space narrowing, and it is typical at 4–6 weeks to see osteolysis adjacent to the endplate. Progressive kyphotic deformity can occur and patients should be followed up with periodic x-ray examinations during treatment. Magnetic resonance imaging with contrast is the study of choice. Computed tomographic (CT) myelogram is 90% sensitive if MRI is contraindicated.

In general, for most severe infections with associated abscess, laboratory markers are sensitive but not specific. Erythrocyte sedimentation rate is elevated in 92–100% of cases [13]; C-reactive protein is nearly uniformly elevated and has been reported in some studies to be prognostic [14]. White blood cell (WBC) count is elevated in 42–90% of cases, while with some atypical or chronic infections the WBC count can often be normal. Blood cultures are positive 24–59% of the time and are most helpful for ruling out infection [12, 13]. If all laboratory markers are negative in a patient with normal immune function, the probability of infection is small [3, 7, 13, 15].

4 Treatment principles

The standard of care is culture-directed IV antimicrobial therapy. Although most infections are caused by *Staphylococcus aureus*, with other skin flora and gram-negative rods making up a lesser proportion, more than 200 organisms have been reported in the literature including fungal and parasitic species. Obtaining an organism via surgical biopsy or CT-guided aspiration is a critical step in guiding antibiotic therapy.

Another important step in treatment is deciding between nonoperative therapy with IV antibiotics alone or with operative intervention. In a retrospective review of 101 patients with hematogenous pyogenic spinal infections, most were spondylodiscitis [15]. Hadjipivlou et al [15] developed an algorithm to help guide surgical decision making (**Fig 12-1**).

4.1 Nonoperative treatment

In patients with spondylodiscitis without sepsis, neurological deficit, abscess, deformity, or spinal instability, the best available evidence indicates nonoperative treatment with culture-directed antibiotics. There is recent literature evidence that supports nonoperative treatment even in the presence of an epidural abscess without sepsis or instability, which have traditionally been compelling indications for surgical intervention. Several small studies [16–20] described encouraging results for medical treatment alone in selected patients with spinal epidural abscesses. In a larger series Adogwa et al [21] concluded that early surgical decompression with antibiotics was not associated with superior clinical outcomes compared with IV antimicrobials alone for patients 50 years and older.

These findings were controversial, however, and two large series [2, 22] reported a 38–41% failure rate with medical management alone in the setting of spinal epidural abscesses. Delayed surgery or failed medical management was also associated with worse neurological outcomes. Predictors of poorer results included increased pain, degree of deficits, dorsal abscess, diabetes mellitus, increased C-reactive protein or WBC on presentation, positive blood cultures, methicillin-resistant *S aureus* infection, patient older than 65 years, and concomitant SCI [2, 21, 22]. A review [15] of pyogenic spinal infections also concluded that patients treated nonoperatively more frequently reported residual back pain than those who underwent operative intervention.

Prognosticators for failure of medical management such as these help guide treatment planning. Nonoperative treatment is typically favored [3] in the setting of complete SCI lasting greater than 24 to 36 hours without sepsis. Treatment decisions are also guided by the degree of deficits and patients; those who have pain alone with subtle deficits and a stable American Spinal Injury Association examination are generally managed nonoperatively [9]. In addition, severity of pain can guide clinicians toward operative intervention as the family and patient may not tolerate medical management alone.

4.2 Operative treatment

Surgical debridement, decompression, and reconstruction are the treatments of choice in the setting of deformity or instability. Other factors that raise consideration for surgery include the presence and degree of neurological findings, evolving deficits, sepsis, or the persistence of infection despite antibiotic therapy. Various relative surgical contraindications have been suggested [2, 9, 16], including multilevel abscess, if the patient is neurologically intact, and a complete SCI for more than 24 hours.

Standard surgical treatment includes incision, drainage, and debridement with culture-directed antibiotics. For patients with substantial tissue involvement or well-established infection, multiple debridements may be required. Identifying these cases or patients with a soft-tissue deficit or difficult wound closures is a challenge. Delayed primary closure, retention of instrumentation, and negative-pressure wound therapy dressing placement has been reported with promising results in some studies [3, 23]. One small series also showed good outcomes using continuous irrigation [24]. Single debridement, primary wound closure, serial debridement, flaps, and negative-pressure dressings are other treatment options [3].

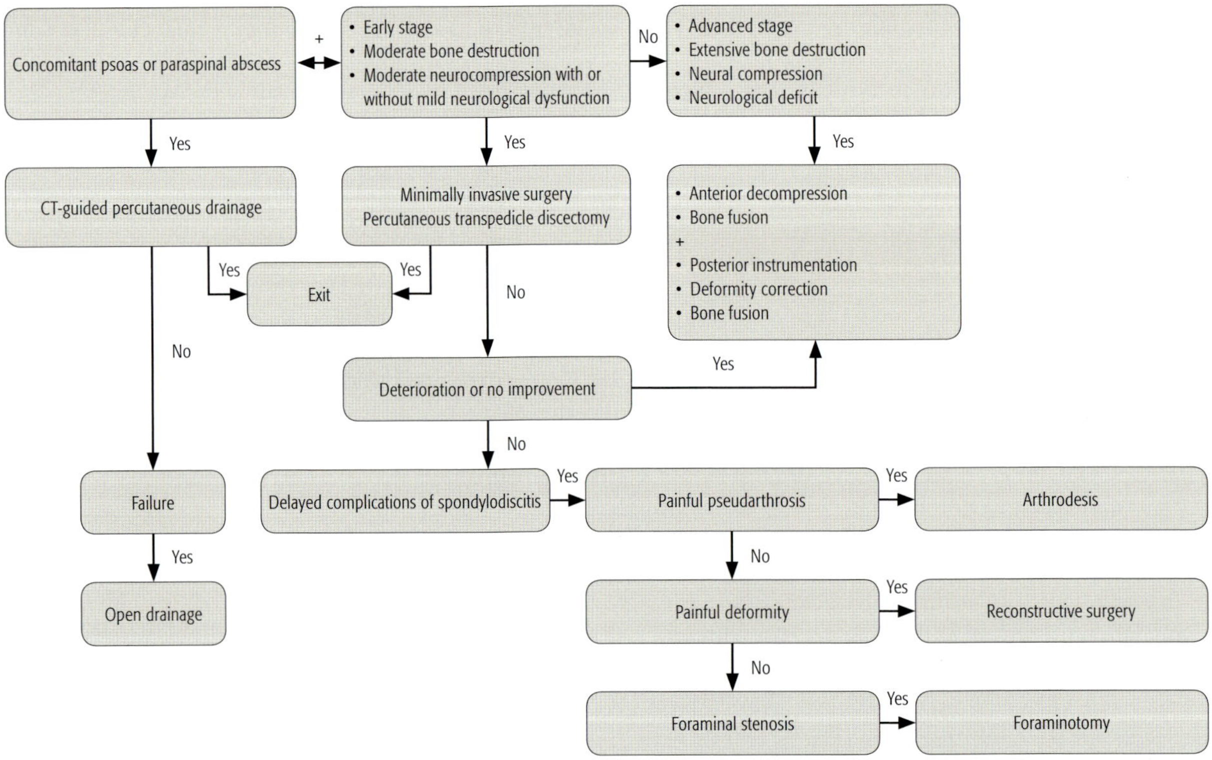

Fig 12-1 Algorithm for surgical management of spondylodiscitis [15].

5 Infection after spine surgery

Surgical-site infections (SSIs) decrease health-related quality of life, increase risk of readmission, prolong the length of hospital stay, and raise hospital charges with a cost estimated in recent literature at USD 34,307 per incident [25]. The incidence varies by study type, region of the spine, and institution ranging from 0.7 to 19%. The high variability is due to differing surgical sites, surgical complexity, and patient factors. Large posterior thoracolumbar surgeries in the setting of trauma have the highest rates of postoperative infection [26].

In addition to cost, infection increases risk to patients and is a source of decreased satisfaction. In studies [27, 28] controlling for pain and other predictors of lower satisfaction, SSI was shown to decrease the perception of surgical success. Infection is also perceived by patients to be a considerably more severe event than by surgeons [27, 28].

Risk factors for infection can be grouped into those that are patient specific, procedure specific, and intraoperative (**Table 12-1**). A CD4 count lower than 200 is a significant risk factor for infection, while patients with CD4 count more than 600 are not at increased risk. For those with diabetes, a glucose level higher than 125 mg/dL is associated with a fivefold increased risk of infection. Malnutrition as indicated by a total lymphocyte count of fewer than 2,000 cells/µL or a serum albumin level below 35 g/L is also associated with increased infection risk. Higher body mass index has been correlated with higher incidence of complications within the orthopedic literature in general, however, recent studies by Mehta et al [29, 30] suggest that the subcutaneous fat thickness may be a better predictor of risk for site SSIs.

As in most other areas of medicine, spine surgery patients receiving transfusion(s) are at increased risk for postoperative SSI. Transfusion-induced immunomodulation is believed to be the underlying mechanism with effects in multiple areas of normal immune response. Transfusions have also been associated with increased risk of sepsis and death. A systems-based approach to transfusion should be adopted by institutions to safely limit unnecessary transfusion given the associated risks. A spine surgical invasiveness index that considers the type of spine surgery and the number of vertebral levels and presence of instrumentation has recently been introduced. The composite index value was defined as the sum of integer values assigned to six procedure elements, such as disc excision, graft material, and instrumentation, based on the number of vertebral levels involved [32]. The index was initially evaluated in the context of transfusion risk, and was later applied to infection and found to be correlated with increased risk. This group in fact showed that the spine surgical invasiveness index was the strongest independent risk factor for infection after adjusting for other risk factors, such as age and medical comorbidities [33, 34].

Factor	OR (95% CI)
Cervical	
Neurological disorder	2.61 (2.43–2.8)
Cardiac disorder (other than HTN)	2.17 (2–2.36)
Drug or EtOH abuse	1.85 (1.6–2.14)
Pulmonary disorder	1.38 (1.31–1.47)
Diabetes	1.28 (1.2–1.36)
Psychiatric disorder	1.22 (1.14–1.31)
HTN	1.09 (1.04–1.14)
Thoracolumbar	
Neurological disorder	2.76 (2.55–3)
Drug or EtOH abuse	1.79 (1.64–1.95)
Cardiac disorder (other than HTN)	1.62 (1.53–1.71)
Pulmonary disorder	1.39 (1.31–1.48)
Cancer	1.31 (1.12–1.54)
Diabetes	1.12 (1.07–1.16)
Psychiatric disorder	1.1 (1.05–1.14)

Table 12-1 Significant patient risk factors for spine surgical-site infection [31].

Abbreviations: CI, confidence interval; EtOH, ethyl alcohol; HTN, hypertension; OR, odds ratio; SSI, surgical-site infection.

Infection severity scores have also been used as predictors of infection in the presence of methicillin-resistant *S aureus*, distant infection sites, presence of instrumentation, posterior surgery, graft materials, and diabetes. A predictive model called the postoperative infection treatment score for the spine (PITSS) was built to help determine which spinal SSI patients would require multiple irrigation and debridement and guide clinical decision making (**Table 12-2**). This criterion was developed from a consecutive series [35] of 128 patients based on 30 variables identified in a literature review and was internally validated against the same.

It is not surprising that trauma patients are at increased risk for infection, with studies [36] reporting a threefold increase in risk for patients undergoing surgery for SCI compared with elective spine surgery. An elevated abbreviated injury scale grade specifically has been correlated with increased risk of infection [37].

Predictors	PITSS score
Spine location:	
• Cervical	1
• Thoracolumbar	2
• Lumbar/sacral	4
Comorbidities:	
• None/other	0
• Cardiovascular/pulmonary	1
• Diabetes	4
Microbiology:	
• Gram positive	2
• Gram negative or polymicrobial without MRSA	4
• Polymicrobial with MRSA or MRSA alone	6
Distant site infection:	
• None	1
• UTI/PNA	3
• Bacteremia alone	5
• Bacteremia +PNA/UTI	6
Instrumentation:	
• Yes	6
• No	2
Bone graft:	
• None	1
• Autograft	3
• Other (allograft, BMP, and synthetic)	6

Table 12-2 Postoperative infection treatment score for the spine to predict likelihood of requiring two-stage reconstruction after postoperative infection [31].

Abbreviations: PITSS, postoperative infection treatment score for the spine; MRSA, methicillin-resistant *Staphylococcus aureus*; PNA, pneumonia; UTI, urinary tract infection; BMP, bone morphogenetic protein; I&D, irrigation and debridement.

The use of minimally invasive techniques has been studied extensively to reduce modifiable risk factors and infection rates. In a review article, Parker et al [38] found minimally invasive transforaminal lumbar interbody fusion associated with reduced infection risk compared to traditional transforaminal lumbar interbody fusion procedures. However, in discectomy procedures, no difference was found using a minimally invasive approach compared to open.

Sterile technique remains a fundamental principle for infection prevention. The sterile field gradually becomes contaminated during surgery, with positive intraoperative cultures demonstrated in some studies [39]. This is supported by literature describing how breaks in technique and microcontamination also occur in the surgical setting [40]. Other investigations have examined regions of C-arm sterility, scrubs, gowns, microscopes, and even graft materials and implants demonstrating varying degrees of impurity, increasing contamination with prolonged operative time, and varying infectivity by region of operating room equipment sampled. Other methods often used to potentially prevent infections include preoperative testing for aggressive pathogens, antibiotic prophylaxis using cefazolin with vancomycin or clindamycin, and direct antibiotic treatment of the operative site using agents such as vancomycin powder [41, 42]. The use of intrawound vancomycin powder with povidone-iodine wound irrigation was shown to significantly reduce rates of SSI by as much as 50%.

When postoperative infection occurs, early diagnosis and aggressive surgical and medical management can lead to successful results. There is significant cost and decreased satisfaction on the part of patients as well as practitioners. Prevention remains the best option with rigorous sterile technique, appropriate antibiotics, adjuvant therapy, medical optimization of patients, and careful decision making regarding the institution of surgical intervention.

6 Outcome

The frequency of relapse is low with 4 weeks of modern antibiotic therapy and close follow-up [13, 43]. The mortality rate is 5–16% depending on a patient's age and comorbidities, and may be higher with *S aureus* than with other pathogens [12]. In patients with epidural abscess, risk factors for permanent neurological sequelae include advanced age, impaired immunity, and concomitant diabetes mellitus or rheumatoid arthritis [3]. The chance of spontaneous vertebral fusion also increases with infections higher in the spine, from 24% in the lumbar region to 75% in the thoracic region and approaching 100% in the cervical spine [44]. Deformities are more common with tuberculosis but can also occur with pyogenic infection.

In terms of outcome measures, patients with vertebral osteomyelitis fare poorly compared to normal controls. According to a study by O'Daly et al [45], the risk of adverse outcomes is around 66%, with resulting significant differences in SF-36 and Oswestry disability index scores and other health measures. Delays in diagnosis and neurological deficit at presentation were risk factors for adverse outcome, defined as persistence of pain, residual disability, or death.

7 Conclusion

Early diagnosis and appropriate treatment of spondylodiscitis with culture-directed antibiotics can avoid the need for further surgery. Failure rates of medical management alone are up to 40%. The keys to success are early identification of the organisms and early initiation of appropriate treatment.

8 References

1. **Mixter WJ, Smithwick RH.** Acute intraspinal epidural abscess. *N Engl J Med.* 1932;207(3):126–131.
2. **Kim SD, Melikian R, Ju KL, et al.** Independent predictors of failure of nonoperative management of spinal epidural abscesses. *Spine J.* 2014 Aug 1;14(8):1673–1679.
3. **Kim CW, Currier BL, Eismont FJ.** Infections of the spine. In: Herkowitz HN, Balderston RA, eds. *Rothman-Simeone the Spine.* 5th ed. Philadelphia: Saunders/Elsevier; 2011:1513–1570.
4. **Hlavin ML, Kaminski HJ, Ross JS, et al.** Spinal epidural abscess: a ten-year perspective. *Neurosurgery.* 1990 Aug;27(2):177–184.
5. **Kaufman DM, Kaplan JG, Litman N.** Infectious agents in spinal epidural abscesses. *Neurology.* 1980 Aug;30(8):844–850.
6. **Khanna RK, Malik GM, Rock JP, et al.** Spinal epidural abscess: evaluation of factors influencing outcome. *Neurosurgery.* 1996 Nov;39(5):958–964.
7. **Reihsaus E, Waldbaur H, Seeling W.** Spinal epidural abscess: a meta-analysis of 915 patients. *Neurosurg Rev.* 2000 Dec;23(4):175–204; discussion 205.
8. **Heusner AP.** Nontuberculous spinal epidural infections. *N Engl J Med.* 1948 Dec 2;239(23):845–854.
9. **Darouiche RO.** Spinal epidural abscess. *N Engl J Med.* 2006 Nov 9;355(19):2012–2020.
10. **Rigamonti D, Liem L, Sampath P, et al.** Spinal epidural abscess: contemporary trends in etiology, evaluation, and management. *Surg Neurol.* 1999 Aug;52(2):189–196; discussion 197.
11. **McHenry MC, Easley KA, Locker GA.** Vertebral osteomyelitis: long-term outcome for 253 patients from 7 Cleveland-area hospitals. *Clin Infect Dis.* 2002 May 15;34(10):1342–1350.
12. **Carragee EJ.** Pyogenic vertebral osteomyelitis. *J Bone Joint Surg Am.* 1997 Jun;79(6):874–880.
13. **Sapico FL, Montgomerie JZ.** Pyogenic vertebral osteomyelitis: report of nine cases and review of the literature. *Rev Infect Dis.* 1979 Sep–Oct;1(5):754–776.
14. **Jaye DL, Waites KB.** Clinical applications of C-reactive protein in pediatrics. *Pediatr Infect Dis J.* 1997 Aug;16:735–746; quiz 746–747.
15. **Hadjipavlou AG, Mader JT, Necessary JT, et al.** Hematogenous pyogenic spinal infections and their surgical management. *Spine (Phila Pa 1976).* 2000 Jul 1;25(13):1668–1679.
16. **Leys D, Lesoin F, Viaud C, et al.** Decreased morbidity from acute bacterial spinal epidural abscesses using computed tomography and nonsurgical treatment in selected patients. *Ann Neurol.* 1985 Apr;17(4):350–355.
17. **Siddiq F, Chowfin A, Tight R, et al.** Medical vs surgical management of spinal epidural abscess. *Arch Intern Med.* 2004 Dec 13–27;164(22):2409–2412.
18. **Xiao BR, Wang CW, Lin JC, et al.** Successful medical treatment of spinal epidural abscess. *J Microbiol Immunol Infect.* 2008 Apr;41(2):180–182.
19. **Godeau B, Brun-Buisson C, Brugières P, et al.** Complete resolution of spinal epidural abscess with short medical treatment alone. *Eur J Med.* 1993 Oct–Nov;2(8):510–511.
20. **Duc C, Grange L, Gaudin P, et al.** Extensive primary epidural abscess. Report of a case. *Joint Bone Spine.* 2002 May;69(3):312–315.
21. **Adogwa O, Karikari IO, Carr KR, et al.** Spontaneous spinal epidural abscess in patients 50 years of age and older: a 15-year institutional perspective and review of the literature: clinical article. *J Neurosurg Spine.* 2014 Mar;20(3):344–349.
22. **Patel AR, Alton TB, Bransford RJ, et al.** Spinal epidural abscesses: risk factors, medical versus surgical management, a retrospective review of 128 cases. *Spine J.* 2014 Feb 1;14(2):326–330.
23. **Canavese F, Krajbich JI.** Use of vacuum assisted closure in instrumented spinal deformities for children with postoperative deep infections. *Indian J Orthop.* 2010 Apr;44(2):177–183.
24. **Jeanneret B, Magerl F.** Treatment of osteomyelitis of the spine using percutaneous suction/irrigation and percutaneous external spinal fixation. *J Spinal Disord.* 1994; 7:185–205.
25. **Shepard J, Ward W, Milstone A, et al.** Financial impact of surgical site infections on hospitals: the hospital management perspective. *JAMA Surg.* 2013 Oct;148(10):907–914.
26. **McGirt MJ, Parker SL, Lerner J, et al.** Comparative analysis of perioperative surgical site infection after minimally invasive versus open posterior/transforaminal lumbar interbody fusion: analysis of hospital billing and discharge data from 5170 patients. *J Neurosurg Spine.* 2011 Jun;14(6):771–778.
27. **Bono CM, Harris MB, Warholic N, et al.** Pain intensity and patients' acceptance of surgical complication risks with lumbar fusion. *Spine (Phila Pa 1976).* 2013 Jan 15;38(2):140–147.
28. **Hart RA, Cabalo A, Bess S, et al.** Comparison of patient and surgeon perceptions of adverse events after adult spinal deformity surgery. *Spine (Phila Pa 1976).* 2013 Apr 20;38(9):732–736.
29. **Mehta AI, Babu R, Karikari IO, et al.** 2012 Young Investigator Award Winner: The distribution of body mass as a significant risk factor for lumbar spinal fusion postoperative infections. *Spine.* 2012 Sep;37(19):1652–1656.
30. **Mehta AI, Babu R, Sharma R, et al.** Thickness of subcutaneous fat as a risk factor for infection in cervical spine fusion surgery. *J Bone Joint Surg Am.* 2013 Feb 20;95(4):323–328.
31. **Radcliff KE, Neusner AD, Millhouse PW, et al.** What is new in the diagnosis and prevention of spine surgical site infections. *Spine J.* 2015 Feb 1;15(2):336–347.
32. **Mirza SK, Deyo RA, Heagerty PJ, et al.** Development of an index to characterize the "invasiveness" of spine surgery: validation by comparison to blood loss and operative time. *Spine.* 2008 Nov 15;33(24):2651–2661; discussion: 2662.
33. **Schwarzkopf R, Chung C, Park JJ, et al.** Effects of perioperative blood product use on surgical site infection following thoracic and lumbar spinal surgery. *Spine (Phila Pa 1976).* 2010 Feb 1;35(3):340–346.
34. **Cizik AM, Lee MJ, Martin BI, et al.** Using the spine surgical invasiveness index to identify risk of surgical site infection: a multivariate analysis. *J Bone Joint Surg Am.* 2012 Feb 15;94(4):335–342.
35. **DiPaola CP, Saravanja DD, Boriani L, et al.** Postoperative infection treatment score for the spine (PITSS): construction and validation of a predictive model to define need for single versus multiple irrigation and debridement for spinal surgical site infection. *Spine J.* 2012 Mar 1;12(3):218–230.
36. **Blam OG, Vaccaro AR, Vanichkachorn JS, et al.** Risk factors for surgical site infection in the patient with spinal injury. *Spine.* 2003 Jul 1;28(13):1475–1480.
37. **Wilson JR, Cadotte DW, Fehlings MG.** Clinical predictors of neurological outcome, functional status, and survival after traumatic spinal cord injury: a systematic review. *J Neurosurg Spine.* 2012 Aug 31;17(1 Suppl):11–26.

38. **Parker SL, Adogwa O, Witham TF, et al.** Post-operative infection after minimally invasive versus open transforaminal lumbar interbody fusion (TLIF): literature review and cost analysis. *Minim Invasive Neurosurg.* 2011 Feb;54(1):33–37.
39. **Nandyala SV, Schwend RM.** Prevalence of intraoperative tissue bacterial contamination in posterior pediatric spinal deformity surgery. *Spine (Phila Pa 1976).* 2013 Apr 15;38(8):E482–486.
40. **Hopper WR, Moss R.** Common breaks in sterile technique: clinical perspectives and perioperative implications. *AORN J.* 2010 Mar;91(3):350–364; quiz 365–367.
41. **Schönbach E, Behrend C.** Surgical Site Infection (SSI) in Spine Surgery. In: Vaccaro AR, Koerner JD, Kim DH, eds. *Recent Advances in Spinal Surgery.* New Delhi: Jaypee Brothers Medical Publishers; 2016:83–98.
42. **Tomov M, Mitsunaga L, Durbin-Johnson B, et al.** Reducing surgical site infection in spinal surgery with betadine irrigation and intrawound vancomycin powder. *Spine (Phila Pa 1976).* 2015 Apr 1;40(7):491–499.
43. **Eismont FJ, Bohlman HH, Soni PL, et al.** Pyogenic and fungal vertebral osteomyelitis with paralysis. *J Bone Joint Surg Am.* 1983 Jan;65(1):19–29.
44. **Collert S.** Osteomylelitis of the spine. *Acta Orthop Scand.* 1977;48(3):283–290.
45. **O'Daly BJ, Morris SF, O'Rourke SK.** Long-term functional outcome in pyogenic spinal infection. *Spine.* 2008 Apr 15;33(8):E246–253.

13 Soft-tissue infections

Sven Hungerer, Mario Morgenstern

1 Basics

The skin is the largest organ and covers the whole body with a surface area of approximately 2 square meters. Besides the skin, soft tissue includes muscles, tendons, ligaments, fascia, fibrous tissues, fat, synovial membranes, nerves, and blood vessels.

Skin and soft-tissue infections (SSTIs) are multifaceted and range from mild superficial infections to deep necrotizing infections with serious systemic complications. These infections can rapidly progress with a fulminant clinical course, requiring immediate recognition, and treatment with proper medical and surgical management [1]. This chapter provides recommendations for diagnosis and treatment of surgically relevant SSTIs in adult patients. Bacterial SSTIs in children and adolescents, eg, impetigo, are not covered in this chapter.

The treatment recommendations are based on the 2014 practice guidelines of the Infectious Diseases Society of America for the diagnosis and management of SSTIs as well as on European guidelines and recent literature and recommendations [2].

This chapter provides a clinical guide to promptly diagnose SSTI, identify life-threatening necrotizing disease patterns, detect causative pathogens, and to use in a timely fashion the appropriate antimicrobial, adjuvant, and surgical treatments.

1.1 Classification of SSTIs

There are various methods to classify and grade SSTIs aiming to direct the appropriate treatment. Regarding the severity of the clinical course, SSTIs can be differentiated in uncomplicated, complicated, or necrotizing SSTIs.

The US Food and Drug Administration (FDA) has categorized SSTIs as uncomplicated and complicated. Uncomplicated SSTIs include erysipelas, cellulitis, furuncles, and simple abscesses; complicated SSTIs include infected burns and ulcers, deep-tissue infections, and major abscesses. The necrotizing SSTIs are their own entity [3]. The terms uncomplicated or complicated SSTIs established by the FDA are not useful clinically and were developed to guide drug company studies [3].

Specific descriptions based on pathogenesis and clinical manifestations are more relevant for clinical use. Therefore, differentiation into categories of nonpurulent and purulent infections has surgical consequences and is more useful for clinical care.

Another clinically relevant classification was described by Kingston et al [4] and is based on urgency of surgical action (**Table 13-1**).

Progress and surgical action	Soft-tissue infections
Slow progressive infections (generally nonsurgical treatment)	• Furuncle • Limited cellulitis • Erysipelas • Impetigo
Progressive infection of moderate rapidity (urgent treatment)	• Abscess (including also: carbuncle, abscess after injection, perirectal abscess) • Septic bursitis • Cellulitis • Paranychia
Rapidly progressive infections: severe life-threatening necrotizing soft-tissue infections (NSTIs)	• Necrotizing fasciitis • Fournier's gangrene • Rabies • Toxic shock syndrome • Gas gangrene with myonecrosis • Other NSTIs

Table 13-1 Classification of soft-tissue infections in terms of clinical progress and urgency of surgical action (modified from Kingston et al [4]).

The severity of the clinical course is mainly correlated to the depth of the SSTI. Therefore, depth of the affected skin layer is another essential criterion in definition and classification of soft-tissue infections (**Fig 13-1**). The terms "cellulitis" and "erysipelas" are often used inconsistently because the clinical differentiation may be difficult [5]. The distinction relates to the depth of inflammation. Erysipelas is defined as an inflammation of the upper layer of the dermis including the superficial lymphatic system. Cellulitis affects the deeper dermis as well as subcutaneous fat.

Clues to severe deep soft-tissue infection are symptoms of systemic illness (eg, fever, hypothermia, tachycardia with heart rate > 100 beats/minute, and hypotension with systolic blood pressure < 90 mm Hg or 20 mm Hg below baseline) and the following clinical signs: pain disproportionate to the physical findings, violaceous bullae, cutaneous hemorrhage, skin sloughing, skin anesthesia, rapid progression of infection, and gas in the soft tissue [5]. However, these signs occur late in the course of a necrotizing soft-tissue infection (NSTI) and are not always present. In these cases immediate surgical evaluation is the primary focus for diagnostic and therapeutic reasons.

In summary, clinical assessment of the severity and extent of the infection is crucial. Therefore, several classifications and algorithms for clinical decision making have been published [5, 6]. In clinical routine, their practicality is controversial and the focus should be the prompt identification of any NSTIs, which require immediate surgical and antibiotic therapy.

1=Epidermis
2=Dermis
3=Superficial fascia
4=Subcutaneous tissue
5=Deep fascia
6=Muscle

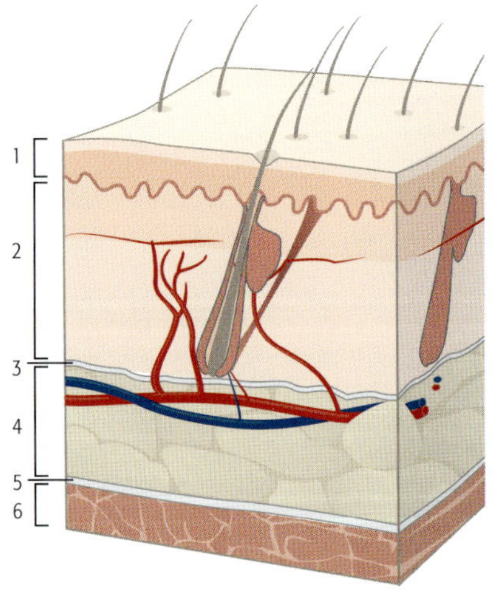

Fig 13-1 Skin and soft-tissue layers.

1.2 Epidemiology

Skin and soft-tissue infections are common with a renewed importance due to dramatically increased frequency and severity of the infections [2]. In the United States, a 27% increase in hospital admissions due to SSTI was recorded from 2000 to 2004. Emergency department visits increased from 1.2 million in 1993 to 3.4 million in 2005. Most patients with a minor and uncomplicated SSTI are seen and treated by the outpatient sector and account for 6.3 million physician visits annually. This increase can be explained by the emergence of antibiotic-resistant organisms, especially community-acquired methicillin-resistant *Staphylococcus aureus* (MRSA) in the United States.

1.3 Risk factors

The presence of risk factors for SSTIs influences the strategy and success of treatment and may portend the clinical course. Risk factors can be divided into two categories: patient-related and etiological risk factors.

Patient-related risk factors for developing SSTI include any condition that results in an immunocompromised state or affection of local blood supply, drainage, and impairment of the skin barrier [7]. Multiple patient-related risk factors correlate with a more rapid progression, worse outcomes and healing, and are also associated with more resistant pathogens [7].

Systemic factors include critical illness, old age, diabetes mellitus, an immune compromised state, obesity, intravenous (IV)/subcutaneous drug use, alcohol abuse, malnutrition, smoking, long-term corticosteroid therapy, chronic immune suppression, cancer, kidney disease, and liver disease. Local factors include peripheral vascular disease, chronic fungal disease such as tinea pedis, skin erosions, or ulcers.

Etiological risk factors encompass the extent of injury. The trauma mechanism and the exposure to the environment increase the likelihood of a later wound or surgical-site infection (SSI).

With SSIs, additional surgery and injury-related risk factors have to be considered. Contributing factors increasing the risk of developing SSI are the extent of microbial contamination at an incision site, duration and performance of the operation, the length of preoperative hospital period, and preoperative procedures like antimicrobial prophylaxis and skin preparation or hair removal [8, 9]. Important systemic patient-related factors increasing the risk of SSI are underlying comorbidities such as diabetes mellitus, rheumatoid arthritis, elevated serum glucose level, low hemoglobin level, as well as acute urinary tract infections, immunosuppressive medications, smoking, malnutrition, or obesity [10]. *Staphylococcus aureus* skin carrier status should not be neglected, which increases SSI twofold to ninefold [10] (see chapter 4 Prevention of intraoperative infection for more SSI information). Specific risk factors for NSTIs are summarized in **Table 13-2**.

Specific risk factors
Renal insufficiency
Diabetes mellitus
Arterial occlusive disease
Intravenous drug abuse
Immunosuppression
Obesity (body mass index > 30 kg/m²)
Age (> 65 years)
Liver disease
Trauma

Table 13-2 Risk factors for necrotizing soft-tissue infections.

1.4 Microbiology and etiology

Soft-tissue infections are typically a bacterial infection caused by various pathogens from gram-positive to gram-negative species. Once bacteria have breached the skin barrier, they can cause SSTI, promoted by above-mentioned predisposing factors. Specific pathogens are responsible for particular clinical conditions, which are discussed in the part of this chapter on each specific condition [5].

1.5 Clinical manifestation

Clinical manifestation differs tremendously depending on the extent of the underlying disease and can range from localized erysipelas or furunculosis to fulminant NSTIs with systemic signs of infection. Nearly all SSTI cases have the classic signs and symptoms of acute inflammation: redness, pain, swelling, and warmth described by Celsus (ca 30 BC–40 AC) and loss of function described by Galen (129–200 AC) [12].

1.6 Diagnosis

These five clinical manifestations or symptoms are highly valid for an on-the-spot diagnosis of soft-tissue infection. The primary aim of clinical evaluation and instrument-based diagnostics is to establish the cause and severity of the infection, to recognize life-threatening infections, and those requiring immediate therapy.

The patient's history must be obtained carefully because soft-tissue infections possess diverse etiologies. The history may provide valuable clues to the likely identity of the pathogen. Information about the patient's immune system, history, medications (especially immunomodulatory therapy), antimicrobial therapy, drug abuse, the geographical location, travel history, recent trauma, recent surgery, animal exposure, bites, and hobbies should be obtained [2].

The physical examination should document the location and extent of the SSTI as well as presence of skin lesions. The above-mentioned classic signs of infection are sought and skin redness can be marked on the skin to monitor the course of disease and the success of therapy. Specific skin findings offer clues to certain etiologies and suggest specific therapy. Palpable crepitus is found in gas-forming infections and should raise suspicion of NSTIs and infections caused by anaerobic organisms, such as *Clostridium perfringens*. Skin necrosis can be a hint for NSTIs or advanced arterial circulatory disorder. Fluctuance suggests abscess formation, which requires surgical intervention. Bullae and purpura are seen in advanced stages of necrotizing infections. The examination should include the arterial pulse status, venous sufficiency, and lymphatic status. The basic vital signs, such as body temperature, pulse rate, blood pressure, respirations, and mental status, are essential elements of every examination.

Imaging studies can be helpful for diagnosis. Ultrasound is a fast, inexpensive, and safe diagnostic tool to detect deep infections, especially abscesses and to estimate the location, size, and extent of the abscess.

Radiographic examinations may detect potential bone involvement, the presence of an orthopedic device-related infection, and to detect the presence of gas or foreign bodies. Magnetic resonance imaging (MRI) or computed tomographic (CT) scans may be helpful in suspected deep infections and is indicated in suspected NSTIs to determine the location and extent of the infection. It can be combined with angiography to evaluate the arterial blood supply. These examinations provide useful information to plan surgery but they should never delay a necessary surgical intervention.

Laboratory examinations are recommended in every suspected SSTI especially in purulent, complicated, and severe SSTI to identify life-threatening disease patterns and to monitor treatment success. Laboratory tests include leukocyte count, C-reactive protein (CRP) level, and erythrocyte sedimentation rate. These basic tests offer a picture of the patient's health status. Routine chemistry tests and coagulation studies identify coagulopathy or diabetes. In NSTIs, further studies such as serum creatine kinase (for monitoring muscle and tissue destruction) and procalcitonin or interleukin-6 may be helpful (see topic 2.7 of this chapter). In severe or necrotizing infections with systemic symptoms, aerobic and anaerobic blood cultures should be taken.

The analysis of microbial growth and the antibiotic susceptibility testing provide important information to refine and direct the definitive antibiotic treatment, which is mandatory in purulent and necrotizing infections. In general, the sampling is performed intraoperatively according to recommendations listed in chapter 7 Diagnostics. Needle aspiration can be useful in certain conditions like bursitis but may be controversial. A superinfection caused by recurrent needle aspiration should be avoided.

1.7 Differential diagnosis

The differential diagnosis of cellulitis and erysipelas includes allergen-triggered (contact) dermatitis, cutaneous inflammation of gout, herpes zoster, and the lipodermatosclerosis, which mainly occurs in obese patients with lower extremity venous insufficiency [5, 13].

1.8 Therapy

Treatment of SSTIs and choice of the appropriate therapy requires evaluation of the local and systemic status of the patient to determine the level of severity and to categorize into nonpurulent or purulent infections. The treatment options include basic principles like rest, ice, and elevation of the affected extremity, a surgical approach, and/or the systemic antibiotic therapy. **Fig 13-2** is a simplified treatment algorithm for SSTI that considers MRSA, adapted from the

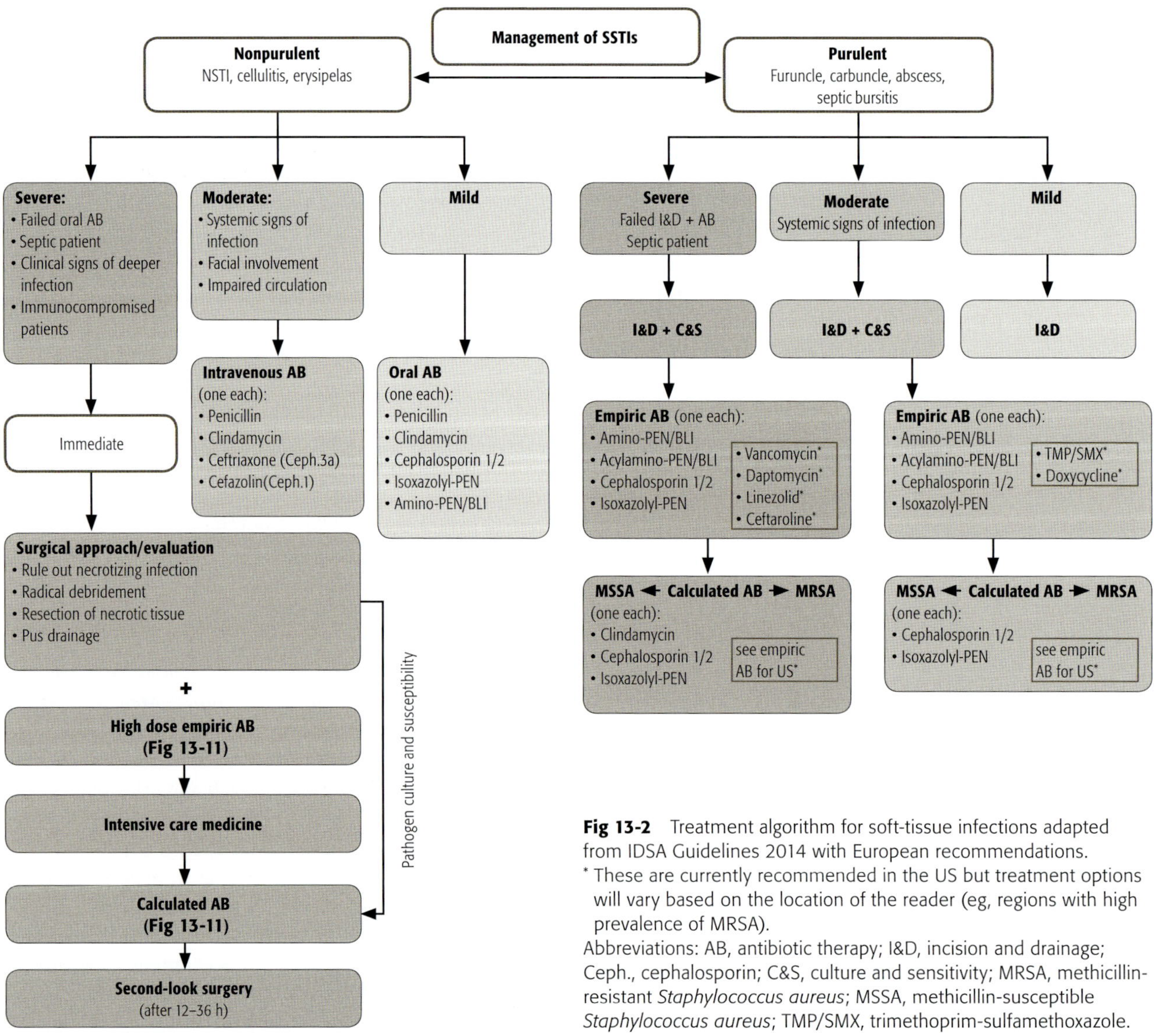

Fig 13-2 Treatment algorithm for soft-tissue infections adapted from IDSA Guidelines 2014 with European recommendations.
* These are currently recommended in the US but treatment options will vary based on the location of the reader (eg, regions with high prevalence of MRSA).
Abbreviations: AB, antibiotic therapy; I&D, incision and drainage; Ceph., cephalosporin; C&S, culture and sensitivity; MRSA, methicillin-resistant *Staphylococcus aureus*; MSSA, methicillin-susceptible *Staphylococcus aureus*; TMP/SMX, trimethoprim-sulfamethoxazole.

2014 practice guidelines of the Infectious Disease Society of America [2] and includes recommendations of the German Paul-Ehrlich Society of Chemotherapy. The German guidelines are developed for regions with a low rate of MRSA.

1.8.1 Antimicrobial therapy

The emergence of antibiotic resistance among the common pathogens causing soft-tissue infections like MRSA and erythromycin resistance in *Streptococcus pyogenes* is commonly observed. Therefore, it is recommended that empiric antibiotic therapy includes agents with activity against resistant strains [5]. Antibiotic therapy is divided into an empiric or targeted regimen. Empiric treatment is used when the identity and susceptibility of the causative pathogen is unknown.

Due to the antibiotic resistance and the variety of microorganisms, an interdisciplinary approach should be used when treating bacterial infections. The surgeon's focus should be immediate diagnosis, application of the treatment algorithm, and initiation of the appropriate empiric antibiotic therapy. In terms of the antibiotic stewardship, antimicrobial medication should be reassessed and adapted to specific pathogens and susceptibility patterns in collaboration with an infectious diseases specialist.

Empiric and calculated antibiotic treatment of soft-tissue infections

Minor SSTIs may be empirically treated with semisynthetic penicillin, first-generation or second-generation oral cephalosporins, macrolides, or clindamycin [5]. If bacterial samples have been taken and analyzed, antibiotic therapy should be started as soon as possible, especially in patients with necrotizing infections, complicated cases, and nonresponders with assistance from an infectious diseases specialist.

Treatment of MRSA soft-tissue infections

In the last two decades, MRSA has emerged as a significant threat within the hospital environment, and also to the healthy population in the community setting. It has shown an increasing prevalence in STIs [14, 15]. Recent estimates suggest MRSA causes more than 11,000 deaths, and 80,000 invasive infections in the United States per year [16]. The current guidelines for antibiotic treatment of MRSA SSTIs are highlighted separately in this chapter. Doxycycline, clindamycin, and trimethoprim-sulfamethoxazole have good antistaphylococcal activities and are recommended as empiric antibiotic therapy in regions with high rates of MRSA STIs and first-line therapy after pathogen identification [17]. Vancomycin, linezolid, and daptomycin have an excellent efficacy against MRSA and should be reserved for patients with severe infections or if previous antibiotic therapy was not effective (**Fig 13-2**) [18, 19].

1.8.2 Surgical and nonsurgical treatment

Surgical and nonsurgical treatment of SSTIs is not a contradiction in terms. Often the nonsurgical treatment is necessary to optimize the patient and his or her health condition to minimize the impact of surgery. Nonsurgical treatment should not delay the surgical treatment if the indication is vital. A rapidly progressive clinical course of SSTI requires early surgical intervention. Slow progress of infection allows more time for diagnosis and nonsurgical treatment.

Nonsurgical treatment

Nonsurgical treatment is often multidisciplinary to reduce risk factors (see topic 1.4 of this chapter) and includes the treatment of the underlying diseases, such as arterial occlusive disease, venous insufficiency, diabetes, neoplastic and paraneoplastic syndromes. Elderly patients may experience intractable pruritus as adverse effect of medications or may develop delirium. Autoimmune and contagious infections of the skin, such as tinea corporis, candida, and scabies, need to be considered in the differential diagnosis.

The multidisciplinary care of SSTIs includes overall internal medicine, dermatology, and surgery. Other disciplines should be consulted as required.

Initial therapy of soft-tissue inflammation is managed according to the PRICE principle, which stands for protection, rest, ice, compression, and elevation, and targets the five classic symptoms of inflammation (see topic 1.5 of this chapter). Protection and rest can be easily achieved by bed rest and wound dressing. Dressings with antiseptic solution are an alternative for ice and avoid thermal injury. Most patients keep their affected extremities elevated by intuition. The extremity can be supported with pillows. Compression and lymph drainage should be done with caution; this might be counterproductive in acute inflammation. The local perfusion can be restricted by compression.

Other treatment options include the hyperbaric oxygen (HBO) therapy for critical wounds. The evidence for HBO is still controversial [20]. In necrotizing fasciitis, HBO is sometimes the last hope and it should not delay surgical therapy [20]. Centers with HBO machines often possess the expertise needed to treat these critically ill patients.

Surgical treatment

The major principles of surgical treatment were described by Hippocrates (460–370 BC): "Ubi pus, ibi evacua," ie, where you find pus, there you should evacuate it. This is the surgical objective to drain the pus, resect necrotic tissue, and reduce the bacterial load. A hesitant surgical strategy results in a prolonged clinical course and worsens the outcome for critically ill patients.

Negative-pressure wound therapy (NPWT) has emerged for wound care of SSTIs over the last two decades [22]. The benefits for NPWT were postulated as reduction of wound volume/size, wound-bed preparation and faster wound healing, decreased drainage time for acute wounds, enhancement of response to first-line treatment, increased patient survival, and reduction of cost (**Fig 13-3**) [23]. The NPWT offers some potential advantages such as patient comfort. It is usually applied in the operating room under sterile conditions and changed after an interval of usually 3–7 days depending on the patient's situation and local conditions.

Plastic surgery needs to be considered after management of the inflammatory process, if local wound closure cannot be achieved. Techniques vary from meshed skin grafts to local or free flaps. The assistance from plastic surgeons is part of the multidisciplinary approach, which is essential in the treatment of patients with infections.

An alternative or additive option is biosurgery. Biosurgery with sterile maggots of the common green bottle fly (Lucilia sericata) is suitable for chronic wounds and patients with high intraoperative risk factors [24, 25]. Maggots are not applicable in wounds with intensive secretion or acute inflammation.

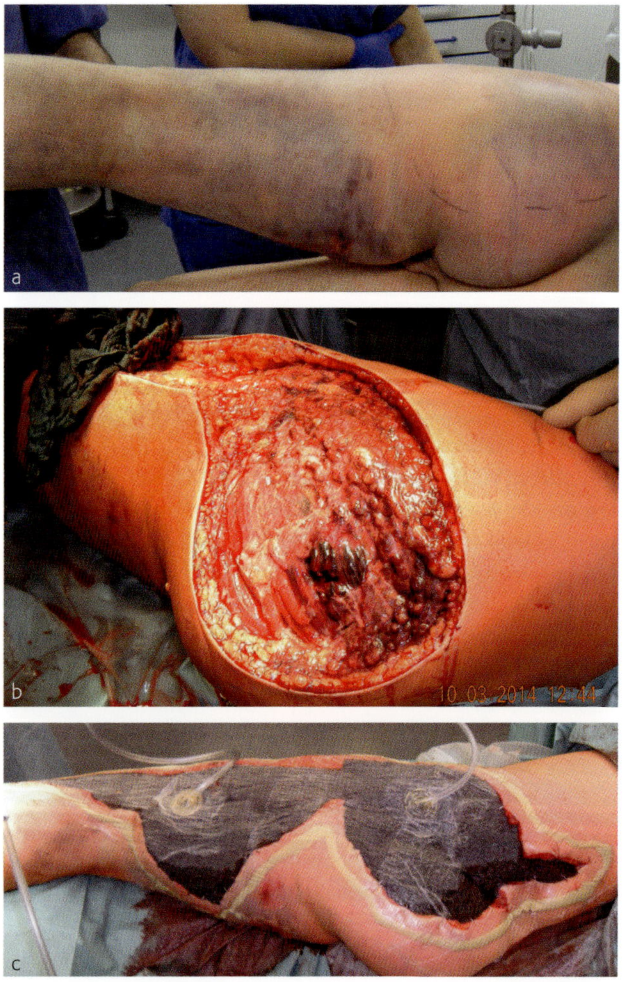

Fig 13-3a–c Necrotizing soft-tissue infections of the lower extremity.
a–b Before and after surgical intervention: incision reveals pus drainage and necrosis of deeper tissue layers, ie, fat and muscle necrosis.
c Wound coverage with negative-pressure wound therapy.

2 Specific clinical manifestations

2.1 Erysipelas

2.1.1 Definition and clinical manifestation

Erysipelas, which means in ancient Greek "red skin", is defined as an acute infection of the upper layers of skin and the superficial lymphatic system. This disease appears as a fiery red, painfully tender plaque with well-demarcated borders [5]. The clear line of demarcation and the elevation of the involved tissue are pathognomonic features of erysipelas [26]. The most frequent location is the lower extremity (**Fig 13-4**) [27].

2.1.2 Etiology and microbiology

Erysipelas is commonly caused by *S pyogenes* (serogroup A) and other β-hemolytic streptococci. Rare causative organisms are group B streptococci and *S aureus* [27].

The portal of pathogen entry is a disrupted area of skin, which is caused by local trauma, ulceration, macerated skin, chronic fungal infections (eg, tinea pedis) or eczema, and other inflammatory skin disorders. Predisposing factors are a compromised local host defence and conditions promoting skin fragility, such as obesity, previous cutaneous trauma, and edema caused, for example, by venous or lymphatic insufficiency [28].

2.1.3 Diagnosis

Erysipelas is diagnosed by the clinical manifestation of well-demarcated rash and inflammation (**Fig 13-4**). Blood cultures are not useful in common erysipelas or cellulitis and are only recommended in cases of severe infection with systemic manifestation [29]. Needle aspiration and skin biopsies are not indicated routinely and may be more beneficial in patients with an impaired immune system or after animal bites [30]. The borders of the erythema can be marked with a waterproof pen to monitor the course of the infection and the success of the initiated antibiotic therapy (**Fig 13-4**).

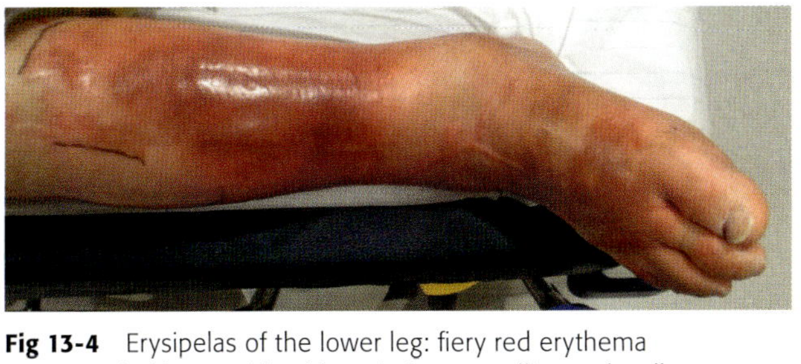

Fig 13-4 Erysipelas of the lower leg: fiery red erythema accompanied by considerable soft-tissue swelling and well-demarcated borders.

2.1.4 Specific treatment

In contrast to purulent infections which require surgical drainage, erysipelas and cellulitis are best treated nonsurgically with antibiotic therapy [2]. This should be accompanied by supportive therapy, such as immobilization and elevation of the affected area, to promote gravity drainage of the edema [5].

Empiric antibiotic therapy for erysipelas and cellulitis should cover streptococci like *S aureus* [5]. Depending on the clinical severity it can be given parenterally or orally. In many cases oral medications can be used, such as antimicrobial agents like penicillin, amoxicillin, amoxicillin-clavulanate, dicloxacillin, cephalexin, or clindamycin (**Fig 13-2**) [2, 5]. Duration of antimicrobial therapy should be individualized depending on clinical response but in general 5–10 days is sufficient [31]. In severely ill patients with systemic signs of infection, parenteral therapy with penicillinase-resistant penicillin or a first-generation cephalosporin should be administered [2, 5]. Severe cases have to be monitored in the hospital setting. In patients with a penicillin allergy, clindamycin or moxifloxacin are alternative choices; cephalexin can be considered if cephalosporins are tolerated [2, 5]. After improvement of local and systemic infection, status parenteral therapy can be switched after 5–7 days to oral antibiotics. Empiric coverage for MRSA should be considered in patients not responding to initial therapy, patients with previous episodes of MRSA infection or MRSA nasal colonization, IV drug abuse, or patients with recurrent skin infections with underlying risk factors. The MRSA treatment recommendations are IV drugs, such as vancomycin, daptomycin, linezolid and telavancin, or oral therapy with doxycycline, clindamycin, or trimethoprim-sulfamethoxazole [2].

Complicating factors that may delay recovery are diabetes, chronic venous insufficiency, tinea pedis, or lymphedema and should be treated by appropriate therapy.

2.2 Cellulitis

2.2.1 Definition

Cellulitis is an acute extensive spreading bacterial infection of the dermis and the subcutaneous fat, which can lead to abscess formation.

2.2.2 Etiology and microbiology

Diffuse cellulitis or infections without a defined portal are mainly related to streptococcal species, especially β-hemolytic streptococci. On the other hand *S aureus* is the most common bacteria in cases of cellulitis associated with furuncles, carbuncles, or abscesses, and those caused by penetrating trauma, injection treatment, and IV drug abuse. Different pathogens are responsible for cellulitis related to trauma, water contact, and animal, insect, or human bites [5]. Cellulitis and erysipelas present corresponding etiology and pathogenesis.

2.2.3 Clinical manifestation

Cellulitis occurs as a rapidly spreading painful area of edema, heat, and redness without sharp borders. It can be accompanied by lymphangitis and inflammation of the regional lymph nodes or thrombophlebitis [32]. On the inflamed skin area, vesicles, bullae, and cutaneous hemorrhage (petechiae) may be present (**Fig 13-5**). Usually systemic signs of infections are mild and may be seen before skin manifestations. In the case of cutaneous hemorrhage in combination with severe signs of systemic infections—high fever, hypotension, tachycardia, leukocytosis, and confusion—a deeper NSTI should be considered [5]. Recurrent attacks of cellulitis can lead to lymphedema.

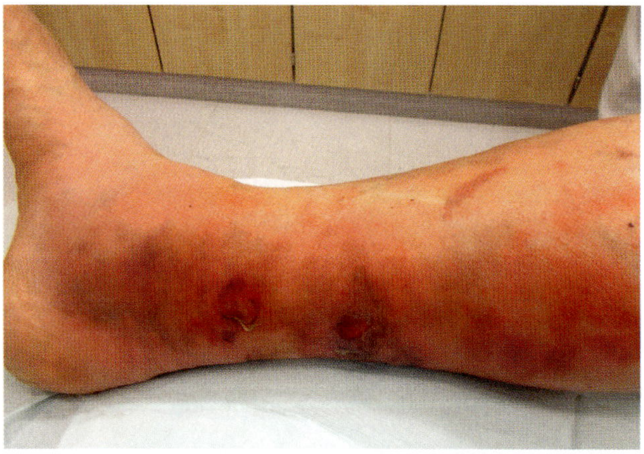

Fig 13-5 Cellulitis of the lower leg; presenting with no sharp borders, vesicles, bullae, and cutaneous hemorrhage.

2.2.4 Diagnosis

Cellulitis is diagnosed by its clinical manifestations with further considerations according to the disease pattern of erysipelas.

2.2.5 Specific treatment

Cellulitis is treated in the same manner as erysipelas.

2.3 Furuncles and carbuncles

2.3.1 Definition

Furuncles are localized dermal or subdermal infections of a hair follicle with a small abscess formation. Coalescent-infected follicles with multiple locations of pus drainage are defined as carbuncle. They occur on hairy skin, particularly in the axilla, inguinal, the upper back, and the neck [5].

2.3.2 Etiology and microbiology

Furuncles and carbuncles are usually caused by *S aureus*. Carbuncles are often seen in patients with diabetes [5]. *Staphylococcus aureus*-related outbreaks of furunculosis may occur in settings of close personal contact associated with skin lesions and inadequate personal hygiene. In such cases the transmission of pathogens is facilitated by fomites [33–35]. Repeated attacks of furunculosis occur in people (especially in children) with a compromised host immune response. In other cases, *S aureus* skin colonization is the only identifiable predisposing risk factor in recurrent furuncles, and it remains unclear why some carriers develop a recurrent skin infection and others do not [36].

2.3.3 Clinical manifestation

Initially, furuncles and carbuncles present as dense and red painful nodules. With time, pus formation with subsequent drainage or scar formation is seen.

2.3.4 Specific treatment

Incision and drainage is required in larger furuncles and carbuncles, since smaller lesions can be treated with moist heat to promote drainage [5]. Systemic antibiotic therapy is solely recommended in case of conjunction with extensive-surrounding cellulitis or sign of systemic infection [5]. In the case of recurrent furunculosis and *S aureus* nasal colonization, one approach is decolonization by mupirocin application [37].

2.4 Cutaneous abscess

2.4.1 Definition

A cutaneous abscess is a collection of pus within the dermis and the deeper skin tissues [38, 39].

2.4.2 Etiology and microbiology

Cutaneous abscesses are mainly polymicrobial and contain skin and adjacent mucous membrane-colonizing bacterial flora [38–40]. *Staphylococcus aureus* is the most common pathogen but only 25% have a single disease-causing pathogen present [41].

2.4.3 Clinical manifestation

Cutaneous abscesses present as painful, tender, and fluctuant nodules, with a central pustule and surrounding erythematous swelling [38, 39].

2.4.4 Diagnosis

The primary step in diagnosing a cutaneous abscess is clinical diagnosis and obtainment of the patient's history with focus on recurrent abscesses or IV drug abuse and further risk factors. In most cases diagnosis is provided by clinical picture. Superficial abscess can be seen or palpated. Ultrasound is a fast, inexpensive, and easy diagnostic tool to confirm the diagnosis, to detect deeper abscesses, and to determine the size and extent of the abscess. Laboratory examination is mandatory but encapsulated abscesses often lack elevated infection parameters. An MRI or CT scan may be helpful in suspected deep abscesses but are not indicated to diagnose simple cutaneous abscesses. Bacterial culture and Gram stain of pus from abscesses are recommended [2].

2.4.5 Specific treatment

Surgical debridement with incision, evacuation of the pus, and exploration of the cavity to detect loculations is the recommended therapy [2]. The surgical site can be packed with gauze or covered with a dry dressing. Larger abscesses can be treated with NPWT, followed by a second-look surgery. Suturing the wound closed is an option but it carries risk of recurrent infection and should be monitored closely [42, 43]. Intravenous antibiotics are recommended for systemic illness, surrounding cellulitis, multiple lesions, cutaneous gangrene, and in the presence of compromised host immune defences, but is rarely necessary in uncomplicated cases [5]. Antimicrobial therapy active against MRSA is indicated in patients with abscesses or carbuncles who have an impaired host immune system and patients with systemic inflammatory response syndrome [2]. Guidelines for antibiotic therapy are listed in **Fig 13-2**, considering in addition recommendations for the US and regions with high prevalence of MRSA.

2.5 Septic bursitis

2.5.1 Definition

A bursa is a soft-tissue cushion lined by a synovial membrane to reduce friction between soft-tissue layers—usually found adjacent to a bony prominence. The most prominent bursae affected by bursitis are the olecranon bursa and prepatellar bursa. Bursitis typically occurs in male patients aged 40–60 years and can be divided into the common nonseptic bursitis (NSB) and septic bursitis (SB). The focus of this chapter is on SB.

2.5.2 Etiology and microbiology

Nonseptic bursitis is mainly related to secondary trauma, crystal deposition (ie, gout or pseudogout), overuse by athletes, or occurs in certain occupational groups. It is due to a mechanical overload resulting in an overproduction of bursal fluid and swelling promoting the cycle of chronic sterile inflammation.

In contrast, SB is an inflammation caused by infection, typically resulting from bacterial inoculation. *Staphylococcus aureus* represents the most frequent causative pathogen in 80% of cases, followed by streptococci [44]. Generally, a skin lesion is the portal of pathogen entry but in rare cases hematogenous seeding or spread from an adjacent cellulitis is responsible. The olecranon and prepatellar bursae are in a superficial and exposed location. Septic olecranon bursitis occurs four times as often as prepatellar bursitis. Other predisposing factors are rheumatoid arthritis, alcohol abuse, immune deficiency, and history of chronic bursitis.

2.5.3 Clinical manifestation

Due to similar clinical presentations, the differentiation between NSB and SB is difficult. The most common symptoms present in NSB as well as SB are bursal swelling, redness, and tenderness. Bursal warmth, fever, skin lesions, or increasing tenderness can be considered as decision criteria for a septic inflammation. Some patients with acute SB may present with a fever [45]. In subacute or chronic cases, differentiation from noninfectious bursitis can be difficult.

2.5.4 Diagnosis

Diagnostic methods include blood testing, x-rays, ultrasound, and bursal fluid aspiration to determine the appropriate treatment. Blood sampling should include the typical infection studies, sedimentation rate, CRP level, and white blood cell (WBC) count. Biplanar x-rays should be obtained to identify underlying bone lesions, foreign bodies, or osteomyelitis. Ultrasound can additionally characterize the bursal structure, enlargement, and content. An MRI or CT scan may be helpful in suspected deep bursal infection (eg, of the pelvis) or in infections involving the adjacent soft tissue [46].

Bursal aspiration is typically recommended to confirm clinical findings. Macroscopic characteristics of the aspirate can suggest the infectious etiology [46]. Purulent aspirates indicate a septic etiology in contrast to the clear, hemorrhagic or milky fluid suggesting a sterile nonseptic inflammation. The laboratory analysis of the aspirate includes Gram stain, bacterial culture, WBC count, and bursal fluid glucose level [47]. The most specific test indicating a bacterial infection is a positive Gram stain or bacterial culture, which also allows targeted antibiotic therapy. A WBC count of more than 3,000 cells/µL and a total bursal fluid glucose lower than 31 mg/dL or fluid-to-serum ratio less than 50% are considered further criteria suggesting SB [48].

Thus, needle aspiration is critical but it bears the risk of a superinfection if not performed properly. When recurrent needle aspiration is used for treatment, a chronic infection situation may become established. From a legal point of view it is hard to prove that the bacterial infection of a bursa is not caused by the aspiration.

2.5.5 Specific treatment

In infected and noninfected bursitis, nonsteroidal antiinflammatory drugs, and the PRICE methods, consisting of protection, rest/immobilization, ice, compression, and elevation are recommended and should be used for 10–14 days [48]. Bursal aspiration is also suggested in both cases to relieve pain, increase range of motion, and to diagnose the etiological pathogens [48]. Aspiration in SB results in both drainage and a reduction of the bacterial load. The initial classification of bursitis remains important to nonoperative or surgical treatment. In SB, the appropriate antibiotic treatment is the keystone and should be started when an infection is suspected. Since *S aureus* is causative in approximately 80% of cases, the empiric antibiotics should have antistaphylococcal activity [48]. In regions with high prevalence of MRSA infections, clindamycin, doxycycline, or oral trimethoprim–sulfamethoxazole is recommended [48].

In mild and moderate cases of SB, ambulatory, oral antibiotic therapy for 2 weeks is recommended and usually sufficient, as the antibiotics have been shown to achieve high intrabursal levels [48]. In severe cases with progression of local findings or accompanying systemic signs of infection, hospitalization and IV antibiotic treatment for 10 days is usually required. In general, the duration of antibiotic therapy should be determined by the clinical course, response to the therapy, culture results, the immune status, and health of the host [48]. Most patients respond to nonsurgical therapy. However, in cases of a recurrent SB after failed nonoperative therapy bursectomy is indicated. Surgical bursectomy should not be performed in an acutely inflamed bursa. In the literature, recurrent needle drainage is described but the authors fear the risk of superinfection and recommend complete bursectomy when needed.

Surgical therapy with bursectomy is indicated in cases of severe systemic infection with involvement of the surrounding tissue or complications, such as cellulitis, abscess formation, or skin necrosis [48]. In these cases, intervention should be performed urgently to reduce the bacterial load and to prevent further spread of infection. Intravenous antibiotics are recommended for 7 days [48] and can be prolonged according to the clinical course in severe cases. In olecranon bursitis, the skin incision should not be placed over the bony olecranon process to avoid wound-healing difficulty and a sensitive scar [49]. In severe inflammation with swelling, induration, and obscured soft-tissue layers, the course of the ulnar nerve should be considered. In prepatellar bursitis a horizontal incision along the skin folds is the standard. Primary wound closure should be achieved and should be performed without skin tension. In cases with skin defects, eg, after excision of necrotic tissue, massive swelling, or suspected necrotizing infection, an NPWT closure for continuous drainage can be used. An early secondary wound closure should be the goal and recurrent debridement with change of the negative-pressure wound sealing is an exception. After open bursectomy, the extremity should be immobilized until proper wound healing has occurred. The upper extremity is splinted in flexion, whereas for the lower extremity a brace is sufficient. Complications include wound-healing problems, development of a subcutaneous hematoma, chronic pain, and in rare cases, recurrent infections [49]. The arthroscopic bursectomy is described in the literature as an alternative method with decreased complications in terms of wound-healing disorders. The authors recommend open bursectomy, especially in cases of acute inflammation to provide complete removal of infected tissue and to avoid pathogen spread in the adjacent tissue.

The key message: in SB, antibiotic therapy is the key element, and should be initiated if an infection is suspected and accompanied by the PRICE scheme. Open bursectomy is recommended if severe systemic infection results from bursitis with involvement of the surrounding tissue or complications, such as cellulitis, abscess formation, or skin necrosis as well as in refractory cases. Recurrent infection and failed nonoperative therapy require surgical intervention, which should not be performed in the setting of acute inflammation. Endoscopic bursectomy is an alternative surgical method that the authors do not recommend.

2.5.6 Prognosis

Especially in cases of inadequate treatment of the infection, either by insufficient antimicrobial therapy or surgical debridement, persistence of pathogens can result in recurrent infections. Most cases of SB resolve with needle aspiration and appropriate antibiotic therapy.

2.6 Soft-tissue infections as complication after trauma and surgery

2.6.1 Surgical-site infection

Surgical-site infection is the most common adverse event in surgical patients and the third most common nosocomial infection with an average incidence of 2.6% [50–52]. The frequency, however, is dependent on the injury pattern and localization, soft-tissue damage, and patient's comorbidities, which allow a categorization from clean and low-risk operations to high-risk procedures [53]. In this part of the chapter the authors focus on SSIs after fracture fixation, joint replacement, and various surgeries of the orthopedic and trauma spectrum that involve solely the soft tissue. Deep SSIs involving the implant are covered in chapters 4 Prevention of intraoperative infection, 9.1 Infection after fracture, 9.2 Infected nonunion, and 10 Infection after joint arthroplasty.

Definition and classification

The definition of SSIs used by the British Nosocomial Infection National Surveillance System is: "A surgical-site infection occurs when micro-organisms get into the part of the body that has been operated on and multiply in the tissue" [54]. The US Centers for Disease Control and Prevention definition states that SSI or wound infections mainly occur within the first 30 days after surgery and they are categorized in superficial incisional SSI, deep incisional SSI, and organ/space SSI [55]. Superficial infections affect the subcutaneous layers, whereas deep incisional infections include the muscular fascia and the muscle [2, 51].

Etiology and microbiology

An important risk factor for subsequent wound infection is the extent of microbial contamination at a surgical site [8]. Therefore, operative wounds are classified based on microbial contamination in the following categories: clean, clean-contaminated, contaminated, and dirty [56].

The most frequent pathogen causing SSI is *S aureus*; however, the spectrum of pathogens varies with the affected body region [2, 57].

Clinical manifestation

Surgical-site infections commonly present with local signs of infection, such as erythema, pain, swelling, and purulent drainage, and can be accompanied by fever and other systemic signs of infection. Early postoperative fever usually arises from noninfectious or unknown causes and is usually not associated with SSI since postoperative wound infections rarely occur within the first 48 hours after incision. Rare cases of SSIs that manifest within the first 2 days after surgery are generally caused by *S pyogenes* and *Clostridium* species [2].

Diagnosis

According to the US practice guidelines, SSIs are diagnosed with at least one of the following symptoms:

- Purulent incision drainage
- Positive culture of aseptically obtained fluid or tissue from the superficial wound
- Local signs and symptoms of pain and tenderness, swelling, and erythema after the incision is opened by a surgeon (unless culture negative)
- Diagnosis of SSI by the attending surgeon or physician based on their experience and expert opinion [2]

Within the UK definition surgeons' opinion is not used as an indicator for infection; the presence of pus is used instead of cultured microorganisms from clinical samples [54].

Postoperative fever or systemic signs of infection should always lead to a direct examination of the wound and be followed by a test of the WBC count and CRP level. Especially in fever occurring within the first few days, signs suggestive of infection due to *S pyogenes* and *Clostridium* species must be ruled out [2].

Numerical scoring systems, such as the Southampton Wound Assessment Scale and ASEPSIS, can help to evaluate the severity of SSIs and to monitor the course of the infection. Magnitude of serous or purulent exudate, erythema, and suppuration of deep tissue are used to evaluate the status of infection [58, 59].

Specific treatment

Early flat erythematous skin changes in the near surrounding of the wound which are not accompanied by swelling or drainage typically will resolve without any specific therapy [2]. Spread of the erythema, wound drainage, and swelling indicate need for treatment. The surgical debridement of the incision to evacuate the detritus and infected tissue is the most important aspect of therapy [2]. The extent of local infection and the presence of systemic signs should be evaluated carefully to initiate the appropriate surgical treatment and launch adjuvant systemic antimicrobial therapy. Adjunctive systemic antibiotic therapy is not necessary if erythema and induration is less than 5 cm and if the patient has minimal systemic signs of infection (ie, temperature < 38.5° C; WBC count < 12,000 cells/μL, and pulse rate < 100 beats/minute) [2, 60]. Especially in subcutaneous abscesses, various studies could not prove a relevant benefit for adjuvant antimicrobial therapy when combined with surgical drainage [2, 61, 62]. Complementary prophylactic antibiotics are not indicated since incision and surgical debridement of superficial abscesses rarely causes bacteremia [63]. An erythema exceeding 5 cm beyond the surgical incision or a systemic inflammatory response with high fever (> 38.5° C) or pulse rate (> 110 beats/minute) require additional therapy—typically a short course of antimicrobial therapy. In the case of a proven MRSA infection or nasal colonization or if the patient had a prior MRSA infection, antimicrobial therapy should include vancomycin, daptomycin, linezolid, telavancin, or ceftaroline [2]. Empiric antibiotic therapy in SSI following surgery of intestinal or genitourinary tract should cover gram-negative and anaerobic pathogens. See chapter 5 Systemic antibiotics, **Table 5-1** and **Table 5-2** for details on antibiotic therapy.

Prevention

Surgical-site infections are associated with increased morbidity and mortality and pose a high economic burden on the healthcare system [64]. Additionally, the emergence of antibiotic resistance has been observed over the last three decades [57]. Therefore, prevention of SSIs by system changes, surveillance, and education is of particular importance [65]. The prevention of perioperative infections for most surgeries in trauma care and orthopedics is discussed in detail in chapter 4 Prevention of intraoperative infection [65–67].

2.6.2 Wound infection after trauma

Skin and soft tissue can be traumatized by blunt or penetrating force, thermally, chemically, or by radiation. Trauma can lead to contamination of the injured tissue and subsequent development of a wound infection. The cause as well as the extent of trauma, the body site, and the host immune status all play a critical role in the development of wound infection. Misunderstanding of trauma can result in inappropriate management, such as missed antibiotic prophylaxis. The most common wound infections are related to penetrating soft-tissue trauma (including burn and bite injuries).

Generally, wound infections are treated according to the treatment principles of SSIs. There are different treatment recommendations for infections following mammalian or human bites. These specific problems are discussed separately.

In every open injury, the tetanus vaccination status of the patient must be validated. A tetanus toxoid booster should be administered to patients with an unknown vaccination status or incomplete vaccination series for clean wounds if more than 5 years elapsed since the last dose and for dirty wounds if 5 years have passed [2].

Animal and human bite wounds

Mammalian bites are most commonly caused by dogs or cats and are colonized by microorganisms found in the animal's oral cavity. The multimicrobial flora is a mixture of aerobic and anaerobic pathogens including streptococci, staphylococci, *Moxarella*, *Neisseria*, *Fusobacterium*, *Bacteroides*, and *Pasteurella* species, a common gram-negative bacterium in cats and dogs [68]. Patients with animal bites in areas with high prevalence of rabies should be considered for rabies vaccination according to regional recommendations [2]. It should be considered that bites caused by bats also pose a high risk of rabies transmission.

Human bites result in bacterial contamination with both aerobic and anaerobic pathogens, the risk of transmitting HIV or hepatitis B/C. Patients should be treated with antibiotic prophylaxis and possible viral transmission.

Treatment principles after bite trauma

Basic principles include both appropriate surgical therapy and antimicrobial prophylaxis. Early antimicrobial prophylaxis for 3–5 days should be administered and is recommended in the following circumstances:

- All cat bites
- Moderate or severe injuries, especially to face and hand
- Injuries that may have penetrated the periosteum or joint capsule
- Immunocompromised patients
- Preexisting or developing edema of affected body area [2]

Surgical debridement and irrigation of the bite wound should be considered. Primary wound closure is solely recommended for wounds to the face [2]. Temporary NPWT is an option to ensure wound drainage and enable a second-look surgery. Major soft-tissue defects or significant soft-tissue swelling that prevents primary wound closure can be covered by NPWT. Local antibiotics used for bite wounds lack the literature support and thus this option is not recommended.

Treatment principles in infection after bite trauma

Amoxicillin-clavulanate, an antimicrobial agent active against aerobic and anaerobic bacteria is the first choice oral therapy in infected animal bite wounds [2]. Other treatment options with aerobic coverage are second- or third-generation cephalosporins (IV usage), levofloxacin, or trimethoprim-sulfamethoxazole, which should be accompanied by anaerobic coverage with clindamycin or metronidazole. Moxifloxacin is an alternative therapy [2]. Surgical therapy is indicated according to the treatment guidelines for SSTIs based on local and systemic factors.

2.7 Necrotizing soft-tissue infections

2.7.1 Definition

Necrotizing soft-tissue infections are characterized by the necrosis of skin and subcutaneous tissue (ie, necrotizing cellulitis), fascia (ie, necrotizing fasciitis), and underlying muscle (ie, myonecrosis), or combinations of these findings [69]. Necrotizing soft-tissue infections are rare bacterial infections with an incidence of 0.4–0.5 cases per 100,000 people [70–72]. They can present in combination with a fulminant and life threatening septic course, such as the necrotizing fasciitis. They differ considerably from superficial infections by clinical presentation and course, coexisting systemic manifestation, and treatment strategies [73, 74]. Necrotizing soft-tissue infections are cross-layer infections with a possible involvement of the fascia and the muscle compartments, which lead to a necrosis of the affected tissue. They were first described in 1871 by Jones and termed "hospital gangrene" [70]. In 1952 Wilson described necrotizing fasciitis as affecting the fascia and subcutaneous tissue [75]. Since then multiple descriptions and classifications of NSTIs were published, which led to some confusion. Therefore, one must emphasize that defining the specific variant is of secondary importance and that NSTIs have common pathophysiological and clinical manifestation with the same principles for diagnosis and treatment [76, 77].

2.7.2 Etiology and microbiology

An NSTI typically develops after injury to the involved site enabling bacteria to breach the skin barrier [5]. Necrotizing fasciitis may be associated with any trauma or incision to the skin including minor lesions, such as insect bites and injection sites [78, 79]. In 20–45% of the cases, no definitive access point can be found because these minor lesions are often forgotten or obscure [5, 80]. Any impairment of the host immune system, obesity, and the risk factors listed in **Table 13-2** predispose to NSTI, although half of the cases occur in previously healthy individuals [81, 82].

Disease-causing pathogens can be aerobic, anaerobic, gram positive and gram negative, or even fungal species [5, 7, 8]. Considering the infecting pathogen, the Giuliano Classification defines two types of necrotizing fasciitis [83]:

Type I: synergistic acting anaerobic-aerobic mixed infections
Type II: group A streptococci possibly combined with *S aureus* or *Staphylococcus epidermidis*

The Giuliano Classification has no impact on the clinical diagnosis or therapy. Type I fasciitis is reported to be less aggressive in the clinical course than type II with *S pyogenes* (group A streptococci) as causative bacteria.

2.7.3 Clinical manifestations

The initial stage of the necrotizing fasciitis lacks major cutaneous signs and resembles a cellulitis, which is generally treated nonoperatively with antibiotics [5, 7, 8]. In patients believed to have cellulitis, the triad of swelling, erythema (**Fig 13-5**), and disproportionately severe pain often precedes skin findings, and should raise suspicion of necrotizing fasciitis [84]. Another clue of a deeper and devastating infection is the rapid spread of erythema, despite systemic antibiotic therapy [85]. As it progresses, warmth and induration of the skin with a woody feeling of the subcutaneous tissues develops. Palpation permits discrimination from cellulitis and erysipelas. In superficial infections, subcutaneous tissues can be palpated and are yielding in fasciitis [5, 78]. In the advanced stages, classic signs of a necrotizing infection of the skin and deeper layers develop (see chapter 5 Systemic antibiotics, **Table 5-1** and **Table 5-2**). Here a primary stage to skin necrosis (**Fig 13-6**) is often an undemarcated marmorated skin with blisters and bullae, which are draining

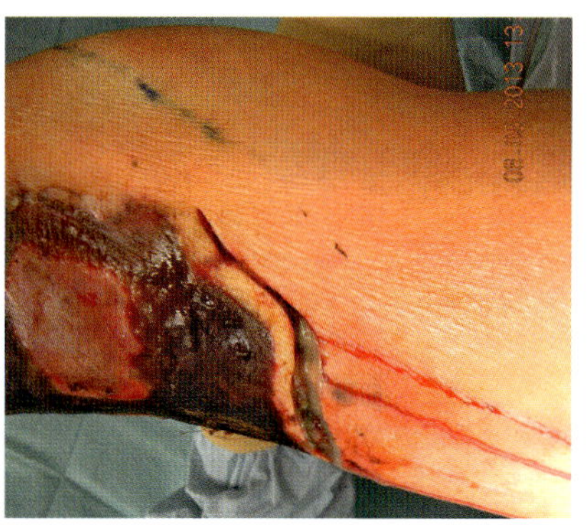

Fig 13-6 Advanced stage of necrotizing soft-tissue infection with skin necrosis. Surgery reveals pus drainage and confirms diagnosis.

serosanguinous and later hemorrhagic fluid (**Fig 13-7**). These are accompanied by signs of systemic infection: fever, hypotension, tachycardia, and altered consciousness [86]. Requiring admission to an intensive care unit, the critically ill patient can develop multiorgan failure with acute renal failure (35%), coagulopathy (29%), liver dysfunction (28%), and acute respiratory distress syndrome (14%) [87]. It is essential to not miss the diagnosis of NSTI because initially classic skin findings are not present and not all patients show a systemic symptom, such as fever [88]. The most sensitive diagnostic symptom, which is present in nearly 100% of cases, is the disproportionately severe pain [89].

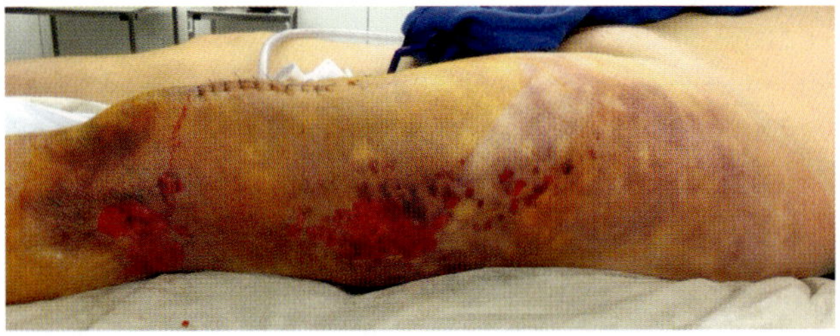

Fig 13-7 Advanced stage of necrotizing soft-tissue infection: undemarcated subcutaneous hemorrhage and infection accompanied by draining bullae and blisters with areas of beginning skin necrosis.

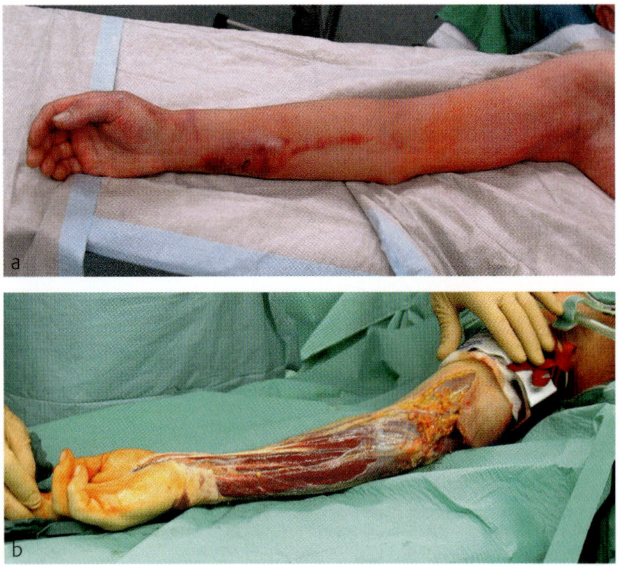

Fig 13-8a–b Initial and preoperative skin findings often do not represent the extent of the underlying infection.

2.7.4 Diagnosis

The diagnosis of NSTI is primarily a clinical diagnosis considering the patient's symptoms and clinical course, risk factors, and the local skin lesions. Clinical judgment is the most important factor when diagnosing NSTI. The next step after clinical diagnosis of NSTI is the immediate radical surgical debridement of the affected soft tissues to reduce morbidity and mortality [26].

Due to the tremendous consequences for the patient's clinical outcome and due to legal considerations, in-person evaluation is the key element and this diagnosis should be made by at least two physicians or surgeons. Any other options for diagnosis of NSTIs should not delay the surgical therapy.

The early clinical diagnosis is difficult because of the initial absence of systemic signs of infection. In the early phase, the minor skin lesions appear which may resemble cellulitis (**Fig 13-8**) [2]. A high index of suspicion is critical and is the most important factor in early diagnosis of NSTIs. Consequently, laboratory and x-ray examinations should be added to support early diagnosis but should never delay surgical intervention [78, 90].

History and examination

Initially, the diagnosis begins with a medical history and detailed examination. The classic signs of NSTIs should raise suspicion and inform the diagnosis of NSTI (**Table 13-3**). Risk factors should be determined (**Table 13-2**). In patients with IV/subcutaneous drug abuse and chronic debilitating diseases, it is important to suspect NSTI [77]. A complete clinical examination can detect the above-mentioned skin manifestations, such as a possible skin lesion or for migrating inflammation and lymph node affection. The vital signs as well as the mental status are also important findings [2].

Signs of necrotizing soft-tissue infections
Severe constant pain (disproportionate to injury or clinical presentation)
Blisters and bullae (draining serosanguineous and later hemorrhagic fluid)
Skin necrosis (preceded by violaceous discoloration)
Superficial fat and fascia necrosis (often foul-smelling)
Crepitus (indicating gas in the soft tissue)
Edema (extending beyond the erythema)
Cutaneous anesthesia
Woody feeling of subcutaneous tissues
Signs of systemic toxicity
Rapid progression (despite antibiotic therapy)

Table 13-3 Classic signs of necrotizing soft-tissue infections.

Radiological evaluation

Plain x-rays may detect gas in the soft tissue. The diagnostic value is low because gas production occurs in advanced stages and is rarely present early on [78]. Imaging by CT or MRI can show edema extending along the fascial plane, but the sensitivity and specificity are low. Ultrasound is quick and immediately available. If epifascial fluid is detected, surgical exploration is mandatory.

Laboratory findings

Important laboratory findings are sepsis parameters, such as leukocytosis, leukopenia, and increase of CRP, procalcitonin, or interleukin-6. Procalcitonin is suitable to assess the success of surgical debridement by calculating the preoperative/postoperative ratio [91].

Fisher et al [92] defined five criteria for the diagnosis of necrotizing fasciitis:

- Moderate to severe systemic toxic reaction
- Absence of major vascular occlusion
- Surgical site: extensive necrosis of the fascia undermining the surrounding tissue and absence of primary muscle involvement (**Fig 13-9**)
- Microbiology: failure to demonstrate clostridia
- Histology: leukocyte infiltration, focal fascia necrosis, and necrosis of the surrounding tissue, microvascular thrombosis

Only the first two criteria are suitable for the immediate diagnosis of NSTI, respective of necrotizing fasciitis. All other criteria are only useful if surgery has already been performed: assessment of fasciitis, myositis, microbiology, or histology. These results can only confirm the diagnosis of NSTI and are therefore not useful parameters in decision making (**Fig 13-9**).

2.7.5 Differential diagnosis

Cellulitis

The crossover from cellulitis to NSTIs is rapid, and this is the challenge. The treatment of cellulitis is nonoperative with antibiotics, immobilization, and local antiseptic dressing. A clinical course with rapid deterioration of the patient's condition must raise suspicion for the diagnosis of NSTI and surgical exploration should be the next step.

Gas gangrene

Gas gangrene is another life-threating infection of the soft tissue often involving the muscles. Gas gangrene is caused by *Clostridium perfringens* or *Bacillus* species. The typical clinical findings are the crepitation of skin and soft tissues and the initial high pain levels. The skin appears to be more livid. Intraoperative findings are bubbles in wound secretion and raspberry-like necrosis of the muscles.

Pyoderma gangrenosum

Pyoderma gangrenosum (PG) is an autoimmune disease that sometimes mimics necrotizing fasciitis to a striking degree [93]. This can be induced by trauma or surgery; the clinical features are purulent necrosis of skin, subcutaneous tissue, and fascia without microbiological findings. It is a diagnosis by exclusion and this is essential to treat PG. Treatment for PG is the diametric opposite to NSTIs. Once PG is suspected, immunosuppression with high-dose cortisol or methotrexate is the therapy of choice. Any further surgery should be avoided or minimized.

Gram-positive toxic shock syndrome

Gram-positive toxic shock syndrome (TSS) is an acute, toxin-induced septic shock syndrome characterized by hypotension [94]. Causative agents are streptococci or staphylococci producing a "superantigen" (eg, TSST-1). One clinical criterion for the diagnosis of TSS is soft-tissue necrosis.

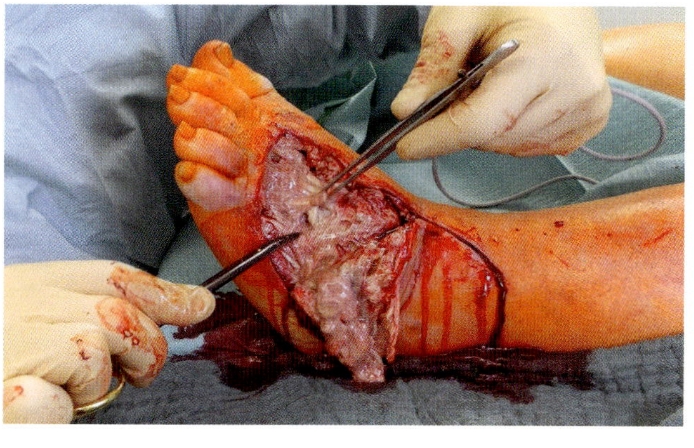

Fig 13-9 Surgery reveals necrotic fascia and subcutaneous fat; the incision must be expanded until no more pus drainage or necrosis is detected.

2.7.6 Specific treatment

The treatment for NSTIs with acute septic inflammatory reaction is based on a three-pillar strategy:

1. Radical surgical debridement: surgical debridement is the primary therapeutic modality and includes resection of necrotic skin, subcutaneous tissue, and fascia. The primary aim is the reduction of bacterial and inflammatory load. The resection of all affected tissue should create a "fire line" to avoid progression of the process to the trunk. The prognosis for the patient decreases rapidly if the trunk is affected. "Life before limb": amputation for life-threating infections with circumferentially affected limbs is necessary in 30–50% of cases. A second-look operation is mandatory after 12–36 hours depending on the clinical course. The patient should return according to systemic and local status to the operating room on regular intervals [2]. Small incisions and inappropriate wound coverage should be avoided because sufficient drainage is not possible and local infection can progress (**Fig 13-10**).
2. Early high-dose antibiotic therapy: current recommendations for empiric antibiotic treatment should include agents active against both aerobes including MRSA and anaerobes [2]. The treatment recommendations are summarized in **Fig 13-11**. The recommendations for the US consider a high prevalence of MRSA and are designed to cover methicillin-resistant staphylococci. This suggestion should be applied in regions with a high-MRSA prevalence. Recommendations for low MRSA infection rates are adapted from the German Paul-Ehrlich Society of Chemotherapy guidelines. As soon as a microbial cause has been determined and susceptibility testing is available, antibiotic therapy should be reevaluated and targeted with the assistance of an infectious diseases specialist. Recommendations for pathogen-guided antimicrobials are listed in **Fig 13-11**. Antibiotics should be given until surgical treatment is completed and no additional debridement is necessary, the patient has improved clinically, and fever has been absent for 48–72 hours [2].
3. Intensive care unit monitoring and treatment of multiorgan failure and fluid management.

For temporary wound closure and conditioning of soft tissues, NPWT is suitable. The NPWT simplifies the fluid management of the patient. It provides an aseptic wound closure even for large wounds or whole extremities or after partial skin removal from the trunk (**Fig 13-3**).

An adjuvant therapy option is hyperbaric oxygen therapy [21]. Even though there is little evidence for hyperbaric oxygen therapy in the treatment of NSTIs in contrast to gas gangrene, it should be considered for patients with necrotizing STIs but it should never delay surgical therapy [95–97].

2.7.7 Prognosis

Even with optimal therapy, NSTI is associated with a high mortality ranging from 21.4% to 50% [70].

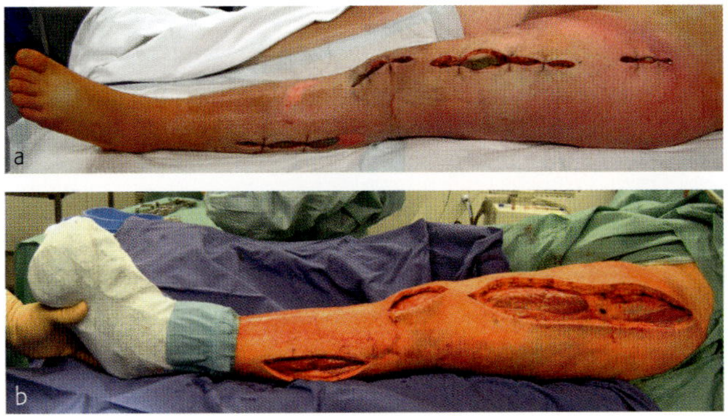

Fig 13-10a–b Radical debridement in necrotizing soft-tissue infections: limited incisions should be avoided to guarantee appropriate drainage.

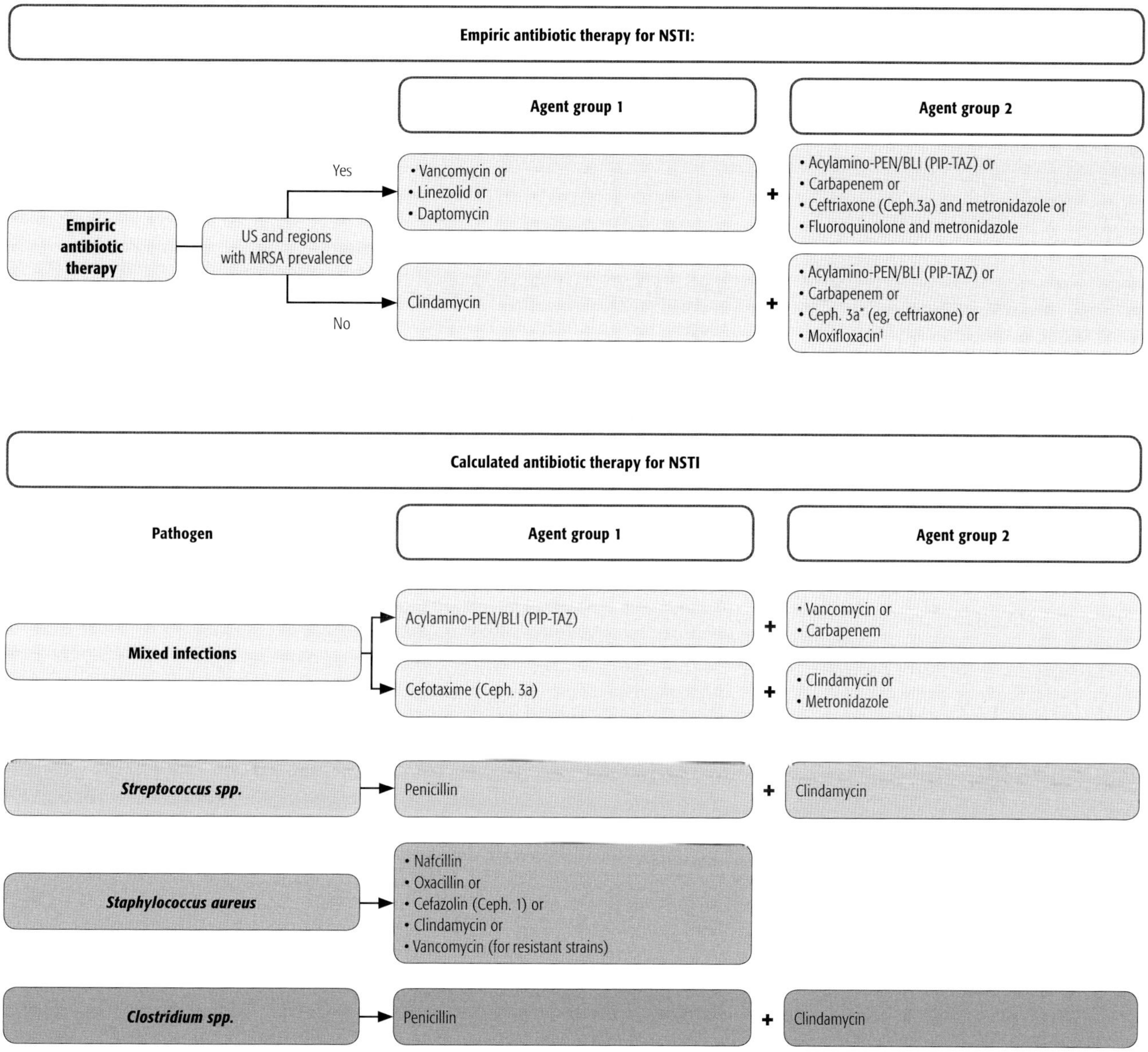

Fig 13-11 Antibiotic treatment of necrotizing soft-tissue infections adapted from IDSA Guidelines 2014 with European recommendations. These are currently recommended in the US but treatment options will vary based on the location of the reader.

* Empiric antibiotic therapy for NSTI in regions with low MRSA prevalence: third-generation cephalosporin can be also combined with metronidazole (instead of clindamycin).

† Moxifloxacin can be also combined with linezolid (instead of clindamycin).

Abbreviations: MRSA, methicillin-resistant *Staphylococcus aureus*; acylamino-PEN/BLI, acylamino-penicillin with a β-lactamase inhibitor; PIP-TAZ, piperacilin tazobactam; Ceph.3a, third-generation cephalosporin; Ceph.1, first-generation cephalosporin; spp., species.

3 References

1. **Brook I.** Microbiology and management of soft tissue and muscle infections. *Int J Surg.* 2008 Aug;6(4):328–338.
2. **Stevens DL, Bisno AL, Chambers HF, et al.** Practice guidelines for the diagnosis and management of skin and soft tissue infections: 2014 update by the Infectious Diseases Society of America. *Clin Infect Dis.* 2014;59 Jul 15;59(2):e10–52.
3. **Rajan S.** Skin and soft-tissue infections: classifying and treating a spectrum. *Cleve Clin J Med.* 2012 Jan;79(1):57–66.
4. **Kingston D, Seal DV.** Current hypotheses on synergistic microbial gangrene. *Br J Surg.* 1990 Mar;77(3):260–264.
5. **Stevens DL, Bisno AL, Chambers HF, et al.** Practice guidelines for the diagnosis and management of skin and soft-tissue infections. *Clin Infect Dis.* 2005 Nov 15;41(10):1373–1406.
6. **Wong CH, Khin LW, Heng KS, et al.** The LRINEC (Laboratory Risk Indicator for Necrotizing Fasciitis) score: a tool for distinguishing necrotizing fasciitis from other soft tissue infections. *Crit Care Med.* 2004 Jul;32(7):1535–1541.
7. **Ki V, Rotstein C.** Bacterial skin and soft tissue infections in adults: A review of their epidemiology, pathogenesis, diagnosis, treatment and site of care. *Can J Infect Dis.* 2008 Jan;19(2):173–84.
8. **Berard F, Gandon J.** Postoperative wound infections: the influence of ultraviolet irradiation of the operating room and of various other factors. *Ann Surg.*1964;160(Suppl 2):1–192.
9. **Culver DH, Horan TC, Gaynes RP, et al.** Surgical wound infection rates by wound class, operative procedure, and patient risk index. National Nosocomial Infections Surveillance System. *Am J Med.* 1991 Sep 16;91(3B):152S–157S.
10. **Uckay I, Harbarth S, Peter R, et al.** Preventing surgical site infections. *Expert Rev Anti Infect Ther.* 2010;8(6):657–670.
11. **Wenzel RP, Perl TM.** The significance of nasal carriage of Staphylococcus aureus and the incidence of postoperative wound infection. *J Hosp Infect.* 1995 Sep;31(1):3–24.
12. **Spencer WG.** Celsus' De Medicina-a learned and experienced practitioner upon what the Art of Medicine could then accomplish. *Proc R Soc Med.* 1926;19(Sect Hist Med):129–139.
13. **Kirsner RS, Pardes JB, Eaglstein WH, et al.** The clinical spectrum of lipodermatosclerosis. *J Am Acad Dermatol.* 1993 Apr;28(4):623–627.
14. **Boucher HW, Corey GR.** Epidemiology of methicillin-resistant Staphylococcus aureus. *Clin Infect Dis.* 2008 Jun 1;46 Suppl 5:S344–349.
15. **Centers for Disease C, Prevention.** Outbreaks of community-associated methicillin-resistant Staphylococcus aureus skin infections--Los Angeles County, California, 2002-2003. *MMWR Morb Mortal Wkly Rep.* 2003 Feb 7;52(5):88.
16. **Dantes R, Mu Y, Belflower R, et al.** National burden of invasive methicillin-resistant Staphylococcus aureus infections, United States, 2011. *JAMA Intern Med.* 2013 Nov 25;173(21):1970–1978.
17. **Liu C, Bayer A, Cosgrove SE, et al.** Clinical practice guidelines by the Infectious Diseases Society of America for the treatment of methicillin-resistant Staphylococcus aureus infections in adults and children: executive summary. *Clin Infect Dis.* 2011 Feb1;52(3):285–292.
18. **Stevens DL, Smith LG, Bruss JB, et al.** Randomized comparison of linezolid (PNU-100766) versus oxacillin-dicloxacillin for treatment of complicated skin and soft tissue infections. *Antimicrob Agents Chemother.* 2000 Dec;44(12):3408–3413.
19. **Stevens DL, Herr D, Lampiris H, et al.** Linezolid versus vancomycin for the treatment of methicillin-resistant Staphylococcus aureus infections. *Clin Infect Dis.* 2002 Jun;34(11):1481–1490.
20. **Eskes A, Vermeulen H, Lucas C, et al.** Hyperbaric oxygen therapy for treating acute surgical and traumatic wounds. *Cochrane Database Syst Rev.* 2013 Dec 16;12:CD008059.
21. **Schmale M, Fichtner A, Pohl C, et al.** [Hyperbaric oxygenation for necrotizing soft tissue infections: pro]. *Chirurg. Chirurg.* 2012 Nov;83(11):973–979.
22. **Willy C.** Breakthrough ideas leading to new futures: prologue. *Int Wound J.* 2013 Dec;10 Suppl 1:1–2.
23. **Hunter JE, Teot L, Horch R, et al.** Evidence-based medicine: vacuum-assisted closure in wound care management. *Int Wound J.* 2007 Sep;4(3):256–269.
24. **Gilead L, Mumcuoglu KY, Ingber A.** The use of maggot debridement therapy in the treatment of chronic wounds in hospitalised and ambulatory patients. *J Wound Care.* 2012;21(2):78, 80, 2–5.
25. **Zarchi K, Jemec GB.** The efficacy of maggot debridement therapy--a review of comparative clinical trials. *Int Wound J.* 2012 Oct;9(5):469–477.
26. **Bisno AL, Stevens DL.** Streptococcal infections of skin and soft tissues. *N Engl J Med.* 1996 Jan 25;334(4):240–245.
27. **Chartier C, Grosshans E.** Erysipelas. *Int J Dermatol.* 1990 Sep;29(7):459–467.
28. **Dupuy A, Benchikhi H, Roujeau JC, et al.** Risk factors for erysipelas of the leg (cellulitis): case-control study. *BMJ.* 1999 Jun;318(7198):1591–1594.
29. **Perl B, Gottehrer NP, Raveh D, et al.** Cost-effectiveness of blood cultures for adult patients with cellulitis. *Clin Infect Dis.* 1999;29(6):1483–1488.
30. **Kielhofner MA, Brown B, Dall L.** Influence of underlying disease process on the utility of cellulitis needle aspirates. *Arch Int Med.* 1988 Nov;148(11):2451–2452.
31. **Hepburn MJ, Dooley DP, Skidmore PJ, et al.** Comparison of short-course (5 days) and standard (10 days) treatment for uncomplicated cellulitis. *Arch Intern Med.* 2004;164(15):1669–1674.
32. **Karakas M, Baba M, Aksungur VL, et al.** Manifestation of cellulitis after saphenous venectomy for coronary bypass surgery. *J Eur Acad Dermatol Venereol.* 2002 Sep;16(5):438–440.
33. **Decker MD, Lybarger JA, Vaughn WK, et al.** An outbreak of staphylococcal skin infections among river rafting guides. *Am J Epidemiol.* 1986 Dec;124(6):969–976.
34. **Sosin DM, Gunn RA, Ford WL, et al.** An outbreak of furunculosis among high school athletes. *Am J Sports Med.* 1989 Nov–Dec;17(6):828–832.
35. **Zimakoff J, Rosdahl VT, Petersen W, et al.** Recurrent staphylococcal furunculosis in families. *Scand J Infect Dis.* 1988;20(4):403–405.
36. **Hedström SA.** Recurrent staphylococcal furunculosis. Bacteriological findings and epidemiology in 100 cases. *Scand J Infect Dis.*1981;13(2):115–119.
37. **Raz R, Miron D, Colodner R, et al.** A 1-year trial of nasal mupirocin in the prevention of recurrent staphylococcal nasal colonization and skin infection. *Arch Intern Med.*1996 May 27;156(10):1109–1112.
38. **Ghoneim AT, McGoldrick J, Blick PW, et al.** Aerobic and anaerobic bacteriology of subcutaneous abscesses. *Br J Surg.* 1981 Jul;68(7):498–500.
39. **Meislin HW, Lerner SA, Graves MH, et al.** Cutaneous abscesses. Anaerobic and aerobic bacteriology and outpatient management. *Ann Intern Med.* 1977 Aug;87(2):145–149.
40. **Brook I, Frazier EH.** Aerobic and anaerobic bacteriology of wounds and cutaneous abscesses. *Arch Surg.*1990 Nov;125(11):1445–1451.

41. **Diven DG, Dozier SE, Meyer DJ, et al.** Bacteriology of inflamed and uninflamed epidermal inclusion cysts. *Arch Dermatol.* 1998 Jan;134(1):49–51.
42. **Llera JL, Levy RC.** Treatment of cutaneous abscess: a double-blind clinical study. *Ann Emerg Med.* 1985 Jan;14(1):15–19.
43. **Macfie J, Harvey J.** The treatment of acute superficial abscesses: a prospective clinical trial. *Br J Surg.* 1977 Apr;64(4):264–266.
44. **Perez C, Huttner A, Assal M, et al.** Infectious olecranon and patellar bursitis: short-course adjuvant antibiotic therapy is not a risk factor for recurrence in adult hospitalized patients. *J Antimicrob Chemother.* 2010 May;65(5):1008–1014.
45. **Valeriano-Marcet J, Carter JD, Vasey FB.** Soft tissue disease. *Rheum Dis Clin North Am.* 2003 Feb;29(1):77–88.
46. **Beltran J.** MR imaging of soft-tissue infection. *Magn Reson Imaging Clin N Am.* 1995 Nov;3(4):743–751.
47. **Stell IM, Gransden WR.** Simple tests for septic bursitis: comparative study. *BMJ.* 1998 Jun;316(7148):1877.
48. **Baumbach SF, Lobo CM, Badyine I, et al.** Prepatellar and olecranon bursitis: literature review and development of a treatment algorithm. *Arch Orthop Trauma Surg.* 2014 Mar;134(3):359–370.
49. **Aaron DL, Patel A, Kayiaros S, et al.** Four common types of bursitis: diagnosis and management. *J Am Acad Orthop Surg.* 2011 Jun;19(6):359–367.
50. **Brennan TA, Leape LL, Laird NM, et al.** Incidence of adverse events and negligence in hospitalized patients. Results of the Harvard Medical Practice Study I. *N Engl J Med.* 1991 Feb 7;324(6):370–376.
51. **Mangram AJ, Horan TC, Pearson ML, et al.** Guideline for prevention of surgical site infection, 1999. Hospital Infection Control Practices Advisory Committee. *Infect Control Hosp Epidemiol.*1999 Apr;20(4):250–278; quiz 79–80.
52. **Emori TG, Gaynes RP.** An overview of nosocomial infections, including the role of the microbiology laboratory. *Clin Micribiol Rev.* 1993 Oct;6(4):428–442.
53. **Gaynes RP, Culver DH, Horan TC, et al.** Surgical site infection (SSI) rates in the United States, 1992-1998: the National Nosocomial Infections Surveillance System basic SSI risk index. *Clin Infect Dis.* 2001 Sep;33 Suppl 2:S69–77.
54. **Cooper RA.** Surgical site infections: epidemiology and microbiological aspects in trauma and orthopaedic surgery. *Int Wound J.* 2013 Dec;10 Suppl 1:3–8.
55. **Horan TC, Gaynes RP, Martone WJ, et al.** CDC definitions of nosocomial surgical site infections, 1992: a modification of CDC definitions of surgical wound infections. *Infect Control Hosp Epidemiol.* 1992 Oct;13(10):606–608.
56. **Cruse PJ, Foord R.** The epidemiology of wound infection. A 10-year prospective study of 62,939 wounds. *Surg Clin North Am.* 1980 Feb;60(1):27–40.
57. **National Nosocomial Infections Surveillance System.** National Nosocomial Infections Surveillance (NNIS) System Report, data summary from January 1992 through June 2004, issued October 2004. *Am J Infect Control.* 2004 Dec;32(8):470–485.
58. **Wilson AP, Treasure T, Sturridge MF, et al.** A scoring method (ASEPSIS) for postoperative wound infections for use in clinical trials of antibiotic prophylaxis. *Lancet.* 1986 Feb;1(8476):311–313.
59. **Bailey IS, Karran SE, Toyn K, et al.** Community surveillance of complications after hernia surgery. *BMJ.* 1992 Feb;304(6825):469–471.
60. **Huizinga WK, Kritzinger NA, Bhamjee A.** The value of adjuvant systemic antibiotic therapy in localised wound infections among hospital patients: a comparative study. *J Infect.* 1986 Jul;13(1):11–16.
61. **Paydar KZ, Hansen SL, Charlebois ED, et al.** Inappropriate antibiotic use in soft tissue infections. *Arch Surg.* 2006 Sep;141(9):850–854; discussion 5–6.
62. **Rajendran PM, Young D, Maurer T, et al.** Randomized, double-blind, placebo-controlled trial of cephalexin for treatment of uncomplicated skin abscesses in a population at risk for community-acquired methicillin-resistant Staphylococcus aureus infection. *Antimicrob Agents Chemother.* 2007 Nov;51(11):4044–4048.
63. **Bobrow BJ, Pollack CV Jr, Gamble S, et al.** Incision and drainage of cutaneous abscesses is not associated with bacteremia in afebrile adults. *Ann Emerg Med.* 1997 Mar;29(3):404–408.
64. **Whitehouse JD, Friedman ND, Kirkland KB, et al.** The impact of surgical-site infections following orthopedic surgery at a community hospital and a university hospital: adverse quality of life, excess length of stay, and extra cost. *Infect Control Hosp Epidemiol.* 2002 Apr;23(4):183–189.
65. **Uçkay I, Hoffmeyer P, Lew D, et al.** Prevention of surgical site infections in orthopaedic surgery and bone trauma: state-of-the-art update. *J Hosp Infect.* 2013 May;84(1):5–12.
66. **Matar WY, Jafari SM, Restrepo C, et al.** Preventing infection in total joint arthroplasty. *J Bone Joint Surg Am.* 2010 Dec;92 Suppl 2:36–46.
67. **Meehan J, Jamali AA, Nguyen H.** Prophylactic antibiotics in hip and knee arthroplasty. *J Bone Joint Surg Am.* 2009 Oct;91(10):2480–2490.
68. **Abrahamian FM, Goldstein EJ.** Microbiology of animal bite wound infections. *Clin Microbiol Rev.* 2011 Apr;24(2):231–246.
69. **Rea WJ, Wyrick WJ Jr.** Necrotizing fasciitis. *Ann Surg.* 1970 Dec;172(6):957–964.
70. **Angoules AG, Kontakis G, Drakoulakis E, et al.** Necrotising fasciitis of upper and lower limb: a systematic review. *Injury.* 2007 Dec;38 Suppl 5:S19–26.
71. **Tang WM, Ho PL, Fung KK, et al.** Necrotising fasciitis of a limb. *J Bone Joint Surg Br.* 2001 Jul;83(5):709–714.
72. **Trent JT, Kirsner RS.** Diagnosing necrotizing fasciitis. *Adv Skin Wound Care.* 2002;15(3):135–138.
73. **Ahrenholz DH.** Necrotizing soft-tissue infections. *Surg Clin North Am.*1988 Feb;68(1):199–214.
74. **Lewis RT.** Necrotizing soft-tissue infections. *Infect Dis Clin North Am.* 1992 Sep;6(3):693–703.
75. **Wilson B.** Necrotizing fasciitis. *Am Surg.* 1952 Apr;18(4):416–431.
76. **Dellinger EP.** Severe necrotizing soft-tissue infections. Multiple disease entities requiring a common approach. *JAMA.* 1981 Oct 9;246(15):1717–1721.
77. **Anaya DA, Dellinger EP.** Necrotizing soft-tissue infection: diagnosis and management. *Clin Infect Dis.* 2007 Mar 1;44(5):705–710.
78. **Bellapianta JM, Ljungquist K, Tobin E, et al.** Necrotizing fasciitis. *J Am Acad Orthop Surg.* 2009 Mar;17(3):174–182.
79. **Friederichs J, Torka S, Militz M, et al.** Necrotizing soft tissue infections after injection therapy: Higher mortality and worse outcome compared to other entry mechanisms. *J Infect.* 2015 Sep;71(3):312–316.
80. **Mulla ZD.** Treatment options in the management of necrotising fasciitis caused by Group A Streptococcus. *Expert Opinion Pharmacother.* 2004 Aug;5(8):1695–1700.
81. **Dufel S, Martino M.** Simple cellulitis or a more serious infection? *J Fam Pract.* 2006 May;55(5):396–400.
82. **Goh T, Goh LG, Ang CH, et al.** Early diagnosis of necrotizing fasciitis. *Br J Surg.* 2014 Jan;101(1):e119–125.
83. **Giuliano A, Lewis F Jr, Hadley K, et al.** Bacteriology of necrotizing fasciitis. *Am J Surg.* 1977 Jul;134(1):52–57.
84. **Simonart T.** Group a beta-haemolytic streptococcal necrotising fasciitis: early diagnosis and clinical features. *Dermatology.* 2004;208(1):5–9.

85. **Wong CH, Chang HC, Pasupathy S, et al.** Necrotizing fasciitis: clinical presentation, microbiology, and determinants of mortality. *J Bone Joint Surg Am.* 2003 Aug;85-A(8):1454–1460.
86. **Kihiczak GG, Schwartz RA, Kapila R.** Necrotizing fasciitis: a deadly infection. *J Eur Acad Dermatol Venereol.* 2006 Apr;20(4):365–369.
87. **Kaul R, McGeer A, Low DE, et al.** Population-based surveillance for group A streptococcal necrotizing fasciitis: clinical features, prognostic indicators, and microbiologic analysis of seventy-seven cases. Ontario Group A Streptococcal Study. *Am J Med.*1997;103(1):18–24.
88. **Rodriguez RM, Abdullah R, Miller R, et al.** A pilot study of cytokine levels and white blood cell counts in the diagnosis of necrotizing fasciitis. *Am J Emerg Med.* 2006 Jan;24(1):58–61.
89. **Young MH, Aronoff DM, Engleberg NC.** Necrotizing fasciitis: pathogenesis and treatment. *Exp Rev Anti Infect Ther.* 2005 Apr;3(2):279–294.
90. **Wong CH, Wang YS.** The diagnosis of necrotizing fasciitis. *Curr Opin Infect Dis.* 2005 Apr;18(2):101–106.
91. **Friederichs J, Hutter M, Hierholzer C, et al.** Procalcitonin ratio as a predictor of successful surgical treatment of severe necrotizing soft tissue infections. *Am J Surg.* 2013 Sep;206(3):368–373.
92. **Fisher JR, Conway MJ, Takeshita RT, et al.** Necrotizing fasciitis. Importance of roentgenographic studies for soft-tissue gas. *JAMA.* 1979 Feb 23;241(8):803–806.
93. **Brooklyn T, Dunnill G, Probert C.** Diagnosis and treatment of pyoderma gangrenosum. *BMJ.* 2006 Jul 22;333(7560):181–184.
94. **Lappin E, Ferguson AJ.** Gram-positive toxic shock syndromes. *Lancet Infect Dis.* 2009 May;9(5):281–290.
95. **Willy C, Rieger H, Vogt D.** [Hyperbaric oxygen therapy for necrotizing soft tissue infections: contra]. *Chirurg.* 2012 Nov;83(11):960–972. German.
96. **Edlich RF, Cross CL, Dahlstrom JJ, et al.** Modern concepts of the diagnosis and treatment of necrotizing fasciitis. *J Emerg Med.* 2010 Aug;39(2):261–265.
97. **Massey PR, Sakran JV, Mills AM, et al.** Hyperbaric oxygen therapy in necrotizing soft tissue infections. *J Surg Res.* 2012 Sep;177(1):146–151.

14 Open wounds

Jorge Daniel Barla, Luciano Rossi, Yoav Rosenthal, Steven Velkes

1 Basics

A wound is a disruption of the normal structure and function of the skin and underlying soft tissue [1]. Wounds are generally classified as acute or chronic. Acute wounds normally heal through an orderly sequence of physiological events that include hemostasis, inflammation, epithelialization, fibroplasia, and maturation [2]. When this process is altered, impeded, or delayed, a chronic wound may develop.

1.1 Phases of wound healing

1.1.1 Inflammation

This phase is characterized by increased vascular permeability and cellular recruitment. Macrophages and stromal mast cells release vasoactive substances that stimulate the chemotaxis of macrophages and polymorphonuclear leukocytes that digest bacteria, foreign debris, and necrotic tissue [3]. The healing progression of chronic wounds is usually arrested in this inflammatory stage.

1.1.2 Migration

Migration or epithelialization refers to basal cell proliferation and epithelial migration occurring in the fibrin bridgework inside a clot [4]. Migration ceases when the layer is replaced; this is normally completed within 48 hours of surgery. The superficial layer of epithelium forms a barrier to bacteria and other foreign bodies. The process of epithelialization is difficult in wounds that are not primarily closed, and may instead heal by secondary intention. In these wounds, the physical distance of epithelial migration is increased across the length and width and depth of the wound.

1.1.3 Fibroplasia

Fibroplasia consists of fibroblast proliferation, accumulation of ground substance, and collagen production [5].

Fibroblasts also synthesize collagen, the primary structural protein of the body. Maximum collagen production begins on day 5 and continues for at least 6 weeks [6]. The developing collagen matrix stimulates angiogenesis. Granulation tissue is the result of the combined production of collagen and growth of capillaries. This exuberant scarring may impede normal organ function or, in the case of skin, may result in keloid formation.

1.1.4 Maturation

Key elements of maturation include collagen cross-linking, collagen remodeling, wound contraction, and repigmentation. As disorganized collagen is degraded and reformed, covalent cross-links are formed that enhance tensile strength [7].

1.2 Complications in wound healing

Following initial successful surgical skin closure, wound dehiscence may result from disruption of the sutured skin, which can be due to technical error, injury, infection, or the presence of foreign material within the wound.

1.3 Risk factors for nonhealing

There are many factors described that can affect wound healing (**Table 14-1**) [8–11]. The most common nonhealing wounds affecting the lower extremities are associated with peripheral artery disease, diabetes, and chronic venous insufficiency [8, 9].

2 Clinical assessment

Any patient with a wound or ulceration should undergo a complete medical history and physical examination. Wound assessment should include:

- Location and number of wounds
- Length, width, depth, and color
- Presence of cellulitis and drainage

Risk factor	Mechanism of action
Peripheral artery disease	Microvascular obstruction decreases arterial blood flow and diminishes the delivery of oxygen and nutrients to the tissues, and impairs removal of metabolic waste products [9, 10].
Diabetes	Multifactorial: vasculopathy, neuropathy, and immunopathy [9].
Chronic venous insufficiency	Congestion and pooling of blood in the superficial veins leads to venous hypertension which, if sustained, is associated with histological changes in the vein wall [12].
Aging	The supply of cutaneous nerves and blood vessels decreases with age, in addition to a general thinning of tissue including dermis and basement membrane. There is a loss of collagen and reduced ability to produce more collagen [13, 14].
Immunosuppressive therapy	Systemic immunosuppression is a risk factor for peripheral wound delay and nonhealing wounds [15, 16].
Sickle cell disease	Caused by dysmorphic red blood cells physically occluding small vessels and vascular shunting [17].
Chemotherapy	Detrimental effect on wound healing, specifically through its effects on vascular endothelial growth factor (VEGF) [19].
Radiation therapy	Irradiated skin in the chronic stage is thin, hypovascular, extremely painful, and easily injured by slight trauma or infection [20].
Spinal cord disease and immobilization	Typically pressure sores, occurring in areas of bony prominence, such as the sacrum, knees, ankle malleoli, and heels [21].
Malnutrition	Prealbumin and albumin should be obtained from patients with nonhealing wounds [22].
Infection	Bacteria produce inflammatory mediators that inhibit the inflammatory phase of wound healing and prevent epithelialization [23].
Smoking and nicotine replacement therapy	Multifactorial with mechanisms that include vasoconstriction causing a relative ischemia of operated tissues, a reduced inflammatory response, impaired bactericidal mechanisms, and alterations of collagen metabolism [24].

Table 14-1 Risk factors for nonhealing.

Symptoms and signs that could suggest the presence of significant infection and the need for hospitalization, intravenous antibiotics, and debridement treatment include:

- Induration, cellulitis extending > 2 cm beyond the wound margins
- Increased local temperature
- Pain on palpation and drainage from the site
- Increasing erythema/cellulitis of the surrounding skin
- Lymphangitis
- Increase in the size of the ulcer
- Large amount of drainage
- Fever

A thorough vascular examination should be performed, including palpation of the radial, femoral, and pedal pulses. Signs of arterial obstruction include lack of peripheral pulses with poor capillary refill, thin atrophic skin, and hypertrophic deformed nails.

Noninvasive diagnostic options for arterial assessment include the ankle-brachial index (results ≤ .9 represent abnormal findings) and Duplex ultrasonography. Noninvasive vascular testing should be performed in patients who present with a wound and have an abnormal pulse examination, and patients with a nonhealing extremity wound or ulcer.

2.1 Laboratory workup

Routine laboratory studies are performed to evaluate for active infection, anemia, nutritional status, and medical conditions that place the patient at risk for nonhealing wounds (**Table 14-1**):

- Complete blood count and differential
- Metabolic panel, liver function tests, albumin, prealbumin, hemoglobin A1c
- Prealbumin and albumin are not perfect markers of nutritional status, but should be evaluated for any patient with a nonhealing wound
- Wound cultures should only be obtained if cellulitis is suspected to help guide antibiotic therapy. If a culture is indicated, the sample should be obtained after a wound has been thoroughly cleansed and debrided [25, 26]

2.2 Differentiation of chronic ulcers

Characteristic clinical location and appearance usually allows for clear distinction between ischemic, venous, and neuropathic ulcers (**Table 14-2**).

Ischemic ulcers

- Pathophysiology: inadequate perfusion due to arterial obstruction
- Obstruction may be caused by atherosclerosis affecting the large or medium arteries, or from other disorders that affect the small vessels (eg, thromboangiitis obliterans or Buerger's disease, vasculitis, scleroderma)
- Pain in the extremity at rest, and increased pain with elevation of the extremity and activity. Pain may be localized to the ulcer or more generalized to the foot
- Location over prominent osseous areas and other areas where there is a potential for pressure and skin shearing including between the toes, on the tips of toes, over phalangeal tufts, at the lateral malleolus

Venous ulcers

- Most common type
- Predisposing factors: deep vein thrombosis and venous valvular incompetence. Medial and lateral malleoli are the most common sites
- Periwound skin: is often eczematous, presenting with erythema, scaling, weeping, and crusting
- Intense pruritus in the region
- Hyperpigmentation and stasis dermatitis of the surrounding skin. Frequently red with granulation tissue
- Calcification in wound base is common

Pressure ulcers

- Pressure ulcers are areas of necrosis and ulceration where soft-tissue structures are compressed between osseous prominences or hard external surfaces
- Ulcer severity ranges from nonblanchable skin erythema (stage I) to full-thickness skin loss with extensive soft-tissue necrosis (stage III) and full-thickness skin/muscle necrosis with exposed structures, such as muscle, tendon, and bone (stage IV). The diagnosis is clinical
- Location over osseous prominences including the medial and lateral metatarsal heads, calcaneus, ischial tuberosities, greater trochanter, fibular head, and sacrum
- Fibrotic tissue including necrotic eschar
- Deep probing to the level of bone and undermining of skin edges
- Surrounding periwound erythema

Diabetic neuropathic ulcers

- Multifactorial: diabetic neuropathy, autonomic dysfunction, and vascular insufficiency
- Characteristics of neuropathic diabetic ulcers include:
  - Location at areas of repeated trauma, such as the plantar metatarsal heads or dorsal interphalangeal joints
  - Overgrowth of hyperkeratotic tissue (corns or calluses) on other regions of the foot. Hyperkeratotic callous formation may imply adequate vascularity
  - Undermined borders
  - Lack of sensation

Malignant ulcers

- Tumors can present with features similar to chronic wounds, and may not be easily distinguished from a venous ulcer
- Skin biopsy should be considered in any nonischemic wound that does not demonstrate signs of healing after approximately 3 months of treatment [28]

Hypertensive ulcers

- Uncommon and can be easily confused with other types of chronic ulcers
- Pathophysiology: calcification that obliterates small arterioles similar to calcific uremic arteriolopathy [29]
- The typical hypertensive ulcer is located in the supramalleolar region of the anterolateral leg or Achilles tendon. Bilateral ulcers are common. These are associated with arterial hypertension in patients with perceptible pulses
- The reduction in tissue perfusion leads to local ischemia and ulcer formation. The ulcer begins as a red patch which becomes cyanotic, forming a painful ulcer with an ischemic wound bed
- Management consists of controlling hypertension and local wound care

Table 14-2 Chronic ulcers.

3 Wound management

3.1 Initial management

Irrigation and debridement—wounds that have devitalized tissue, contamination, or residual suture material require debridement before further wound management. These materials impede the body's attempt to heal by stimulating the production of abnormal metalloproteases and consuming the local resources necessary for healing [30].

Irrigation helps to decrease the bacterial load and remove loose material, and should be a part of routine wound management [31]. Warm, isotonic (normal) saline is typically used at low pressure. The addition of dilute iodine or other antiseptic solutions (eg, chlorhexidine and hydrogen peroxide) is generally unnecessary. These solutions have minimal effect against bacteria and could potentially impede wound healing through toxic effects on normal tissue (see chapter 6 Local delivery of antibiotics and antiseptics for additional information) [32]. Low pressure irrigation is usually adequate to remove material from the surface of most wounds. Removing large areas of necrotic tissue is indicated whenever there is any evidence of infection (ie, cellulitis, sepsis). Surgical debridement is also indicated in the management of chronic nonhealing wounds to remove infectious debris, handle undermined wound edges, or obtain deep tissue for culture and pathology [33]. Serial surgical debridement in a clinical setting, when appropriate, appears to be associated with an increased likelihood of healing [34].

3.2 Topical therapy

Growth factors—use of growth factors important for wound healing includes platelet-derived growth factor (PDGF), fibroblast growth factor, and granulocyte-macrophage colony stimulating factor (GM-CSF):

- Platelet-derived growth factor: platelet-derived growth factor is a gel preparation that promotes cellular proliferation and angiogenesis, and thereby improves wound healing [35]. It is indicated for noninfected diabetic foot ulcers that extend into the subcutaneous tissue and have an adequate vascular supply [35].
- Epidermal growth factor: topical application of human recombinant epidermal growth factor was associated with a greater reduction in ulcer size and higher ulcerhealing rate compared with placebo [36].
- Granulocyte-macrophage colony stimulating factor—intradermal injections of GM-CSF promote healing of chronic leg ulcers, including venous ulcers [37].

3.3 Wound dressings

The dressing can have a significant impact on the speed of wound healing [38].

Some general principles for chronic wound management are [39]:

- Hydrogels for the debridement stage
- Foam and low-adherence dressings for the granulation stage
- Hydrocolloid and low-adherence dressings for the epithelialization stage
- Human studies showed that moist wounds heal more rapidly compared with dry wounds [38]

Acute wound fluid is rich in platelet-derived growth factor, basic fibroblast growth factor, and has a balance of metalloproteases serving a matrix custodial function [40]. In addition to faster wound healing, wounds treated with occlusive dressings are associated with less prominent scar formation [41].

Dressings can be classified by their water-retaining abilities as open, semiopen, or semiocclusive (**Table 14-3**).

Open dressings	Gauze is typically moistened with saline before placing it into the wound. Wet-to-moist gauze dressings are useful for packing large soft-tissue defects until wound closure or coverage can be performed. Advantage: • Inexpensive Disadvantage: • Require frequent dressing changes
Semiopen dressings	Typically consist of fine mesh gauze impregnated with petroleum, paraffin wax, or other ointment. This initial layer is covered by a secondary dressing of absorbent gauze and padding, then finally a third layer of tape or other method of adhesive. Advantage: • Low cost and ease of application Disadvantages: • Does not maintain a moisture-rich environment or provide good exudate control • Need for frequent changing
Semiocclusive dressings	Semiocclusive dressings include films, foams, alginates, hydrocolloids, and hydrogels.
Films	Polymer films are transparent sheets of synthetic self-adhesive dressing that are permeable to gases, such as water vapor and oxygen, but impermeable to larger molecules including proteins and bacteria. This property enables insensible water loss to evaporate, traps wound fluid enzymes within the dressing, and prevents bacterial invasion. Transparent film dressings were found to provide the fastest healing rates, lowest infection rates, and to be the most cost-effective method for dressing split-thickness skin graft donor site [42]. Advantages: • Ability to maintain moisture • Encourage rapid reepithelization • Transparency and self-adhesive properties Disadvantage: • Limited absorptive capacity
Foams	They consist of two layers: a hydrophilic silicone or polyurethane-based foam, which lies against the wound surface, and a hydrophobic, gas-permeable backing to prevent leakage and bacterial contamination [43]. Advantages: • Highly absorbent • Conform to the shape of the wound and can be used to pack cavities. Disadvantages: • Opacity of the dressings • Need to be changed each day
Alginates	Natural complex polysaccharides from various types of algae form the basis of alginate dressings. Their activity as dressings is unique because they are insoluble in water but in the sodium-rich wound fluid environment these complexes exchange calcium ions for sodium ions and form an amorphous gel that packs and covers the wound [44]. More appropriate for moderately to heavily exudative wounds. Advantages: • Augmentation of hemostasis • Can be washed away with normal saline to minimize pain during dressing changes • Can stay in place for several days Disadvantages: • Require secondary dressing that must be removed to monitor the wound • Unpleasant odor
Hydrocolloids	A gel or foam on a carrier of self-adhesive polyurethane film. The colloid composition of this dressing traps exudate and creates a moist environment. Bacteria and debris are also trapped, and washed away with dressing changes in a gentle, painless form of mechanical debridement. Advantage: • Ability to use them for packing wound Disadvantages: • Malodor • Potential need for daily dressing changes, and allergic contact dermatitis has been reported [45]
Hydrogels	A matrix of synthetic polymers with > 95% water formed into sheets, gels, or foams that are usually sandwiched between two sheets of removable film. The inner layer is placed against the wound, and the outer layer can be removed to make the dressing permeable to fluid. These unique matrices can absorb or donate water depending on the hydration state of the tissue that surrounds them. Hydrogels are most useful for dry wounds. Advantage: • They initially lower the temperature of the wound environment they cover, which provides cooling pain relief for some patients [46] Disadvantage: • They have been found to selectively permit gram-negative bacteria to proliferate [47]
Hydroactive	Polyurethane matrix that combines the properties of a gel and foam. Hydroactive selectively absorbs excess water while leaving growth factors and other proteins behind [48].

Table 14-3 Wound dressings.

4 Wound coverage

4.1 Skin grafts

Skin grafts are the most basic biological dressings and consist of skin taken from a donor site and grafted onto a wound on the same patient. Skin grafts are used for wound closure, to prevent fluid and electrolyte loss, and reduce bacterial burden and infection [49, 50].

4.2 Full-thickness skin grafts

Full-thickness skin grafts contain the epidermis and dermis, and thus retain more of the characteristics of normal skin, including color, texture, and thickness compared with split-thickness skin grafts. Full-thickness skin grafts are limited to relatively small, uncontaminated, well-vascularized wounds. The skin used for full-thickness skin grafts is obtained from areas of redundant and pliable skin, such as the groin, lateral thigh, lower abdomen, or lateral chest. Donor sites are usually closed primarily. The main disadvantages of full-thickness skin grafts include limited availability of donor skin and the potential for fluid accumulation beneath the graft [49, 50].

4.3 Split-thickness skin grafts

Split-thickness skin grafts are commonly used tissue for wound coverage.

Compared with full-thickness skin grafts, split-thickness skin grafts tolerate a less than ideal wound bed and have a broader range of applications. Split-thickness skin grafts can be meshed to provide coverage of a greater surface area at the recipient site, with expansion ratios generally ranging from 1:1 to 6:1. Split-thickness skin graft donor sites heal spontaneously with cells supplied by the remaining epidermal appendages. Donor sites can be reharvested once healing is complete.

Split-thickness grafts have disadvantages. They are more fragile, especially when placed over areas with little underlying soft-tissue bulk for support. Split-thickness grafts contract more during healing, do not grow with the individual, and tend to be smoother and shinier than normal skin because of the absence of skin appendages in the graft. They also tend to be abnormally pigmented, either pale or white, or alternatively, hyperpigmented, particularly in darker-skinned individuals. For these reasons, split-thickness skin grafts are more widely used for control of infection and prevention of fluid/electrolyte loss rather than cosmesis [51]. **Fig 14-1** is an example of a posttraumatic skin defect managed with a split-thickness skin graft.

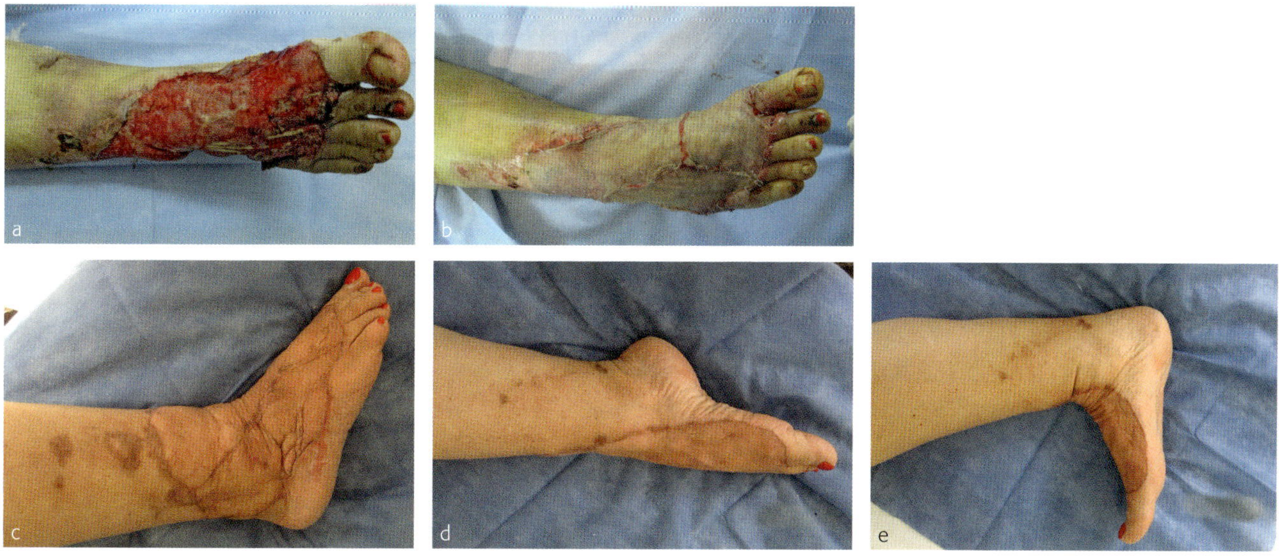

Fig 14-1a–e An example of a posttraumatic skin defect managed with a split-thickness skin graft.
a Preoperative image.
b Intraoperative image shows split-thickness skin graft.
c–e Postoperative images show a healed split-thickness skin graft on the dorsum of the foot and anterior ankle. The patient has regained excellent range of dorsi flexion and plantar flexion with this coverage technique.

4.4 Biological (cell-based dressings)

Biological (cell-based dressings) are composed of a live-cell construct that contains at least one layer of live allogenic cells.

Cell-based dressings can be used when traditional dressings have failed or are deemed inappropriate [52]. Cell-based dressings are ideal for the treatment of chronic ulcers because additional cells and growth factors are added to a deficient wound-healing environment. Accelerated wound healing reduces the risk of wound infection.

5 Adjunctive therapies

5.1 Hyperbaric oxygen therapy (HBOT)

This has been shown in vitro to have effects on wound healing [53, 54]. Endothelial progenitor cells play an important role in wound healing because they participate in the formation of new blood vessels in areas of hypoxia [53, 54]. Hyperbaric oxygen therapy may improve the survival of skin grafts and reconstructive flaps that have compromised blood flow, thereby preventing tissue breakdown and the development of wounds.

5.2 Flaps

High-energy trauma can be associated with severe soft-tissue injury. Wide areas of necrosis require aggressive debridement and lead to large defects that can require flap coverage. Besides using negative-pressure wound therapy (NPWT) as a temporary device, all the above-described available methods may not be suitable in this scenario. It is known that complete wound coverage before 1 week improves results, thus reducing complications like infection and bone healing [55, 56].

Depending on the type, size, and wound location, a local pediculated or a distant microvascularized flap may be used. Wounds associated with a fracture at the same level usually require a muscle flap followed by a split-thickness skin graft, skin plus subcutaneous tissue, or some combination of them [57–59]. A vascular evaluation must to be done prior to any flap. Angiography, computed tomographic angiography, and/or Doppler ultrasound can be used.

Fig 14-2 shows a large plantar defect secondary to an open calcaneal fracture treated with a sural flap. In **Fig 14-3** an open type IIIB tibial fracture managed using an anterolateral thigh flap is presented.

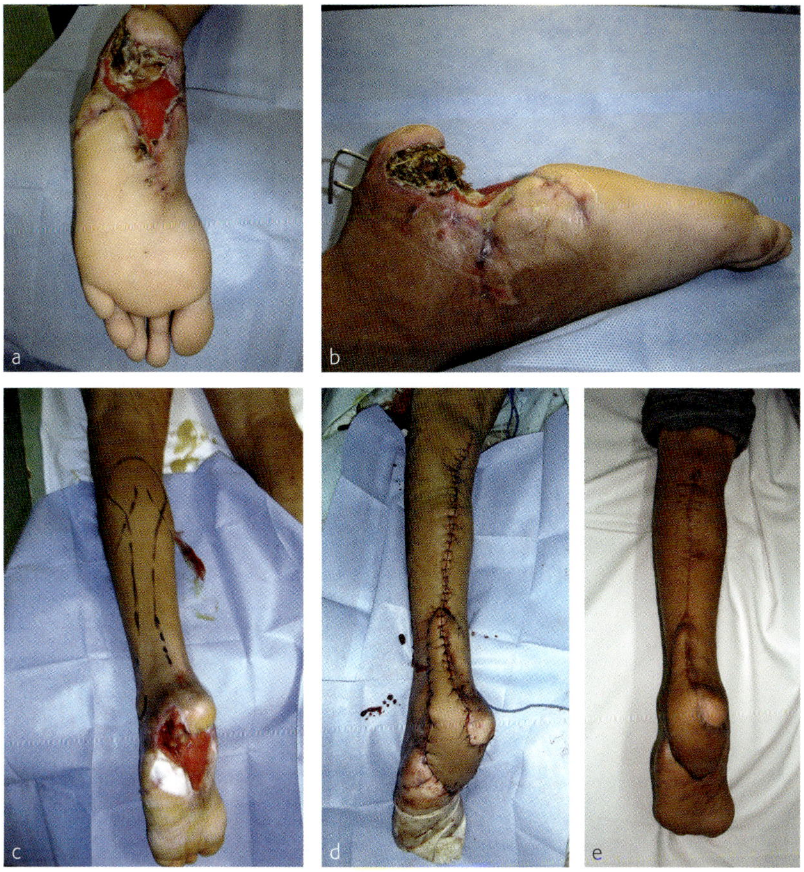

Fig 14-2a–e A large plantar defect secondary to an open calcaneal fracture treated with a sural flap.
a–b Preoperative images.
c Intraoperative image before sural flap coverage.
d Intraoperative image after sural flap coverage.
e Postoperative healing.

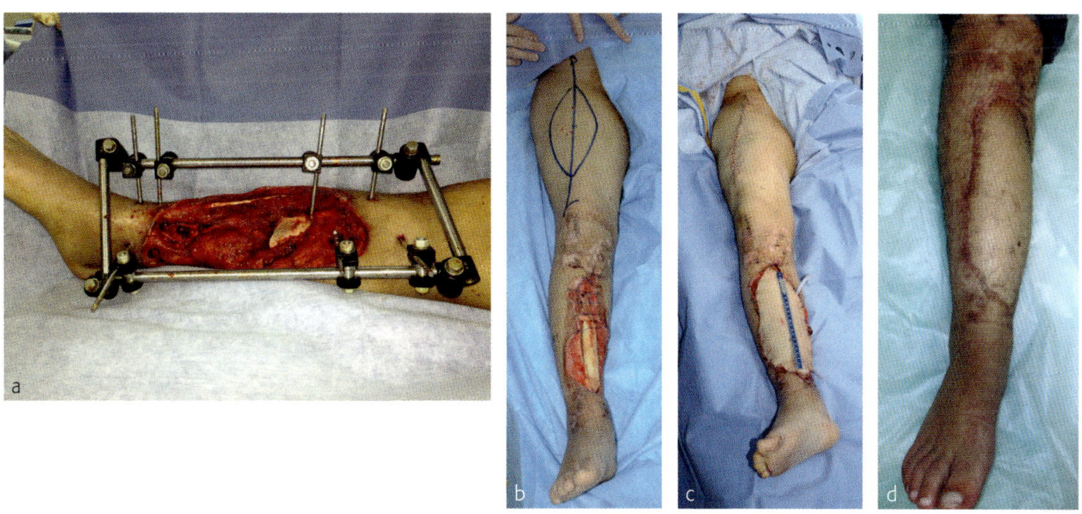

Fig 14-3a–d Open type IIIB tibial fracture managed using an anterolateral thigh flap.
a Preoperative image with external fixator.
b Intraoperative image showing marked out anterolateral thigh flap.
c Intraoperative image showing placement of anterolateral thigh flap.
d Postoperative healing.

6 Negative-pressure wound therapy for the treatment of open wounds

6.1 Introduction

Due to high rates of military and civilian trauma, physicians are often faced with challenging high-energy soft-tissue wounds and fractures, demanding complex surgical procedures. The aging population and the increasing prevalence of obesity and diabetes mellitus contribute to the rise in the incidence of chronic wounds that are becoming an increasing burden to our healthcare system. Better, cost-effective methods of closing difficult wounds efficiently will reduce the pain and amputation rates associated with these wounds [60].

Negative-pressure wound therapy has been used since 1940, but with the introduction of vacuum-assisted closure (VAC), a form of topical negative pressure, in 1996, it has gained increasing popularity [61]. This innovative method has improved and revolutionized wound care treatment. The technique involves an open cell-foam dressing put into the wound cavity, connecting it to a vacuum pump with a tube and covering it with an adhesive drape. A controlled continuous or intermittent subatmospheric pressure of 125 mm Hg is applied [62]. An illustrative case in **Fig 14-4** demonstrates the efficacy of NPWT to facilitate wound healing of an infection after removal of infected hardware.

Lower extremity wounds with exposed tendon, bone, or fixation device present a difficult treatment challenge. DeFranzo et al [63] showed greatly reduced tissue edema, diminished circumference of the extremity, and thus decreased wound's surface area by using NPWT. This method led to a profuse granulation tissue response that rapidly covered bone and hardware, allowing successful primary closure, without complications in roughly 95% of patients [63].

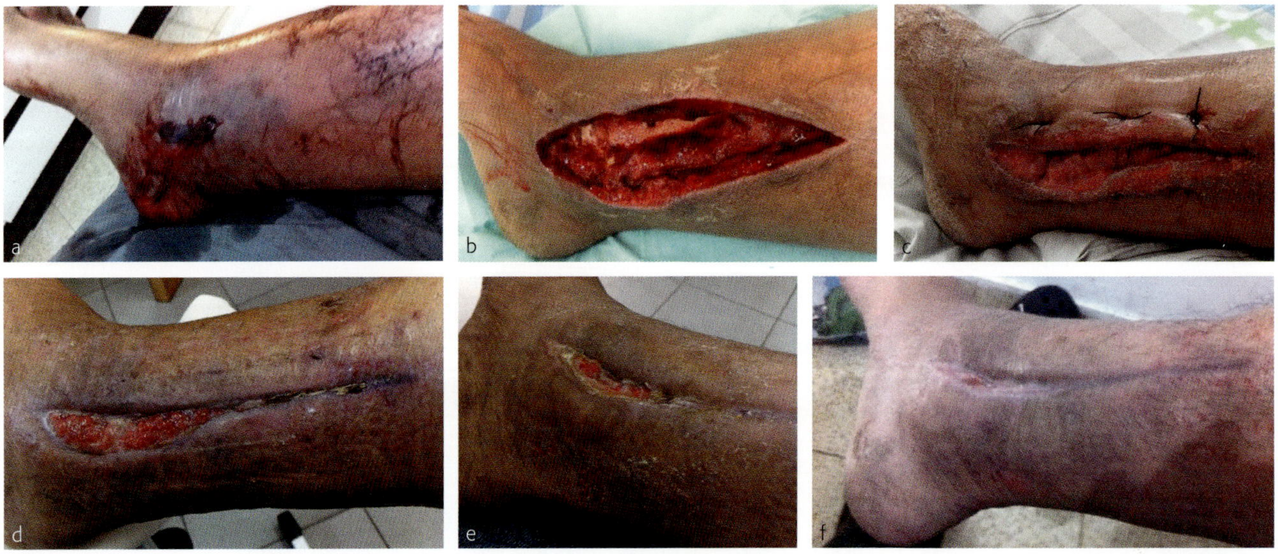

Fig 14-4a–f Clinical example: treatment of a surgical wound infection with a difficult wound closure. A 58-year-old man with diabetes was admitted with a closed distal metaphyseal fracture of the tibia. He underwent open reduction and internal fixation with a plate.

a–b Six months later he developed a wound infection (**a**) that was treated with surgical incision, drainage and implant removal (**b**). His wound was treated with three cycles of negative-pressure wound therapy (NPWT) dressings.

c He then underwent approximation of the edges of the wound using nylon sutures.

d Following closure, he had three additional cycles of NPWT.

e–f This was followed by local dressing till secondary closure that was achieved within a few weeks.

6.2 Mechanism of action

Negative-pressure wound therapy facilitates wound healing through multiple mechanisms of action both at the macroscopic and microscopic levels. There are four primary mechanisms of action of the NPWT device described in the literature:

- Contraction of the wound (macrodeformation): maintaining approximation of tissues during wound healing allows earlier closure by delayed primary or secondary granulation. The open-pore polyurethane foam that is used with the NPWT device efficiently transmits pressure and evacuates exudates. For deformable wounds, cutting the foam in a strategic fashion will facilitate wound closure by allowing the wound edges to come together more quickly [60, 64].
- Stabilization of the wound environment: NPWT provides an isolated, warm, and moist environment. The NPWT device uses a semiocclusive polyurethane drape that has limited permeability to gases and water vapor and impermeability to proteins and microorganisms. The dressing is typically changed every 2–3 days, which eliminates the discomfort of the daily dressing changes typically associated with traditional gauze-based dressings [60, 64].
- Removal of extracellular fluid: edema impedes healing and thus elevation and compression of extremities to decrease edema and facilitate healing is recommended. Application of a distributed suction allows evacuation of fluid directly from the extracellular space and appears to decrease edema. Furthermore, it assists by removing inflammatory mediators and cytokines [60, 64].
- Microdeformation at the foam-wound interface: computer models have shown that NPWT produces 5–20% strain across the healing tissues. In vivo models showed stimulation of wound healing through promotion of cell division and proliferation, growth factor production, and angiogenesis [65].

Wang et al [66] showed that NPWT significantly increased the expression of ICAM-1, MIF, VEGF and collagen I and therefore, indicate that NPWT therapy is an effective method for treating severe traumatic wounds, as it increases the expression of cytokines in wounds. Furthermore, studies have shown that a controlled subatmospheric pressure of 125 mmHg to porcine wounds increased blood flow in the area fourfold and bacteria levels decreased significantly in four days [67].

There are six secondary effects:

- Speed of wound healing: Eginton et al [68] witnessed a significant reduction of wound volume by using NPWT in comparison with normal saline dressings. Furthermore, microscopic analysis of wound cross-sections showed a significant increase in the granulation tissue amount per wound unit length in NPWT-treated compared with occlusive dressings [69–71]. However, the Cochrane review [68] found no evidence to support the effectiveness of NPWT to reduce time to complete healing.
- Granulation tissue formation: the application of NPWT results in an impressive granulation tissue response. This may be contributed to by microdeformation, which induces localized hypoxia near the wound surface that upregulates the HIF-1α-VEGF pathway [60, 72].
- Cell proliferation: at least three of the primary mechanisms are likely to contribute to proliferation, including microdeformation, fluid removal, and maintenance of a warm and moist wound environment [60, 72].
- Modulation of inflammation: mast cells, for example, play an important role in wound healing, as in mast cell-deficient mice, granulation tissue response has been shown to be muted, suggesting that mast cells are critical for NPWT success [73].
- Change in neuropeptides: NPWT resulted in a significant increase in dermal and epidermal nerve fiber densities and in substance P, calcitonin gene-related peptide, and nerve growth factor expression was seen in NPWT-treated wounds, suggesting that NPWT can modulate nerve fiber and neuropeptide production in the wound [69].
- Change in bacterial levels: reducing the bacterial loads of a wound improves its healing capacity because the body can then concentrate on healing rather than fighting an invasion by bacteria, virus, or yeast. Various studies have shown both increased and decreased bacterial levels following the use of NPWT. For instance, Moues et al [70] compared NPWT to moist gauze dressings in 54 patients and found stable bacterial load in both groups. However, nonfermentative gram-negative bacilli showed a significant decrease in NPWT-treated wounds, whereas *Staphylococcus aureus* showed a significant increase in NPWT-treated wounds.

6.3 Indications and contraindications

Meeting the correct indications and avoiding the contraindications is crucial for usage of NPWT. Before the application of NPWT, the patient and wound must be assessed for the appropriateness of the treatment. In 1995 the US Federal Drug Administration (FDA) approved VAC for NPWT for the treatment of nonhealing wounds and expanded the indications in 2000 to include chronic, acute, traumatic and subacute wounds, flaps, and grafts (**Table 14-4**) [74].

6.4 Utilization of NPWT in the setting of acute orthopedic trauma

Regardless of the use of NPWT, the primary surgical treatment of an open fracture must always begin with thorough debridement and stabilization of the fracture before addressing the soft-tissue defects [75].

Parrett et al [76] examined the trends in the management of soft-tissue injuries in open tibial fractures. They demonstrated a change in practice with a trend down the reconstructive ladder. In 1997, the authors began using NPWT and now use it in nearly half of all open fractures. On the other hand, they use fewer free flaps. Despite this trend, there has been no change in infection, amputation, or malunion/nonunion rates and a decrease in reoperation rate with at least 1-year follow-up [76].

DeFranzo et al [63] reported 100% closure rates of challenging wounds (eg, over exposed bones, tendons, or implants) with use of NPWT.

Indications
• Chronic wounds • Acute wounds • Traumatic wounds (soft-tissue injuries) • Infected wounds (necrotizing fasciitis) • Subacute wounds • Dehisced wounds • Partial-thickness burns • Ulcers and pressure sores • Flaps and grafts
Contraindications
• Wounds with necrotic tissue • Untreated osteomyelitis • Fistulas to organs or body cavities • Placement directly over exposed veins, arteries, or nerves • Malignancy within the wound • Sensitivity to silver (in the case of silver impregnated dressings only)

Table 14-4 Indications and contraindications for the use of negative-pressure wound therapy.

Stannard et al [77] ran two parallel studies regarding the efficacy of NPWT. The first study was an evaluation of the use of NPWT to assist in evacuation of a draining hematoma and in closure of the surgical incision. The group found that NPWT reduced the hematoma draining time and infection rate by nearly half (from 3.1 to 1.6 days). The second study was an evaluation of NPWT as an adjunct to healing of surgical incisions after fractures that are at high risk for wound-healing problems (ie, patients with one of three high-risk fractures after high-energy trauma—calcaneus, pilon, and Schatzker IV through VI tibial plateau fractures). Again, draining time was significantly reduced but not the infection rate.

In a different study [78], the same authors investigated 263 trauma patients with one of three high-risk fracture types (tibial plateau, pilon, calcaneal) requiring surgical stabilization and showed a decreased incidence of wound dehiscence and total infections after high-risk fractures when patients have NPWT applied to their surgical incisions after closure in comparison with standard postoperative dressings.

Labler and Trentz [79] examined 13 patients with traumatic pelvic injuries and concluded that the application of NPWT as temporary coverage of large-tissue defects in pelvic regions supports wound conditioning and facilitates the definitive wound closure.

Another study was conducted in the Himalayan Institute of Medical Sciences by Sinha et al [80], involving 30 patients with open musculoskeletal injuries in extremities requiring coverage procedures. The authors compared NPWT with standard saline dressings and found the following:

- There was significant decrease in wound size from day 0 to day 8 in the NPWT group compared with the saline group.
- There was significant decrease in the bacterial growth in the NPWT group compared with the saline group.

However, Dedmond et al [81] examined 50 grade III open tibial shaft fractures, which did not show NPWT superiority in reducing infection and nonunion rates compared with historical controls, but concluded that this technique may be beneficial in decreasing the need for free tissue transfer or rotational muscle flap coverage.

Negative-pressure wound therapy is being widely used and is supported for use for a range of surgical applications. However, there is no evidence to support or refute the effectiveness of NPWT to improve healing rates or to reduce time to complete healing from a large-scaled Cochrane review, examining five studies, following 280 patients [82].

In the case of pediatric patients, Halvorson et al [83] compared the use of NPWT with historical controls, and concluded that the use of NPWT therapy for pediatric open fractures in various locations appears to be an equally safe and effective modality to help reduce infection in pediatric open fractures.

6.5 Tips and precautions

Preventive measures include [72]:

- Negative-pressure wound therapy is not a substitute for adequate debridement or reconstructive techniques, such as a skin graft or flap.
- Placing only one piece of foam into a single wound, when possible, is highly recommended. If more than one piece of foam is placed, physicians and nurses should carefully document the number of foam pieces placed to reduce the chance of a forgotten piece.
- Due to some case reports of bleeding while using NPWT, when placing NPWT over blood vessels or organs, a nonadherent dressing or a thick layer of tissue should cover the vessels or organ to reduce the risk of bleeding. Furthermore, care must be taken when using NPWT immediately after a large debridement or when a patient is receiving anticoagulation therapy.
- When the clinician anticipates wound adhesion to the dressing, a wound contact layer can be placed under the wound. The use of a nonadherent wound contact layer prevents the growth of tissue into foam, thus facilitating dressing changes, although this may slightly reduce the formation of granulation tissue.
- Another strategy to reduce the degree of wound-bed adhesion is by increasing the frequency of dressing changes, thus reducing the pain during dressing changes. Another frequently used method is to instill saline into the wound through the wound filler 15–30 minutes before gently removing the dressing [84].

6.6 Evaluation of treatment

Regular review progress is essential, especially with an accurate and reproducible method of wound measurement. As long as there is a substantial reduction in wound area after 1 or 2 weeks, continuation of NPWT is strongly indicated with frequent reassessments. However, if improvement has ceased, NPWT ought to be discontinued.

In chronic wounds, an effective general assessment measure is to assess the:

- Wound margins for inflammation after the first application of NPWT therapy. Increased inflammation may be an indication for treatment discontinuation.
- Wound margins for a thin white epithelium after the second and subsequent applications, which indicates healing.
- Overall appearance of the wound bed. A beefy, granular appearance is a positive outcome, while a dusky bed indicates inadequate tissue perfusion. Granulation tissue should increase by around 3–5% per day.

6.7 Complications of NPWT

Although the introduction of NPWT was a breakthrough in wound management and has significantly improved wound healing, no method is perfect, and NPWT is no exception; complications are infrequent but can be serious. These include pain, trauma, or skin damage, bleeding, infection, anxiety, impaired quality of life, and malnutrition [85].

6.7.1 Pain

In addition to the effects on a patient's well-being, high levels of pain have also been linked to delayed healing and therefore prolonged treatment [86]. Patients treated with NPWT encounter pain, particularly during start-up suction and dressing removal [87]. Webster et al [82] reported that pain levels were lower in patients who received hospital-based NPWT in comparison to patients who had commercial NPWT closure.

6.7.2 Trauma or skin damage

This may occur when tissue grows into the foam on the dressing. One trial [84] has encountered a high incidence of fracture blisters in the NPWT group (62.5%) compared with the standard dressing group (8.3%).

Bleeding has been reported in some studies of NPWT, but the number of cases is small [86].

6.7.3 Infection

Clinically, NPWT powered by continuous electricity-removed exudate kept the wound clean and facilitated wound healing. When power was off, sponges covering the wound were foreign and acted as the source of infection. If the sponges fell out of place, the wound bed was open to the environment and the risk of infection increased. This does not seem to be the case in central negative pressure [85].

6.7.4 Anxiety

It has been found that the stress associated with wound dressing-change pain, or with the anticipation of pain, can be related to delayed wound healing [88]. Patients receiving NWPT experienced significantly increased anxiety scores in comparison with those receiving standard treatment [89].

6.7.5 Quality of life

Whether NPWT improves or hurts a patient's quality of life is controversial and studies vary between benefit and impairment. The treatment powered by central negative pressure or a portable machine may limit the activities of patients. Other decreases in quality of life included poor appetite, sleep problems, and even a change of cognitive status [85].

6.7.6 Malnutrition

Exudates extracted from patients with an open abdomen or soft-tissue wounds treated with NPWT comprise a significant loss of protein, which should be considered when assessing protein requirements. Immunoglobulins and electrolytes losses were noted as well [90].

6.8 Cost-effectiveness

The cost-effectiveness was inspected in a few trials that concluded the following: usage of NPWT results in reduction in consumption of nursing time; reduction in pain scores (after week 5 of treatment); reduction in complexity and number of surgical procedures/adverse events; reduction in length of treatment and hospital stay/number of hospitalizations; reduction of total wound care cost; improved comfort for the patient and nurses; and improvement in clinical outcome [61, 71, 91].

The daily cost of NPWT was compared with a negative-pressure system developed in the hospital. The mean cost to supply equipment for NPWT therapy was nearly 25 times more expensive than the latter. For those who cannot afford the expense of hiring the equipment required for NPWT, using the hospital's aspiration system to achieve negative pressure is probably as safe as NPWT. There are clear cost benefits when noncommercial systems are used to create the negative pressure required for wound therapy, with no reduction in clinical outcome [82].

7 Conclusion

Open wounds represent a significant challenge to the managing clinicians. It is essential to perform a thorough assessment of the nature and etiology of the open wound and to thoroughly comprehend comorbidities that may complicate its healing. There are many therapies available to manage the open wound. A comprehensive approach to the problem is needed. In some cases, the wound can be managed with local wound care, whereas in other cases more aggressive interventions including hyperbaric oxygen therapy, NPWT, or surgical treatment may be required. In many cases, frequent assessments and a multidisciplinary approach to the problem will prove beneficial to the patient.

8 References

1. **Atiyeh BS, Ioannovich J, Al-Amm CA, et al.** Management of acute and chronic open wounds: the importance of moist environment in optimal wound healing. *Curr Pharm Biotechnol.* 2002 Sep;3(3):179–195.
2. **Schultz GS, Sibbald RG, Falanga V, et al.** Wound bed preparation: a systematic approach to wound management. *Wound Repair Regen.* 2003 Mar;11 Suppl 1:S1–28.
3. **Diegelmann RF, Evans MC.** Wound healing: an overview of acute, fibrotic and delayed healing. *Front Biosci.* 2004 Jan 1;9:283–289.
4. **Darby IA, Hewitson TD.** Fibroblast differentiation in wound healing and fibrosis. *Int Rev Cytol.* 2007;257:143–179.
5. **Doillon CJ, Dunn MG, Bender E, et al.** Collagen fiber formation in repair tissue: development of strength and toughness. *Coll Relat Res.* 1985 Dec;5(6):481–492.
6. **Haukipuro K.** Synthesis of collagen types I and III in reincised wounds in humans. *Br J Surg.* 1991 Jun;78(6):708–712.
7. **Dodson MK, Magann EF, Meeks GR.** A randomized comparison of secondary closure and secondary intention in patients with superficial wound dehiscence. *Obstet Gynecol.* 1992 Sep;80(3 Pt 1):321–324.
8. **Morbach S, Furchert H, Groblinghoff U, et al.** Long-term prognosis of diabetic foot patients and their limbs: amputation and death over the course of a decade. *Diabetes Care.* 2012 Oct;35(10):2021–2027.
9. **Mills JL, Sr.**, Conte MS, Armstrong DG, et al. The Society for Vascular Surgery Lower Extremity Threatened Limb Classification System: risk stratification based on wound, ischemia, and foot infection (WIfI). *J Vasc Surg.* 2014 Jan;59(1):220–234 e1–2.
10. **Santilli JD, Santilli SM.** Chronic critical limb ischemia: diagnosis, treatment and prognosis. *Am Fam Physician.* 1999 Apr 1;59(7):1899–1908.
11. **Singh N, Armstrong DG, Lipsky BA.** Preventing foot ulcers in patients with diabetes. *JAMA.* 2005 Jan 12;293(2):217–228.
12. **Brem H, Tomic-Canic M.** Cellular and molecular basis of wound healing in diabetes. *J Clin Invest.* 2007 May;117(5):1219–1222.
13. **Reddy M.** Skin and wound care: important considerations in the older adult. *Adv Skin Wound Care.* 2008 Sep;21(9):424–436; quiz 37–38.
14. **Fore J.** A review of skin and the effects of aging on skin structure and function. *Ostomy Wound Manage.* 2006 Sep;52(9):24–35; quiz 6–7.
15. **Bosanquet DC, Rangaraj A, Richards AJ, et al.** Topical steroids for chronic wounds displaying abnormal inflammation. *Ann R Coll Surg Engl.* 2013 May;95(4):291–296.
16. **Hofman D, Moore K, Cooper R, et al.** Use of topical corticosteroids on chronic leg ulcers. *J Wound Care.* 2007 May;16(5):227–230.
17. **Trent JT, Kirsner RS.** Leg ulcers in sickle cell disease. *Adv Skin Wound Care.* 2004 Oct;17(8):410–416.
18. **Minniti CP, Eckman J, Sebastiani P, et al.** Leg ulcers in sickle cell disease. *Am J Hematol.* 2010 Oct;85(10):831–833.
19. **Erinjeri JP, Fong AJ, Kemeny NE, et al.** Timing of administration of bevacizumab chemotherapy affects wound healing after chest wall port placement. *Cancer.* 2011 Mar 15;117(6):1296–1301.
20. **Regan MA, Teasell RW, Wolfe DL, et al.** A systematic review of therapeutic interventions for pressure ulcers after spinal cord injury. *Arch Phys Med Rehabil.* 2009 Feb;90(2):213–231.
21. **Wu SC, Crews RT, Armstrong DG.** The pivotal role of offloading in the management of neuropathic foot ulceration. *Curr Diab Rep.* 2005 Dec;5(6):423–429.
22. **Raffoul W, Far MS, Cayeux MC, et al.** Nutritional status and food intake in nine patients with chronic low-limb ulcers and pressure ulcers: importance of oral supplements. *Nutrition.* 2006 Jan;22(1):82–88.
23. **Lipsky BA, Berendt AR, Cornia PB, et al.** 2012 Infectious Diseases Society of America clinical practice guideline for the diagnosis and treatment of diabetic foot infections. *Clin Infect Dis.* 2012 Jun;54(12):e132–173.
24. **Sorensen LT.** Wound healing and infection in surgery: the pathophysiological impact of smoking, smoking cessation, and nicotine replacement therapy: a systematic review. *Ann Surg.* 2012 Jun;255(6):1069–1079.
25. **Lipsky BA.** A report from the international consensus on diagnosing and treating the infected diabetic foot. *Diabetes Metab Res Rev.* 2004 May-Jun;20 Suppl 1:S68–77.
26. **Armstrong DG, Lipsky BA.** Advances in the treatment of diabetic foot infections. *Diabetes Technol Ther.* 2004 Apr;6(2):167–177.
27. **O'Meara S, Al-Kurdi D, Ovington LG.** Antibiotics and antiseptics for venous leg ulcers. *Cochrane Database Syst Rev.* 2008 (1):CD003557.
28. **Senet P, Combemale P, Debure C, et al.** Malignancy and chronic leg ulcers: the value of systematic wound biopsies: a prospective, multicenter, cross-sectional study. *Arch Dermatol.* 2012 Jun;148(6):704–708.
29. **Senet P, Vicaut E, Beneton N, et al.** Topical treatment of hypertensive leg ulcers with platelet-derived growth factor-BB: a randomized controlled trial. *Arch Dermatol.* 2011 Aug;147(8):926–230.
30. **Smith F, Dryburgh N, Donaldson J, et al.** Debridement for surgical wounds. *Cochrane Database Syst Rev.* 2013;9:CD006214.
31. **Fernandez R, Griffiths R.** Water for wound cleansing. *Cochrane Database Syst Rev.* 2012;2:CD003861.
32. **Moore ZE, Cowman S.** Wound cleansing for pressure ulcers. *Cochrane Database Syst Rev.* 2013;3:CD004983.
33. **Armstrong DG, Lavery LA, Nixon BP, et al.** It's not what you put on, but what you take off: techniques for debriding and off-loading the diabetic foot wound. *Clin Infect Dis.* 2004 Aug 1;39 Suppl 2:S92–99.
34. **Wilcox JR, Carter MJ, Covington S.** Frequency of debridements and time to heal: a retrospective cohort study of 312 744 wounds. *JAMA Dermatol.* 2013 Sep;149(9):1050–1058.
35. **Fang RC, Galiano RD.** A review of becaplermin gel in the treatment of diabetic neuropathic foot ulcers. *Biologics.* 2008 Mar;2(1):1–12.
36. **Falanga V, Eaglstein WH, Bucalo B, et al.** Topical use of human recombinant epidermal growth factor (h-EGF) in venous ulcers. *J Dermatol Surg Oncol.* 1992 Jul;18(7):604–606.
37. **Da Costa RM, Ribeiro Jesus FM, Aniceto C, et al.** Randomized, double-blind, placebo-controlled, dose- ranging study of granulocyte-macrophage colony stimulating factor in patients with chronic venous leg ulcers. *Wound Repair Regen.* 1999 Jan-Feb;7(1):17–25.
38. **Svensjo T, Pomahac B, Yao F, et al.** Accelerated healing of full-thickness skin wounds in a wet environment. *Plast Reconstr Surg.* 2000 Sep;106(3):602-12; discussion 13–14.
39. **Paddle-Ledinek JE, Nasa Z, Cleland HJ.** Effect of different wound dressings on cell viability and proliferation. *Plast Reconstr Surg.* 2006 Jun;117(7 Suppl):110S-8S; discussion 9S–20S.

40. **Armstrong DG, Jude EB.** The role of matrix metalloproteinases in wound healing. *J Am Podiatr Med Assoc.* 2002 Jan;92(1):12–18.
41. **Dyson M, Young S, Pendle CL, et al.** Comparison of the effects of moist and dry conditions on dermal repair. *J Invest Dermatol.* 1988 Nov;91(5):434–439.
42. **Rakel BA, Bermel MA, Abbott LI, et al.** Split-thickness skin graft donor site care: a quantitative synthesis of the research. *Appl Nurs Res.* 1998 Nov;11(4):174–182.
43. **Thomas DR, Goode PS, LaMaster K, et al.** A comparison of an opaque foam dressing versus a transparent film dressing in the management of skin tears in institutionalized subjects. *Ostomy Wound Manage.* 1999 Jun;45(6):22–24, 7–8.
44. **Lalau JD, Bresson R, Charpentier P, et al.** Efficacy and tolerance of calcium alginate versus vaseline gauze dressings in the treatment of diabetic foot lesions. *Diabetes Metab.* 2002 Jun;28(3):223–229.
45. **Grange-Prunier A, Couilliet D, Grange F, et al.** [Allergic contact dermatitis to the Comfeel hydrocolloid dressing]. *Ann Dermatol Venereol.* 2002 May;129(5 Pt 1):725–727.
46. **Coats TJ, Edwards C, Newton R, et al.** The effect of gel burns dressings on skin temperature. *Emerg Med J.* 2002 May;19(3):224–225.
47. **Menaker GM.** Wound dressings for office-based surgery. *Facial Plast Surg.* 2004 Feb;20(1):91–105.
48. **Achterberg V, Meyer-Ingold W.** Hydroactive dressings and serum proteins: an in vitro study. *J Wound Care.* 1996 Feb;5(2):79–82.
49. **Hogsberg T, Bjarnsholt T, Thomsen JS, et al.** Success rate of split-thickness skin grafting of chronic venous leg ulcers depends on the presence of Pseudomonas aeruginosa: a retrospective study. *PLoS One.* 2011;6(5):e20492.
50. **Simon DA, Dix FP, McCollum CN.** Management of venous leg ulcers. *BMJ.* 2004 Jun 5;328(7452):1358–1362.
51. **Puttirutvong P.** Meshed skin graft versus split thickness skin graft in diabetic ulcer coverage. *J Med Assoc Thai.* 2004 Jan;87(1):66–72.
52. **Blok CS, Vink L, de Boer EM, et al.** Autologous skin substitute for hard-to-heal ulcers: retrospective analysis on safety, applicability, and efficacy in an outpatient and hospitalized setting. *Wound Repair Regen.* 2013 Sep-Oct;21(5):667–676.
53. **Thom SR.** Hyperbaric oxygen: its mechanisms and efficacy. *Plast Reconstr Surg.* 2011 Jan;127 Suppl 1:131S–41S.
54. **Kranke P, Bennett M, Roeckl-Wiedmann I, et al.** Hyperbaric oxygen therapy for chronic wounds. *Cochrane Database Syst Rev.* 2004 (2):CD004123.
55. **Godina M.** Early microsurgical reconstruction of complex trauma of the extremities. *Plast Reconstr Surg.* 1986 Sep;78(3):285–292.
56. **Patzakis MJ, Wilkins J, Moore TM.** Considerations in reducing the infection rate in open tibial fractures. *Clin Orthop Relat Res.* 1983 Sep(178):36–41.
57. **Hallock GG.** Utility of both muscle and fascia flaps in severe lower extremity trauma. *J Trauma.* 2000 May;48(5):913–917.
58. **Afifi AM, Mahboub TA, Losee JE, et al.** The reverse sural flap: modifications to improve efficacy in foot and ankle reconstruction. *Ann Plast Surg.* 2008 Oct;61(4):430–436.
59. **Schierle CF, Rawlani V, Galiano RD, et al.** Improving outcomes of the distally based hemisoleus flap: principles of angiosomes in flap design. *Plast Reconstr Surg.* 2009 Jun;123(6):1748–1754.
60. **Orgill DP, Manders EK, Sumpio BE, et al.** The mechanisms of action of vacuum assisted closure: more to learn. *Surgery.* 2009 Jul;146(1):40–51.
61. **Braakenburg A, Obdeijn MC, Feitz R, et al.** The clinical efficacy and cost effectiveness of the vacuum-assisted closure technique in the management of acute and chronic wounds: a randomized controlled trial. *Plast Reconstr Surg.* 2006 Aug;118(2):390–397; discussion 398–400.
62. **Morykwas MJ, Faler BJ, Pearce DJ, et al.** Effects of varying levels of subatmospheric pressure on the rate of granulation tissue formation in experimental wounds in swine. *Ann Plast Surg.* 2001 Nov;47(5):547–551.
63. **DeFranzo AJ, Argenta LC, Marks MW, et al.** The use of vacuum-assisted closure therapy for the treatment of lower-extremity wounds with exposed bone. *Plast Reconstr Surg.* 2001 Oct;108(5):1184–1191.
64. **Putnis S, Khan WS, Wong JM.** Negative pressure wound therapy - a review of its uses in orthopaedic trauma. *Open Orthop J.* 2014;8:142–147.
65. **Saxena V, Hwang CW, Huang S, et al.** Vacuum-assisted closure: microdeformations of wounds and cell proliferation. *Plast Reconstr Surg.* 2004 Oct;114(5):1086–1096; discussion 97–98.
66. **Wang W, Pan Z, Hu X, et al.** Vacuum-assisted closure increases ICAM-1, MIF, VEGF and collagen I expression in wound therapy. *Exp Ther Med.* 2014 May;7(5):1221–1226.
67. **Morykwas MJ, Argenta LC, Shelton-Brown EI, et al.** Vacuum-assisted closure: a new method for wound control and treatment: animal studies and basic foundation. *Ann Plast Surg.* 1997 Jun;38(6):553–562.
68. **Eginton MT, Brown KR, Seabrook GR, et al.** A prospective randomized evaluation of negative-pressure wound dressings for diabetic foot wounds. *Ann Vasc Surg.* 2003 Nov;17(6):645–649.
69. **Younan G, Ogawa R, Ramirez M, et al.** Analysis of nerve and neuropeptide patterns in vacuum-assisted closure-treated diabetic murine wounds. *Plast Reconstr Surg.* 2010 Jul;126(1):87–96.
70. **Moues CM, Vos MC, van den Bemd GJ, et al.** Bacterial load in relation to vacuum-assisted closure wound therapy: a prospective randomized trial. *Wound Repair Regen.* 2004 Jan-Feb;12(1):11–17.
71. **Vuerstaek JD, Vainas T, Wuite J, et al.** State-of-the-art treatment of chronic leg ulcers: A randomized controlled trial comparing vacuum-assisted closure (V.A.C.) with modern wound dressings. *J Vasc Surg.* 2006 Nov;44(5):1029–1037; discussion 38.
72. **Orgill DP, Bayer LR.** Negative pressure wound therapy: past, present and future. *Int Wound J.* 2013 Dec;10 Suppl 1:15–19.
73. **Younan GJ, Heit YI, Dastouri P, et al.** Mast cells are required in the proliferation and remodeling phases of microdeformational wound therapy. *Plast Reconstr Surg.* 2011 Dec;128(6):649e–658e.
74. **Karlakki S, Brem M, Giannini S, et al.** Negative pressure wound therapy for managementof the surgical incision in orthopaedic surgery: A review of evidence and mechanisms for an emerging indication. *Bone Joint Res.* 2013;2(12):276–284.
75. **A N, Khan WS, J P.** The evidence-based principles of negative pressure wound therapy in trauma & orthopedics. *Open Orthop J.* 2014;8:168–177.
76. **Parrett BM, Matros E, Pribaz JJ, et al.** Lower extremity trauma: trends in the management of soft-tissue reconstruction of open tibia-fibula fractures. *Plast Reconstr Surg.* 2006 Apr;117(4):1315–1322; discussion 23–24.
77. **Stannard JP, Robinson JT, Anderson ER, et al.** Negative pressure wound therapy to treat hematomas and surgical incisions following high-energy trauma. *J Trauma.* 2006 Jun;60(6):1301–1306.
78. **Stannard JP, Volgas DA, McGwin G, 3rd, et al.** Incisional negative pressure wound therapy after high-risk lower extremity fractures. *J Orthop Trauma.* 2012 Jan;26(1):37–42.

79. **Labler L, Trentz O.** The use of vacuum assisted closure (VAC) in soft tissue injuries after high energy pelvic trauma. *Langenbecks Arch Surg.* 2007 Sep;392(5):601–609.
80. **Sinha K, Chauhan VD, Maheshwari R, et al.** Vacuum Assisted Closure Therapy versus Standard Wound Therapy for Open Musculoskeletal Injuries. *Adv Orthop.* 2013;2013:245940.
81. **Dedmond BT, Kortesis B, Punger K, et al.** The use of negative-pressure wound therapy (NPWT) in the temporary treatment of soft-tissue injuries associated with high-energy open tibial shaft fractures. *J Orthop Trauma.* 2007 Jan;21(1):11–17.
82. **Webster J, Scuffham P, Sherriff KL, et al.** Negative pressure wound therapy for skin grafts and surgical wounds healing by primary intention. *Cochrane Database Syst Rev.* 2012;4:CD009261.
83. **Halvorson J, Jinnah R, Kulp B, et al.** Use of vacuum-assisted closure in pediatric open fractures with a focus on the rate of infection. *Orthopedics.* 2011 Jul;34(7):e256–260.
84. **Malmsjo M, Gustafsson L, Lindstedt S, et al.** Negative pressure wound therapy-associated tissue trauma and pain: a controlled in vivo study comparing foam and gauze dressing removal by immunohistochemistry for substance P and calcitonin gene-related peptide in the wound edge. *Ostomy Wound Manage.* 2011 Dec;57(12):30–35.
85. **Li Z, Yu A.** Complications of negative pressure wound therapy: a mini review. *Wound Repair Regen.* 2014 Jul-Aug;22(4):457–461.
86. **Upton D, Andrews A.** Pain and trauma in negative pressure wound therapy: a review. *Int Wound J.* 2013 Mar 12.
87. **Vuolo JC.** Wound-related pain: key sources and triggers. *Br J Nurs.* 2009 Aug 13-Sep 9;18(15):S20, S2–5.
88. **Upton D, Solowiej K, Hender C, et al.** Stress and pain associated with dressing change in patients with chronic wounds. *J Wound Care.* 2012 Feb;21(2):53–54, 6,8 passim.
89. **Upton D, Stephens D, Andrews A.** Patients' experiences of negative pressure wound therapy for the treatment of wounds: a review. *J Wound Care.* 2013 Jan;22(1):34–39.
90. **Hourigan LA, Linfoot JA, Chung KK, et al.** Loss of protein, immunoglobulins, and electrolytes in exudates from negative pressure wound therapy. *Nutr Clin Pract.* 2010 Oct;25(5):510–516.
91. **Schwien T, Gilbert J, Lang C.** Pressure ulcer prevalence and the role of negative pressure wound therapy in home health quality outcomes. *Ostomy Wound Manage.* 2005 Sep;51(9):47–60.

Section

3 Cases

Section 3
Cases

15.1 Acutely infected tibial nail

James F Kellam

1 Case description

A 35-year-old male helicopter mechanic fell from the top of a helicopter onto the tarmac. He had an open tibial diaphyseal fracture. His initial treatment involved administration of a cephalosporin antibiotic, debridement of the open wound 6 hours after the injury, and stabilization of the tibia with a reamed locked nail. At debridement the bone was not contaminated but he had approximately 50% of his anterior compartment debrided due to necrotic muscle from the injury. He also had a 6 x 8 cm anteromedial skin and subcutaneous defect. It was a Gustilo-Anderson type IIIB open tibial fracture. The patient required three more debridements with negative-pressure wound therapy over the next 2 weeks. An ipsilateral free latissimus dorsi flap was performed at 3 weeks after the initial debridement (**Fig 15.1-1**).

2 Indications

Two weeks following the flap coverage, the patient had necrosis of the split-thickness skin over the flap and the flap was of questionable viability. The flap was regrafted with split-thickness skin and observed. At this time his foot was plantigrade, he had no vascular insufficiency, and sensation and motor function to the foot were normal. He presented at 8 weeks from his injury with cloudy drainage emanating from under the free flap. The flap was viable and the skin graft had taken completely. His x-rays showed some fracture-site bony resorption but no evidence of healing (**Fig 15.1-2**). The white blood cell count was elevated with a left shift; the erythrocyte sedimentation rate was 80 mm/h (normal range: 0–23 mm/h), and C-reactive protein was 4.2 mg/L (normal range: less than 5 mg/L). He was afebrile but felt generally unwell. Cultures were deferred in favor of a deep biopsy for tissue culture.

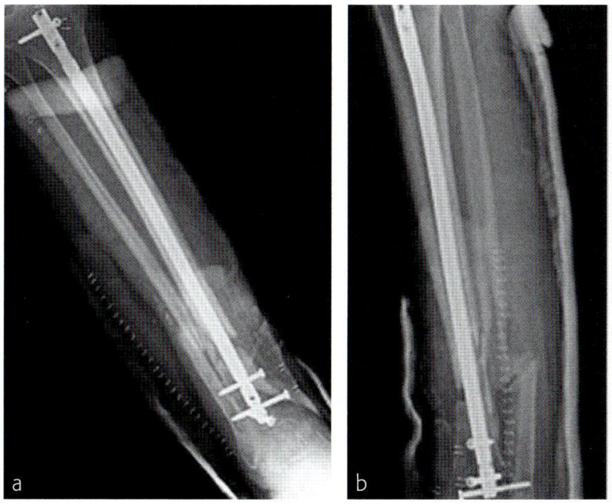

Fig 15.1-1a–b X-rays of the lower limb following the initial debridement and nailing.
a AP view.
b Lateral view.

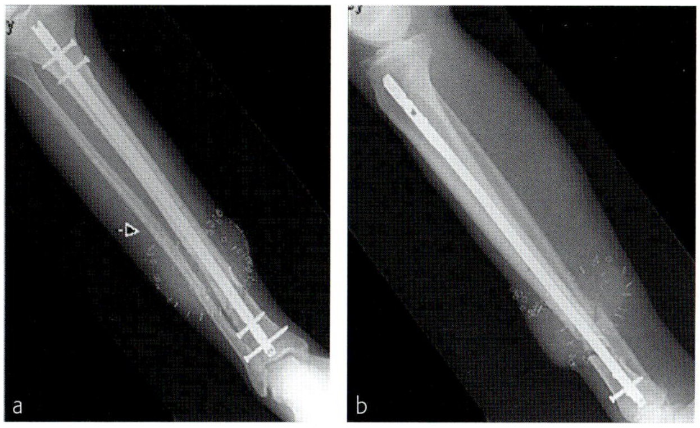

Fig 15.1-2a–b X-rays of the lower leg at the time of drainage from the flap. The fracture appears to be resorbing, which is indicative of an infective process.
a Lateral view.
b Internal rotation oblique view.

3 Preoperative planning

The patient will not receive any preoperative antibiotics so the preoperative staff and anesthetists need to be notified that this is an infected case and cultures will be taken intraoperatively. A radiolucent operative table is needed. A tourniquet is placed on the thigh but not inflated due to the potential for heat necrosis during intramedullary (IM) canal reaming. Standard operative sterile preparation of the skin will be used. Prior to entering the room, the IM nail removal equipment is checked to ensure it is complete. A 32 French chest tube, ball-tipped reaming guide, two packs of polymethylmethacrylate (PMMA), and 2 g of gentamicin powder must be present in the operating room. The patient is prepared and draped in a standard fashion. The nail is removed through the prior incisions. The canal is reamed to two sizes above the nail removed. The prior distal locking screw holes will act as vents for the reamings. After reaming the canal, it is irrigated with saline solution using a total hip IM irrigator aspirator to ensure that all the debris from the most caudal part of the reaming tract is removed. The PMMA nail (see below) is made and inserted. The guide wire is cut at the entry to the IM canal and bent past a right angle to prevent it from falling into the canal. The incision is closed and the leg splinted. Postoperatively the leg will be placed in a short leg cast and the patient allowed to bear weight as tolerated.

4 Surgical approach

The prior fracture site was approached by elevating the flap based on its vascular pedicle. The nail was removed through the previous medial parapatellar incision and the locking screw removed through the old stab wounds.

5 Surgical debridement

The patient underwent re-exploration: the flap was elevated on its pedicle. The fracture site was debrided and specimens from bone, fibrous fracture-site tissue, and muscle were taken for culture. The bone ends were debrided of any necrotic nonbleeding bone. It was noted that there was pus tracking up and down the medullary canal. This indicated that the IM canal was contaminated by the infection and would require a debridement by IM reaming.

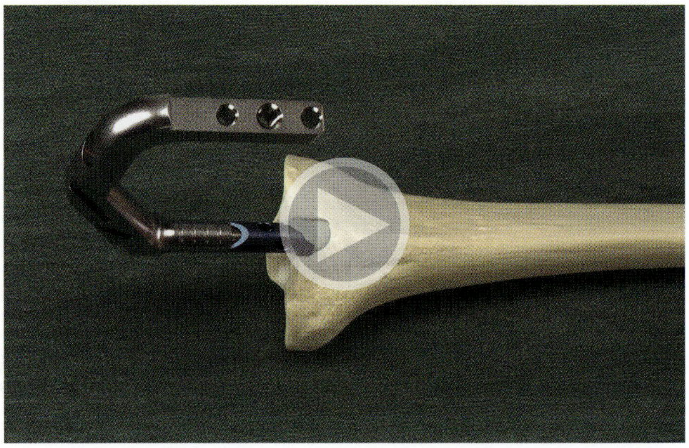

Video 15.1-1 Preparing an antibiotic-loaded cement nail for the tibia.

6 Implant removal and temporary fixation

The intramedullary nail was removed, the canal reamed 2 mm above the nail size and thoroughly irrigated with saline using a total hip medullary irrigator aspirator. Using the largest chest tube (32F) and a beaded reaming guide wire inserted into the chest tube, it was filled with PMMA with 2 g of gentamicin and allowed to solidify (**Video 15.1-1**). Once hard, the chest tube was cut away and the PMMA nail inserted into the medullary canal to provide some fracture stability and deliver local antibiotics (**Fig 15.1-3**). The flap was replaced and closed. The tissue cultures grew methicillin-resistant *Staphylococcus aureus* sensitive to vancomycin.

7 Postoperative management (1)

The infectious diseases physician was consulted to help manage the infection medically. The infectious diseases specialist recommended 1 g of vancomycin intravenously twice daily for 6 weeks. A percutaneous intravenous central catheter was inserted for the delivery of antibiotics. The wound was checked and the lower leg placed in a patellar tendon-bearing cast to allow weight bearing as tolerated. At 2 weeks the cast was removed, the flap was viable, and the incision had healed. The lower leg remained in the patellar tendon-bearing cast. At 6 weeks the erythrocyte sedimentation rate and C-reactive protein had returned to normal and the incision had no drainage and was healed.

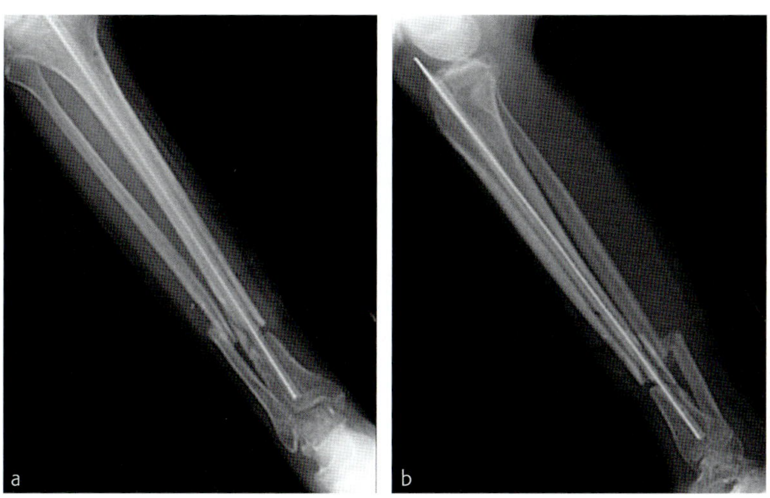

Fig 15.1-3a–b X-rays of the lower leg following nail removal, reaming, debridement, and the insertion of an antibiotic polymethylmethacrylate nail.

a AP view.

b Lateral view.

8 Reimplantation

The patient had the PMMA nail removed, the canal reamed, and a static locked IM nail inserted (**Fig 15.1-4**). The reamings were sent for culture. Following nailing, an anterior iliac crest autogenous cancellous bone graft was inserted by the central technique. This technique exposes the lateral aspect of the tibia anterior to the intermuscular membrane, which is excised from its tibial insertion to allow the bone graft to be placed posteriorly to the tibia as well as lateral and extending to the fibula [1, 2].

9 Postoperative management (2)

Postoperatively, the patient was allowed to bear weight as tolerated. The culture was negative for growth. At 2 weeks the incisions were healed with no further drainage.

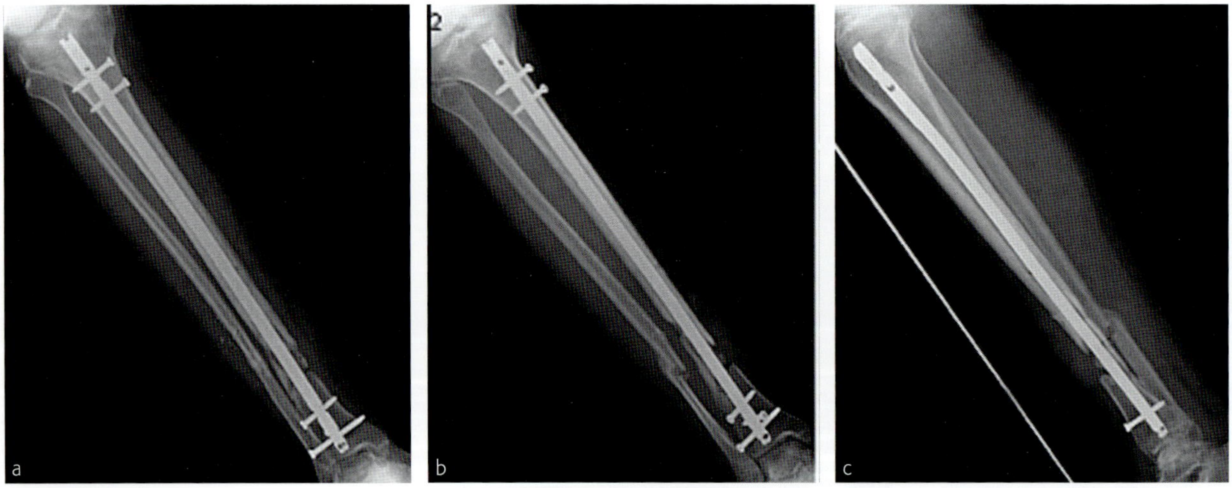

Fig 15.1-4a–c X-ray of the lower leg nail at 6 weeks following antibiotic polymethylmethacrylate nail and the insertion of an new statically locked nail.

a AP view.
b Internal oblique view.
c Lateral view.

10 Outcome

By 5 months postoperatively, the patient was bearing full weight and returned to his job as a helicopter mechanic (**Fig 15.1-5**).

11 Pitfalls

- The delay in obtaining viable coverage increased risk for infection.
- The failure to appreciate the potential issue with flap coverage led to wound breakdown and infection.

12 Pearls

- Administration of antibiotics as soon as possible from the time of injury.
- Thorough assessment of the wound and aggressive debridement.
- Must achieve early (within 3–5 days) coverage of the wound.
- Recognition of flap problems early demands an aggressive response such as redebridement and assessment for revision of coverage.

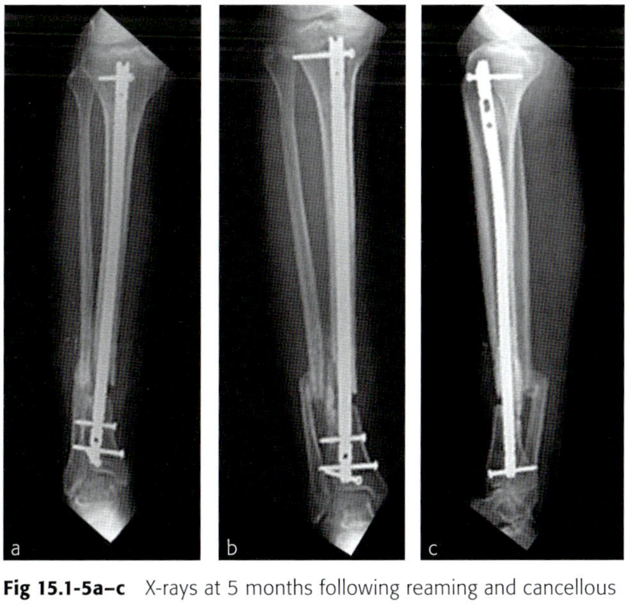

Fig 15.1-5a–c X-rays at 5 months following reaming and cancellous bone grafting via the central route.
a AP view.
b Internal rotation oblique view.
c Lateral view.

13 Reference

1. **Ryzewicz M, Morgan SJ, Linford E, et al**. Central bone grafting for nonunion of fractures of the tibia: a retrospective series. *J Bone Joint Surg Br. 2009 Apr;*91(4):522–529.
2. **Rijnberg W.J. and Van Linge B.** Central grafting for persistent nonunions of the tibia. *J Bone Joint Surg (Br) 1993;* 75B:926–931.

15.2 Acutely infected lateral malleolar fracture

A Samuel Flemister Jr

1 Case description

A 66-year-old man with a history of rheumatoid arthritis presented with a 3-day history of increased pain, redness, and warmth about the lateral aspect of the right ankle. The patient denied any fevers, chills, or night sweats. The patient had undergone open reduction and internal fixation for an ankle fracture 2 years before (**Fig 15.2-1**). Eight months after the initial operation, the patient had the lateral plate and screws removed secondary to a draining wound. Two broken syndesmotic screws were not removed from the tibia (**Fig 15.2-2**). Cultures taken at that time revealed methicillin-sensitive *Staphylococcus aureus*. The patient had been treated with oral antibiotics consisting of cephalexin 500 mg orally four times per day and trimethoprim/sulfamethoxazole double strength 500 mg orally twice per day. The patient had not had any problems with the wound or the ankle since the time of this hardware removal. The patient had recently started use of etanercept and prednisone to treat his rheumatoid arthritis.

2 Indications

Relatively urgent surgical debridement was indicated to avoid sepsis and decompensation. The patient was elderly and immunocompromised. He presented with a draining wound that was obviously infected. Laboratory studies revealed an erythrocyte sedimentation rate of 78 mm/h (normal range: 0–23 mm/h), white blood cell (WBC) count 8,700 (normal range: 4,000–10,000 cells/μL), and C-reactive protein 27 mg/L (normal range: less than 5 mg/L). Although these markers were not very elevated given the patient's relative immunocompromised state, they were felt to be significant.

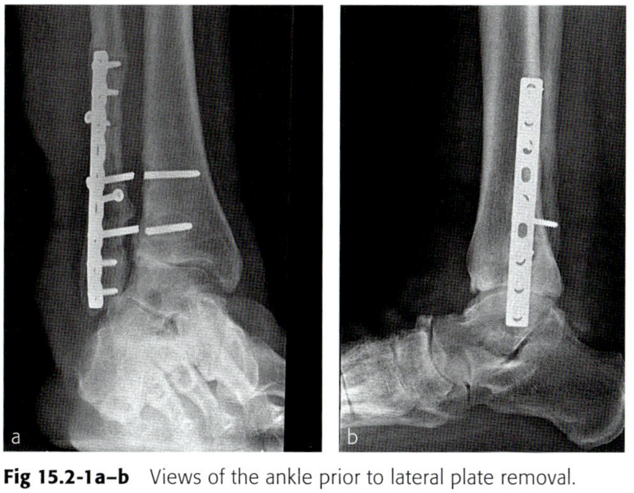

Fig 15.2-1a–b Views of the ankle prior to lateral plate removal.
a AP view.
b Lateral view.

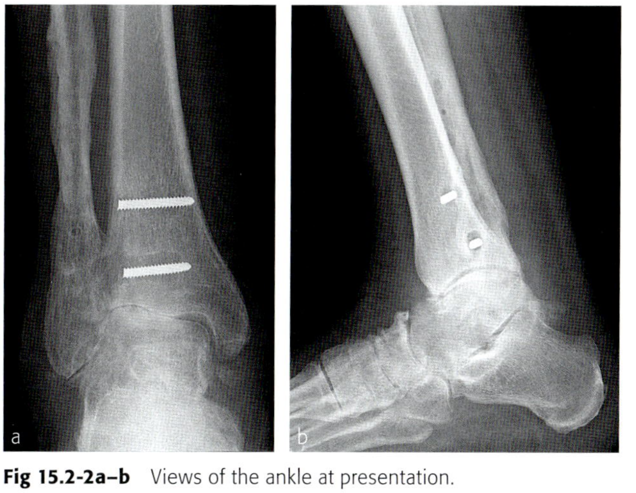

Fig 15.2-2a–b Views of the ankle at presentation.
a AP view.
b Lateral view.

3 Preoperative planning

This immunocompromised patient was admitted to the hospital and started on ampicillin/sulbactam 1.5 g intravenously every 6 hours. A radiolabeled WBC scan suggested a focus of osteomyelitis in the fibula (**Fig 15.2-3**). Both bone debridement and removal of residual hardware were planned. A broken-screw removal set was made available.

4 Surgical approach

The patient was placed in the supine position with a sandbag under the ipsilateral hip. The previous lateral incision was used. Antibiotics had been administered on the schedule determined at the time of admission. A pneumatic tourniquet was applied to the thigh but not inflated. The patient was given a general anesthetic. This was his third operation in this area so significant scarring was anticipated. Care was taken to avoid injury to the superficial peroneal nerve and maintain full-thickness skin flaps.

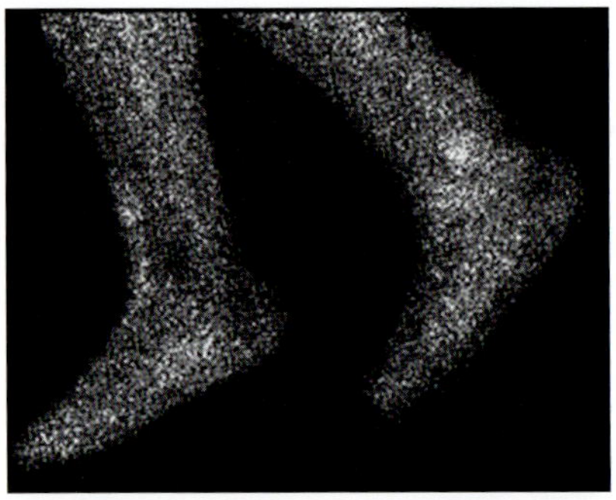

Fig 15.2-3 Tagged white blood cell scan of the ankles.

5 Surgical debridement

The skin edges and subcutaneous tissue associated with the draining wound were excised. All necrotic-appearing soft tissue was removed. The wound was then irrigated with normal saline solution. The tagged WBC scan had isolated an area of osteomyelitis to the most proximal syndesmotic screw hole. This area was overdrilled with a hollow core reamer and the screw hole cored out. The remainder of the bone was then inspected for any compromised areas and debrided as needed. Once adequate debridement and removal of hardware had been accomplished, the wound was once again irrigated and then loosely closed with a single layer of nylon suture.

6 Implant removal

A centering guide was placed through the original syndesmotic screw hole in the fibula and passed to the adjacent screw hole in the tibia until it engaged the broken screw. A hollow reamer slightly larger than the screw was then placed over the centering guide and the centering guide withdrawn. The reamer was used to overdrill the screw. This permitted placement of an extraction bolt over the screw for removal.

7 Temporary fixation

No temporary fixation was required given that adequate stability remained after resection of a compromised area of the fibula.

8 Postoperative management

The patient was placed into a removable short leg splint and kept nonweight bearing for approximately 2 weeks until the wound had healed. The wound was inspected every 1 or 2 days to be monitored for resolution of infection. After 2 weeks he was then allowed to bear weight as tolerated in a regular shoe that would not irritate the wound. A compressive stocking was used to reduce edema. An infectious diseases physician was consulted for advice. Surgical cultures again grew methicillin-sensitive *S aureus* and the patient received a 6-week course of intravenous cefazolin (1 g every 8 hours).

9 Reimplantation

No implant was required as the fracture had healed.

10 Outcomc

The wound healed well and the inflammatory markers decreased. The patient eventually developed significant ankle arthrosis due to a combination of posttraumatic osteoarthritis and rheumatoid arthritis versus infection (**Fig 15.2-4**). However, the patient also developed peripheral neuropathy and had a minimal amount of pain. Therefore, no further surgery was required.

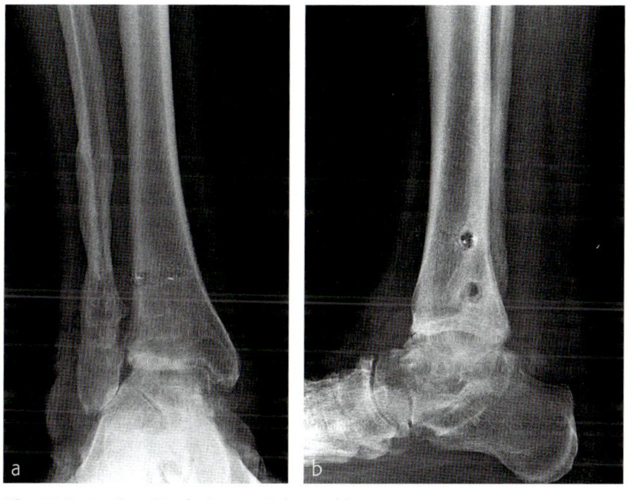

Fig 15.2-4a–b Final views of the ankle.
a AP view.
b Lateral view.

11 Pitfalls

- In this case, making an accurate diagnosis of the amount of bone that needed to be resected was essential. Underresection of infected bone would lead to recurrent problems and overresection could possibly cause instability necessitating ankle arthrodesis.
- This case illustrates the importance of removing all hardware in cases of infection.

12 Pearls

- Advanced imaging such as the combination of bone scan and labeled WBC scan can help to localize the involved areas of osteomyelitis and help guide the surgical approach.
- All infected hardware should be removed especially if the fractures are healed.
- Temporary fixation is required if instability develops.
- Culture-specific antibiotics should be used for an adequate length of time to eradicate the infection.
- An infectious diseases consultant is an important team member.
- If enough resection of the fibula was required that the tibiotalar joint became unstable, then an ankle arthrodesis would be required.

15.3 Acutely infected proximal humerus after soft-tissue repair

Matthias A Zumstein

1 Case description

A 66-year-old man complained of a 3-day history of an acute onset of pain and increased stiffness in his right shoulder. Four weeks previously he had undergone rotator-cuff repair with an arthroscopic procedure for an acute traumatic tear of the rotator-cuff tendons. He had no fever, chills, or malaise. On clinical examination there was no indication of an infection (eg, warmth, erythema). The C-reactive protein (CRP) was elevated at 223 mg/L (normal range: less than 5 mg/L), as was the white blood cell count (WBC) at 12.5 g/L (normal range: 4–10 g/L). A magnetic resonance imaging (**Fig 15.3-1**) including intravenous contrast application showed multiple-fluid collections along the anterosuperior portal, involving the joint and the bone of the proximal humerus. Synovial fluid leukocyte count showed 25 x 10^9/L with 80% neutrophils.

2 Indications

The symptoms of acute pain combined with these laboratory and radiographic findings strongly suggested an acute surgical-site infection involving the anterolateral portal and bone of the proximal humerus. Hence, the decision for an arthroscopic debridement was taken. Additionally, the potential for subsequent interventions was discussed, depending on the extent of intraoperative findings and microbiological results.

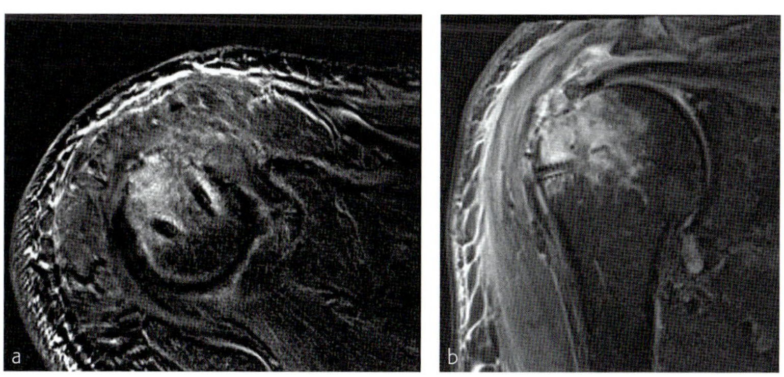

Fig 15.3-1a–b Preoperative magnetic resonance images.
a Contrast axial view.
b Contrast coronal view.

3 Preoperative planning

The most important point to discuss in this section is the amount of debridement necessary and removal of implants. The author suspected an acute infection of the subacromial bursa, the joint, and the bone. Complete synovectomy, removal of all suture material and anchors, if easily feasible, were planned. However, if the anchors were deeply fixed in the bone, they would have not been removed due to the possible osseous damage.

A standard arthroscopic setup was chosen with a beach-chair position including a limb positioner (**Fig 15.3-2**). Arthroscopic scissors were prepared to cut the sutures, and closed as well as open clamps were prepared to remove tissue.

No antibiotics were given to the patient prior to microbiological sampling. General anesthesia was chosen in this case.

4 Surgical approach

Standard posterior, anteromedial, anterolateral, and lateral portals were chosen to address all areas of the shoulder intraarticularly and subacromially (**Fig 15.3-3**).

The surgeon starts with the posterior portal, which should be conducted with the arm in internal rotation to penetrate the muscle fibers and not the tendon. The author prefers to make the portals outside to control the angles and the accessibility with the instruments. Alternatively and especially in case of excessive inflammation and inadequate intraarticular vision, the anteromedial portal can be made inside out using a switching stick.

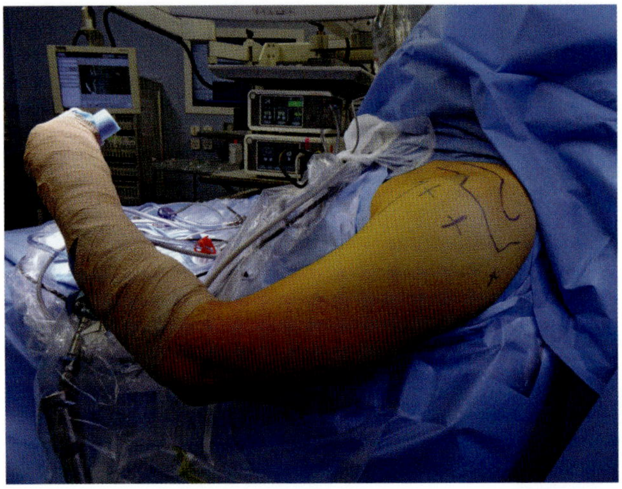

Fig 15.3-2 A standard arthroscopic setup was chosen with a beach-chair position including a limb positioner.

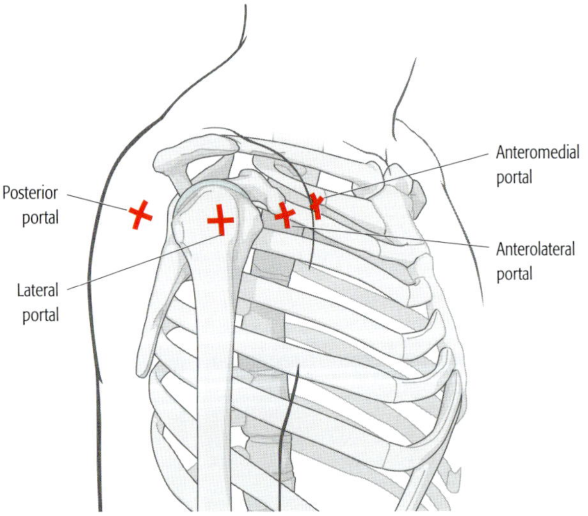

Fig 15.3-3 Portals for surgical approach.

5 Surgical debridement

5.1 Intraarticular debridement (synovial and optional capsule)

After establishing the posterior and anteromedial portals, a meticulous intraarticular synovectomy and debridement should be made. Starting from anterosuperior by removing the rotator interval until the subscapularis tendon inferiorly and the coracohumeral ligament superiorly, the synovium can be resected easily until the inferior 6 o'clock position. Using a switching stick, the bursa below the coracoid can be dissected to be sure that there is no abscess in the subcoracoid bursa. Attention should be paid at the medial border below the acromion as the acromial branch of the thoracoacromial artery emerges medially.

If there are potential abscesses in the subscapular fossa, this area is rinsed by spreading the layer between the middle glenohumeral ligament and the glenoid labrum using the switching stick and going down into the fossa. Then, the scope and the working instruments are switched and the synovectomy is completed posteriorly and posteroinferiorly. Again, in case of abscesses in the fossa infraspinata, the same procedure can be performed posteriorly with a switching stick going in between the labrum and the capsule in front of the infraspinatus.

The author tenotomizes the long head of the biceps if it is not yet performed by the previous intervention. There is no evidence that patients have negative side effects following tenotomy or tenodesis of the long head of the biceps at midterm. In case of a partially or totally healed tendon of the posterosuperior cuff and if there are sutures visible that came out of the medial anchors, the author prefers to cut them at this stage. Alternatively and without healing, the sutures can be easily cut from the lateral view.

5.2 Subacromial debridement (bursa, adhesions)

After putting the scope in the lateral portal and establishing the anterolateral portal by triangulation and the help of a spinal needle, a complete subacromial bursectomy is performed until the spine of the scapula and the complete acromion is visible. Anteriorly the coracoacromial ligament can be incised, excised to gain full access to the anterior compartment. If needed, the transverse ligament can be incised to debride potential abscesses in the bicipital groove.

6 Anchor removal

The author decided to remove all the sutures. This was done by cutting the medial sutures during the intraarticular arthroscopy. However, complete removal of the sutures was performed from the subacromial approach. As the tendon was partially healed to the greater tuberosity, the author removed only the lateral anchors. This was made with the arm in abduction to access the anchors recess with a conical extraction screw. After placing the tip of the conical extraction screw into the anchors' recess, it is held as vertical as possible and a gentle tapping on the extraction screw is made. Turn it counterclockwise, exerting pressure, until the extraction screw grasps into the anchor and continue to turn counterclockwise to remove the anchor.

After removing all implants, empiric intravenous antimicrobial therapy (amoxicillin/clavulanate 2.2 g every 6 hours) was started immediately.

7 Temporary fixation

The most anterior part (3 mm width) of the tendon of the rotator cuff had not completely reattached to the greater tuberosity. As minor cuff lesions may not predispose to further tendon retraction, fatty infiltration, and atrophy, nor to inferior clinical results, no additional implants were used.

8 Postoperative management

Immediately postoperatively, the arm was protected in a sling during the day and a Gilchrist bandage at night. Two days postoperatively, *Staphylococcus aureus* grew from all samples. The intravenous treatment was changed to flucloxacillin (2 g every 6 hours) for a further 5 days (ie, total intravenous treatment 7 days). After the wounds were dry, and the CRP had fallen to 5 mg/L, the antimicrobial treatment was switched to oral rifampin (450 mg twice daily) and levofloxacin (500 mg twice daily) for a total treatment duration of 3 months.

Mobilization was allowed without restriction immediately postoperatively. The postoperative course was uneventful, as were follow-up investigations after 6 and 12 weeks.

9 Outcome

At the 6-month follow-up, the patient was very satisfied with the final result. After intensive rehabilitation, his examination showed flexion of 160°, active external rotation of 50°, and internal rotation at L5.

10 Pitfalls

Particular pitfalls to avoid include performing arthroscopic debridement on hemiarthroplasty, total shoulder replacement, or reverse shoulder replacement joints. It is also a contraindication to manage a shoulder with arthroscopic treatment if bony involvement is noted on preoperative imaging. Relative contraindications to this procedure would be patients in whom the desired positioning for shoulder arthroscopy is not possible.

11 Pearls

11.1 Surgical approach

Both arthroscopic and open surgery are options for a complete debridement of the shoulder. However, the authors believe they can address more precisely all areas within the joint as well as the fossa subscapularis and the fossa infraspinata using an arthroscopic procedure. All viewing and working portals can be switched in both the subacromial as well as the intraarticular space so therefore all options are possible. Furthermore, going far posterior in the subacromial space is less difficult with an arthroscopic procedure. Only experienced shoulder arthroscopists should perform this surgery.

11.2 Implant removal

This case is a typical "debridement and implant retention" case: this treatment option is mainly considered in acute infections with a short duration of symptoms, and in early postoperative infections. The following principles are essential for such a case:

- Surgery must be performed rapidly.
- Irrigation and debridement should be meticulous, and are easily performed by arthroscopy.
- Mobile elements, such as sutures, should be removed.
- The soft-tissue damage is not severe (eg, sinus tract or multiple or large abscess and necrotic material).
- There is absence of a difficult-to-treat pathogen (eg, rifampin-resistant staphylococci, fungi).

With correct patient selection, the outcome of this procedure has been reported to be good with an infection-free interval ranging from 85% to 100%.

15.4 Infected tibial delayed union with broken implants

Christoph Sommer

1 Case description

A 23-year-old driver was involved in a car crash and sustained a grade IIIA open intraarticular distal lower-leg fracture (pilon fracture) AO/OTA Classification 43-C3 (**Fig 15.4-1**). The first step in surgery consisted of initial debridement of the wound, revealing a large metadiaphyseal fragment with small articular component (**Fig 15.2-2a**), which was completely detached from the soft tissue and therefore avascular. Due to only minimal contamination, this fragment was cleaned and preserved in the refrigerator at 4° C. The fracture was stabilized with a joint-bridging external fixator (**Fig 15.4-2b**). A postoperative computed-tomographic (CT)

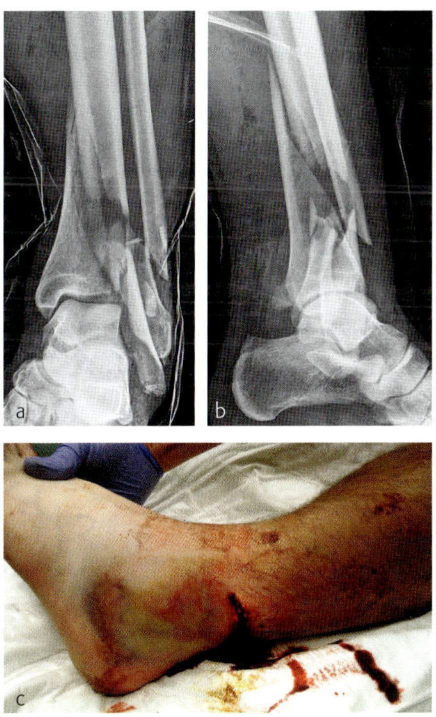

15.4-1a–c Initial x-rays after the accident showing a pilon fracture with a relatively simple fracture pattern, but massively displaced and large anterolateral articular fragment.

- **a** AP view.
- **b** Lateral view.
- **c** Clinical aspect from lateral showing the wound at the level of the fibula fracture.

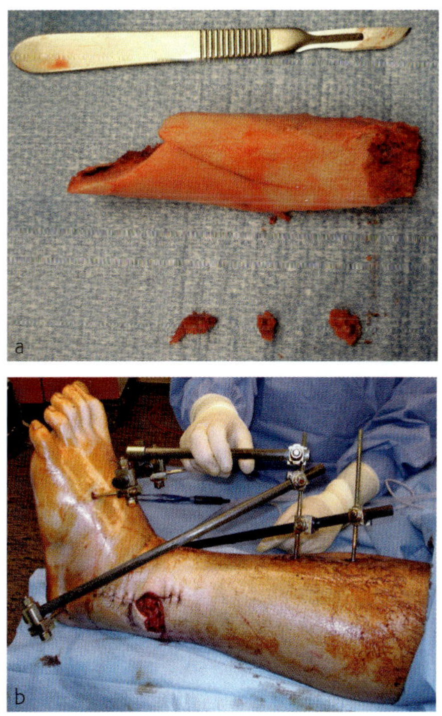

15.4-2a–b Initial operation 2 hours after admission.

- **a** Removed and temporarily preserved large epimetadiaphyseal fragment.
- **b** Ankle bridging external fixator and partially open wound treatment, lateral.

scan was used for further planning (**Fig 15.4-3**). Two days later a second look with irrigation was performed, and 5 days later definitive reconstruction was accomplished using a small posteromedial approach for reduction and antiglide plate fixation of the diaphyseal component (**Fig 15.4-4a**), and a primary lateral extended approach for articular reconstruction and fixation. The large preserved bone fragment was reinserted, anatomically reduced, and rigidly fixed using lag screws and a neutralization plate (**Fig 15.4-4b–d**). Postoperative x-rays demonstrated correct alignment and hardware position of the open reduction and internal fixation (**Fig 15.4-5**). Wound healing was uneventful and there were no signs of infection after 6 weeks (**Fig 15.4-6**).

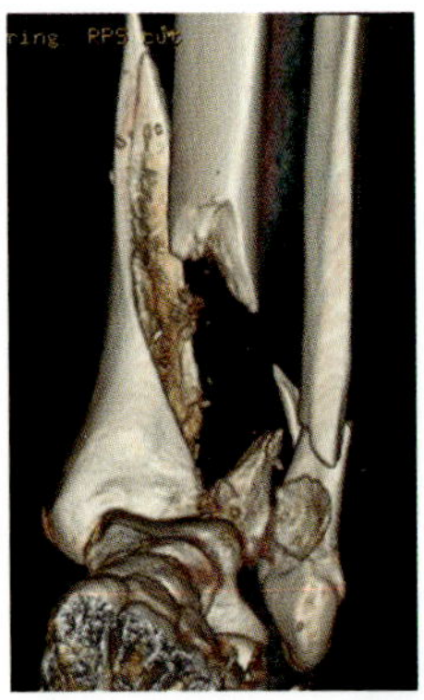

15.4-3 Computed tomographic scan after the initial operation reveals the fracture pattern and shows the large bone defect, anterolateral.

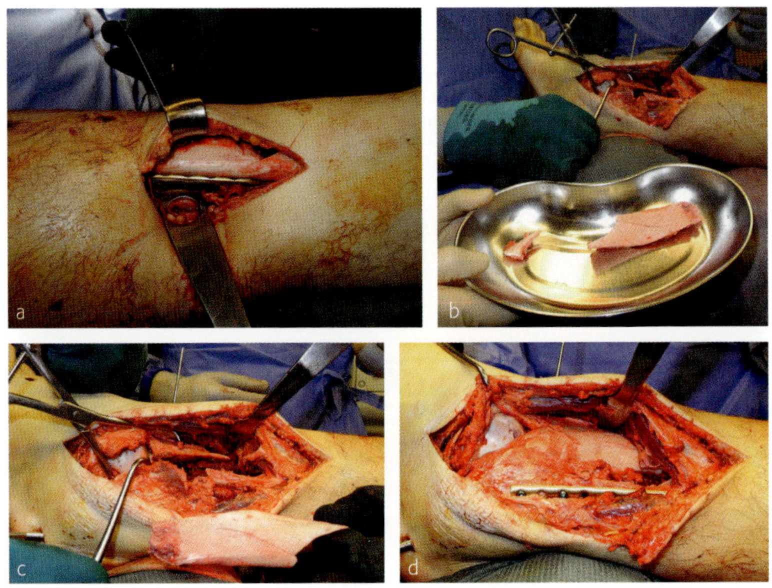

15.4-4a–d Definitive reconstruction of the bone 7 days after injury.
- **a** Small posteromedial incision at the level of the distal diaphysis with small antiglide plate.
- **b** Preserved anterolateral fragment before reimplantation.
- **c** Lateral extended approach demonstrating the lateral defect with corresponding fragment.
- **d** Large fragment reduced and fixed with lag screws. Plate fixation of the fibula.

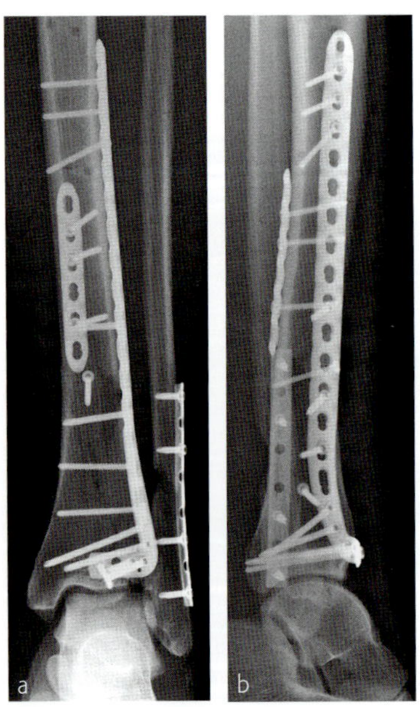

15.4-5a–b Postoperative x-rays showing an anatomical reconstruction with stable plate fixation of the tibia and fibula.
- **a** AP view.
- **b** Lateral view.

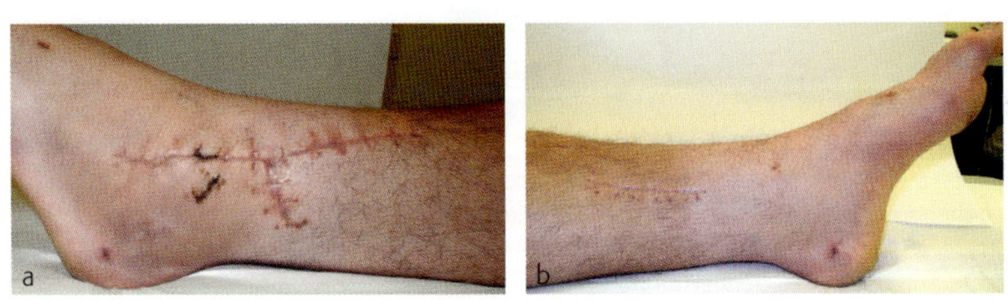

15.4-6a–b Soft-tissue situation 6 weeks after injury shows a clean and calm situation without any signs of infection.
- **a** Lateral aspect.
- **b** Medial aspect.

Three and a half months after injury, the plate broke (**Fig 15.4-7**) and the patient was readmitted. The posteromedial wound was slightly inflamed suggesting a possible low-grade infection in the diaphyseal region. Clinically there were no signs of articular infection and no intraarticular effusion was detected by sonography. The C-reactive protein (CRP) level was normal (4.0 mg/L). The clinical diagnosis of a delayed union with implant failure due to a bone vascularity problem (with possible low-grade infection) was made.

2 Indications

Delayed union in a case of implant failure in the distal tibia 4 months after initial management is a clear indication for surgical treatment. Due to the low index of suspicion clinically (no redness, only minimal swelling, and warmth of the skin), normal CRP level, and no radiographic signs of a deep infection, no further diagnostic studies were performed prior to reoperation.

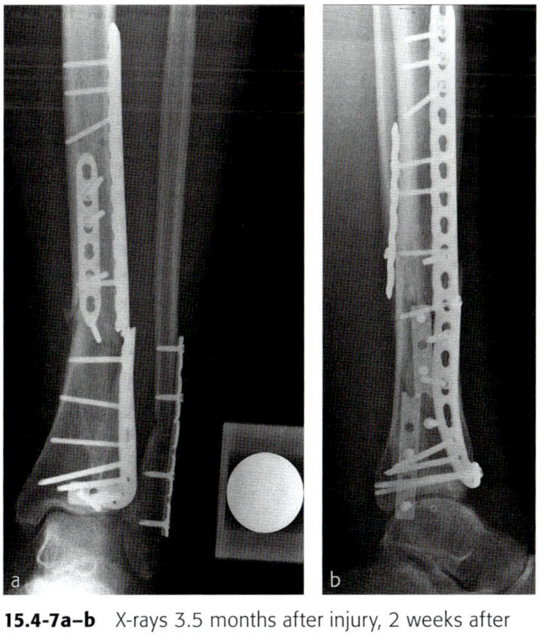

15.4-7a–b X-rays 3.5 months after injury, 2 weeks after the patient started full weight bearing.
a AP view.
b Lateral view.

3 Preoperative planning

A staged procedure was planned. The first step consisted of:

- Removal of the failed implants (lateral plate and screws of the medial tibial plate, fibular plate)
- Bone debridement as necessary with several biopsies for cultures
- Fracture stabilization (tibia and fibula) based on the intraoperative findings

Fixation options included an external fixator, or a combination with one or several plates.

After this first step, a broad-spectrum antibiotic prophylaxis was planned until the definitive microbiological results were available. As an additional step, bone grafting seemed to be necessary.

The patient was positioned supine with a pillow under the left buttock (**Fig 15.4-8**). A thigh tourniquet was placed and inflated at the beginning to permit better inspection of the operative field and to decide if any signs of an infection were present. During surgery, after initial debridement, the tourniquet was deflated to judge the vitality of the remaining bone to decide if further bone debridement might be necessary.

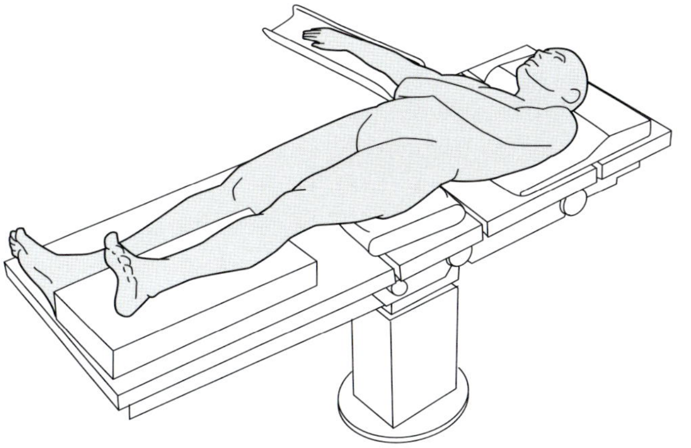

15.4-8 Positioning for reoperation: supine with a pillow under the left buttock.

4 Surgical approach

To remove the failed implants and to inspect and debride the delayed union zone, both old incisions (anterolateral as primary and posteromedial as second smaller approaches) were opened. The anterolateral (extended) approach followed the anterior border of the fibula with a slight anterior curve distally to extend 4–5 cm over the anterolateral ankle joint (**Fig 15.4-4d, Fig 15.4-9a–b**). The superior extensor retinaculum and fascia were incised longitudinally just in front of the fibula. Elevation of the extensor tendons/muscles permits surgical exposure of the anterolateral part of the tibia. At joint level, the anterolateral edge (tubercle of Tillaux-Chaput) of the tibia with the intact anterior syndesmotic ligament is visualized. The distal part of the anterolateral plate was mobilized and removed. This approach permits exposure of 8 cm of the distal tibia. Further proximally, there exists a "taboo" zone (**Fig 15.4-9a**) because at that level the neurovascular bundle (anterior tibial artery and vein and deep peroneal nerve) crosses the distal tibia from proximal posterior to distal anterior and therefore is in danger. A small separate anterolateral stab incision more proximally at the level of the proximal part of the plate is used to deliver these implants (visible at the end of the operation in **Fig 15.4-9f**). For the medial plate, a small posteromedial approach at the level of the existing plate was performed. The approach exposes the posteromedial edge of the tibia in a straightforward way without endangering any vital structures (visible at the end of the operation in **Fig 15.4-9g**).

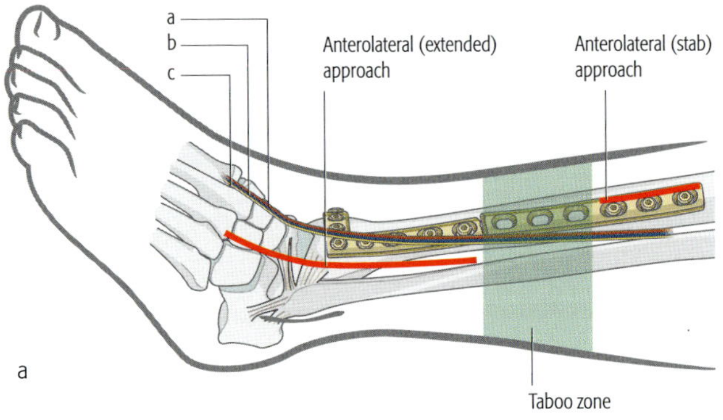

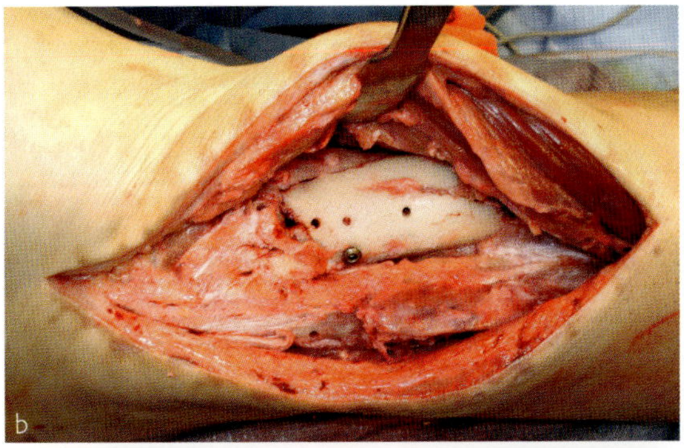

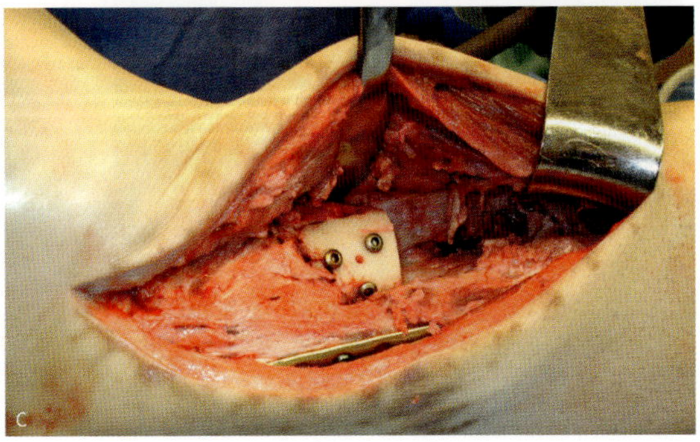

Fig 15.4-9a–c First revision surgery after plate breakage, 3.5 months after initial injury.

- **a** Preoperative plan.
- **b** First aspect from lateral revealing the large reimplanted, avascular metadiaphyseal fragment of the tibia.
- **c** After subtotal removal of this fragment, leaving the articular part of the fragment in situ (the distal end of the segmental resection).

5 Surgical debridement, implant removal, and temporary fixation

After removal of the broken lateral tibial plate distally, the initially reimplanted large osseous fragment (**Fig 15.4-4b–d**) was clearly visible as "white", avascular cortical bone (**Fig 15.4-9b**). On the lateral side, no signs of an infection were noted, but on the medial side a small amount of purulent fluid was found around the nonunion zone. Therefore, it was quite clear that an infected nonunion was present in combination with a large avascular bone fragment. At this time, the decision was made to aggressively debride the avascular bone, which consisted of a large area of the distal tibia. Considering the large size of the bony defect, the author decided to excise the entire involved bone segment (10 cm in length) and to reconstruct this using a segmental transport (**Fig 15.4-9c–e**). Before doing this, the broken plate on the fibula (one-third tubular plate) was replaced by a new (stronger) locking compression plate (LCP) 3.5, and an ankle bridging external fixator was applied. The left distal anterolateral avascular fragment (involved a small part of the articular surface of the ankle) was retained and revised with three new 3.5 mm cortical lag screws (**Fig 15.4-9c**). The defect zone was cleaned by jet lavage using 5 L of lactated Ringer's solution. Both wounds were closed over a suction drain (**Fig 15.4-9f–g**). No dead space filler was inserted; an early segmental transport was planned for some days later.

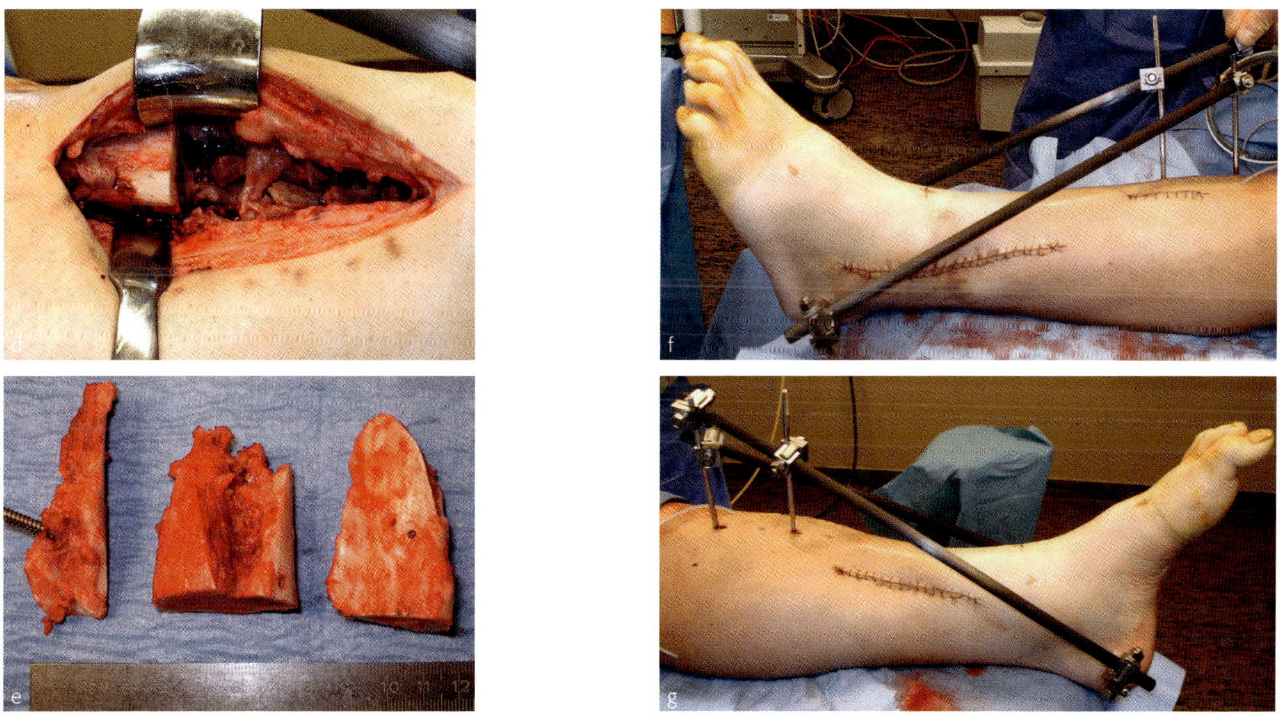

Fig 15.4-9d–g First revision surgery after plate breakage, 3.5 months after initial injury (cont).
d Aspect from posteromedial at the level of the distal diaphysis (proximal end of the segmental resection).
e Removed avascular bone pieces.
f–g End of surgery demonstrating the ankle-bridging external fixator: lateral aspect (**f**) and medial aspect (**g**).

6 Postoperative management

Broad-spectrum intravenous antibiotic treatment with coamoxicillin 2.2 g three times per day and gentamicin 300 mg per day was started intraoperatively immediately after debridement and performance of tissue biopsies for microbiological cultures. The patient was not mobilized, x-rays showed the large segmental defect with the two suction drains inside (**Fig 15.4-10**). Two days later, a second-look operation with reopening of all wounds, repeat jet lavage, and biopsies for cultures with wound closure was performed. The definitive results of the initial biopsies revealed penicillin-resistant but otherwise sensitive *Staphylococcus epidermidis* and *Staphylococcus hominis,* which were treated with coamoxicillin, 3 x 2.2 g daily intravenously for 14 days, and later clindamycin 3 x 600 mg daily by mouth for 5 months until the surgical treatment was finished. The CRP level remained normal (< 5.0 mg/L) during the entire treatment period. The biopsies taken at the second-look operation were culture negative. One week after the second-look operation, all the wounds appeared healthy and no signs of infection existed (**Fig 15.4-11**). Segmental transport using an anteromedially placed monolateral transport external fixator was applied (**Fig 15.4-12**). The corticotomy was placed proximally in the diaphyseal part of the tibia which was not involved in the initial trauma and surgery. One week after corticotomy transport of the segment was started with 1 mm per day using four 0.25 mm steps every 6 hours. The patient was followed with x-rays every 2–3 weeks (**Fig 15.4-13**) until the docking site was reached 100 days later (**Fig 15.4-14**).

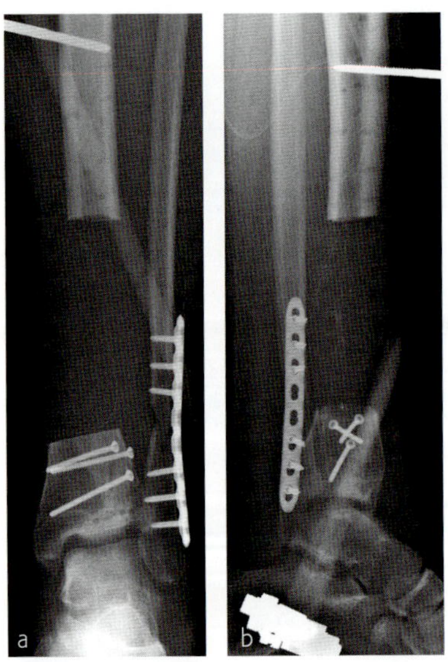

15.4-10a–b X-rays after first revision surgery demonstrating the 10 cm segmental defect and the refixed fibula (locking compression plate 3.5) and tibia (external fixator) in correct alignment.
a AP view.
b Lateral view.

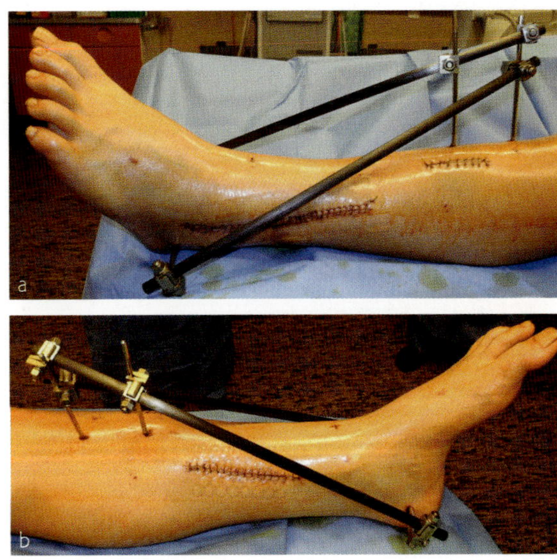

15.4-11a–b Clinical aspect of the leg 9 days after first revision and 7 days after second-look surgery.
a Lateral aspect.
b Medial aspect.

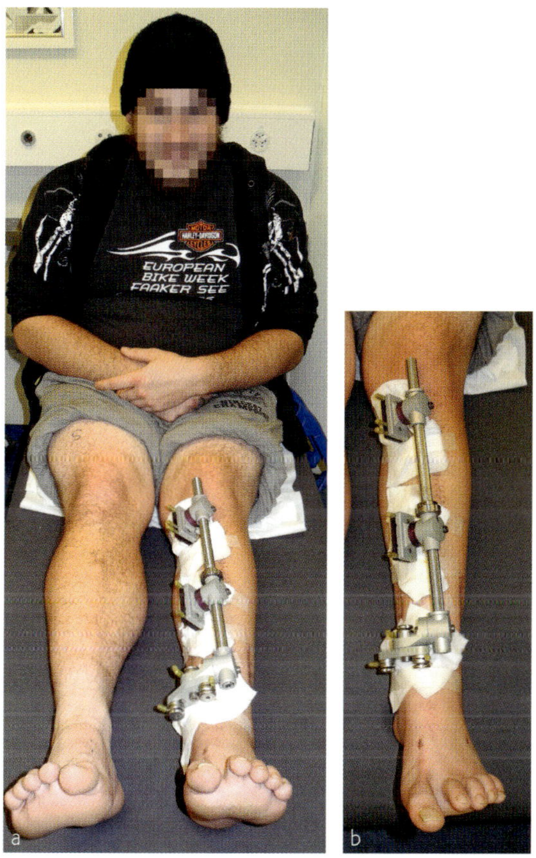

15.4-12a–b Situation after application of the unilateral transport fixator (proximal to distal) demonstrating correct overall alignment (length, axis, rotation) with a highly motivated patient.

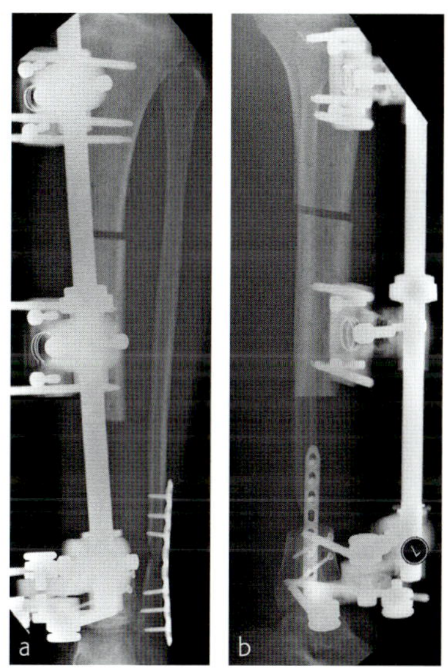

15.4-13a–b X-rays 1 week after the transport had started

a AP view.

b Lateral view.

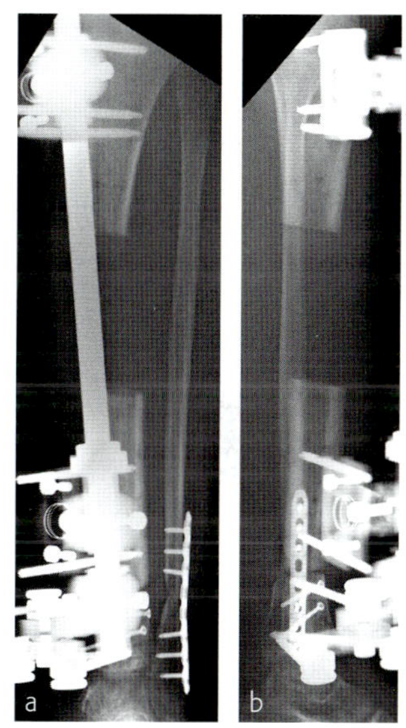

15.4-14a–b X-rays after 100 days of transport time (1 mm/day, in four steps of 0.25 mm each).

a AP view.

b Lateral view.

7 Reimplantation and definitive fixation

One week after completion of the segmental transport, definitive internal fixation was applied. On one side, a strong anterolateral locking compression plate proximal lateral tibia (LCP-PLT) 4.5/5.0 was inserted using a minimally invasive plate osteosynthesis (MIPO) technique for the proximal diaphyseal part to stabilize the newly generated bone in the distraction site in a bridging construct. The docking site was similarly fixed using an LCP distal medial tibial plate 3.5 via a MIPO technique in a compression mode using the transport fixator to maximize the compression at the docking site. A small, interposed bony fragment from the original fracture unfortunately hindered the desired broad contact of the two horizontal bone ends (**Fig 15.4-15**).

Although the patient was mobilized with only 10–15 kg partial weight bearing, 6 weeks later the LCP-PLT was found to be bent in 10–15° of varus, most likely caused by one unintended fully loaded step which created a single overload event for this strong plate (patient's weight: 125 kg) (**Fig 15.4-16**). This malalignment was not tolerable and it had to be corrected by application of a further plate medially (LCP 4.5 narrow), which was again inserted using a MIPO technique after bending the lateral plate back into correct alignment using manual force with a medially applied femoral distractor (**Fig 15.4-17**).

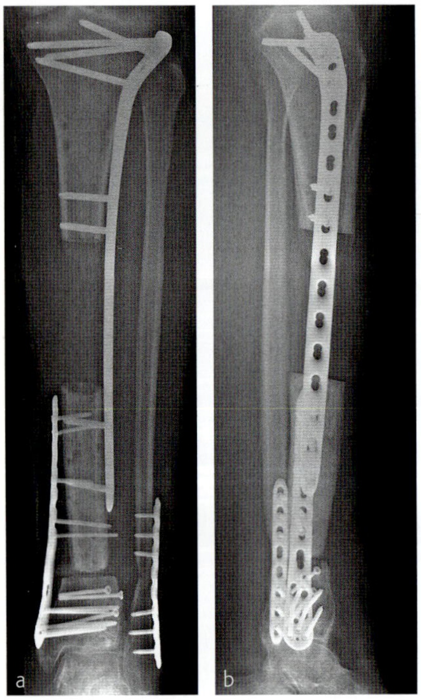

15.4-15a–b X-rays after change from transport external fixator to internal stabilization: locking compression plate proximal lateral tibia 4.5/5.0 anterolateral for the distracted part and locking compression plate 3.5 distal medial tibial plate in compression plate technique for the distal docking site, both inserted using a minimally invasive plate osteosynthesis technique.
- **a** AP view.
- **b** Lateral view.

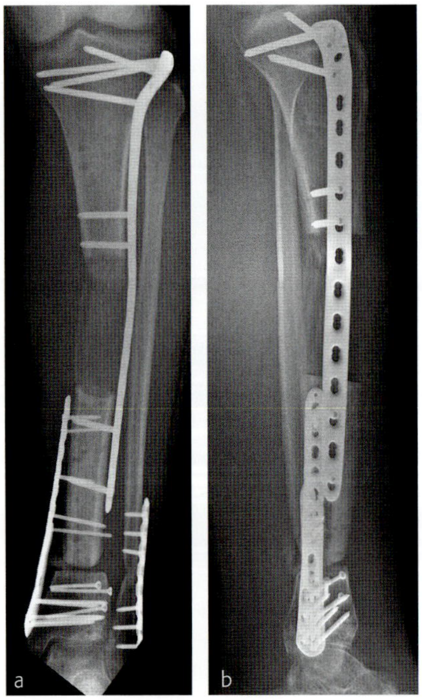

15.4-16a–b X-rays 6 weeks after internal fixation show a bent locking compression plate proximal lateral tibia, which must have been caused by one single (or multiple) overload(s) by the patient standing with full weight on this leg.
- **a** AP view demonstrating a varus deformity of 15°.
- **b** Lateral view.

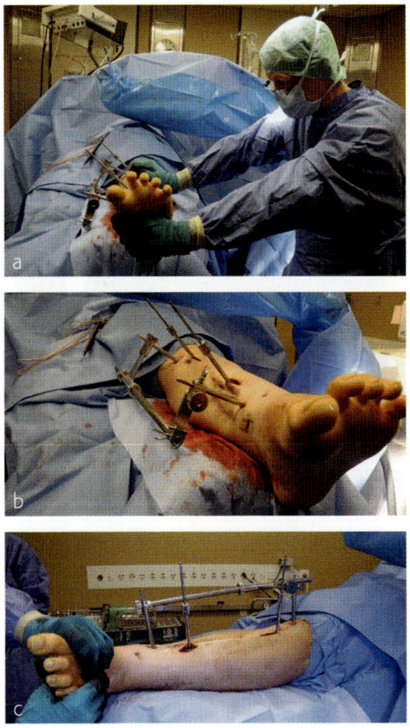

15.4-17a–c Revision of a bent plate.
- **a** Bending back of the plate (in situ) by manual force.
- **b** In combination with the large distractor on the medial side.
- **c** Applying a second (antero) medial plate (locking compression plate 4.5 narrow) using minimally invasive plate osteosynthesis technique.

8 Outcome

After this last operation, correct alignment was documented on x-rays (**Fig 15.4-18**). Further healing was uneventful with timely mineralization of the newly generated bone at the distraction site and primarily endosteal bone healing at the docking site 6 weeks later (**Fig 15.4-19**). The antibiotics were discontinued 6 weeks after the last surgery.

At 1-year follow-up after the initial injury (and 3 months after the last operation), the patient was able to walk without crutches but was still limping due to a moderate pes equinus caused by Achilles tendon shortening (**Fig 15.4-20**). Clinically the infection seemed to be cured, the wounds all closed and benign in appearance. On x-rays (**Fig 15.4-21**), the distracted diaphyseal segment of the tibia showed an increasing mineralization and remodeling, and the fibula was fully united. The distal docking site was still not completely bridged but further healing was expected.

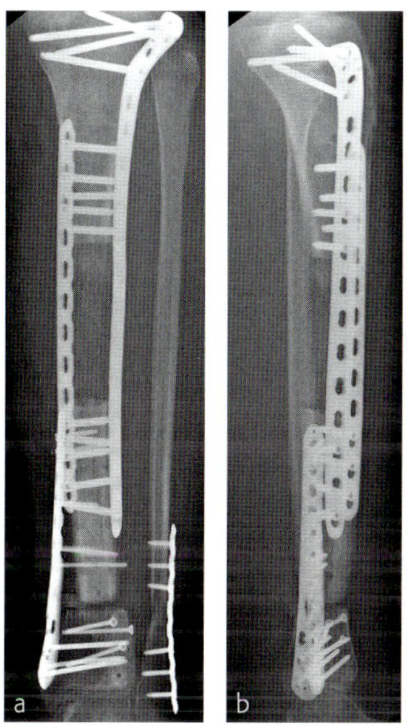

15.4-18a–b X-rays after bending the plate back and adding a further medial plate demonstrating correct alignment as in **Fig 15.4-15a**.
a AP view.
b Lateral view.

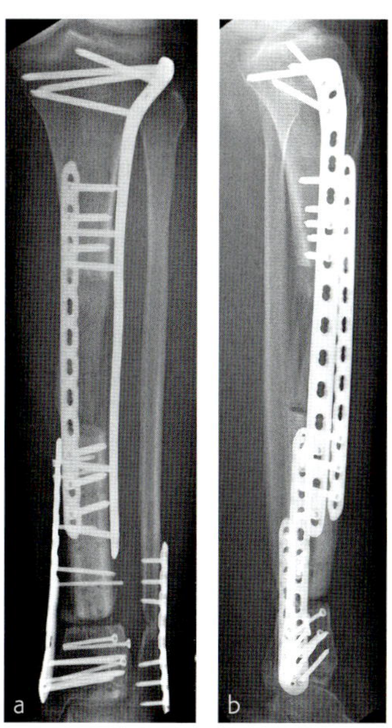

15.4-19a–b X-rays 6 weeks later demonstrate increasing mineralization of the distracted diaphyseal segment but only minimal healing at the distal docking site.
a AP view.
b Lateral view.

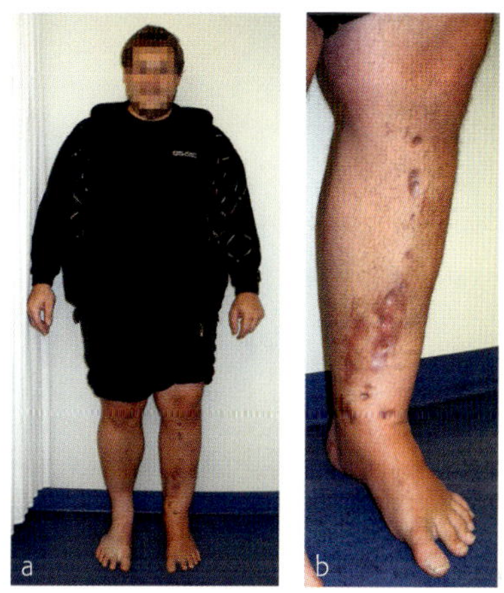

15.4-20a–b One-year follow-up after injury (3 months after last surgery).
a Clinical aspect of the still highly motivated patient.
b Dry and fully healed, but broad scars with remaining moderate soft-tissue swelling at the lower leg and ankle.

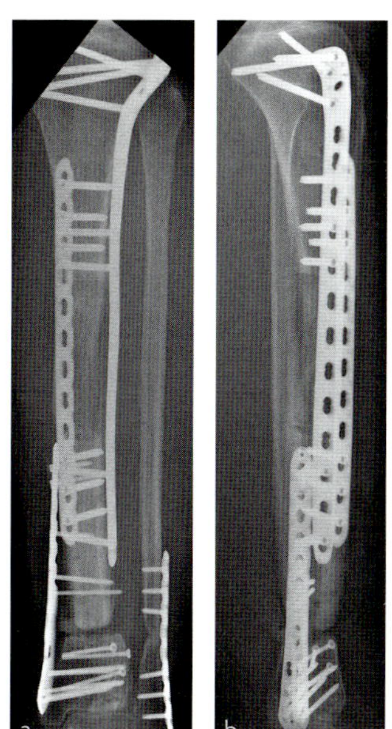

15.4-21a–b One-year follow-up after injury (3 months after last surgery) demonstrates ongoing and increasing mineralization of the distracted segment, but still limited (and questionable) endosteal healing at the docking site.
a AP view.
b Lateral view.

Two months later the patient returned with increased pain and local tenderness at the docking site. Revision surgery revealed an atrophic nonunion with a sequestrum and some surrounding fluid suspicious for low-grade infection. The distal medial plate was removed, the nonunion excised and cleaned with jet lavage. Biopsies were taken for cultures and broad-spectrum intravenous antibiotics (coamoxicillin and gentamicin) were started. An external fixator was applied. Two days later a second look revealed macroscopically clean and vital tissues (**Fig 15.4-22**). The bone defect was replaced by gentamicin polymethylmethacrylate (Masquelet technique). The microbiological cultures revealed a resistant *S epidermidis*, which was treated with long-term intravenous antibiotics (vancomycin 2 x 1.5 g daily). The next operative step was performed 6 weeks later: removal of the cement spacer, defect filling with two autogenous tricorticocancellous bone blocks and additional cancellous bone grafting (iliac crest), and restabilization of the tibia with a distal medial tibial locking plate 3.5 (**Fig 15.4-23**, **Fig 15.4-24**). The last microbiological cultures taken were negative and the long-term antibiotic treatment (intravenous vancomycin) was continuing at the time of writing. Further bone healing under this treatment continues to improve. The CRP level returned to normal after the last operation, and clinically the soft-tissue situation is calm. The most recent x-rays, 8 months after the last surgery, showed slow but progressive bone healing, with remodeling and intact implants without loosening or bone resorption around the screws (**Fig 15.4-25**). The patient is walking pain-free without crutches suggesting a stable (at least partially) healed bone situation.

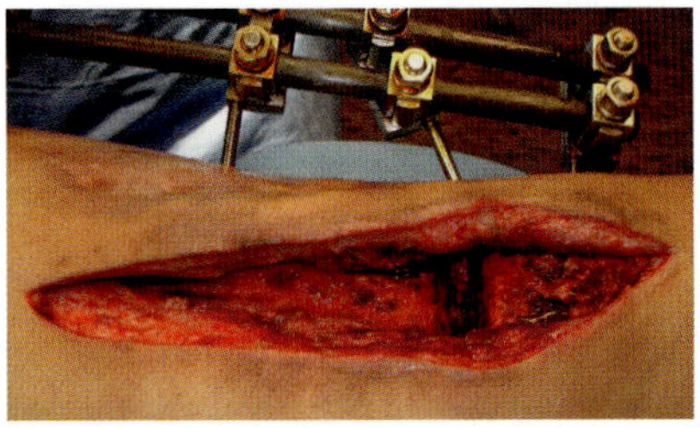

15.4-22 Intraoperative situation after revision (second look) 5 months after the last operation, due to a clinically reactivated infection at the docking site. The bone defect is macroscopically clean and shows vital borders. At that time, the defect was filled with gentamicin polymethylmethacrylate and the wound closed (Masquelet technique).

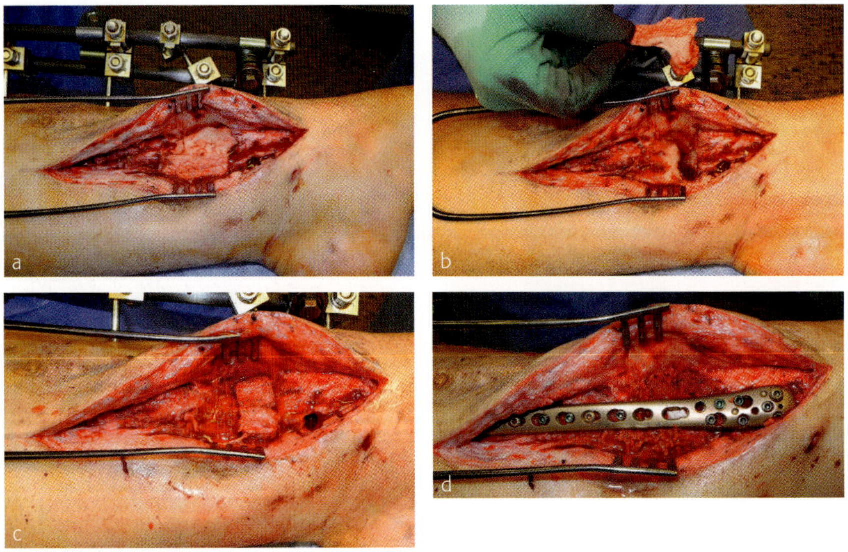

15.4-23a–d Operative pictures 6 weeks later.

- **a** Clean, dry situation.
- **b** Removal of the cement spacer.
- **c** Defect filled with autogenous tricorticocancellous bone blocks (iliac crest).
- **d** Restabilization of the tibia with an LCP distal medial tibial plate 3.5, and further cancellous bone grafting added anteriorly and posteriorly to the plate.

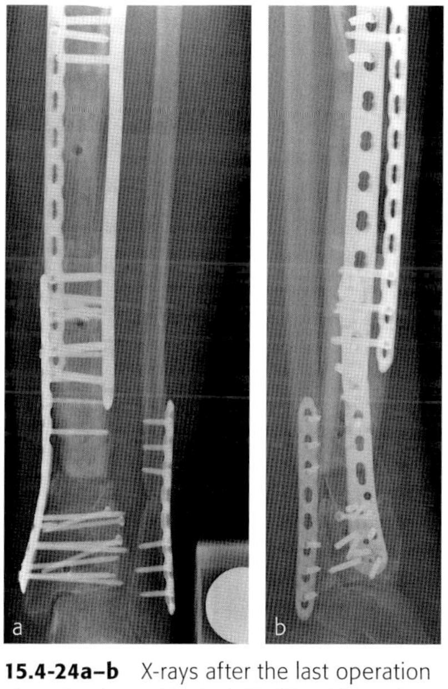

15.4-24a–b X-rays after the last operation show the bone blocks fully filling the defect at the former docking site.

a AP view.

b Lateral view.

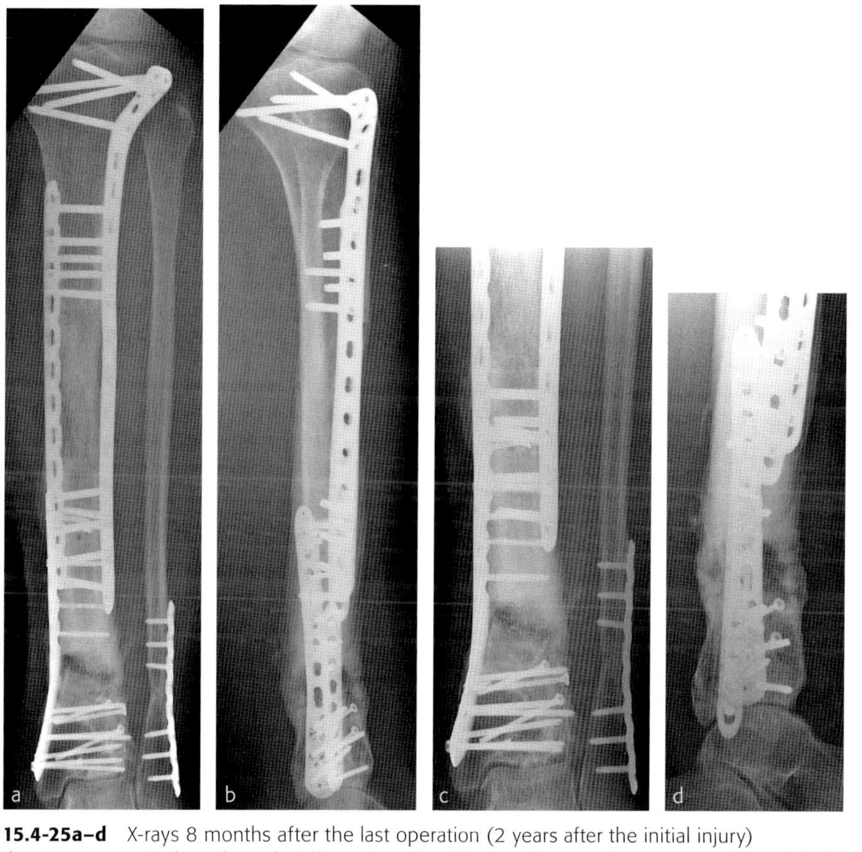

15.4-25a–d X-rays 8 months after the last operation (2 years after the initial injury) demonstrate a nicely and nearly fully remineralized former distracted segment at the midshaft and a slow but progressive healing of the distal docking site with bridging callus posteriorly and laterally. The implants are all intact; all screws are stable in the bone with intact interfaces to the surrounding bone.

a AP view (total).

b Lateral view (total).

c AP view (detail distally).

d Lateral view (detail distally).

9 Pitfalls

9.1 Diagnosis and decision making

- It may be difficult to diagnose a low-grade infection in the setting of delayed union and/or implant failure after fracture treatment. Tissue biopsies for cultures are important in these cases.
- The presence of devitalized bone in cases of (low-grade) infected bone can harbor ongoing chronic bone infection. Intraoperative judgment of vitality of the bone is important, and may lead to under- or overestimation of the amount of resection needed even by an experienced surgeon. There are no preoperative imaging procedures available to localize and quantify the devitalized bone in a precise way.
- Large segmental bone debridement and reconstruction with segmental transport can be risky in cases of poor patient compliance. The decision for this treatment option must be made together with the patient (and the relatives).

9.2 Surgical approach

The anterolateral extended approach to the distal tibia can endanger the superficial and deep peroneal nerve and the anterior tibial artery and vein.

9.3 Implant removal

In case of implant failure and infection, all the implants must be removed. Broken screws can be difficult to extract.

9.4 Temporary fixation

- External fixation is easy to apply in the distal tibia bridging the ankle joint. The unilateral frame might be insufficient in large bone defect with high instability as in this case.
- The Schanz pins should be outside the infected zone.

9.5 Reimplantation

Premature removal of external fixation and conversion to internal fixation after segmental transport critically relies upon patient compliance. One single step with full loading of the construct can bend the plate and lead to further surgery. It may be better to either leave the external fixator in place longer or to stabilize a long-distracted segment with a double-plate fixation or an intramedullary nail.

9.6 Failure of therapy

In cases of critical soft-tissue envelope around the location of the corticotomy or other risk factors leading to an impaired vitality of this region, these might endanger the normal evolution and maturing of the new bone formation at the distraction site.

10 Pearls

10.1 Decision making

- Segmental transport can be an excellent, safe, and overall a useful technique to reconstruct large segmental bone defects in the tibia, if no complications occur. The compliant patient should be educated continuously over the duration of the treatment.
- In most cases, segmental transport leads to a very good new bone quality similar to the normal diaphyseal bone.

10.2 Surgical approach

The anterolateral extended approach to the distal tibia provides good access to the distal tibia and is easier to perform compared to the anterolateral approach. Risk of neurovascular damage is low.

10.3 Implant removal

Failed plates and screws may be easier to remove compared to a failed (broken) nail.

10.4 Temporary fixation

Ankle bridging external fixation is easy to apply and has a low morbidity.

10.5 Definitive revision—second stage

The early exchange of external (transport) fixator to internal fixation is well received by the patient. He or she is finally "rid" of the hated external device. Inserting a strong "plate" as internal fixation (eg, LCP) usually provides sufficient stability even with very early surgery immediately after finishing the transport.

15.5 Acutely infected proximal femoral fracture—dynamic hip screw

Stephen L Kates

1 Case description

An 81-year-old man presented with an intertrochanteric hip fracture treated with a dynamic hip screw at another hospital 3 months prior. He initially fell from a standing height while walking in a casino. He presented with intractable right hip pain and a sacral pressure sore, with exposed bone growing methicillin-resistant *Staphylococcus aureus*.

He had previously been ambulatory but could not walk at the time of presentation. He had remained in a nursing home since he was discharged from the other hospital. He was rendered nonweight bearing by the original surgeon and developed a postoperative deep vein thrombosis after the hip fracture.

Past medical history includes: hypertension, diabetes, coronary artery disease with stents, atrial fibrillation, mild dementia, depression, spinal stenosis, esophageal reflux, and ulcerative colitis.

Medications include: warfarin, methadone for pain, oxycontin, oxycodone immediate release, acetaminophen, imdur, lopressor, cymbalta, prevacid, insulin, avandia, and aspirin.

Laboratory workup revealed: white blood cell count: 10,500 cells/µL, erythrocyte sedimentation rate: 66 mm/h, C-reactive protein: 61 mg/L.

2 Indications

Presumably, this man had developed a surgical-site infection following surgical repair of the right hip fracture (**Fig 15.5-1**). He continually experienced pain including nighttime pain. His systemic inflammatory markers were elevated, supporting a presumed diagnosis of infection. Progressive pain and disability prompted a plan for surgical exploration of the site and removal of the dynamic hip screw.

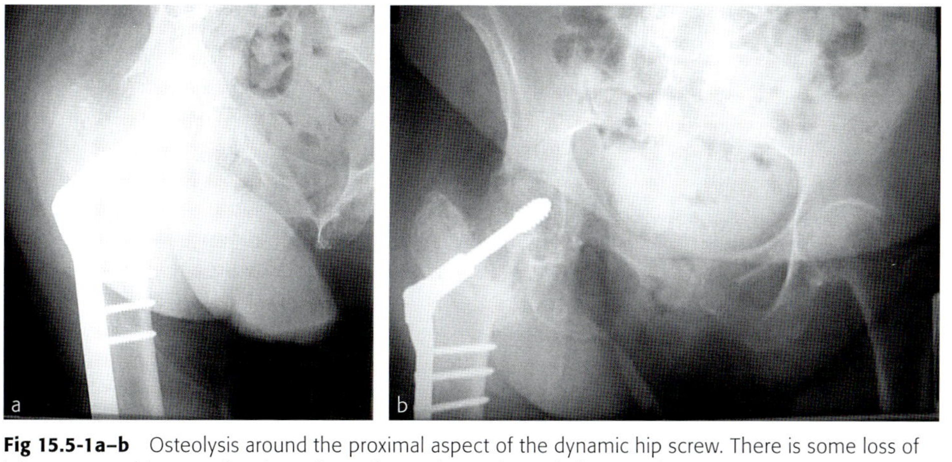

Fig 15.5-1a–b Osteolysis around the proximal aspect of the dynamic hip screw. There is some loss of joint space and increased periosteal reaction at the trochanteric fracture site.

3 Preoperative planning

Preoperative planning included a general medicine and cardiology outpatient consultation to assess the patient's fitness for surgical intervention. Both the cardiologist and medical physician had recommended that surgery be performed under general anesthesia. It was suggested that his warfarin be discontinued 5 days prior to surgery without bridging anticoagulation. This recommendation was based on the fact that he experienced a significant postoperative bleed at the surgical site following the insertion of the dynamic hip screw.

When planning the surgery, the appropriate removal instruments for the dynamic hip screw were ordered. Additionally, a broken-screw set was made available and plans were made to obtain pathology, culture, and sensitivity from the surgical site.

Positioning was planned on the fracture table with availability of the image intensifier in the event that removal of the implants proved to be difficult. General anesthesia was planned with the attending anesthesiologist.

4 Surgical approach

The surgical approach was planned to use his old incision, which was a long lateral hip incision. The incision itself was well healed. The plan was to open the old incision down to the fascia lata, split the fascia lata in line with its fibers and retract it, and then incise the vastus lateralis muscle fascia, splitting the muscle down to the plate. Use of a Charnley self-retaining retractor for exposure was planned. Additionally, angled Weitlaner retractors were made available for exposure.

During the actual surgical exposure, a large abscess was encountered, which was described as thick creamy pus. Culture and sensitivity was taken of this liquid and of tissue surrounding the implants.

5 Surgical debridement

Surgical debridement was carried out after removal of the implants. The wall of the abscess cavity was excised. The underlying bone was noted to be covered with granulation tissue. The cavity occupied by the hip screw was curetted free of biofilm and slimy biological membranes. All areas of devitalized bone were mechanically removed with a rongeur and curette. Bone biopsies were sent to the pathology lab for a permanent section as well as culture and sensitivity. Soft-tissue culture was also sent to the laboratory. **Fig 15.5-2** shows the pathology results.

After managing the patient's hip infection, his sacral pressure sore was debrided back to healthy tissue and a moist sterile normal saline dressing was applied.

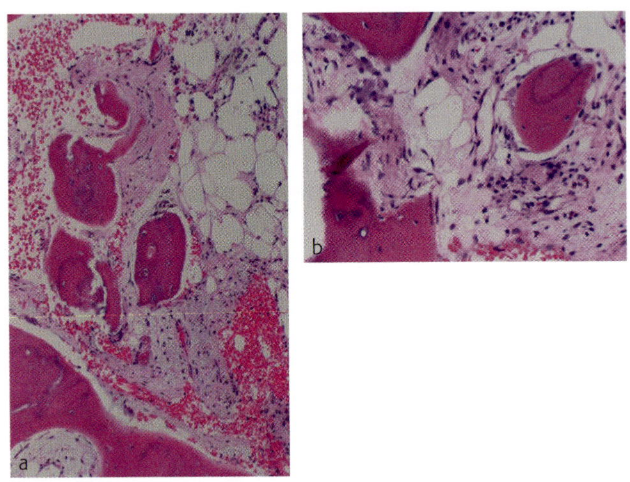

Fig 15.5-2a–b Hematoxylin and eosin stained sections of the infected right femoral bone. Acute and chronic osteomyelitis is demonstrated.

6 Implant removal

Implant removal was readily carried out by removing all the 4.5 mm screws and the plate. The plate implant was found to be somewhat loosened and was readily removed by pulling it off the sliding hip screw. The sliding hip screw was removed with the wrench provided by the manufacturer. No broken implants were encountered and the implant was easily explanted. **Fig 15.5-3** demonstrates the implant removal and condition of the bone.

7 Temporary fixation

In this case, it was decided not to place any additional implants in the bone or large abscess cavity. A decision was made to await further laboratory and culture information.

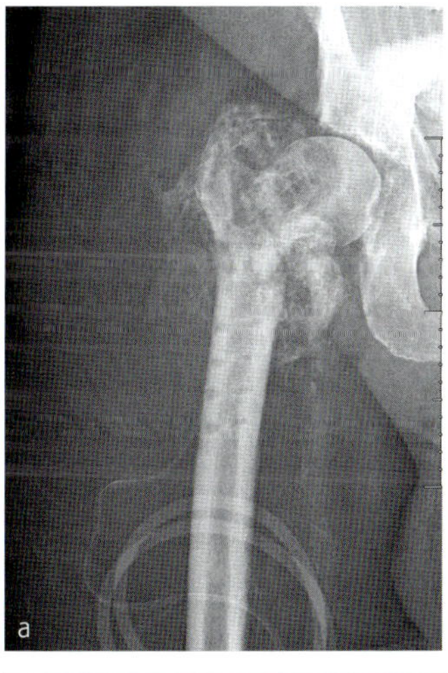

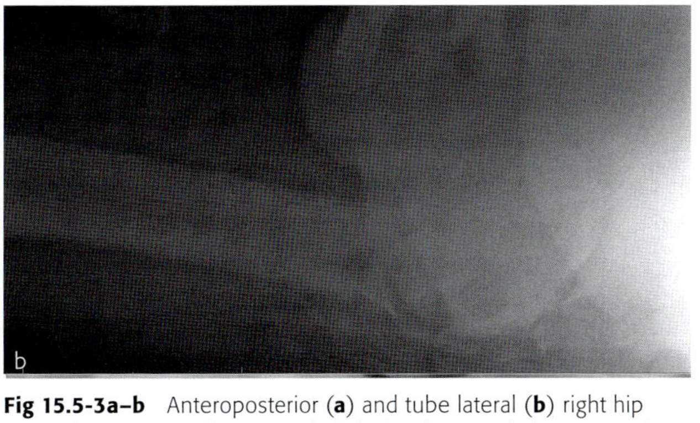

Fig 15.5-3a–b Anteroposterior (**a**) and tube lateral (**b**) right hip x-rays demonstrate the removal of the implants and placement of a suction drain.

8 Postoperative management

The patient was allowed to bear weight as tolerated on the right hip. Unfortunately, he had persistent pain that did not resolve after his wound had healed. His cultures grew *Peptostreptococcus* and *Staphylococcus epidermidis* sensitive to vancomycin. A consultation was requested from the infectious diseases service. He was started on intravenous vancomycin. He was also treated with imipenem to cover previously cultured *Peptostreptococcus*. His postoperative course was marked by persistent pain with weight bearing that was in the hip area rather than the incisional area.

Due to his persistent pain and difficulty with weight bearing, it was decided to reoperate and perform a Girdlestone procedure (**Fig 15.5-4**). The Girdlestone procedure was carried out by extending his lateral incision into a posterior lateral exposure of the hip. The bone was noted to be soft with significant changes consistent with chronic osteomyelitis of the proximal femur. The acetabulum was curetted free of inflamed membranes and the entire head and neck of the femur was resected. His wound was closed over a suction drain. No additional purulent material was noted at the time of surgery, but chronic granulation tissue was present. His postoperative bone cultures again grew *Peptostreptococcus*.

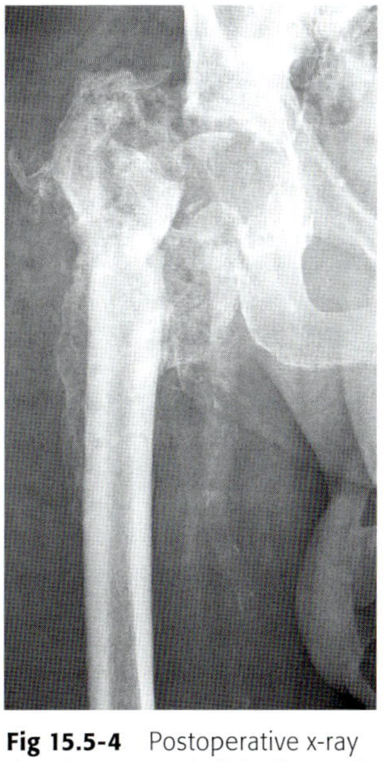

Fig 15.5-4 Postoperative x-ray showing removal of the femoral head and neck and subsequent debridement—the Girdlestone procedure.

9 Reimplantation

The patient's condition was discussed in detail with his daughter and the patient as well as his primary care doctor. A decision was made not to attempt to implant a total hip replacement based on his extremely difficult postoperative course after the hip fracture surgery. He was permitted to bear weight as tolerated on his Girdlestone situation.

10 Outcome

X-rays 5 years postoperatively are shown in **Fig 15.5-5**. At the present time, a 9-year follow-up is available, demonstrating the patient's ability to ambulate without difficulty on his Girdlestone situation. He mostly walks with a walker frame and uses a 3 cm shoe lift in his right shoe. He has experienced no recurrence of infectious symptoms and is generally pleased with his outcome. He is essentially pain free. He still resides in a residential home with nursing assistance.

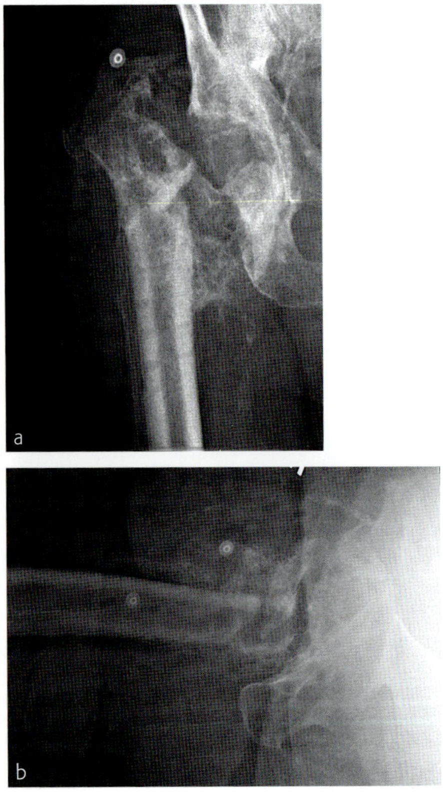

Fig 15.5-5a–b Anteroposterior (**a**) and tube lateral (**b**) x-ray views show the long-term result of a Girdlestone procedure of the right hip.

11 Pitfalls

- Diagnosis and decision making: a painful hip after dynamic hip screw surgery should prompt concern for infection and trigger a workup for infection.
- Surgical approach: infected tissue is typically stiffer and more difficult to mobilize.
- Implant removal: it is important to have the correct instrument set available to remove the lag screw. A broken-screw removal set should be available in the event that a screw has broken.
- Temporary fixation: this may be difficult to achieve, especially in elderly patients
- Rehabilitation: weight bearing as tolerated is important to prevent the sequelae of immobility. Many older adults will have difficulty mobilizing after implant removal unless the fracture has already united.
- Reimplantation: depending on the chronicity, definitive fixation or replacement may be options. Resection arthroplasty is the other reasonable option for debilitated patients.
- Failure of therapy: failure of therapy may result from failure to control the infection. Removal of all devitalized bone and implants are essential to help control the infection. Multiple surgeries should be avoided in elderly patients if possible. Reinfection after revision surgery should prompt concern for retained necrotic bone.

12 Pearls

- Decision making: intervene early when infection is diagnosed. Request an infectious diseases consultation to determine the best drug therapy.
- Surgical approach: use the prior incision and extend it as needed.
- Implant removal: have the correct implant-specific removal set available.
- Temporary fixation: an antibiotic nail or antibiotic-coated temporary hip replacement are two reasonable options for temporary fixation in these cases.
- Definitive revision—second stage: early revision should be planned when medically stable and the infection has been controlled.
- Antibiotic management: use bacteriocidal antibiotics if possible with the help of an infectious diseases consultant.

15.6 Acutely infected proximal femoral fracture—proximal femoral nail

Michael J Zegg, Christian Kammerlander

1 Case description

In early January 2011, a 33-year-old patient presented to the authors' department with a pertrochanteric fracture of the right femur after a fall from 4 m (**Fig 15.6-1**). While the patient had not had prior surgery, multiple falls were documented due to chronic drug and alcohol abuse. At admission, the patient was participating in a methadone program and had a Hepatitis C infection.

Surgical treatment with closed reduction and implantation of a short trochanteric entry nail was performed (**Fig 15.6-2**). Despite the patient's noncompliance, the immediate postsurgical period passed without complications, and the patient was discharged 8 days postoperatively.

The patient subsequently fell again 4 weeks postoperatively due to alcohol and drug intoxication, resulting in a periimplant fracture and fracture of the implant (**Fig 15.6-3**). Revision surgery was performed at the beginning of February, 2011.

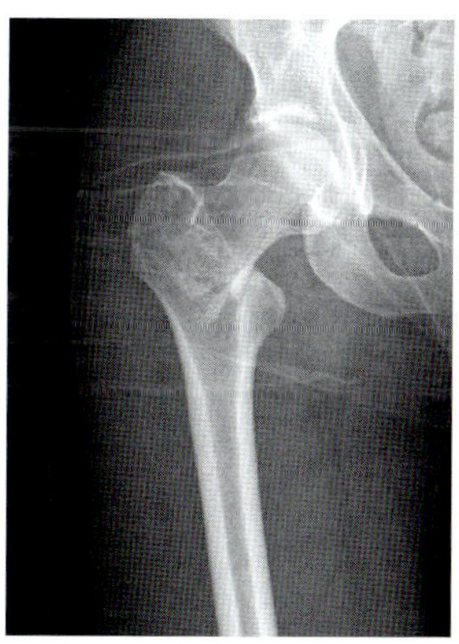

Fig 15.6-1 AP x-ray shows a pertrochanteric fracture of the right femur.

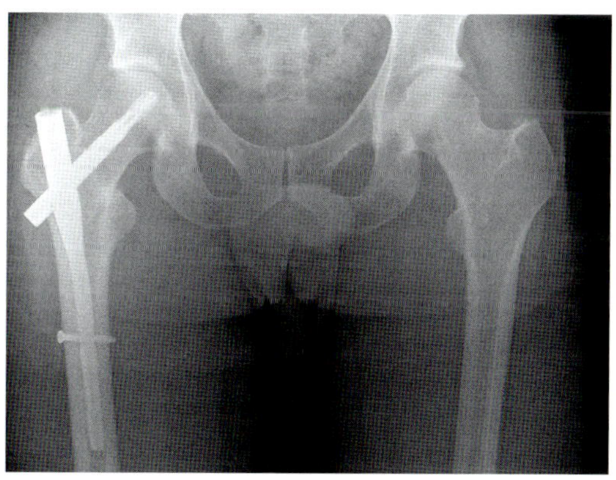

Fig 15.6-2 Postoperative AP x-ray with implanted proximal femoral nail.

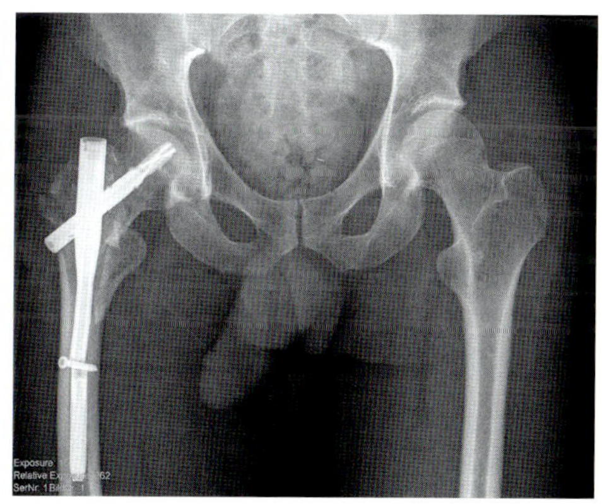

Fig 15.6-3 X-ray control after another fall showing an implant fracture through the locking screw hole.

The short broken implant was removed (**Fig 15.6-4**) and a long nail was implanted (**Fig 15.6-5**). The immediate postsurgical course was without complications, and the patient was discharged after 5 days.

Eight days after the second discharge, the patient presented to the outpatient clinic with severe pain and pronounced signs of local infection at the right hip. Furthermore, x-rays showed a cutout of the helical blade (**Fig 15.6-6**). A computed tomographic scan showed fluid retention in the soft tissue at the previous operation site (**Fig 15.6-7**).

Due to the cutout of the blade and both local (redness, pus at the proximal operation wound) and systemic infection signs with C-reactive protein (CRP) 29.81 mg/dL and leukocyte count of 17,400 cells/µL (**Fig 15.6-8**), revision surgery was indicated.

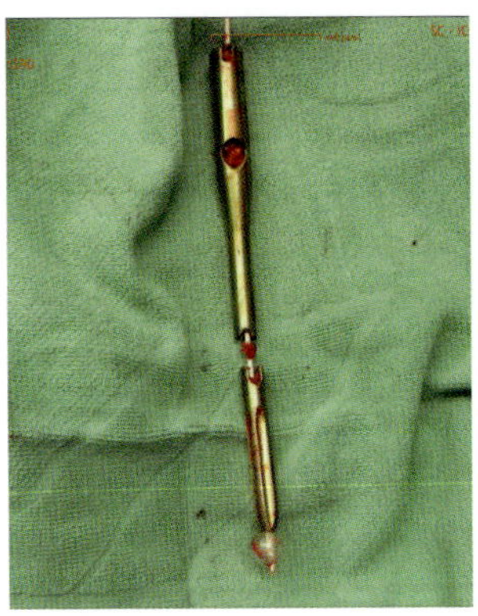

Fig 15.6-4 Removed proximal femoral nail with mounted urinary catheter.

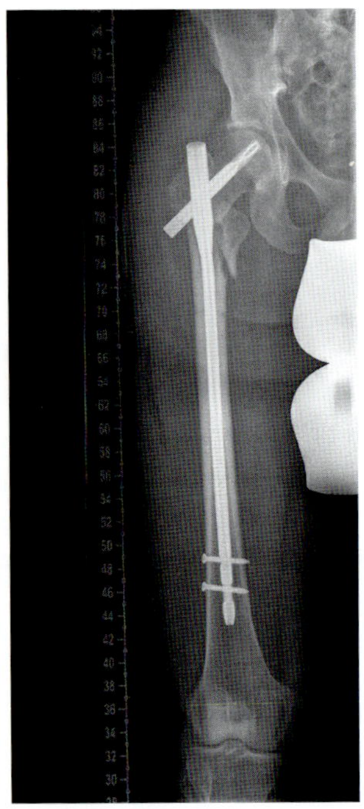

Fig 15.6-5 AP x-ray after the second operation with implanted proximal femoral nail, long.

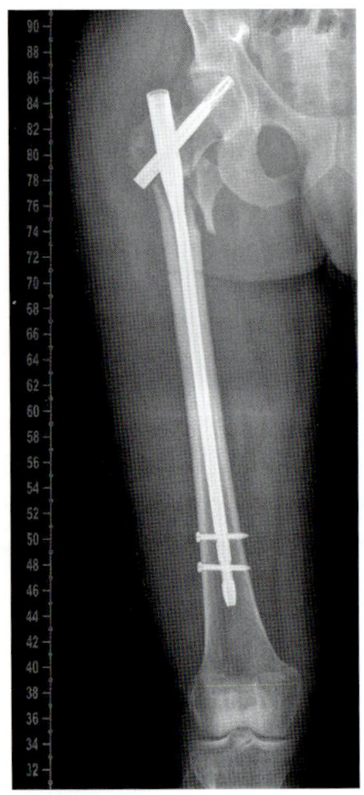

Fig 15.6-6 Control x-ray shows blade cutout.

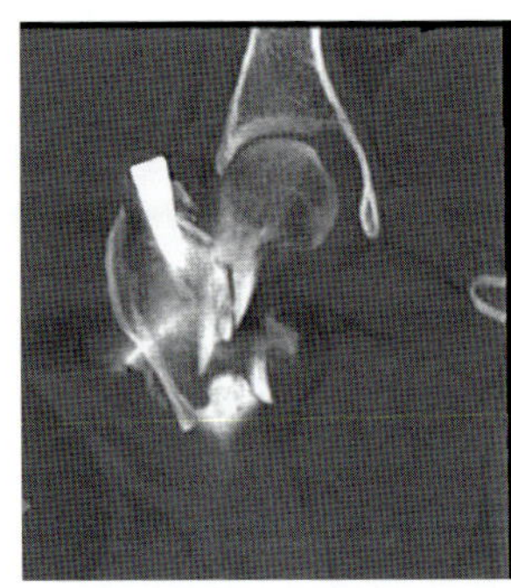

Fig 15.6-7 Computed tomographic scan shows soft-tissue fluid retention at the operative site.

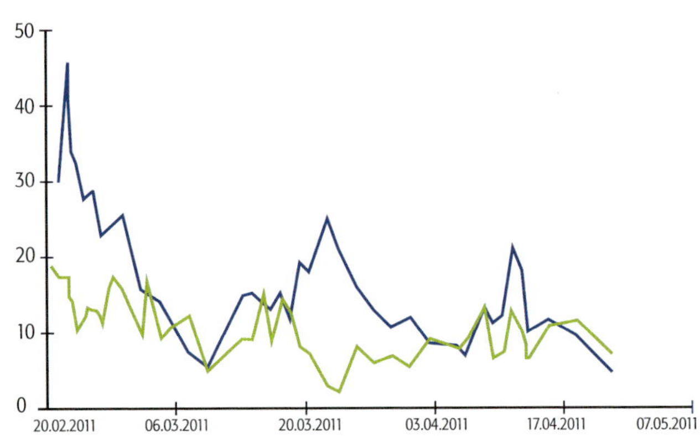

Fig 15.6-8 Systemic infection signs. Blue: C-reactive protein; green: leukocyte count.

Early surgical intervention was performed after planning. First, operative revision and debridement of the soft tissue was performed. The patient was placed in supine position and the approach was performed through the prior incisions. Sutures were removed and a large quantity of pus was found with a subcutaneous connection between the existing proximal and distal incisions. After extensive debridement, signs of infection were also present around the greater trochanter at the entry point of the nail. There was a large amount of pus found and evacuated. After ample lavage, a silver-impregnated negative-pressure wound therapy dressing was applied. During the revision operation many tissue samples were collected for microbiological assessment. After taking the tissue samples, parenteral antibiotic therapy with a second-generation cephalosporin was started.

On the next day, a further revision was performed. To manage the pronounced infection, implant removal was indicated. The patient was placed in true lateral position to enable operative exposure if needed. During removal of the implant, pus was also found inside the bone. Therefore, the femoral head was removed and intramedullary curettage and reaming (11.5 mm diameter) were performed (**Fig 15.6-9**). Further tissue samples were collected. In addition, a cement spacer with gentamicin was formed and implanted. Then three large drains were inserted and the operative wound was closed (**Fig 15.6-10**).

Culture of the tissue samples revealed an infection caused by *Streptococcus dysgalactiae* and coagulase-positive *Staphylococcus*. In accordance with the antibiogram, antibiotic therapy was adapted with amoxicillin/clavulanic acid and vancomycin.

Three days later another septic revision was performed. Once again in true lateral position, the previous incision was opened and resection of necrotic tissue was conducted. The cement spacer was also removed and intramedullary reaming up to 12 mm was performed. Furthermore, a lateral window of the distal femoral shaft was cut out. After ample debridement and lavage, a new cement spacer was inserted. Then two drains proximally and one drain distally, were placed through the resected window inside the femoral shaft before closing the operation wound.

Further bacteriological tests revealed additional contamination with *Escherichia coli*. Therefore antibiotic therapy was adapted once again with piperacillin/tazobactam instead of amoxicillin/clavulanic acid in concordance with the antibiogram.

Four additional revision operations were performed over the next 4 weeks with replacement of cement spacer and repeated intramedullary insertion of polymethylmethacrylate bead chains and minichains loaded with gentamicin sulphate. Negative-pressure wound therapy was initiated to address the loss of soft-tissue coverage following the abovementioned repeated resections of soft tissue. During the last revision, 6 weeks after readmission to the authors' clinic, the antibiotic bead chains were removed, another cement spacer was inserted, and the operation wound closed.

Due to further bacteriological results and repeatedly elevated CRP and leukocyte count, antibiotic therapy was adapted with parenteral administration of imipenem combined with fluconazole.

After nearly 10 weeks with no further local or systemic infection signs present (**Fig 15.6-8**), the patient was discharged once again. Further oral antibiotic therapy with fluconazole was prescribed and short-term follow-up at the outpatient clinic was scheduled.

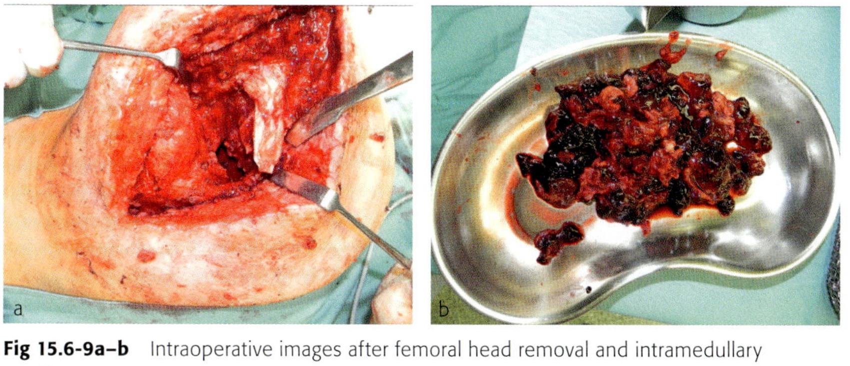

Fig 15.6-9a–b Intraoperative images after femoral head removal and intramedullary curettage.

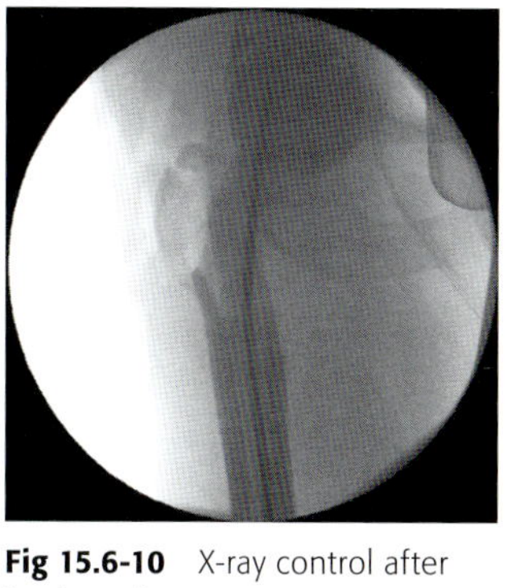

Fig 15.6-10 X-ray control after implanted cement spacer.

One week after discharge the patient reappeared at the outpatient clinic because of pain at the right hip. X-rays showed a broken cement spacer (**Fig 15.6-11**). Blood samples showed alcohol and drug intoxication yet no systemic increase of infection signs. Also no local infection signs around the operation wound were present.

After thorough discussion, and considering the previous extensive infection, revision operations, and noncompliance of the patient due to chronic drug and alcohol abuse, no further revision was planned. Mobilization was possible with crutches and also the pain lessened and so the patient was discharged after 5 days.

Ambulatory follow-up visits showed a promising course with no signs of infection recurrence. Therefore revision surgery with removal of the cement spacer and implantation of an arthroplasty was considered. The patient passed away due to drug intoxication 5 months after discharge.

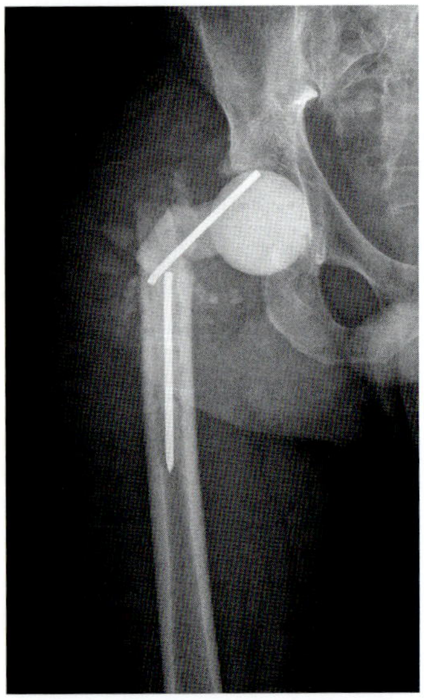

Fig 15.6-11 AP x-ray with broken cement spacer.

2 Indications

- Local infection signs: pain, swelling, reddening, healing disturbance of previous operation wound, pus
- Systemic infection signs: fever, high blood-level CRP, elevated leukocyte count, interleukin-6, high erythrocyte sedimentation rate
- X-ray: loosening, movement of implant

3 Preoperative planning

- Blood samples, local culture
- X-rays
- Computed tomographic scan for further planning: magnitude of revision
- Implant removal set, culture kits, and containers for tissue samples for bacteriological testing

4 Surgical approach

Reuse of the previous incisions and extension if required.

5 Surgical debridement

- Radical debridement is necessary with removal of pus, resection of infected or necrotic soft tissue and of infected or necrotic bone until only healthy soft tissue or bleeding bone is left.
- Reaming intramedullary canal for removal of necrotic and infected bone.
- At least five different tissue samples should be collected for further bacteriological testing.
- Drains should be inserted to prevent fluid retention.
- If the radical debridement does not permit primary closure of the surgical wound, negative-pressure wound therapy should be conducted.

6 Implant removal

- Implant removal is usually required.
- With the removal set an intramedullary nail is straightforward to remove.

7 Temporary fixation

- Cement spacer with correct diameter.
- Antibiotic bead chains.

8 Postoperative management

- After first soft-tissue samples are gathered for bacteriological testing, parenteral antibiotic therapy should be started.
- Adaptation of antibiotic therapy due to the antibiogram is essential.
- Further operative revisions should be planned depending on local and systemic infection signs, and further debridement could be necessary.
- Mobilization is encouraged: partial weight bearing with crutches due to the cement spacer.
- After no systemic or local infection signs after 6 months (or even earlier), removal of the spacer and an arthroplasty may be performed.

9 Outcome

A poor outcome resulted due to noncompliance; drug and alcohol abuse.

10 Pitfalls

- Insufficient diagnostics and planning before revision.
- Only opening of the previous incisions without exposure of the whole infected area.
- Insufficient debridement of soft tissue.
- Not removing the implant in the early stages of revision.
- No temporary stabilization leading to further disability for the patient.
- Early full weight bearing and stopping of antibiotic therapy.
- Too early reimplantation without resolved infection.
- No ambulatory follow-up, noncompliance.

11 Pearls

- If an infection is suspected, blood samples, cultures, x-rays, and optionally a computed tomographic scan are needed to provide all the information needed for decision making.
- Previous incisions need to be reopened and enlarged to enable sufficient assessment of the infection site and radical debridement.
- Implant removal is usually necessary to provide the possibility of healing by means of destroying a biofilm extracellular polymeric substance and to allow intramedullary debridement.
- Implant removal can be tricky especially if the implant is broken. Small hooks or even a urinary catheter (**Fig 15.6-4**) can be helpful.
- Because of removal of the femoral head, in this case a cement spacer was needed; the appropriate diameter of this spacer is essential.
- During rehabilitation, ambulatory check-ups are crucial to identify complications as early as possible.
- An adequate amount of time without infection is needed before arthroplasty or reimplantation of intramedullary nails.
- In this case the removal of the femoral head was necessary due to the advanced infection of the bone although preservation of bone should be a priority.

16.1 Chronically infected distal tibial fracture

Zhao Xie

1 Case description

A 23-year-old man was involved in a motor vehicle accident and sustained grade IIIB open distal tibial and fibular open fractures. He was transferred to the author's institution 13 months after the initial injury. Debridement and muscle tendon repair were performed at the local hospital. Infection developed postoperatively and debridement surgeries were repeatedly performed with negative-pressure wound therapy, but the infection was still not under control.

On admission to the author's institution, physical examination demonstrated external fixation and exposure of the distal end of the tibia with active drainage (**Fig 16.1-1**).

Initial x-ray and computed tomographic examination demonstrated a comminuted nonunited fracture of the distal tibia, with necrotic and infected bone distally (**Fig 16.1-2**).

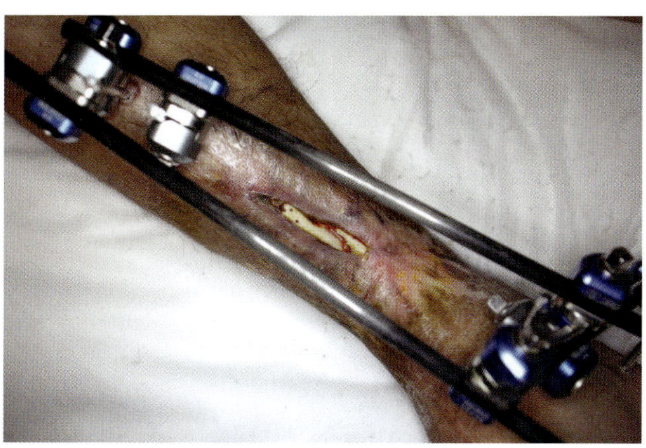

Fig 16.1-1 Clinical appearance.

2 Indication

Nonunion of a tibial comminuted fracture with skin defect and exposed necrotic bone are indications for surgical revision. The surgical plan is to completely remove the necrotic bone and soft tissue, stabilize the fracture, and achieve wound coverage.

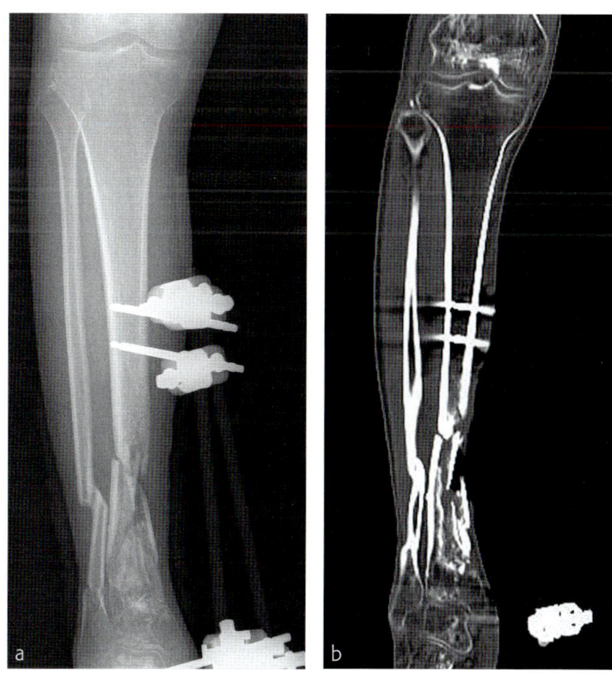

Fig 16.1-2a–b Radiological images.
a X-ray.
b Computed tomographic scan.

3 Preoperative planning

Instruments:

- Pulsed irrigator
- Power drill
- Reamer
- Osteotome
- Bedside x-ray machine
- Locking compression plate

Other:

- Position (supine)
- Tourniquet
- Topical antibiotics (vancomycin 10 g, gentamicin 0.55 g)
- Bone cement
- Antibiotics were selected according to test results taken from the wound sample (*Staphylococcus haemolyticus*) and piperacillin/tazobactam administered 30 minutes before surgery

4 Surgical approach

The surgical approach is from the distal tibia (**Fig 16.1-3**). Necrotic tissue and bone should be debrided. The incision was made over the previous scar, but the margin of the wound had to be resected. All ischemic bone was eliminated including a suspected sequestrum, as biofilm is usually present, resulting in reinfection and further debridement surgery.

5 Surgical debridement

The external fixation was partially removed before the surgery. All granulation tissue, sequestra, and scar tissue were completely removed during surgery. Necrotic bone was completely removed until hemorrhagic spots were seen. The medullary cavity was reamed and thoroughly washed with a pulsed irrigator, and the bone defect was created (**Fig 16.1-4**). The dead space was then filled with antibiotic-loaded bone cement. Cultures were obtained during the surgical debridement.

6 Implant removal

No implant was used during this surgery. The primary external fixator was replaced by a locking plate.

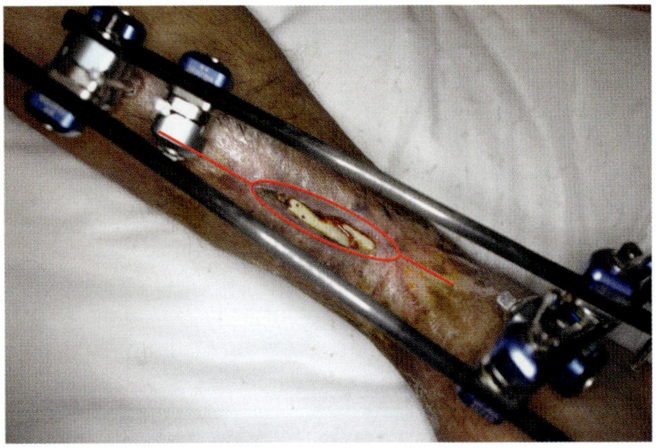

Fig 16.1-3 Distal tibial surgical approach.

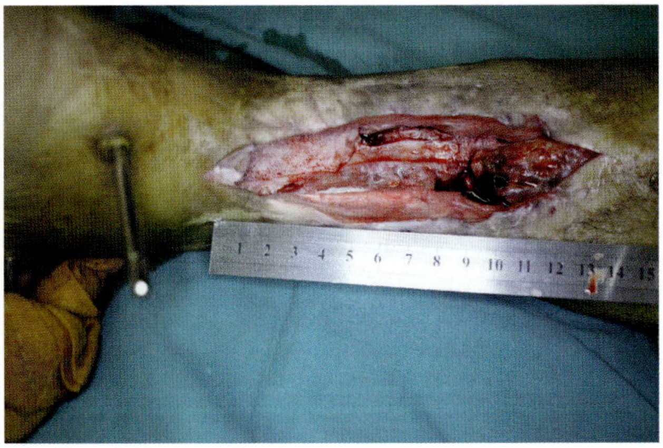

Fig 16.1-4 Bone defect after debridement.

7 Temporary fixation

Antibiotic bone cement was implanted into bone defects (**Fig 16.1-5**), incisions were closed (**Fig 16.1-6**), and external fixation was rebuilt.

Tips:

- To reach fracture-end stabilization, the plate axis should be accordant with the longest axis of the fracture end.
- High-speed drilling should be avoided in case of tissue thermal necrosis injury.
- In trying to close the wound during the hardening of the bone cement, add or decrease the volume of bone cement accordingly.

8 Postoperative management

Micrococcus luteus was found in the intraoperative sample taken during bone graft surgery (while the patient was antibiotics) and cefmenoxime was selected. The patient was given intravenous antibiotics for 2 weeks after surgery and encouraged to perform functional exercises. Less than 20 kg of weight bearing is acceptable. Full weight bearing was prohibited until evidence of callus formation was visible on x-rays.

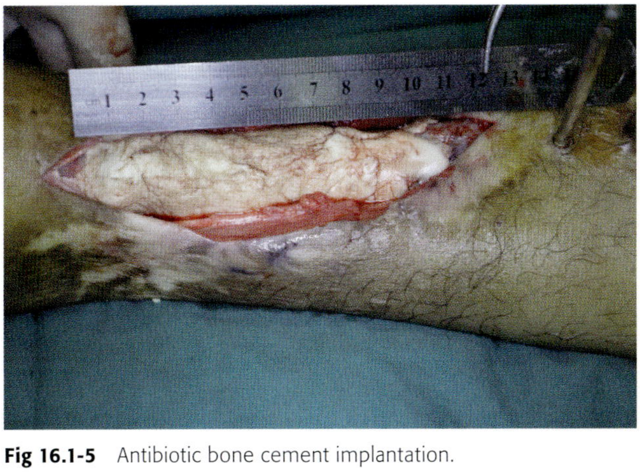

Fig 16.1-5 Antibiotic bone cement implantation.

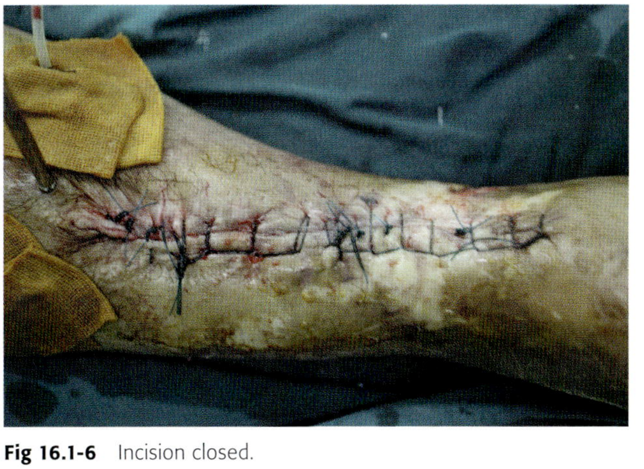

Fig 16.1-6 Incision closed.

9 Reimplantation

There is no consensus on diagnosis of infection after osteomyelitis [1]. In the author's experience, if there is no sign of clinical infection after 2 months of recovery, C-reactive protein and erythrocyte sedimentation rate are normal. The bone graft surgery was performed. First, the fibula was fixed with a locking plate (**Fig 16.1-7**), then the bone grafting was carried out. Autogenous cancellous bone was harvested from the iliac crest (**Fig 16.1-8**) and was placed in the cavity after the bone cement was removed (**Fig 16.1-9**).

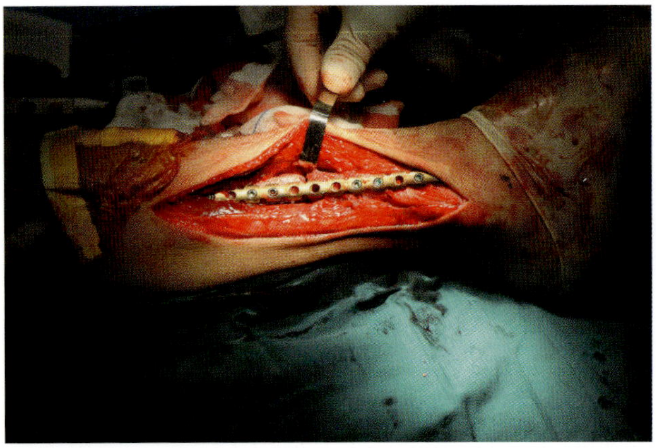

Fig 16.1-7 The fibula was fixed with a locking plate.

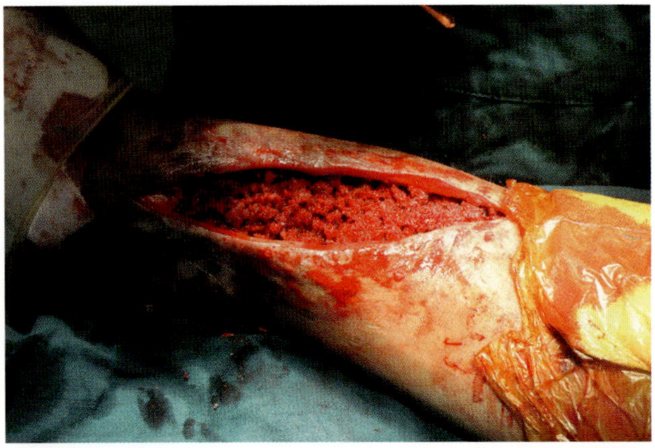

Fig 16.1-8 Autogenous bone grafting.

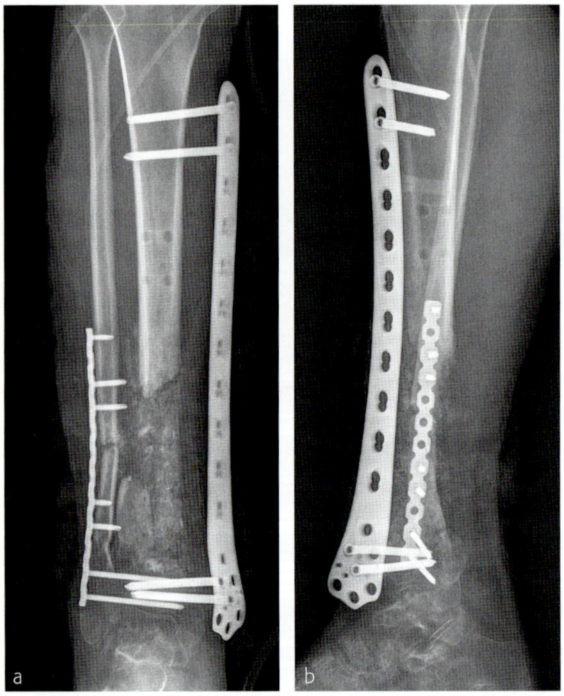

Fig 16.1-9a–b X-rays after bone grafting.
a AP view.
b Lateral view.

10 Outcome

From the clinical appearance of the patient, there is no sign of infection after the surgery (**Fig 16.1-10**). The external fixator was removed 1 year after surgery. Bone corticalization was completed (**Fig 16.1-11**), and the patient was able to fully bear weight.

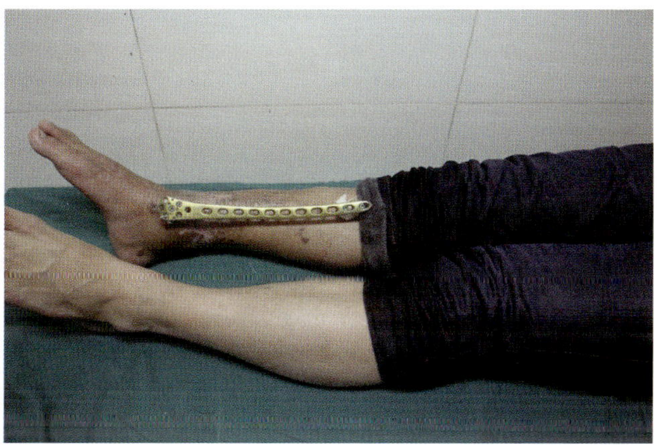

Fig 16.1-10 Postoperative clinical appearance.

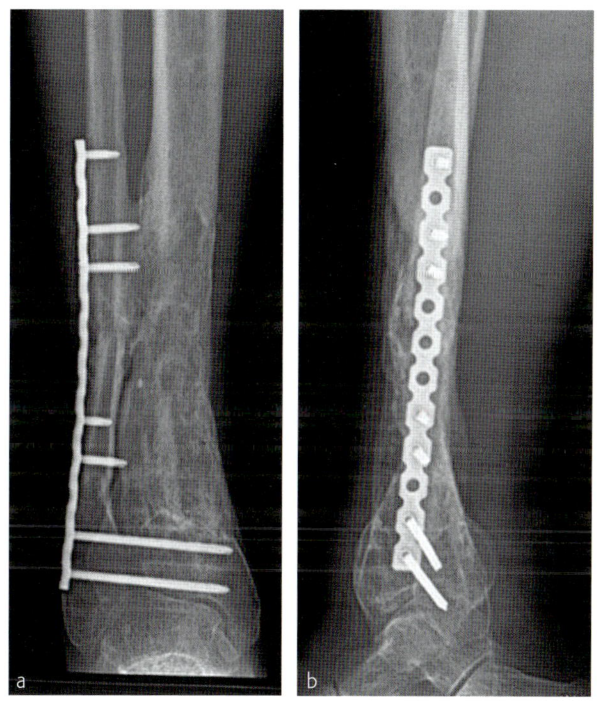

Fig 16.1-11a–b X-rays 18 months postoperatively.
a AP view.
b Lateral view.

11 Pitfalls

- Traditional bacterial culture leads to high false-negative results that might affect the diagnosis of bone infection.
- This surgical approach requires a broad excision of soft tissue and, therefore, may lead to difficulty of wound healing. Flap design should be planned before surgery if primary wound closure cannot be achieved.
- Rehabilitation exercises should be limited due to relatively stable plates. The patient is required to have good compliance and delayed weight bearing.
- Insufficiency of bone cortex formation, bone resorption, and refracture are the risks of cancellous bone grafting.

12 Pearls

- The surgical approach allows for good exposure of the bone infection site for complete debridement.
- External fixation using the locking compression plate is aesthetic and convenient for the patients to get dressed.
- Topical antibiotic administration inhibits bacterial growth in the dead space. The amount and dosage of systemic antibiotics usage can be reduced.

13 Reference

1. **Walter G, Kemmerer M, Kappler C, et al.** Treatment algorithms for chronic osteomyelitis. *Dtsch Arztebl Int.* 2012 Apr;109(14):257–264.

14 Acknowledgements

The author acknowledges the contributions of Professor Jian Zhong Xu and Dr Wei Li.

16.2 Chronically infected proximal tibial fracture

Zhao Xie

1 Case description

A 19-year-old man had a left tibial plateau fracture with proximal fibular fracture caused by a motor vehicle accident. Before he was referred to the author's hospital, he was treated with internal fixation and allograft. On initial examination, he had wound drainage with purulent exudate and a lateral exposed tibial plate (**Fig 16.2-1**, **Fig 16.2-2**).

2 Indication

The plate exposure with purulent exudate served as an obvious indication for bone infection surgery. The fracture should be stabilized, wounds covered, and infection focus controlled with surgery.

3 Preoperative planning

Instruments:

- Pulsed irrigator
- Power drill
- Reamer
- Osteotome
- Bedside x-ray machine
- Hybrid fixator and locking compression plate (LCP)

Other:

- Position
- Tourniquet
- Topical antibiotics (vancomycin 10 g, gentamicin 0.55 g)
- Bone cement
- Antibiotics were selected according to drug test results on the wound sample (*Escherichia coli* and *Acinetobacter baumanii*); third-generation cephalosporin cefmenoxime is administered 30 minutes before surgery

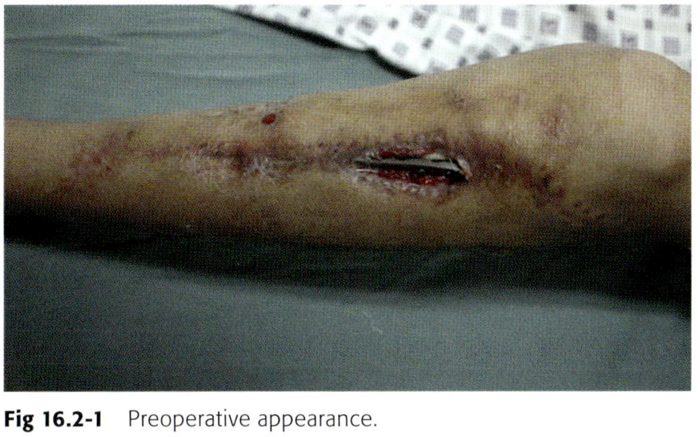

Fig 16.2-1 Preoperative appearance.

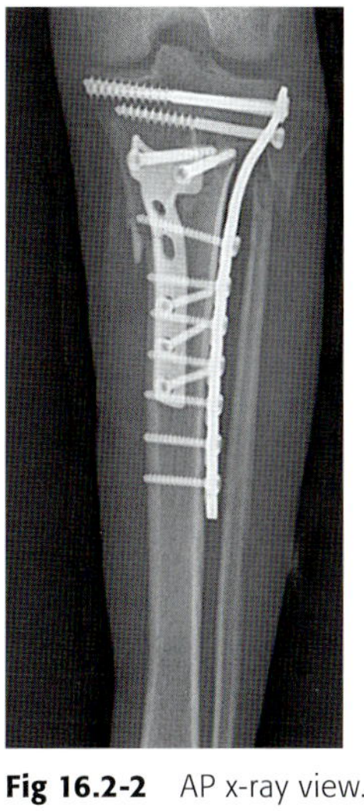

Fig 16.2-2 AP x-ray view.

4 Surgical approach

The incision followed the previous scar, but the margin of the wound had to be resected (**Fig 16.2-3**).

5 Surgical debridement

All granulation tissue, sequestra, and scar tissue were completely removed during surgery. Suspicious necrotic bone should be removed until hemorrhagic spots are seen [1]. Any dead tissue and scar tissue are removed to enhance the recovery of blood supply. The medullary cavity is reamed and washed thoroughly with pulsed irrigator. Segmental ischemic bone (white, beneath the tibial plateau) was retained after the first debridement (**Fig 16.2-4**).The dead space was then filled with antibiotic-loaded bone cement (vancomycin 10 g and gentamicin 0.55 g). The clinical appearance after the first debridement 3 months later showed an active sinus tract (**Fig 16.2-5**). The planned bone grafting was aborted; the patient underwent another debridement and the external fixator was replaced (**Fig 16.2-6**).

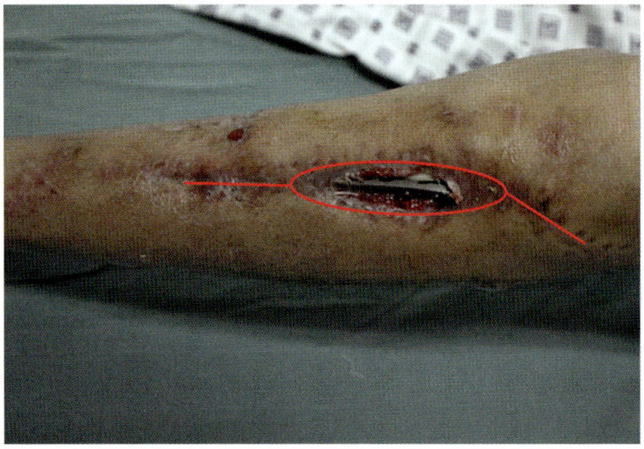

Fig 16.2-3 Surgical approach.

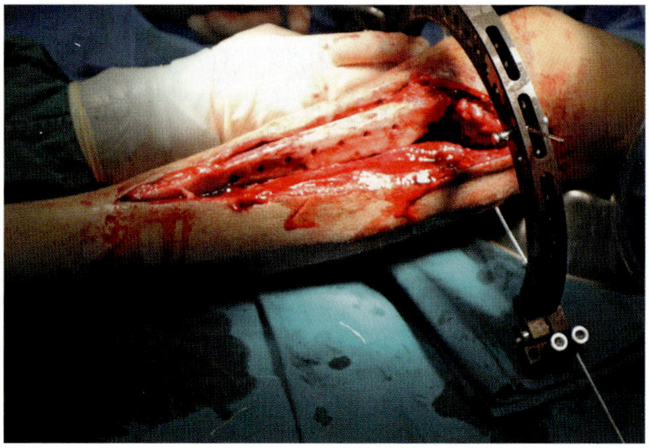

Fig 16.2-4 Bone defect after first debridement.

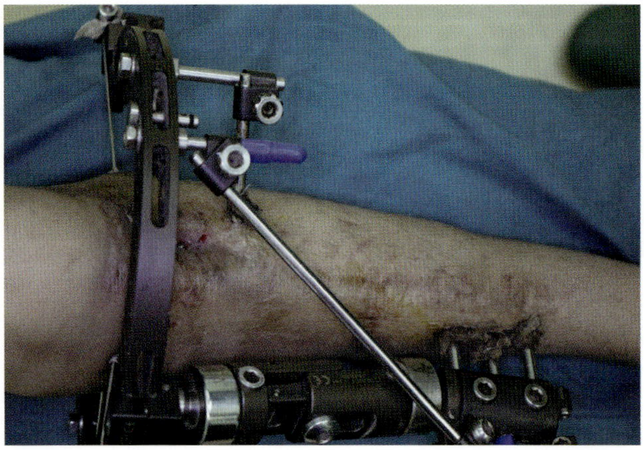

Fig 16.2-5 Clinical appearance 3 months after first debridement.

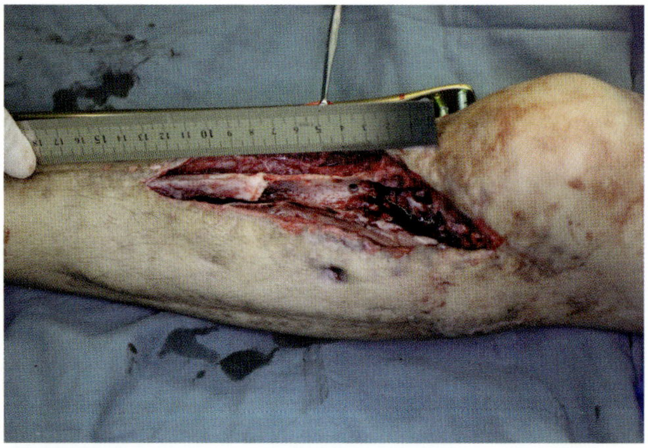

Fig 16.2-6 Bone defect after second debridement. The necrotic segment of bone has now been removed. In retrospect, it should have been removed during the initial debridement.

6 Implant removal

The plate and screws were completely exposed and the screws of the anterolateral and internal plates were removed during the first debridement (**Fig 16.2-7**).

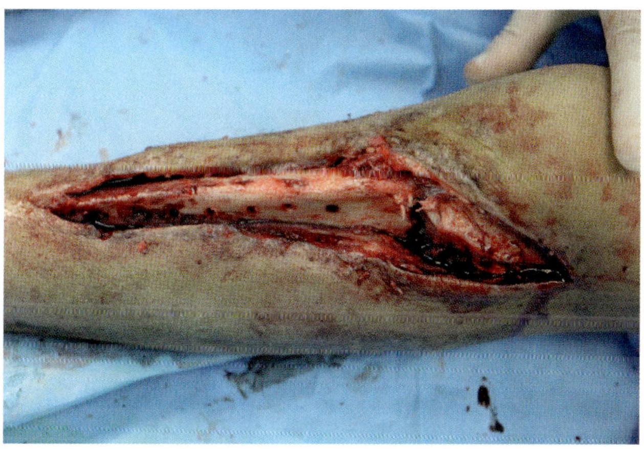

Fig 16.2-7 Implants have been removed.

7 Temporary fixation

Fixation of the bone infection site is usually external. Considering the compliance of the patient, an LCP was used for this external fixation (**Fig 16.2-8**, **Fig 16.2-9**).

Tips:

- The locking plate is more compact compared with the hybrid fixator, but careful postoperative management is important.
- Suspicious necrotic bone should be removed at initial debridement to avoid the need for a second debridement (**Fig 16.2-4**, **Fig 16.2-6**).

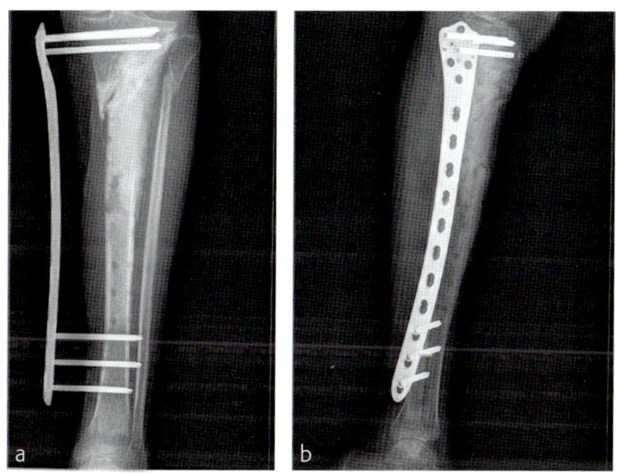

Fig 16.2-8a–b X-rays after debridement show external fixation and the cement spacer.
a AP view.
b Lateral view.

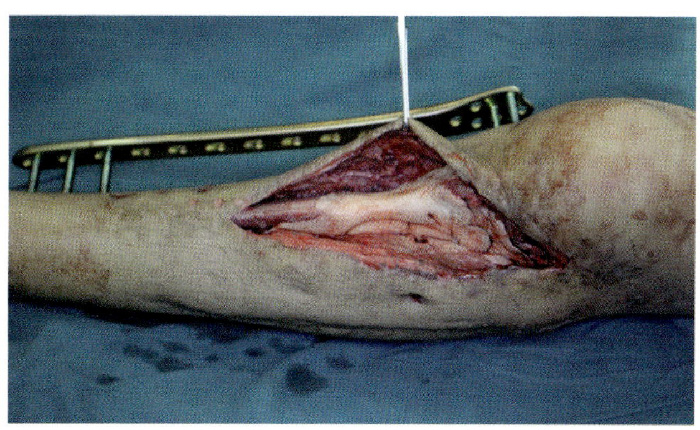

Fig 16.2-9 Antibiotic bone-cement wrapped bone defects (Masquelet technique) [2].

8 Postoperative management

Acinetobacter baumanii was cultured from the intraoperative sample during bone grafting surgery and antibiotic regimen consisting of piperacillin/tazobactam was selected. The patient was given intravenous antibiotics for 2 weeks after surgery and encouraged to perform functional exercises. Less than 20 kg of weight bearing was recommended. Full weight bearing was prohibited until evidence of callus formation was visible on x-rays.

9 Definitive fixation

Accurate diagnosis of infection can be a problem [3]. There were no clinical infection signs after 2 months of recovery; C-reactive protein and erythrocyte sedimentation rate were normal, so the bone graft surgery was carried out (**Fig 16.2-10**). Autogenous cancellous bone was harvested from the iliac crest. At the patient's request the external plate was not changed.

10 Outcome

The external fixator was removed 1 year after surgery. Bone corticalization was completed at the last follow-up (**Fig 16.2-11**), and the patient was able to fully bear weight.

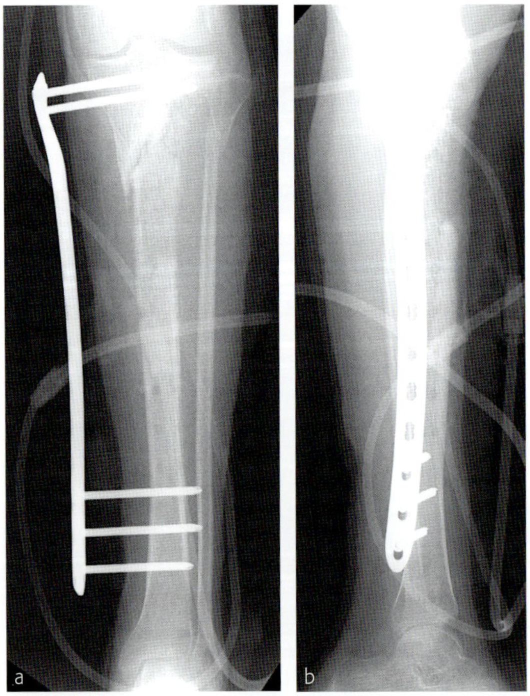

Fig 16.2-10a–b Postoperative bone graft x-rays.
a AP view.
b Lateral view.

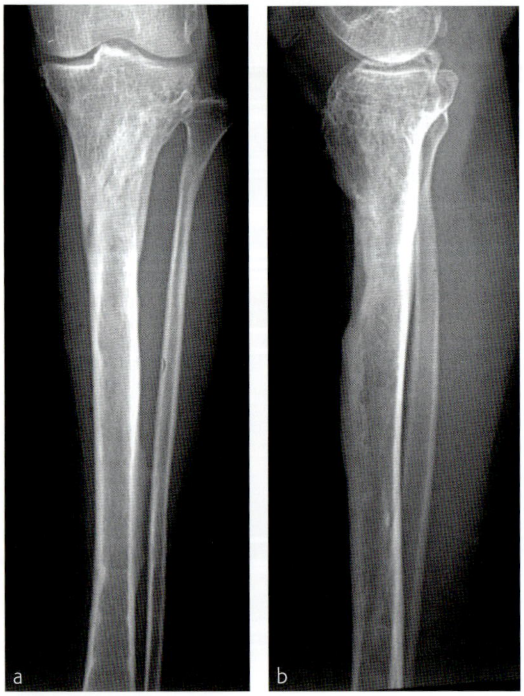

Fig 16.2-11a–b X-rays taken 18 months postoperatively.
a AP view.
b Lateral view.

11 Pitfalls

- Traditional bacterial culture leads to high false-negative results that might affect the diagnosis of bone infection. This is often the result of empiric antibiotic treatment. Cultures should be made from deep specimens obtained when the patient is not receiving antibiotics for at least 2 weeks.
- This surgical approach requires a broad excision of soft tissue and, therefore, may lead to difficulty in wound healing.
- Rehabilitation exercises should be limited due to the relatively stable plate. The patient is required to have good compliance and delayed weight bearing.
- Insufficiency of bone cortex formation, bone resorption, and refracture are the risks of cancellous bone grafting.

12 Pearls

- The surgical approach allows for good exposure of the bone infection site for complete debridement.
- External fixation of LCP is aesthetically acceptable and convenient for patients to get dressed.
- Topical antibiotics administration inhibits bacterial growth in the dead space. The amount and dosage of systemic antibiotics usage can be reduced.

13 References

1. **Tetsworth K, Cierny G 3rd.** Osteomyelitis debridement techniques. *Clin Orthop Relat Res.* 1999 Mar;(360):87–96.
2. **Masquelet AC, Begue T.** The concept of induced membrane for reconstruction of long bone defects. *Orthop Clin North Am.* 2010 Jan 41(1):27–37.
3. **Walter G, Kemmerer M, Kappler C, et al.** Treatment algorithms for chronic osteomyelitis. *Dtsch Arztebl Int.* 2012 Apr;109(14):257–264.

14 Acknowledgements

The author of this chapter acknowledges the contributions of Professor Jian Zhong Xu and Dr Ke Huang.

16.3 Chronically infected distal femoral fracture

Chang-Wug Oh

1 Case description

A 56-year-old man sustained a Gustilo-Anderson comminuted type IIIB fracture of the right distal femur (33-C2) during a motor vehicle accident (**Fig 16.3-1**). The following day a thorough debridement was performed followed by internal fixation with plate and screws (**Fig 16.3-2**). A deep infection developed 4 days postoperatively.

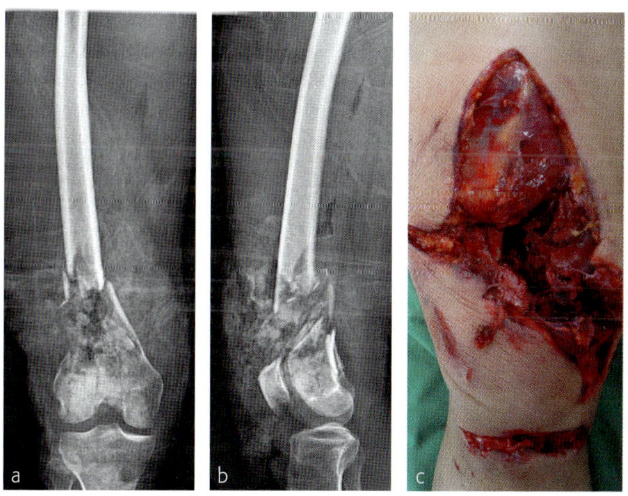

Fig 16.3-1a–c A comminuted open type IIIB fracture of the right distal femur (33-C2).
- **a** AP x-ray.
- **b** Lateral x-ray.
- **c** Clinical appearance.

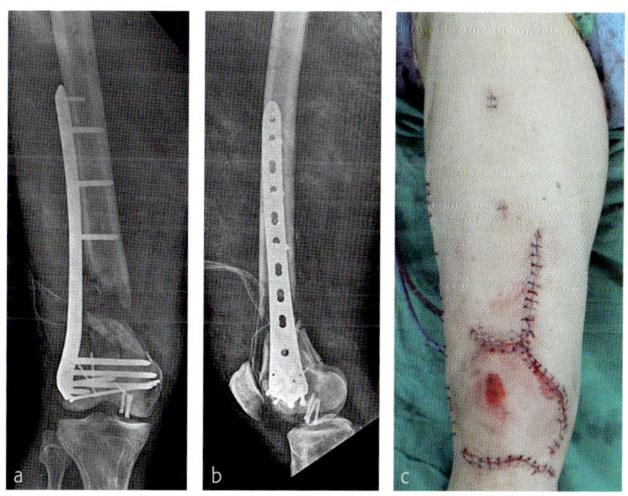

Fig 16.3-2a–c After meticulous debridement of the dirty wound, internal fixation was performed.
- **a** AP x-ray.
- **b** Lateral x-ray.
- **c** Clinical appearance.

2 Indications

Acute infection was strongly suspected with elevated laboratory test results and the clinical findings of redness and warmth (**Fig 16.3-3a**), so wound exploration and debridement was deemed necessary (**Fig 16.3-3b–c**).

3 Preoperative planning

Several debridements were performed to achieve control of this deep infection. The implant should be retained unless there is infection surrounding it. At the time of debridement, radical resection of all necrotic bone was performed until viable bone margins were visualized proximally and distally to the fracture site. Samples were obtained for bacterial and fungal cultures and a frozen-section pathological examination was conducted during debridement. Any dead space should be filled with antibiotic-loaded cement beads or spacers. In a second procedure, the bone defect can be managed by autogenous bone graft or bone transport according to its size.

4 Surgical approach

The lateral parapatellar approach was used. This approach may provide a good view of the articular surface of the distal femur, which may help in removal of any remaining sources of infection. With a longitudinal division of the quadriceps tendon and extensor mechanism, the patella was dislocated medially. A tourniquet was used to minimize blood loss and to improve the view of the articular surface.

5 Surgical debridement

Every 1 or 2 weeks, debridement, wound irrigation, changing of the antibiotic mixed-cement spacer (gentamicin and first-generation cephalosporin—cefalozin 1 g), and negative-pressure wound therapy was performed, while the plate was retained. The organism cultured was *Enterobacter aerogenes*. With several repeated debridements of necrotic bone and soft tissue, a 5 cm bone defect was created in the distal metadiaphyseal area. Eight weeks after initial trauma, the wound was closed without evidence of infection (negative cultures) (**Fig 16.3-4**). Bone transport was planned for when

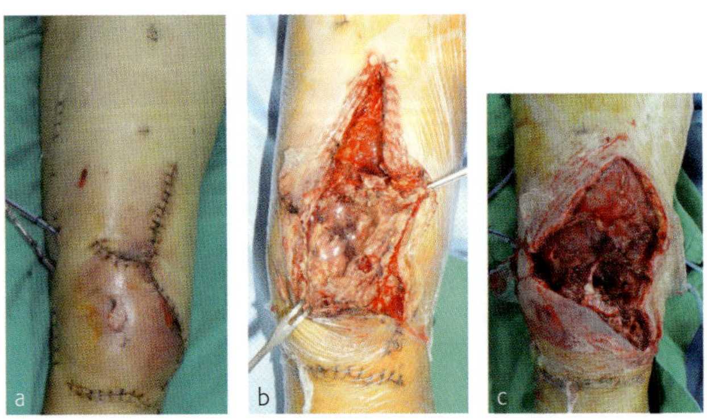

Fig 16.3-3a–c
a On postoperative day 3, postoperative infection was suspected with the localized redness and heat.
b–c The wound was then debrided again and cleaned.

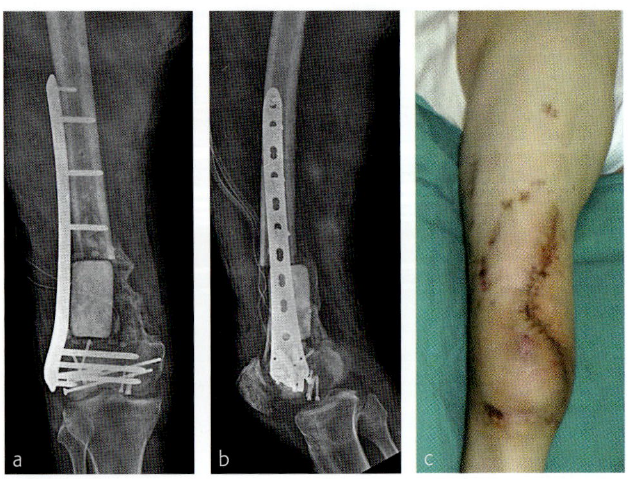

Fig 16.3-4a–c After several rounds of wound debridement and resection of dead bone, the antibiotic-cement spacer was inserted at the segmental bone defect of the distal femur.
a AP x-ray.
b Lateral x-ray.
c Clinical appearance. At 8 weeks after initial injury, the infection was controlled, with stabilization of infectious signs from the laboratory.

there was no clinical or laboratory evidence of infection, based on the findings of erythrocyte sedimentation rate and C-reactive protein investigations. A frozen-section biopsy of the soft tissue taken from the defect should also be performed at the time of the bone transport procedure. If polymorphonuclear leukocytes are less than 3 per high-power field, the reconstructive procedure (either bone graft or bone transport) can be performed with minimal risk of recurrent infection [1, 2].

6 Bone transport procedure

No infection was found around the locking plate so it was retained; it was planned to use a bone transport with external fixator and a locking plate (BTLP) for a large-bone defect of the distal femur [1, 3]. This technique comprises three stages, two operations, and the intervening transport period. **Fig 16.3-5** shows diagrammatically the planned procedure.

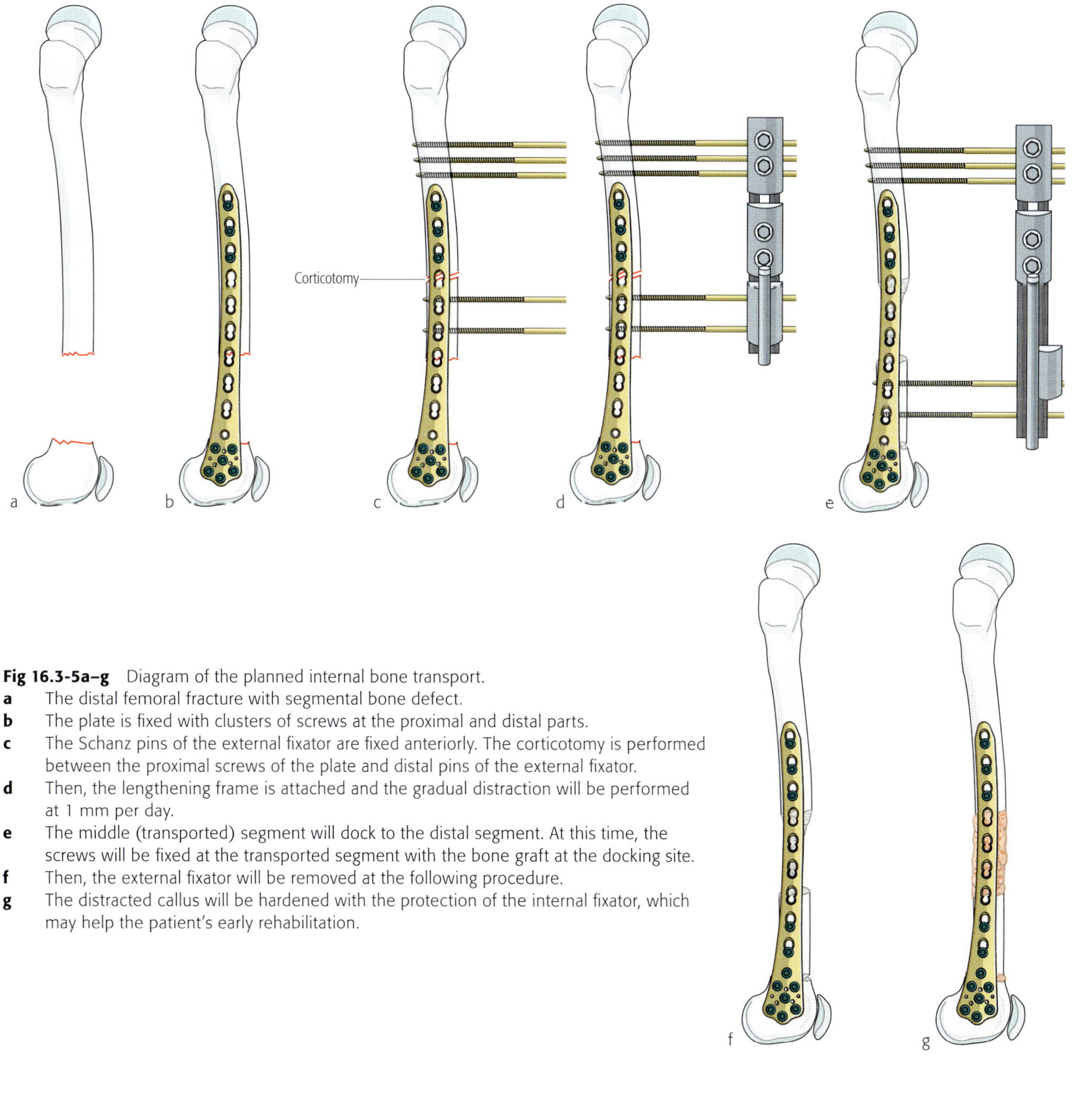

Fig 16.3-5a–g Diagram of the planned internal bone transport.

- **a** The distal femoral fracture with segmental bone defect.
- **b** The plate is fixed with clusters of screws at the proximal and distal parts.
- **c** The Schanz pins of the external fixator are fixed anteriorly. The corticotomy is performed between the proximal screws of the plate and distal pins of the external fixator.
- **d** Then, the lengthening frame is attached and the gradual distraction will be performed at 1 mm per day.
- **e** The middle (transported) segment will dock to the distal segment. At this time, the screws will be fixed at the transported segment with the bone graft at the docking site.
- **f** Then, the external fixator will be removed at the following procedure.
- **g** The distracted callus will be hardened with the protection of the internal fixator, which may help the patient's early rehabilitation.

The first stage involves plate fixation, external fixation, and osteotomy. In this case, the screw location at the proximal segment was changed while the screws at the distal condylar segment were not removed. Three screws were fixed at the uppermost area. A unilateral external fixator was chosen in this case. It was applied at the proximal segment, in which three Schanz pins were fixed above to the proximal end of the plate and two pins were fixed below to the proximal screws of the plate. All Schanz pins were inserted anteriorly, such that they did not contact the locking plate or its screws. Finally, a percutaneous osteotomy was performed using multiple drill holes and an osteotome (**Fig 16.3-6**).

The second stage concerns bone transport. Distraction started at a rate of 1 mm/day (0.25 mm per time, four times per day) after 10 days of latency, to permit regeneration of the periosteal blood supply at the corticotomy sites. Transport was performed in an antegrade direction (from proximal to distal). AP and lateral x-rays were taken weekly or biweekly to assess the formation of callus.

The third stage was conducted after the middle segment approached its docking position, around 3 months after the index procedure (**Fig 16.3-7**). This stage consisted of screw fixation at the transported segment, and removal of the

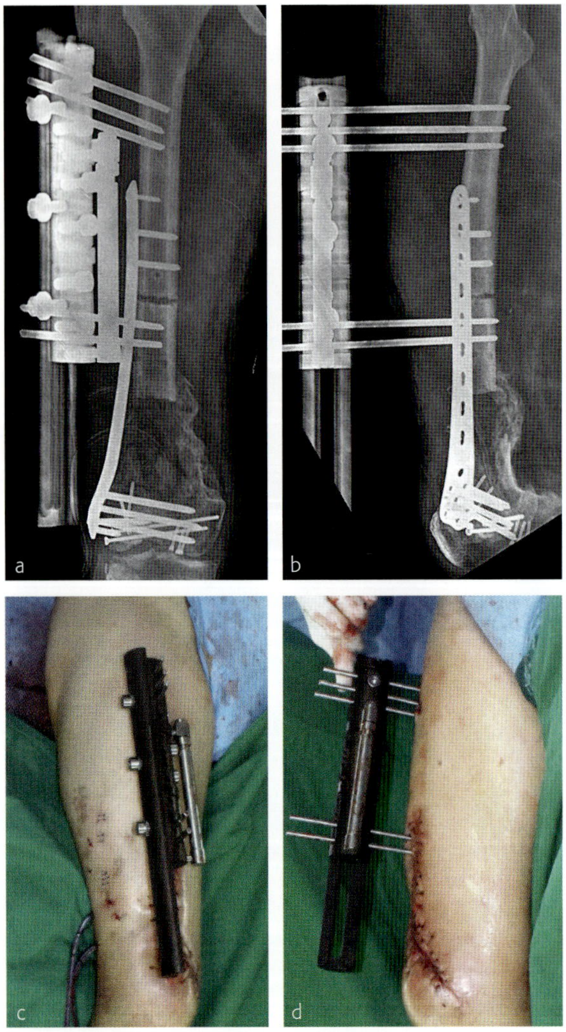

Fig 16.3-6a–d Postoperative x-rays and clinical appearance.
a–b Unilateral external fixator fixed anteriorly and locking plate fixed laterally. Note the osteotomy site.
c–d Clinical appearance after the operation (bone transport with locking plate and external fixator).

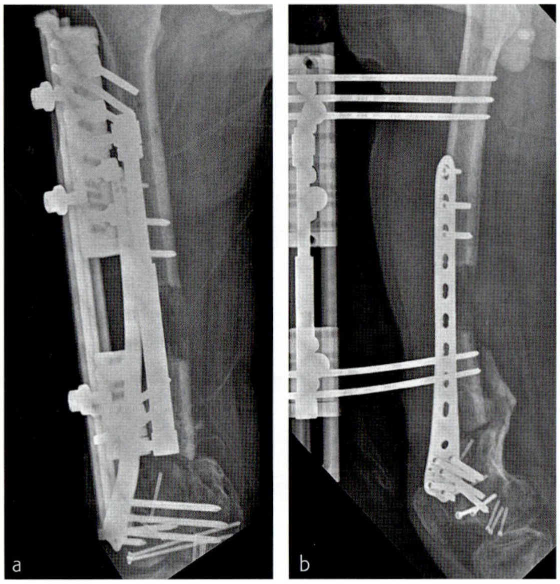

Fig 16.3-7a–b X-rays showing the middle segment approaching the distal segment.
a AP view.
b Lateral view.

external fixator. Screw fixation of the middle segment was performed prior to removing the fixator. Under image intensifier guidance, the empty plate holes on the middle segment are marked for the planned screw fixation. After making stab incisions over the holes, three screws were placed percutaneously. The fixator and its pins were then removed and the wounds created were thoroughly cleaned. Then, autogenous bone graft was performed with additional use of bone substitute (calcium sulfate) at the docking site (**Fig 16.3-8**).

7 Postoperative management

X-rays were taken every 4 weeks until the callus was fully consolidated. Mobilization of the joints was encouraged and partial weight bearing started immediately after removal of the fixator. When signs of bony consolidation were observed in at least three cortices on AP and lateral x-rays, the patient was allowed to walk bearing full weight with crutches, and then slowly weaned off the crutches as tolerated.

8 Outcome

After 15 months, both the docking and distraction sites were healed (**Fig 16.3-9**). The right leg was 25 mm shorter than the left leg, with a slight varus deformity. As the quadriceps muscle was severely damaged, the patient had limited motion of the knee (**Fig 16.3-10**).

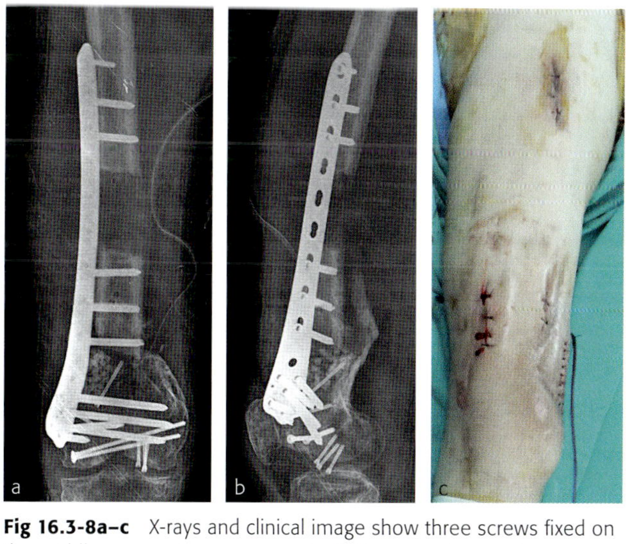

Fig 16.3-8a–c X-rays and clinical image show three screws fixed on the middle segment percutaneously. At the same time, autogenous bone graft was performed with additional use of bone substitute (calcium sulfate) at the docking site. Then external fixator and pins were removed.

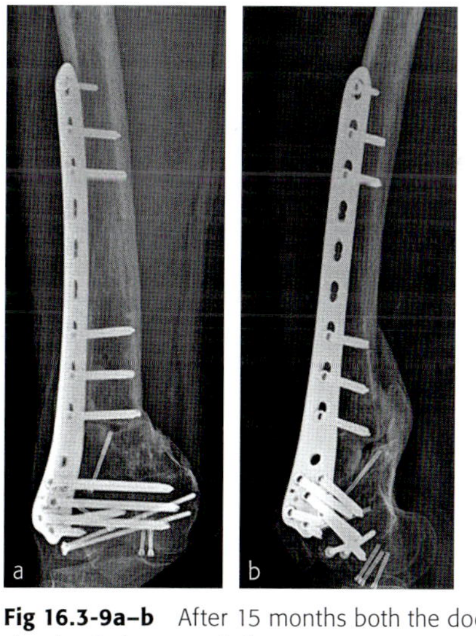

Fig 16.3-9a–b After 15 months both the docking and distraction sites healed uneventfully.

a AP view.

b Lateral view.

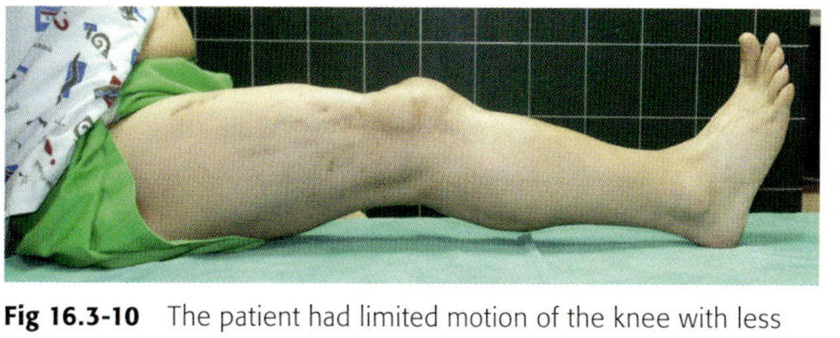

Fig 16.3-10 The patient had limited motion of the knee with less than 30° of flexion. This may have been a result of the initially severely damaged quadriceps muscle.

9 Pitfalls

The timing of closure of open fracture wounds has been controversial. The recent trend in the literature indicates that meticulous debridement by an experienced surgeon followed by primary wound closure is safe in many circumstances including type III open fractures [4]. However, as in this case, there are several factors contributing to wound infection. These were failures of omission such as not recognizing a fracture as open may cause the fracture to be treated or debrided less aggressively, which may favor infection. Although the optimal timing for the treatment of open fractures remains a matter of controversy, timely debridement is still favored by most surgeons. Local factors such as bone or soft-tissue loss, vascular or nerve injury, or compartment syndrome may all influence the potential for complications.

10 Pearls

One of the greatest advantages of BTLP technique is the early removal of the external fixator. Although distraction osteogenesis provides a highly satisfactory means of reconstructing segmental tibial defects, prolonged use of an external fixator is difficult for patients and complications, such as pin-track infections, pin breakage, pin loosening, and joint contractures are almost inevitable [5]. Trifocal and tetrafocal methods of bone transport with multiple osteotomies and two or three levels of bone regeneration have been reported to shorten treatment times. However, the consolidation of distraction callus and docking sites, which represent the longest phase of the bone transport technique, are little reduced with an external fixator as the means of stabilization. Bone transport with locking plate technique needs minimal time with external fixation, which may reduce related complications as seen in the similar procedure for limb lengthening [6].

Loss of axial alignment and distraction callus fractures are not uncommon when transport is performed using only an external fixator. The addition of a preinserted locking plate protects distraction and transport segments, minimizing the incidence of malalignment when BTLP is performed. It also protects the distraction callus sufficiently while permitting early mobilization. The locking plate is also helpful when nailing is difficult in juxtaarticular bone defects with a short remaining segment [3, 7].

11 References

1. **Oh CW, Apivatthakakul T, Oh JK, et al.** Bone transport with an external fixator and a locking plate for segmental tibial defects. *Bone Joint J.* 2013 Dec;95-B(12):1667–1672.
2. **Apivatthakakul T, Arpornchayanon O.** Minimally invasive plate osteosynthesis (MIPO) combined with distraction osteogenesis in the treatment of bone defects. A new technique of bone transport: a report of two cases. *Injury.* 2002 Jun;33(5):460–465.
3. **Oh CW, Song HR, Roh JY, et al.** Bone transport over an intramedullary nail for reconstruction of long bone defects in tibia. *Arch Orthop Trauma Surg.* 2008 Aug;128(8):801–808.
4. **Jenkinson RJ, Kiss A, Johnson S, et al.** Delayed wound closure increases deep-infection rate associated with lower-grade open fractures: a propensity-matched cohort study. *J Bone Joint Surg Am.* 2014 Mar 5;96(5):380–386.
5. **Papakostidis C, Bhandari M, Giannoudis PV.** Distraction osteogenesis in the treatment of long bone defects of the lower limbs: effectiveness, complications and clinical results; a systematic review and meta-analysis. *Bone Joint J.* 2013 Dec;95-B(12):1673–1680.
6. **Oh CW, Song HR, Kim JW, et al.** Limb lengthening with a submuscular locking plate. *J Bone Joint Surg Br.* 2009 Oct;91(10):1394–1399.
7. **Kocaoglu M, Eralp L, Rashid HU, et al.** Reconstruction of segmental bone defects due to chronic osteomyelitis with use of an external fixator and an intramedullary nail. *J Bone Joint Surg Am.* 2006 Oct;88(10):2137–2145.

16.4 Chronically infected hip hemiarthroplasty

Tak-Wing Lau

1 Case description

An 82-year-old woman was admitted to hospital following a simple fall on level ground resulting in left hip pain. The patient had been in good health and only took an antidepressant. She required a cane for walking before this injury.

After admission, she was found to have impaired glucose intolerance. X-rays of her left hip showed a displaced left femoral neck fracture (**Fig 16.4-1**).

On day 2 after admission, she received a left Austin Moore (AM) hemiarthroplasty under spinal anesthesia (**Fig 16.4-2**).

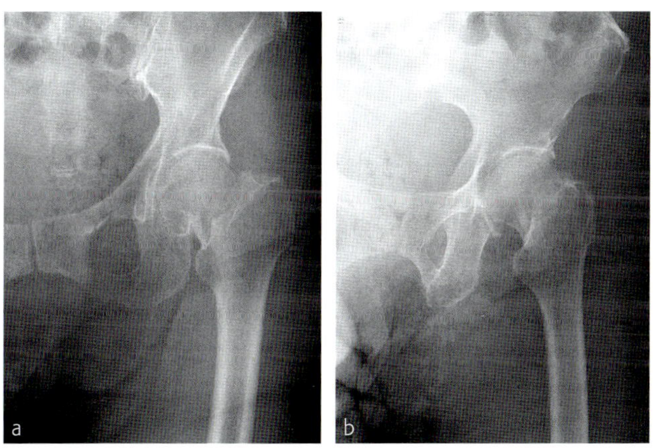

Fig 16.4-1a–b X-rays of the left hip show a displaced left femoral neck fracture.
a AP view of the pelvis shows that the displaced femoral neck fracture has shortened.
b Lateral view of the left hip shows the displaced fracture is in retroversion.

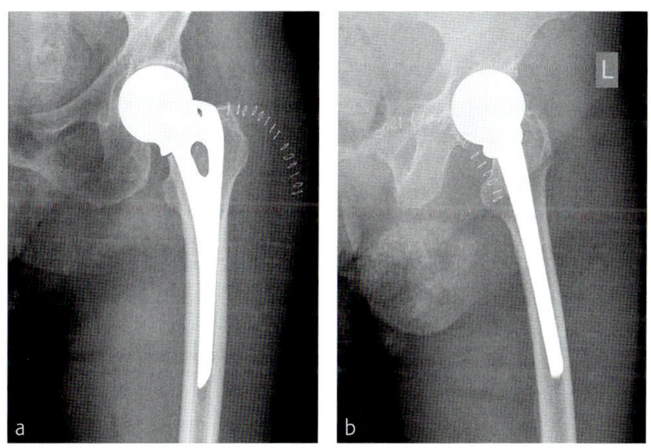

Fig 16.4-2a–b On day 2 after admission, the patient received a left Austin Moore hemiarthroplasty under spinal anesthesia.
a AP view.
b Lateral view.

The procedure was uneventful. She was readmitted to hospital 2 months later with a low-grade fever and increasing left hip pain for 1 month. She was able to walk independently with a walker. Repeated x-rays of the left hip showed no obvious loosening of stem or erosion of the acetabulum (**Fig 16.4-3**).

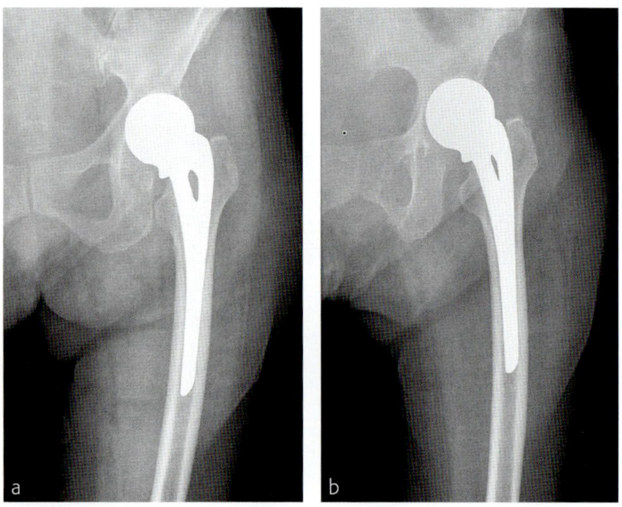

Fig 16.4-3a–b Repeated x-rays of the left hip showed no obvious loosening of the stem or erosion of the acetabulum.
a AP view shows loss of joint space only.
b Lateral view shows the stem without obvious changes.

Laboratory testing showed elevated erythrocyte sedimentation rate (ESR) > 140 mm/h and C-reactive protein (CRP) > 20 mg/L. The patient also reported acute weight loss of 9 kg in the preceding 2 months. In view of the clinical situation, she was referred for a positron-emission tomography computed tomography (PET-CT) scan to rule out underlying malignancy (**Fig 16.4-4**). The PET-CT scan demonstrated an abscess in the left hip region with involvement of the acetabulum and ilium as well. A hip joint aspirate was performed and showed no growth. Exploration, debridement, and revision to a temporary prosthesis of vancomycin-loaded acrylic cement were performed 1 week later (**Fig 16.4-5**). Culture of the synovium showed methicillin-sensitive *Staphylococcus aureus* infection. Intravenous cloxacillin and oral rifampin were given for 1 week then cloxacillin was also given orally. However, the patient developed gastrointestinal side effects after 6 weeks of treatment. Cloxacillin and rifampin were stopped and oral clarithromycin was then given for another 6 weeks.

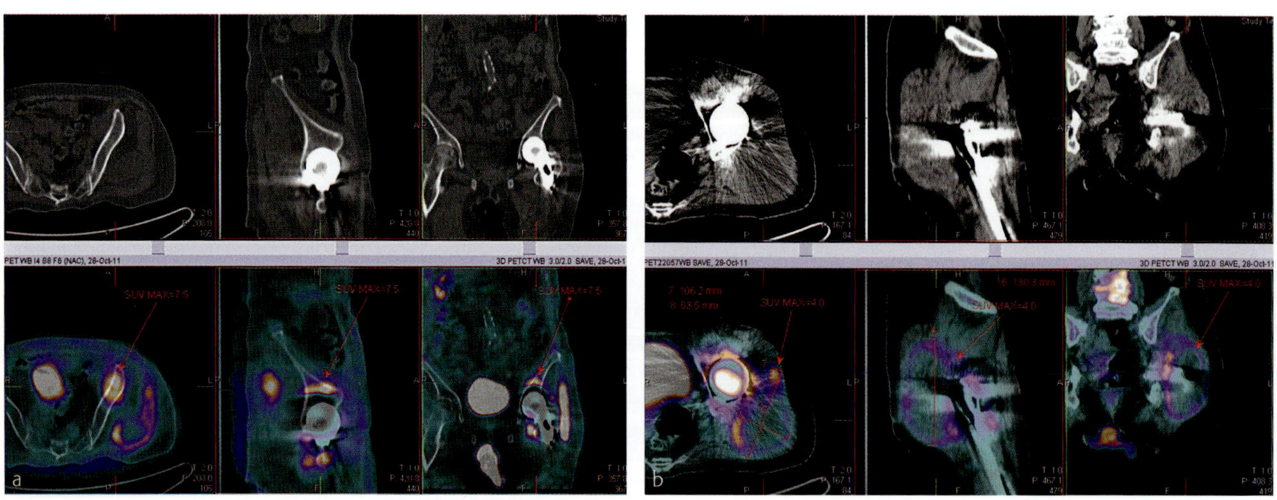

Fig 16.4-4a–b In view of the clinical situation, the patient was referred for a positron-emission tomography computed tomography (PET-CT) scan to rule out underlying malignancy.
a PET-CT shows evidence of inflammation abscess around the ilium.
b PET-CT shows evidence of inflammation abscess around the implants.

Six months later, the patient was walking with a frame. There was persistent hip pain but it was improving. The ESR and CRP also improved significantly. The antibiotic spacer prosthesis was then successfully revised to a total hip replacement (**Fig 16.4-6**) without reinfection. Eighteen months later, the x-ray showed femoral stem loosening. Although loosening due to chronic infection was suspected, serial blood tests including ESR and CRP showed no evidence of reinfection. Hip aspiration showed normal cell count and negative culture. Therefore, a second revision surgery of the loosened femoral stem was performed. Cephazolin was used as a prophylactic antibiotic. No antibiotics were given after the operation. The patient was by now ambulatory with a frame with mild hip pain. Her x-ray and blood tests showed no loosening of the prosthesis or evidence of reinfection (**Fig 16.4-7**).

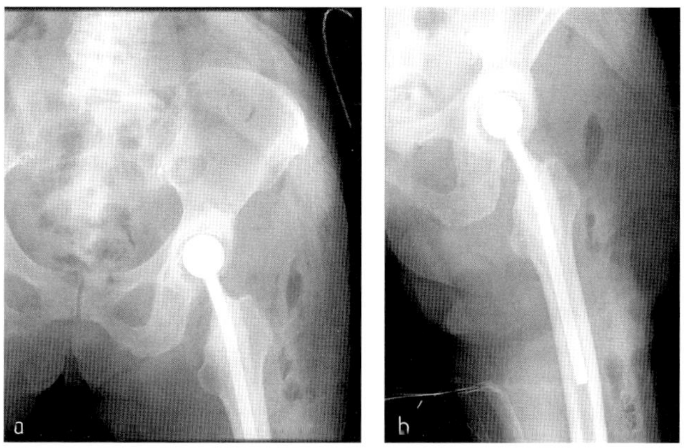

Fig 16.4-5a–b The positron emission tomography-computed tomography scan demonstrated an abscess in the left hip region with involvement of the acetabulum and ilium as well. A hip joint aspirate was performed and showed no growth. Exploration, debridement, and revision to a temporary prosthesis of antibiotic loaded acrylic cement were performed 1 week later.

- **a** AP pelvic view shows temporary prosthesis in place.
- **b** AP femoral view shows the implant in the femur.

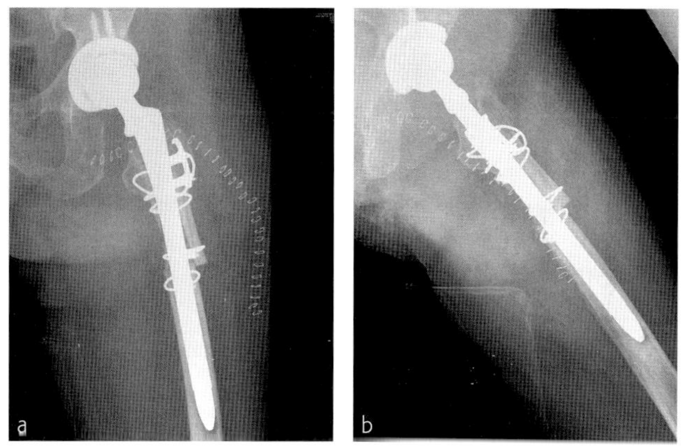

Fig 16.4-6a–b The antibiotic spacer prosthesis was then successfully revised to a total hip replacement.

- **a** The total hip is seen in place. A trochanteric osteotomy was used and cables are back in place.
- **b** Lateral view of the revised prosthesis in place. A monoblock stem was used.

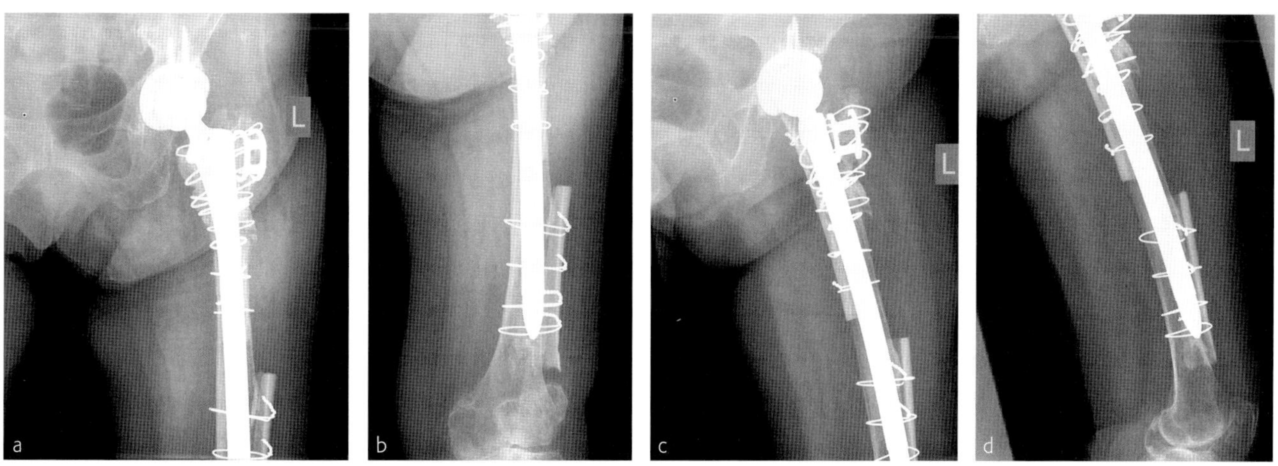

Fig 16.4-7a–d The femoral stem required a second revision 18 months later because of aseptic loosening. Blood tests showed no evidence of reinfection.

- **a** AP femoral view: exchange with a longer stem, supplemented with cables and allograft struts.
- **b** AP femur: the straight long stem did not fully match the femur bowing. A femoral allograft was required distally.
- **c** Lateral view proximally shows cables and allografts.
- **d** Lateral view distally shows cables and allografts.

2 Indications

2.1 Indications for surgical treatment

- A symptomatic left hip hemiarthroplasty infection, which presents with increasing pain and systemic symptoms, ie, fever, weight loss.
- X-rays may show features of implant loosening and rapid bone loss, acetabular erosion, and periosteal reaction.
- Hip joint aspiration is the standard technique for diagnosis, which may show increased fluid white blood cell (WBC) count (> 3,000/mL), or positive Gram stain or cultures.
- A PET-CT scan, technetium bone scan, WBC scan, or gallium scan may be useful to aid diagnosis in indicated situations.
- Laboratory results showed grossly elevated inflammatory markers: ESR and CRP.

2.2 Expected outcome

- Eradication of hip joint infection in the first stage.
- Maintenance of patient mobility, limb length, and hip joint muscle function.
- Provide an aseptic environment for conversion to a second-stage total hip arthroplasty for long-term mobility.
- An infected prosthesis at more than 8 weeks after initial surgery is very unlikely to be cleared by a single debridement. Resolution rate using a two-stage revision procedure with antibiotic prosthesis in this situation is around 78–95%.

3 Preoperative planning

3.1 Removal of AM prosthesis, replaced with antibiotic spacer (first stage)

- General anesthesia (expect operation > 2 hours)
- Lateral position
- Type and screen of blood
- First-generation cephalosporin on induction
- Austin Moore prosthesis removal slide hammer
- Bone chisel for trochanteric osteotomy in case of difficult AM prosthesis removal
- Antibiotic prosthesis preparation:
  - Cemented cup
  - Unreamed tibial nail as femoral stem
  - 28 mm cobalt-chrome metal femoral head
  - Vancomycin plus gentamicin-loaded cement
  - Postoperative systemic broad-spectrum antibiotics, usually in the form of combination therapy, eg, cloxacillin and rifampin
  - Specific antibiotics will be given according to the bacteriological sensitivity test for at least 6 weeks

3.2 Removal of antibiotic spacer; total hip replacement (second stage after 3–6 months)

- General anesthesia
- Lateral position
- Type and screen of blood
- First-generation cephalosporin on induction (or alternative with coverage of the primary pathogen)
- Cement chisel and curettes
- Ultrasound cement-removal device
- Bone saw and osteotome for preparation of extended trochanteric osteotomy
- Trochanteric grip plate
- Cable system
- Cemented acetabulum and femoral stem component for first-stage revision
- Postoperative antibiotics are not routinely prescribed in the author's institution

3.3 Prosthesis templating

- A customized hip, self-fabricated from intramedullary nails and cemented to a metallic hip ball can be a cost-effective approach.
- Alternatively, a commercially available cemented femoral component may be used.
- The acetabular component is preferably cemented.
- Vancomycin- plus gentamicin-loaded cement may be used.
- Prosthesis planning should aim at restoring normal acetabular center position, neck offset, and neck length.
- A large surface area of cement allows effective influence of antibiotics.

4 Surgical approach

A posterolateral approach using a more extensile Kocher-Langenbeck incision was used for both operations. The sciatic nerve must be carefully identified and protected in all cases of revision surgery through this approach.

5 Surgical debridement

5.1 Skin and subcutaneous layer

Drainage of serous fluid and debridement of granulation and necrotic tissue with specimens for microbiological investigations.

5.2 Hip joint and femoral canal debridement

- Radical synovectomy will reduce infectious load. The inflamed synovial tissue has a tendency to bleed but this is usually also controlled by removal.
- Reaming of the acetabulum using acetabular reamers to remove infected cartilage and areas of osteomyelitis in the acetabulum.
- Reaming of femoral canal using flexible reamer to remove infected tissue in intramedullary cavity.
- Pulsatile saline lavage using a tube in the intramedullary canal from retrograde manner can significantly dilute the infectious load.
- There is controversy over the use of antiseptics locally in the wound.
- Surgical instruments and gloves should be exchanged after completion.

6 Implant removal

The specific technique in removing the AM prosthesis is straightforward since it is usually loosened. A slide hammer with hook is typically employed for this removal. In a well-fixed infected prosthesis careful removal of obstructions from the femoral neck is first performed. The prosthesis may be gently reverse hammered by using specific removal tools. An extended trochanteric osteotomy may be used if the above technique fails.

7 Temporary fixation (first stage)

There is preparation of an antibiotic-laden prosthesis that works as a hip joint as well as an antibiotic spacer where limb length and motion are preserved.

Antibiotic cement preparation should be performed using no vacuum and using first-generation cementing techniques (finger packing, no cement restrictor, and no pressurization) for increase of porosity and thus total surface area.

The acetabular side should be cemented in the usual alignment after gentle reaming but without excessive pressurization allowing for easy removal, yet with sufficient temporary stability.

The femoral component should be implanted with minimal cement in the deep canal and mostly filled at the metaphyseal area with finger packing and no pressurization. To increase surface area, cement can cover the implant up to the trunnion.

The implant is gently wobbled in rotation during cement curing to allow a slightly loose fit at the cement-bone interface for easy removal at the second stage.

Hip stability is tested with soft-tissue layers carefully opposed to reduced dead space. Good hemostasis is obtained and a deep drain is not required. The local antibiotic concentration is increased by not placing a deep drain.

8 Postoperative management

Specific antibiotics, according to the culture and sensitivity testing, are given for a minimum of 6 weeks. In this case, clarithromycin was used to treat methicillin-sensitive *S aureus* infection. The duration of antibiotics may be longer than 6 weeks, depending on the clinical response and the serum inflammatory parameters. If there is evidence of residual infection after completion of the whole course of antibiotics, another debridement is performed and the prosthetic spacer may need to be exchanged with systemic antibiotics according to the most updated sensitivity test.

This patient was allowed full weight-bearing walking on the spacer after the surgery. She was advised to mobilize as soon as possible to minimize the complications on prolonged immobilization and disuse atrophy. During the follow-up period, the clinical signs and symptoms are regularly checked to look for reactivation of infection. Regular checking of inflammatory parameters including ESR and CRP is required to monitor the progress. A hip joint aspiration is performed after 3–6 months if there are no clinical or serological signs of residual infection to confirm eradication. The second stage should be withheld if joint fluid WBC count is still more than 3,000 cells/µL. A further course of antibiotics or even a further intermediary spacer exchange may be required.

9 Reimplantation (second stage)

It is safe to proceed to the second stage if a joint aspirate shows negative culture and WBC count of < 3,000 cells/µL (for nonreplaced joints, this is 50,000 cells/µL).

General anesthesia is usually preferred as the second stage is expected to be technically more demanding. The author's usual approach to the hip is a posterolateral approach. The patient is positioned in a lateral position. Usually, first-generation cephalosporin is used for antibiotics on induction, but it should also cover the previous offending organism. After the skin incision, the sciatic nerve is carefully identified and protected. Removal can be difficult if the spacer is very secure in the first stage. An ultrasound cement remover together with an extended trochanteric osteotomy is sometimes required to remove the femoral component and cement completely. A trochanteric stabilization implant with cable system should be ready in case this osteotomy is needed. The acetabular side will usually have significant bone defects either due to previous infectious process or due to debridement. Proper preoperative planning and experience with management of such defects is necessary. Various techniques are used to deal with the defect depending on size, location, and how the acetabular component can be well contained. Small defects may be filled with reamed bone. A large-sized acetabular shell with screws is usually preferred if both the anterior and posterior columns remain intact to provide adequate support. Alternatively, allografts, trabecular metal inserts, or reconstruction cages should be prepared for cases with significant defects.

In this case, a noncemented total hip replacement is performed. For the femur, a revision stem with full-length porous coating is preferred, since there will be significant bone loss proximally. Significant proximal femoral defects are filled with tricalcium phosphate granules mixed with reamed bone harvested from the acetabular side. The distal porous portion of the stem must be secured with "scratch fit" to a length of at least three times that of the femoral diameter. A deep drain is placed and skin is closed in layers to prevent dead space.

10 Outcome

There was eradication of infection and the patient regained her mobility without pain (**Fig 16.4-6a–b**).

11 Pitfalls

11.1 Diagnosis and decision making

- An infected hip prosthesis may not present as an acute infection but can be very subtle in clinical signs and symptoms. A high index of suspicion is required especially if:
  - The patient has low-grade fever without known cause.
  - The patient has unexplained persistent hip or thigh pain.
  - The patient is immunocompromised (diabetic or steroid user).
  - There is radiological evidence of loosening of prosthesis.
  - The patient has persistently elevated ESR without another cause of infection.
- Radioisotope scans provide supplemental anatomical location information to serological tests. These tests are sensitive but may not be specific.
- Patients with fragility hip fractures usually have impaired cognitive status and are unable to fully express their symptoms leading to delay in diagnosis.

11.2 Surgical approach

- Posterolateral approach is the usual approach for hip replacement in the author's center. During revision surgery, extra care must be taken to identify the sciatic nerve because of the extensive scarring after the inflammatory process. Revision surgery without the identification of the sciatic nerve could lead to sciatic nerve injury.
- Hemostasis is always important especially in debridement surgery. Actively inflamed tissues are prone to bleeding. Radical debridement is also essential. Therefore, extra effort in hemostasis is usually required. The anesthetist should also be informed about the possibility of more bleeding than a "typical" hip replacement.

11.3 Implant removal

- The infected prosthesis is often loose but not always. Failure to acknowledge intraoperative difficulty in removing the prosthesis may result in iatrogenic fracture of the acetabulum or the femur. This may complicate the management process of using a spacer.
- Radical debridement is essential to the success of infection eradication. However, it may also cause extra bone loss and weakening of bone stock.

11.4 First-stage temporary replacement

The temporary prosthesis is an antibiotic-loaded cement spacer with hip joint function (**Video 10-1**). In this case it is self-made but its stability must be good for a limited period of time. Some of the common pitfalls in a self-fabricated prosthesis include:

- Loosening of the femoral head from the stem
- Incorrect neck offset and leg length
- Incorrect femoral neck version
- Spacer implanted too securely
- Cement placed too distally in canal

11.5 Rehabilitation

The patient is allowed to bear full weight on the spacer. Since the spacer is a temporary self-made prosthesis its stability would be suboptimal. Hip and thigh discomfort would be common, which may mimic the symptom of infection reactivation. Patients with revision hip replacements, especially after hip fracture, are at higher risk of dislocation.

11.6 Second-stage revision total hip replacement

- Although the infection parameters may be optimal before the definitive surgery, preoperative joint-fluid microscopy is essential to decide if definitive total joint replacement should proceed. Failure to confirm a sterile hip joint before the definitive surgery may result in reactivation of prosthetic infection.
- Defects in the acetabulum and femur can be difficult to deal with. If unaware, soft bone, especially in the acetabulum, can be excessively removed. Careful preoperative planning and knowledge of revision total hip replacement techniques are essential. Aseptic loosing after second-stage revision seems to be commonplace.

11.7 Failure of therapy

- The spacer may be exchanged as an intermediate stage if there is:
  - No improvement in clinical features of infection.
  - Persistent elevation of infection parameters despite appropriate antibiotics.
  - Persistent positive hip joint aspiration infection.
  - Loosening of spacer before the second stage.
- Infection may not be successfully treated if:
  - A new microorganism becomes established or the organism develops resistance during the treatment.
  - The patient develops complications from the antibiotic treatment which in turn need to be changed or stopped.
  - Debridement of sequestrum or infected material is incomplete.
  - There is failure to give a full course of antibiotics of at least 6 weeks.

12 Pearls

12.1 Decision making

The surgeon must have a high index of suspicion in clinical signs and symptoms, radiological evidence, and blood parameters:

- Clinical signs and symptoms:
  - Persistent hip or thigh pain
  - Low-grade fever
  - General malaise and cachexia
  - Failure to improve during rehabilitation
  - Spontaneous dislocation of a hip prosthesis
- Radiological evidence:
  - Presence of radiolucent lines around femoral stem
  - Presence of radiolucent lines around acetabular cup
  - Early subsidence or change of prosthesis position
  - Periosteal reaction
- Blood parameters:
  - WBC count may be normal
  - CRP > 10 mg/L
  - ESR > 30 mm/h

12.2 Surgical approach

- Radical debridement is essential for the success of the treatment.
- Soft tissue: complete synovectomy and removal of granulation tissue.
- Femoral canal: debridement using flexible reamer and retrograde pulsatile lavage of the canal.
- Acetabulum: careful removal of cartilage and necrotic subchondral bone until good bone bleeding is present. Avoid excessive reaming in soft bone as this may lead to significant bony defects.
- Pulsatile lavage of the surgical area improves the success of the debridement.

12.3 Implant removal

Extended trochanteric osteotomy is not usually required for a grossly infected prosthesis but it should be kept in mind in case of difficult removal especially if a noncemented prosthesis must be removed.

12.4 Temporary fixation (replacement)

- Antibiotics added in cement should best be used according to the sensitivity. Commercially available gentamicin- or tobramycin-loaded cement is commonly mixed with vancomycin powder in the ratio of not more than 4 g to 40 g (10% by weight) of cement for effective coverage of gram-positive organisms with minimal detrimental effect to its mechanical properties.
- Use of first-generation cementing technique to increase porosity, increase surface area, and reduce excessive implant locking to bone for easier removal.
- Use of self-fabricated femoral components by using cement to secure a metallic hip ball to an intramedullary nail with a bend can be a cost-effective alternative to commercially available molded implants.
- Definitive revision (replacement).

12.5 Antibiotic management

Six weeks of antibiotics may not be sufficient to treat the infection. Continued use of the appropriate antibiotics is usually required until ESR, CRP, and hip joint aspiration return to normal before definitive replacement.

16.5 Chronically infected distal radial fracture

Peter JL Jebson, David C Ring, George SM Dyer

1 Case description

A 43-year-old healthy woman with no comorbidities presented with progressive wrist pain and swelling 6 months after undergoing open reduction and internal fixation of a closed comminuted left distal radial fracture. She sustained the fracture following a 4.5 meter fall on an obstacle course (**Fig 16.5-1**). A palmar approach was used and a palmar locking plate and screw system were used for fixation (**Fig 16.5-2**). The postoperative course was uneventful and she eventually returned to her occupation and hobbies with no loss of wrist or forearm motion or complications. At 6 months

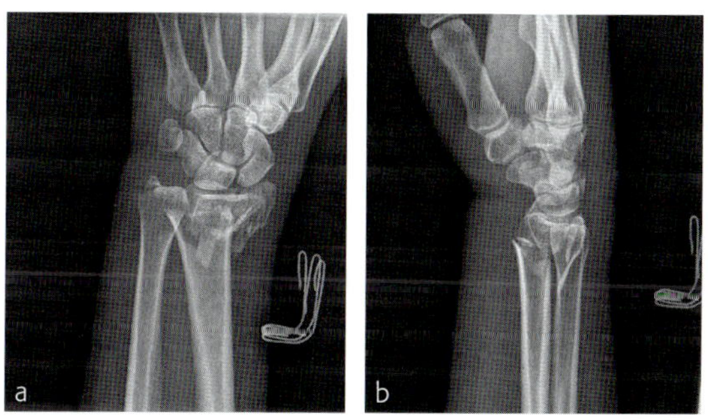

Fig 16.5-1a–b Injury x-rays demonstrate an unstable comminuted intraarticular distal radial fracture.
a Posterolateral view.
b Lateral view.

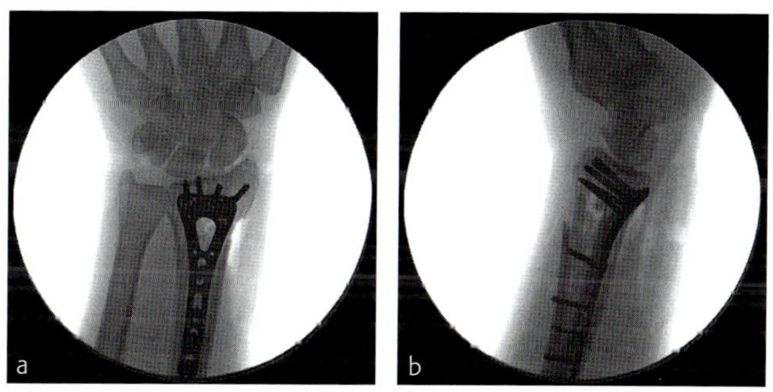

Fig 16.5-2a–b Intraoperative image intensification demonstrates satisfactory reduction and fixation of the fracture using a palmar locking plate and screw system. Note the amount of dorsal metaphyseal comminution.
a Posterolateral view.
b Lateral view.

postoperatively, she noted the spontaneous onset of progressive pain and swelling at the surgical site. There was no history of trauma, wound drainage, fevers, chills, or weight loss. X-rays revealed a questionably healed fracture stabilized with a palmar plate. There was a lucency beneath the plate in the metaphyseal region, possible lysis around the implant, and a loose screw in the palmar soft tissues (**Fig 16.5-3**). She complained of hand numbness. Diminished sensibility was noted in the median nerve distribution.

These findings indicated the need for exploration and removal of all hardware and possible carpal tunnel release depending on operative findings. Surgical exploration was performed using the same incision. Purulent material was encountered when the plate and loose screw were removed. The fracture was healed, but there were several cavities within the radius that required extensive debridement of all infected bone (**Fig 16.5-4**). The carpal tunnel was not released because it was clear that swelling around the median nerve was directly related to the presence of the loose screw and the obvious infection. Wound cultures revealed *Enterobacter cloacae*. Treatment consisted of a 6-week course of oral ciprofloxacin and sulfamethoxazole/trimethoprim DS.

2 Indications

The indication to perform surgical management in this patient was based on the wound status, swelling at the operative site, x-ray findings, and suspected infection. Deep infection following operative treatment of a closed distal radial fracture is extremely rare [1, 2]. It is seen more commonly with open fractures of the distal radius with an overall incidence of 5–7% [3–6]. Deep infection can also occur in the setting of an external fixator pin-track infection, intramedullary nailing, or closed reduction and percutaneous pinning [7].

Indications for surgical management in general include infected nonunion or malunion, sepsis or bacteremia, hardware failure, wound drainage, or neuropathy as noted in this patient [8, 9].

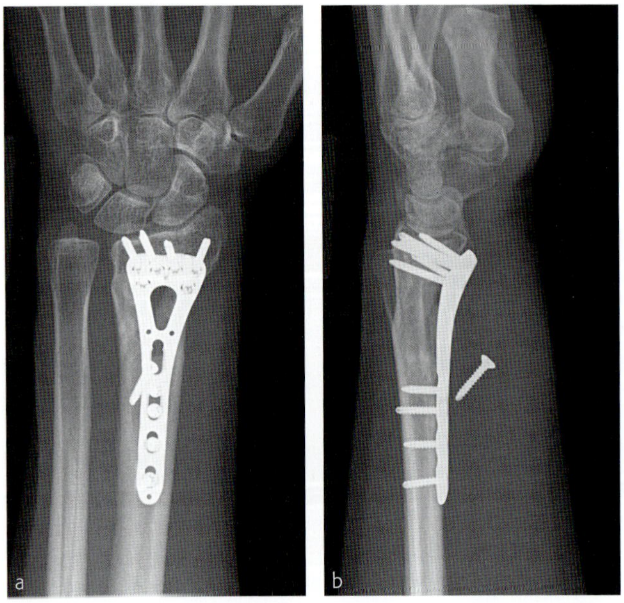

Fig 16.5-3a–b X-rays reveal a questionably healed fracture. Note the lucency beneath the plate in the metaphyseal region, possible lysis around the implant, and a loose screw in the palmar soft tissues.
a Posterolateral view.
b Lateral view.

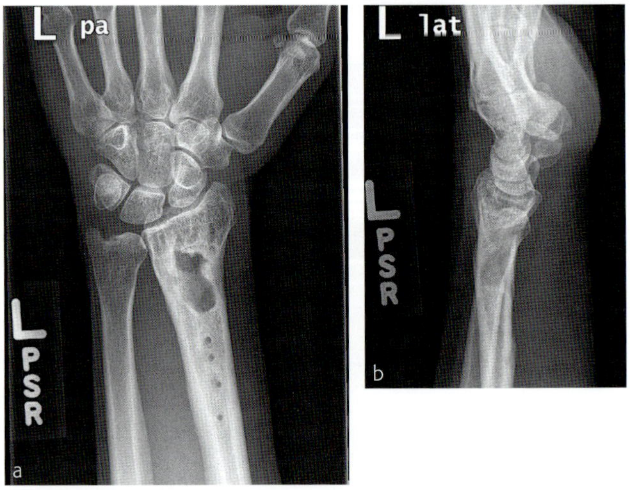

Fig 16.5-4a–b X-rays following implant removal and debridement.
a Posterolateral view.
b Lateral view.

3 Preoperative planning

The goals of treatment are to eradicate the infection, obtain fracture healing, and restore function. Preoperative workup should include serological testing (erythrocyte sedimentation rate, C-reactive protein (CRP), white blood cell count with differential) and plain x-rays of both the involved and uninvolved wrist to determine the normal anatomy. Computed tomography (CT) can be particularly helpful in determining the extent of fracture healing and presence of a nidus and/or sequestrum. Review of the previous operative note(s) is imperative to determine the type of implant used if applicable. Appropriate equipment that should be available in the operating room includes curettes, osteotomes, a screw removal set, external fixation, burr, and antibiotic-laden polymethylmethacrylate cement, which may be used as a temporary spacer. A negative-pressure wound dressing may be necessary if the operative wound is too large to close immediately.

4 Surgical approach

The incision type and location are based on the location of any prior incision(s), associated nerve compression, hardware location, wound status, presence of draining wounds/sinus tracts, and the location of the infection locus/nidus. This decision can be determined after careful physical examination and critical review of diagnostic imaging.

General or regional anesthesia may be used. The patient is positioned supine, an arm board is used, a pneumatic tourniquet is applied but only used without Esmarch exsanguination to avoid forcing infectious material proximally within the forearm. Prophylactic antibiotics are held until intraoperative wound cultures have been obtained.

The surgical approach is often tedious and can be challenging because of scarring and a loss of normal tissue planes and anatomical landmarks. If the fracture has shortened significantly as a result of hardware failure, releasing the brachioradialis and mobilizing the dorsal periosteum and soft tissues can be helpful in restoring length. Occasionally, Z-lengthening of the wrist flexors may be necessary in severely shortened and infected malunions.

5 Surgical debridement

All nonviable devitalized bone and soft tissue should be debrided while preserving nerves and arteries. Debridement is performed using a combination of a number 15 scalpel blade, tenotomy scissors, rongeur, curettes, and osteotomes. Although classic teaching emphasizes the use of a round burr to thoroughly debride infected cortical bone, the bone in the distal radius is often soft enough to debride without power equipment [10]. Additionally, the proximity of the median nerve and radial artery can make burr use dangerous. Following adequate debridement, copious wound irrigation should be performed. Representative bone and tissue should be sent for microbiology (aerobic, anaerobic, fungal cultures, Gram stain) and for histopathology examination. For severe infections, serial debridements may be necessary.

6 Implant removal

This case was straightforward. The implant was somewhat loose but the majority of the fracture had healed and was deemed stable. If there is inadequate fracture healing, the implant may need to be replaced/retained and only removed after adequate union has been confirmed on x-rays and CT scan. If the implant is well fixed, use the correct instrument set associated with the particular implant. In some cases, implant removal can be challenging. Stripped screw heads may be removed with an "easy-out" or by taking the screw head off with an osteotome then overdrilling the remaining screw shaft with a cannulated drill followed by extraction with a fine needle-nose pliers, locking vice grips, or large needle holder. Broken screws may be removed in a similar fashion. Plates may be elevated with an osteotome or key elevator. If hardware is broken, all pieces must be removed if possible and accounted for. Portable image intensification can be helpful in this regard.

7 Temporary fixation

Following debridement and implant removal, the radius may be unstable necessitating immobilization. A carefully applied and appropriately molded cast may be sufficient. Temporary use of an external fixator is a helpful alternative to maintain length and stabilize the soft tissues. Care must be taken when applying the fixator such that the pins are inserted outside of the zone of infection. Insertion of an antibiotic-laden polymethylmethacrylate spacer for large bone resection preserves length, fills the defect, and delivers antibiotics in high concentration.

8 Postoperative management

Postoperatively, the limb is splinted for comfort and elevated. The patient is encouraged to perform immediate finger and thumb range-of-motion exercises. If a wound drain was placed, it should be removed 24–48 hours postoperatively. The limb is not used for weightbearing activities. Consultation with an infectious diseases specialist is highly recommended to determine the treatment regimen, method of antibiotic delivery (intravenous, oral, or combination), and follow the patient response including routine serological testing (for CRP). Supplemental below-elbow bracing may be necessary if a cast is not used. If applicable, the patient is instructed on and initiates external fixator pin-site care when the sutures are removed 2 weeks postoperatively. The patient is encouraged to perform frequent exercises to reduce edema, improve range of motion, and hand function. Patients that need more teaching and coaching, or additional camaraderie can work with a hand therapist.

9 Reimplantation

Reimplantation or revision internal fixation is usually performed a minimum of 6 weeks postoperatively but the exact timing is based on the patient's overall health status, the status of the soft tissues, the response to the antibiotic regimen, and following a discussion with the infectious diseases consultant. Reimplantation should only occur after the infection has been eradicated, the wound has healed, and soft-tissue homeostasis is apparent with minimal or no edema and good finger and thumb motion. The patient should not have any systemic symptoms such as persistent fever, their nutritional status must be optimized, and a normal CRP confirmed. The erythrocyte sedimentation rate can be persistently elevated for several months and should not be used to determine timing of reimplantation.

When reimplantation is performed, the type of prophylactic antibiotics used should be based on the prior wound culture results and recommendations of the infectious diseases consultant. Antibiotics are usually continued until drain removal at 48 hours postoperatively. The continued use of "suppressive" antibiotics following revision internal fixation is not typically necessary if the infection has been completely eradicated. However, the need for use is determined by the treating surgeon and infectious diseases consultant.

The type of surgical approach is based on several factors including the location of any prior incisions, the status of those incisions, the presence and location of any draining sinus, and the type of implant selected. An extensile exposure is necessary and may involve a dorsal, palmar, or a combination of approaches. The surgeon should consider the use of a locking plate or plates because of disuse osteopenia. The plate needs to be long enough to provide adequate fixation in the distal metaphysis and subchondral regions. If a corticocancellous graft is used, screws may be inserted through the plate and into the graft. If there is not enough bone distally for implant purchase or if the radiocarpal joint is damaged, wrist fusion is recommended [11].

For metaphyseal bone defects less than 5 cm, autogenous corticocancellous or cancellous bone graft from the iliac crest is preferred. The iliac crest should be prepped but the graft is harvested only after the distal radius has been exposed and debrided and no active infection confirmed. The surgical team should use separate gloves, gowns, and instruments to avoid cross-contamination. If the defect is larger, a vascularized-free fibula graft is preferred [12].

Intraoperative wound cultures with a tissue Gram stain should be obtained. The authors recommend a minimum of three samples obtained from different wound locations. The need for continued postoperative antibiotics is based on the operative findings, intraoperative culture results, prior response to the antibiotic regimen, and recommendations of the infectious diseases consultant.

10 Outcome

The patient was doing well at the 4-month follow-up after the last surgery when she came in for an unrelated reason. She continued to experience occasional aching in the wrist. She had full range of motion of the fingers, wrist, and forearm, and no numbness. There was no recurrence of the infection and the fracture eventually healed (**Fig 16.5-5**).

11 Pitfalls

- One of the most common pitfalls in the management of the patient with an infected distal radial fracture is a delay in the diagnosis and initiation of appropriate treatment. The surgeon often fails to consider or recognize a deep infection or treats the patient with a course of oral antibiotics for an incorrectly diagnosed "cellulitis" in lieu of aggressive debridement, wound culture, and possible hardware removal.
- Another pitfall is the failure to perform an adequate debridement. All devitalized infected bone and soft tissues should be excised preserving important nerves, arteries, and veins. The surgical team must remember to obtain appropriate tissue specimens for microbiology and histopathology.

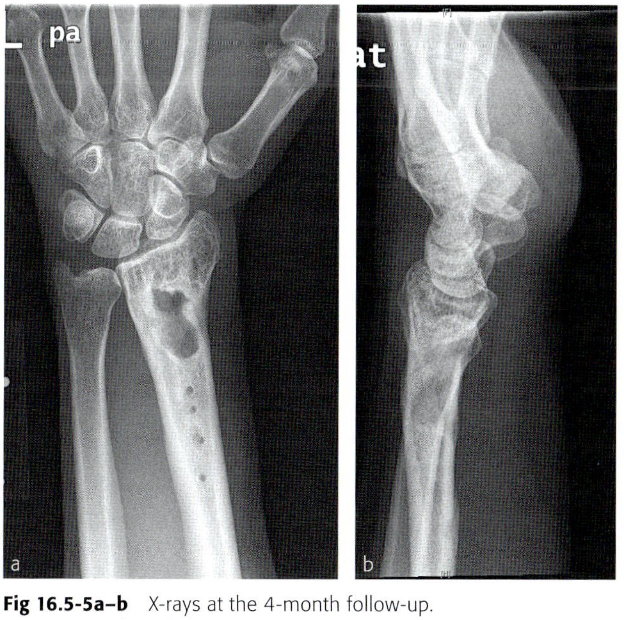

Fig 16.5-5a–b X-rays at the 4-month follow-up.
a Posterolateral view.
b Lateral view.

- A common mistake is to leave the hardware in when stability is questionable or not have the correct equipment to facilitate removal. Failure to adequately support the unstable wrist following implant removal and debridement results in further soft-tissue trauma, may be painful with movement, and fails to maintain limb length and alignment with resultant myotendinous shortening, loss of motion, and contracture development.
- Inadequate rehabilitation may result in a stiff, swollen hand with significant functional loss.
- Unrecognized and untreated nerve compression may result in complex regional pain syndrome.
- Additional pitfalls at reimplantation include using too short a plate with inadequate stability and loss of fixation, using a nonlocking plate in osteopenic bone with resultant poor screw purchase and stability, not using an adequate volume of bone graft, and not using autogenous bone graft.

12 Pearls

- Always have a high index of suspicion of the patient who presents with "cellulitis" or draining sinus after a distal radial fracture particularly if the fracture was open and contaminated, underwent open reduction internal fixation, or had an infected percutaneously inserted K-wire.
- The authors recommend consultation with an infectious diseases specialist.
- The surgical approach should be based on the location of the:
  - Prior incision(s)
  - Draining sinus, if present
  - Nidus identified on plain x-rays or CT scan
- An extensile approach is particularly helpful. Review the previous operative note(s) to determine the type of implant and make sure you have all appropriate equipment ordered and available in the operating theater before you begin the procedure.
- Adequate debridement consists of the removal of all infected devitalized avascular bone and soft tissue except important structures such as the radial and ulnar arteries and median and ulnar nerves.
- Always obtain adequate and representative specimens for microbiological analysis, including a Gram stain (aerobic and anaerobic), and fungal cultures.

- The decision to remove any hardware is based on the fracture and wound status. If the fracture is fully healed or the implant is loose, removal of all hardware is recommended. If the fracture is not healed and the implant is well fixed, the implant may be replaced or retained. These implants are typically coated with a biofilm.
- Multiple debridements may be necessary and should be performed every 48–72 hours.
- The decision to perform reimplantation is based on several factors and should be done in conjunction with the infectious diseases consultant.
- If temporary external fixation is used, the pins should be inserted outside of the surgical/infection zone. Restore length after hardware removal.
- The use of a postoperative drain should be considered if significant bleeding and/or edema is anticipated following debridement. Hematoma formation should be avoided.
- Consider a prophylactic carpal tunnel release if the patient has any symptoms of median nerve compression or a history of carpal tunnel syndrome in the past that was treated nonoperatively.
- When performing definitive fixation, a locking plate and screws are recommended if the bone is osteopenic or a large bone defect is noted following debridement. Careful preoperative planning is imperative to make sure that the plate is long enough. Alternatively, consider dorsal bridge plating to completely avoid the former zone of infection and to minimize reliance on osteopenic metaphyseal periarticular bone.
- If the radius is shortened, release the brachioradialis and dorsal periosteum to mobilize the distal fragment. The use of intraoperative temporary external fixation to restore length prior to plate application may be helpful. Despite these measures, you may not be able to recover full radial length and the distal radioulnar joint and ulna itself may need to be addressed to avoid impaction, symptomatic instability, or incongruency.
- The authors' preference for filling defects less than 5 cm is autogenous corticocancellous or cancellous bone graft from the iliac crest. Larger defects may require a vascularized-free fibular graft.
- The need for postoperative antibiotics is usually determined in conjunction with the infectious diseases specialist and is based on several factors including the: type of infecting organism(s), response to the preoperative antibiotic regimen, intraoperative findings, and patient's overall health status.

13 References

1. **Esenwein P, Sonderegger J, Gruenert J, et al.** Complications following palmar plate fixation of distal radius fractures: a review of 665 cases. *Arch Orthop Trauma Surg.* 2013;133(8):1155–1162.
2. **Tarallo L, Mugnai R, Zambianchi F, et al.** Volar plate fixation for the treatment of distal radius fractures: analysis of adverse events. *J Orthop Trauma.* 2013;27(12):740–745.
3. **Glueck DA, Charoglu CP, Lawton JN.** Factors associated with infection following open distal radius fractures. *Hand.* 2009;4(3):330–334.
4. **Zumsteg JW, Molina CS, Lee DH, et al.** Factors influencing infection rates after open fractures of the radius and/or ulna. *J Hand Surg Am.* 2014;39(5):956–961.
5. **Rozental TD, Beredjiklian PK, Steinberg DR, et al.** Open fractures of the distal radius. *J Hand Surg Am.* 2002;27(1):77–85.
6. **Kurylo JC, Axelrod TW, Tornetta P 3rd, et al.** Open fractures of the distal radius: the effects of delayed debridement and immediate internal fixation on infection rates and the need for secondary procedures. *J Hand Surg Am.* 2011;36(7):1131–1134.
7. **Botte MJ, Davis JL, Rose BA, et al.** Complications of smooth pin fixation of fractures and dislocations in the hand and wrist. *Clin Orthop Relat Res.* 1992;(276):194–201.
8. **Shields DW, Elson DW, Marsh M, et al.** Catastrophic osteomyelitis following percutaneous wire fixation of a distal radial fracture: a cautionary tale of poor patient selection followed by surgical mishap. *BMJ Case Reports.* 2013;1–3.
9. **Birdsall PD, Milne DD.** Toxic shock syndrome due to percutaneous Kirschner wires. *Injury.* 1999; 30(7):509–510.
10. **Tetsworth K, Cierny G 3rd.** Osteomyelitis debridement techniques. *Clin Orthop Relat Res.* 1999;(360):87–96.
11. **Prommersberger KJ, Fernandez DL, Ring D, et al.** Open reduction and internal fixation of un-united fractures of the distal radius: does the size of the distal fragment affect the result? *Chir Main.* 2002 Mar;21(2):113–123.
12. **Chin KR, Spak JI, Jupiter JB.** Septic arthritis and osteomyelitis of the wrist: reconstruction with a vascularized fibular graft. *J Hand Surg Am.* 1999;24(2):243–248.

17 Acute osteomyelitis of the femur

Peter E Ochsner

1 Case description

A 34-year-old female physiotherapist had experienced some weakness in her left leg for some time. She suffered from insomnia and loss of appetite. An evening of jazz dancing was followed by worsening pain in the thigh muscles. An examination by ultrasound of the thigh suggested a muscle tear and bleeding. Ten days later the patient noted a slight fever that was accompanied by shivers after 3 days.

She went to the hospital emergency department with a temperature of 40.1° C; her erythrocyte sedimentation rate was 31 mm/h and leukocyte count 7,300 cells/µL with 87% granulocytes. According to the admission note, the thigh was found to have lateral tenderness without inflammation. It was thought to be a traumatic event unrelated to the actual inflammatory process. Two blood cultures were taken followed by intravenous antibiotic therapy with cefazolin (2 g every 6 hours) and gentamicin (80 mg every 8 hours). Hepatomegaly and splenomegaly were also noted on ultrasound examination. A liver biopsy showed signs of inflammation probably triggered by a general infection. The C-reactive protein increased to 108 mg/L two days after beginning treatment with antibiotics. After a second episode of fever of 39.1° C was recorded on the third hospital day, the temperature remained ~ 37.4° C. One blood culture grew out *Streptococcus milleri* on the fifth day.

Eventually, the patient complained only of pain in the left thigh. X-rays and a computed tomographic scan of the femur were performed (**Fig 17-1**). The density of the bone marrow was elevated indicating an infection of the medullary canal. Computed tomography with iodinated contrast medium also revealed surrounding soft-tissue enhancement. Osteomyelitis rather than a malignant tumour was suggested, which was concordant with the history and examination findings.

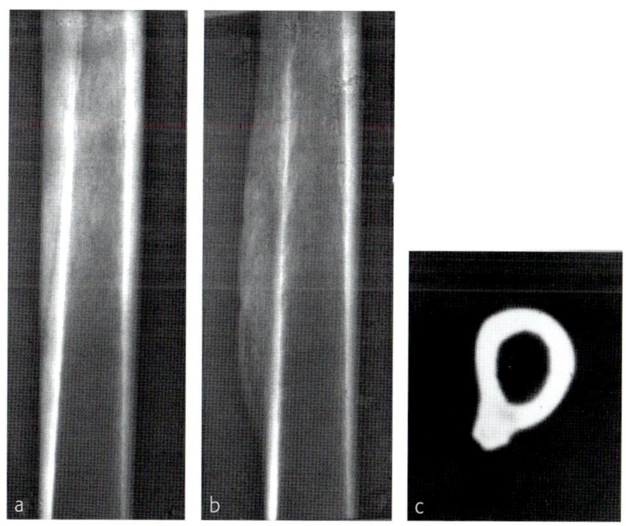

Fig 17-1a–c The left femur.
a–b AP and lateral x-ray: distinct thickening of the lateral cortex and the linea aspera over a length of 12 cm combined with signs of osteoporosis.
c Central section of the computed tomography: local osteolytic area in the centre of the linea aspera.

2 Indications

On hospital day 6, the orthopedic surgeon was consulted. The findings suggested the diagnosis of an acute infection on the basis of a primary chronic intracortical osteomyelitis with possible extension in the medullary cavity and adjacent soft tissues leading to an acute infection. Surgical removal of the nidus and drainage of the medullary canal was planned.

3 Surgical procedure

Exposure was obtained using a lateral incision. The linea aspera was exposed where a 15 mm diameter abscess was found. The linea aspera was softened and thickened. The most prominent part was removed with a chisel exposing where some yellow pus emerged (**Fig 17-2**). A fenestration of the femur from the posterior side was performed. Four drill holes (3.2 mm diameter) were placed at the site of the planned corners of the cortical window, which were then connected with an oscillating saw (**Fig 17-3a**). In the medullary cavity, pus was present and therefore drained. Additional pus was evacuated. The medullary cavity was curetted, irrigated, and extensively drained. The pus and two intra-operative tissue samples were harvested. All microbiological testing remained negative.

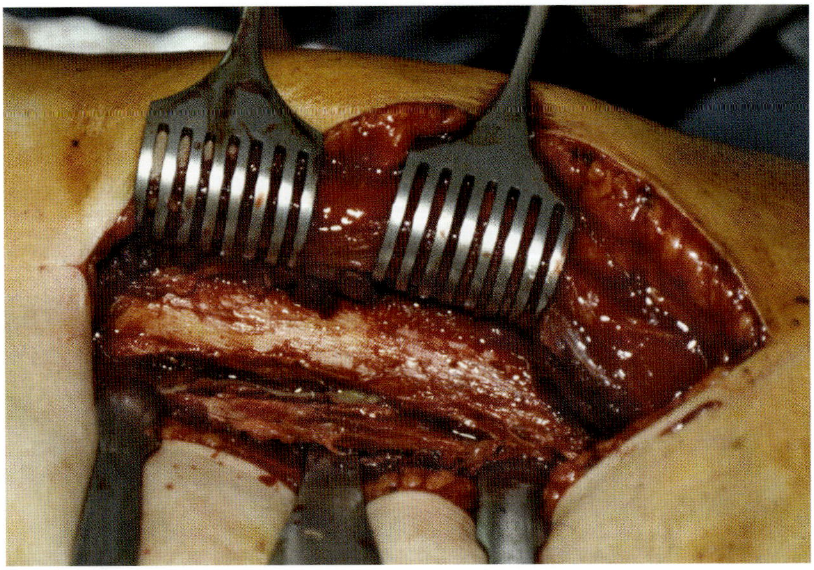

Fig 17-2 The posterior aspect of the femur after chiselling away the thickened linea aspera. In the centre yellow granulation tissue becomes visible.

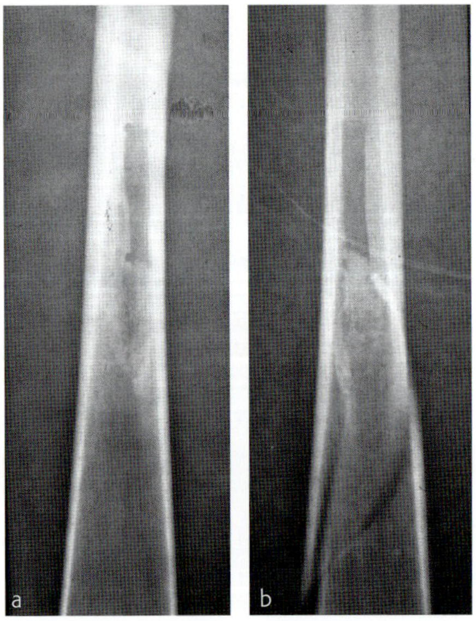

Fig 17-3a–b Postoperative follow up x-rays:
- **a** The bone window with drill holes in the four edges.
- **b** Fracture through the lower end of the window 18 days postoperatively.

4 Histological analysis

The histological samples were processed without decalcification. The thickened linea aspera was osteoporotic (**Fig 17-1a**, **Fig 17-4a**). It contained numerous wide longitudinal channels with signs of active enlargement (**Fig 17-4b**). Inflammatory cells were present diffusely. Together, these findings suggested an acute infection superimposed on chronic infection (**Fig 17-4b–c**).

5 Postoperative management

Antibiotic therapy with intravenous cefazolin for 6 weeks was given using a port-à-cath system thus allowing ambulatory intravenous therapy. C-reactive protein normalized within 2.5 weeks. Full weight bearing using crutches was allowed for 8 weeks.

6 Complication

Eighteen days after fenestration the patient tried to stand up from a low sofa and felt a crack, accompanied by severe pain. The x-ray presented a slightly displaced spiral femoral fracture through the window (**Fig 17-3b**). Open reduction and internal fixation was then performed. The intraoperative reduction was held using two Weber clamps and fixed with two 3.5 mm lag screws protected by a plate osteosynthesis. Mobilization was allowed with 15 kg using two crutches. Full weight bearing was permitted after 3 months.

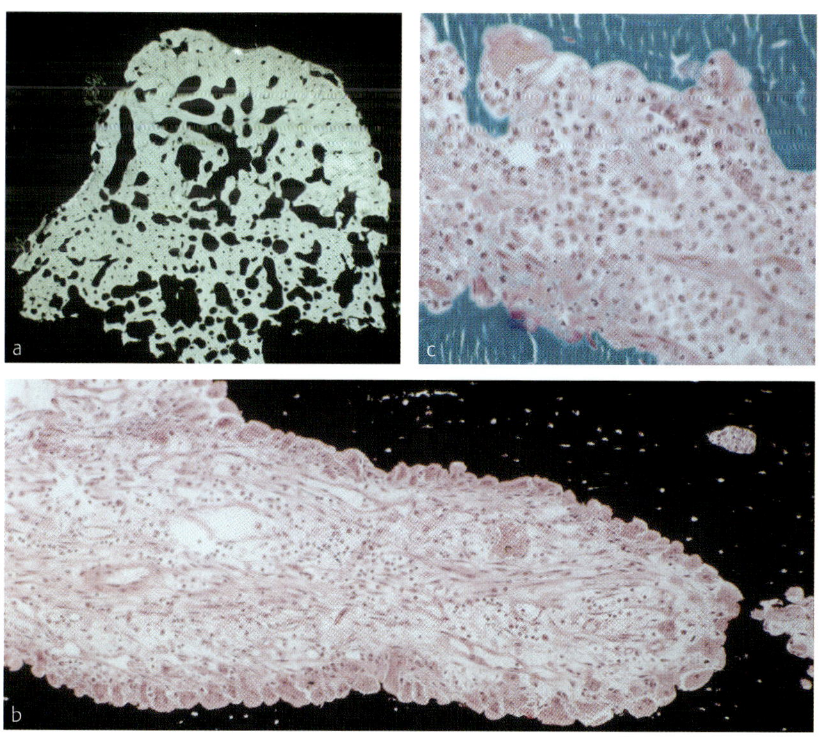

Fig 17-4a–c Histological analysis using a technique without decalcification.

a Microradiograph of a transverse section of the linea aspera at the level of the most radiolucent aspect (**Fig 17-1c**): chronic changes with rarefaction of the osseous structure. There is no real central "nidus" comparable with an osteoid osteoma.

b Longitudinal section adjacent to the section in **Fig 17-4a** (von Kossa stain section): newly formed wide longitudinal channel lined with many osteoclasts eating away the cortical bone structure. The center contains only chronic inflammatory cells.

c Magnified detail (Goldner stain) with distinct acute infection containing many segmented granulocytes.

7 Outcome

The 11-year follow-up demonstrated full reconstruction of the femur, but a defect remained in the area of the linea aspera (**Fig 17-5**). The patient noted slight recurrent pain for several years. Twenty-three years after onset, the patient is completely pain free, remarking a slight weakness of the left leg.

8 Comment

An acute infection occurred in a patient that presented with a very short history of local tenderness at the thigh, primarily not being considered as the source of the acute general infection, accompanied by hepatosplenomegaly and impressive serum inflammatory markers. The local infection must have developed over a period of months judging by the histological changes (**Fig 17-4**) and the osteoporotic changes found in the linea aspera. The cause of the acute onset of infection was unclear.

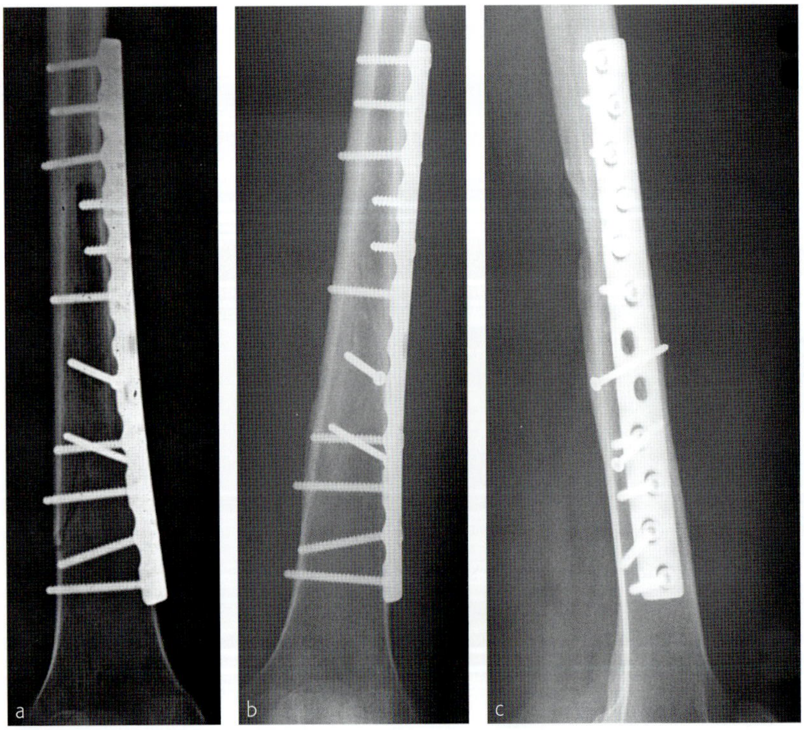

Fig 17-5a–c X-rays showing the situation after osteosynthesis.
a Postoperatively.
b–c After 11 years.

9 Pitfalls

- During the clinical presentation of infection, the osseous origin of the infection was missed.
- The weakening of the bone structure by the posterior bone window was such that a fatigue fracture through the inferior part of the bone window occurred. In the following years the author therefore changed the technique to an oval-shaped bone fenestration beginning with two drill holes of a larger diameter (8–10 mm diameter), which are then interconnected with an oscillating saw (**Fig 17-6**).

10 Pearls

- It is remarkable how a small local area of bone infection with histological signs of chronic primary development can provoke such an acute infection.
- This is a very rare case of intracortical infection leading to an acute development.
- The clinical picture of acute infection helped to rule out a malignant bone tumour.

11 Acknowledgements

The histological sections were carried out by Peter Zimmermann in the laboratory for undecalcified histology run by the author's department for orthopedic surgery at the Kantonsspital Liestal, and Stratec AG, Oberdorf, Switzerland.

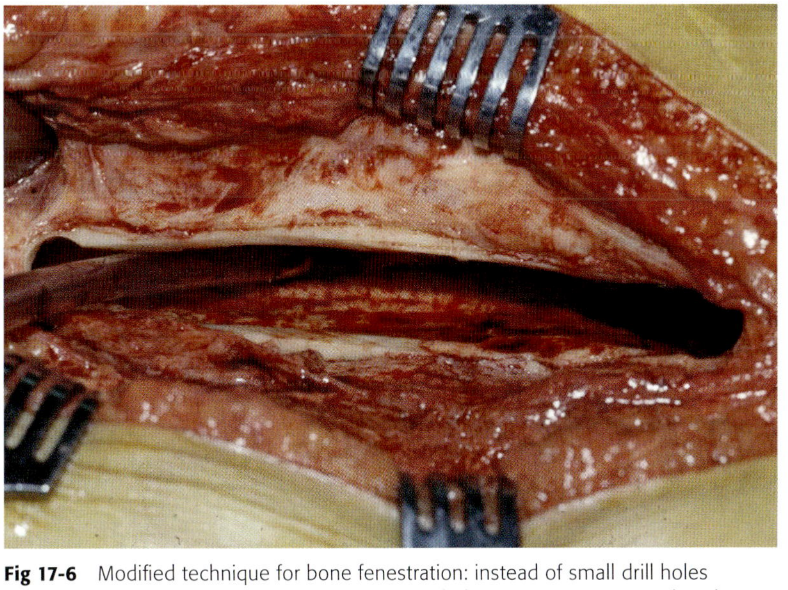

Fig 17-6 Modified technique for bone fenestration: instead of small drill holes (3.5 mm diameter) in the corners, two large drill holes (Ø 8–10 mm) are placed at the end of the planned window significantly diminishing the risk of fracture.

18 Chronic osteomyelitis of the tibia

Peter E Ochsner

1 Case description

A 34-year-old man developed swelling in the forearm and the lower leg. A tenderness of the anterior leg compartment was noted. Six weeks later, erythrocyte sedimentation rate (ESR) was 10 mm/h and hemoglobin (Hb) 147 g/L. Homeopathic therapy was attempted with partial pain relief after. Two-and-a-half months after the onset of symptoms, local swelling and warmth were more prominent. An x-ray of the distal tibia showed suspicious cortical changes (**Fig 18-1a**). A magnetic resonance imaging study demonstrated an osteolysis of the lateral and posterior cortical bone with periosteal swelling along the whole tibial shaft in this area. The radiologist suggested a differential diagnosis of telangiectatic osteosarcoma, malignant fibrous histiocytoma, non-Hodgkin's lymphoma, and Ewing sarcoma. The patient therefore was referred to the musculoskeletal oncology department for further diagnosis. Three-phase bone scintigraphy showed activity in the distal part of the tibia; angiography did not show pathological vessels; computed tomographic scan of the thorax and abdomen were negative. A second x-ray of the lower tibia presented a slight progression of the periosteal ossification (**Fig 18-1b**). In the absence of clear signs of infection, a biopsy was proposed but rejected by the patient. The patient attempted treatment with homeopathic drugs.

Six months after onset, ESR was 7 mm/h. A new x-ray of the tibia presented a sharp delimitation of the cortical bone (**Fig 18-1c**). The radiologist added chronic osteomyelitis as a further option to the original differential diagnosis of malignant tumours. One month later the patient presented with a progressive swelling with ESR 52 mm/h, Hb 133 g/L, leukocytes 14,400 cells/µL, including 9,550 granulocytes.

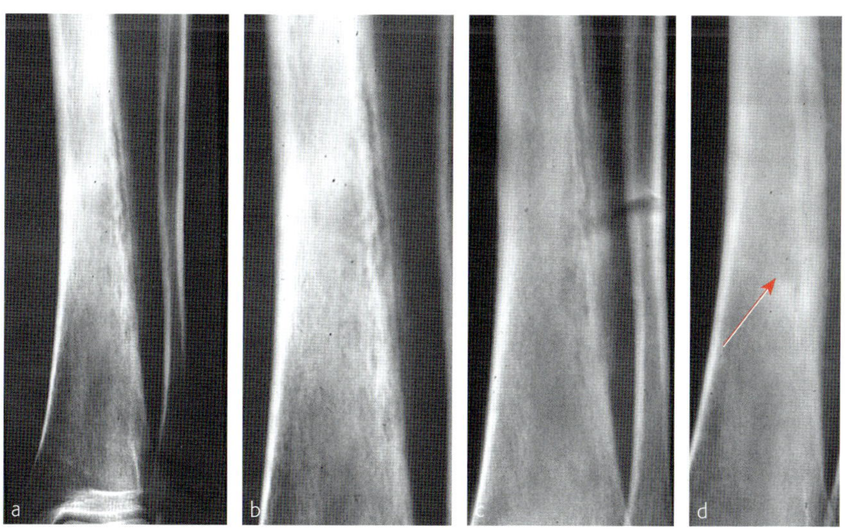

Fig 18-1a–d Development of the radiological changes in the left tibia.
a–b Overview (**a**) and detail (**b**) of the first x-ray, 2.5 months after onset. Localized thickening of the lateral cortex by new periosteal bone formation without a clear-cut borderline. Thinning of the original cortex.
c Two weeks later the periosteal bone is thickened.
d Four months later the periosteal thickening of the cortex is consolidated with sharp demarcation. The arrow indicates anterolateral cortical perforation (**Fig 18-2c**).

2 Indications

Two weeks later, 7.5 months after the onset of swelling, acute progression was observed. At hospitalization a local area of fluctuation was evident (**Fig 18-2**). The patient presented with fever of 38.2° C, Hb 12 g/L, leukocytes 19,100 cells/μL (80% granulocytes), C-reactive protein 147 mg/L, ESR 122 mm/h. Incision of the swelling evacuated about 200 cc of pus. Treatment was started with amoxicillin/clavulanic acid 2.2 g three times per day intravenously. A plaster splint was applied. The microbiological analysis presented α-haemolytic streptococci and coagulase-negative staphylococci after 4 days.

3 Surgical procedure

The plan for surgery was to evacuate the intramedullary abscess with any sequestra. The intention was to create a lateral cortical window (**Fig 18-3**) and curette the medullary cavity. The surgical approach was chosen from lateral in the area of the most evident radiological changes giving a view of the anterior perforation (**Fig 18-2c**) and the planned window. From the bone surface a thin new periosteal bone layer was removed together with the periosteum. After drilling four holes (3.2 mm diameter) the window was created with an oscillating saw. Through this opening, curettage of the medullary cavity followed including reaming away the inner parts of the cortex to remove sequestered bone.

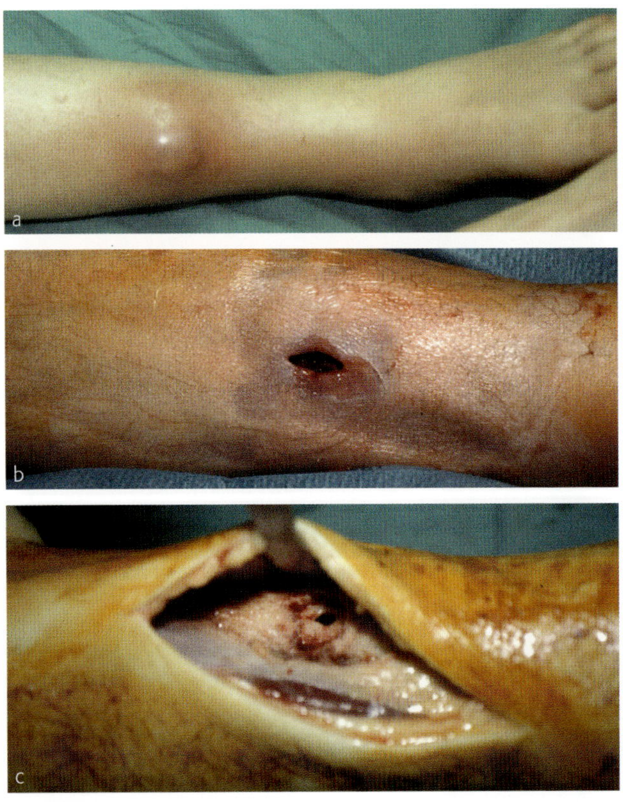

Fig 18-2a–c Patient images.
a Lower leg immediately prior to incision.
b Two days later.
c Lateral incision, presenting the anterior spontaneous perforation of the cortex allowing the pus to reach the subcutaneous region.

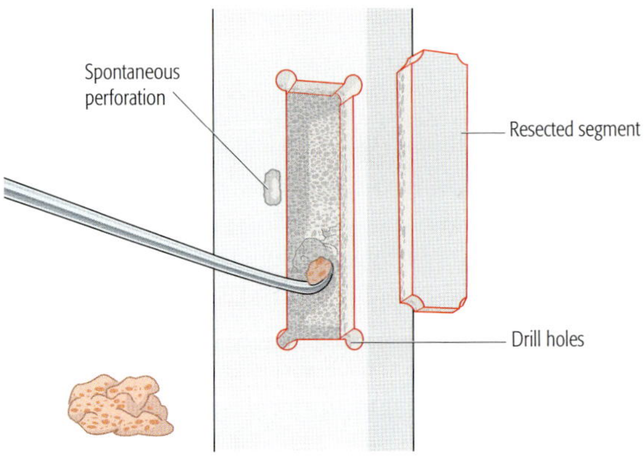

Fig 18-3 Surgical plan: a lateral segment is resected after placing drill holes in the four edges. Then a thorough curettage of the cavity follows. The removed segment then undergoes histological analysis.

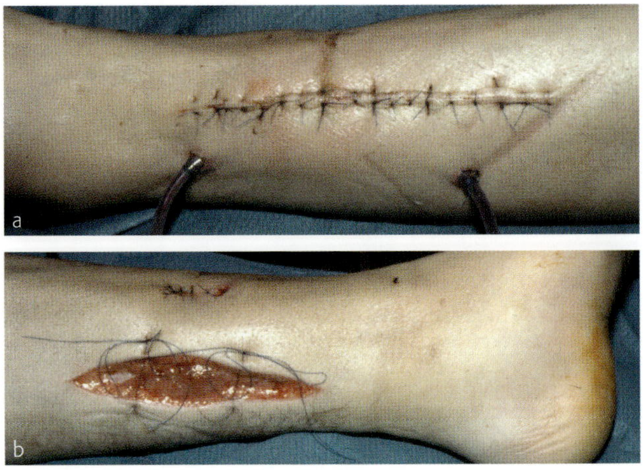

Fig 18-4a–b Approach and additional incision.
a Sutured lateral approach and drainage.
b Medial view of the sutured anterior incision and an additional posterior incision to relax the skin tension, ready for later closure.

Three tissue specimens were obtained and all were negative. Because of the local swelling, an additional dorsomedial incision prepared for delayed closure was placed to relax the local tension when the wounds were closed (**Fig 18-4a–b**).

4 Histological analysis

The resected bone segment and some curettage material of the medullary cavity underwent undecalcified histological analysis. The bone removed with the periosteum consisted of newly formed bone areas containing a great percentage of osteoid and osteoblasts. Then followed a thick layer of compact periosteal bone, richly vascularized (**Fig 18-5**, **Fig 18-6a**), arranged more in a radial manner not showing a classic composition with osteons. From the original cortical bone only dead-bone islands remained, having a brittle aspect, presenting only empty osteocyte cavities (**Fig 18-5**, **Fig 18-6b**). Inside this dead bone new osteons are visible; partially under formation, partially mature. In the area of lacunae (**Fig 18-5**) the soft-tissue content does not show any signs of infection. Towards the center of the medullary cavity there is partially chronic inflammation with many plasma cells and local acute infection containing small sequestra and granulocytes (**Fig 18-7**). An infection membrane surrounds the intramedullary abscess cavity.

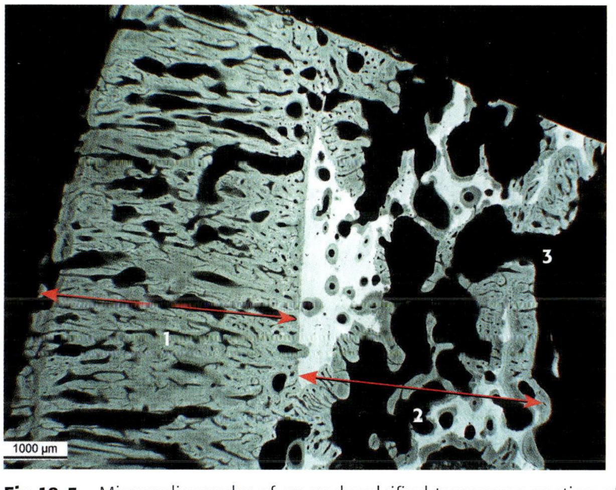

Fig 18-5 Microradiography of an undecalcified transverse section of the removed cortical segment (see **Fig 18-3**):

1. Layer of newly formed periosteal bone (see also **Fig 18-6a**).
2. Area of the original cortex. The dead remnants appear completely white (see also **Fig 18-6b**). Most of the cortex is removed by osteoclastic activity, partially forming empty lacunae, partially being replaced by gray new bone formation.
3. Location of **Fig 18-7**.

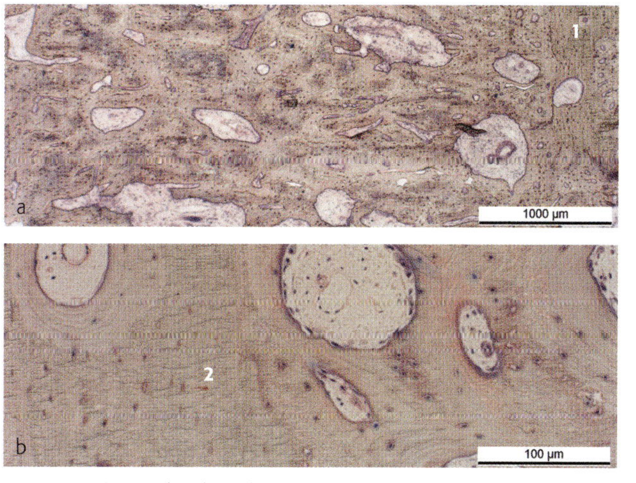

Fig 18-6a–b Undecalcified sections stained according to Romanowski.

a New periosteal bone adjacent to the dead remnants of the original cortical bone (**1**). It contains numerous channels containing vessels.

b Dead remnants of the old cortex (**2**) with empty osteocyte holes. The dead, brittle elements are fragmented. New vital osteons with central vessels partially mature (left) partially in formation presenting a blue osteoid ring and osteoblasts lining it.

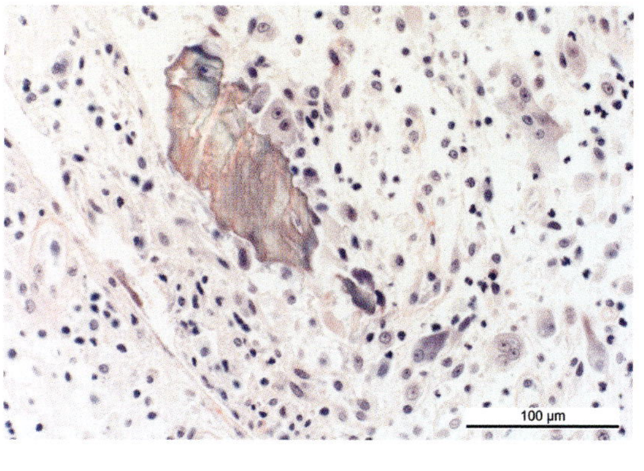

Fig 18-7 Detail of the inner limit of the cortical area (see also **Fig 18-5**). Undecalcified section, stained according to Romanowski. Numerous granulocytes with segmented nuclei indicate an acute infection. One little brittle sequestrum with an attached osteoclast containing two nuclei.

5 Further development

Antibiotic treatment with amoxicillin/clavulanic acid 2.2 g three times daily intravenously was continued for 6 weeks, followed by 6 weeks of oral treatment. C-reactive protein was < 5 mg/L after 2 weeks, ESR 8 mm/h after 3 months. Partial weight bearing was followed for 5 months using crutches. Two weeks later the patient slipped on ice and suffered a bone fracture from the bone window in a distal direction necessitating a plaster cast for 6 weeks. From then on the patient was pain free without recurrence of infection. At the 10-year follow-up, the x-ray presented thickened borders of the bone window but no closure of the gap (**Fig 18-8**). Twenty-five years after the treatment the patient was without inflammatory symptoms or pain.

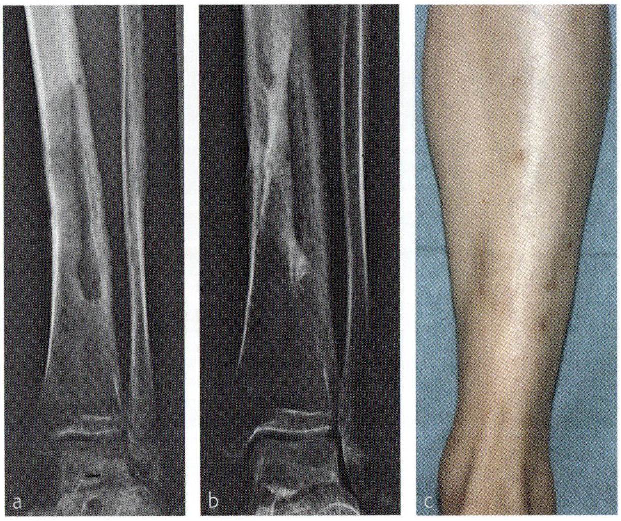

Fig 18-8a–c Postoperative development.
a X-ray at 3 months.
b X-ray taken 10 years after operative revision. Lateral cortical window still visible. No recurrence, no pain.
c Clinical photo taken 10 years after operative revision.

6 Comment

This osteomyelitis developed without clear signs of infection, initially even without any elevation of the ESR. It is comprehensible that the first x-ray (**Fig 18-1a**) suggested a diagnosis of a malignant bone tumour leading to a magnetic resonance imaging supporting this idea. A biopsy would have been indicated and capable of revealing the correct diagnosis. Because the patient refused a biopsy and any therapy, the spontaneous development could be observed, which turned to an acute abscess formation after 7.5 months. In this period the radiological picture became typical for osteomyelitis with a clear-cut external delimitation of the cortical thickening. Any formation of an involucrum or bulky sequestrum was missing confirming the primary chronic development.

7 Pitfalls

- In the differential diagnosis, a chronic osteomyelitis was not included.
- The cortical window led to a very slow consolidation. A slip on the ice provoked a bone fracture. A better technique to cut the window using an oval hole with a rotary burr is advisable to avoid this complication (**Fig 17-6**).

8 Pearls

- The spontaneous development of a primary chronic osteomyelitis in an adult can occur without extended sequestrations. A primary remodeling can occur in living bone with periosteal new bone formation and remodeling of the earlier cortical area can occur spontaneously.
- Exceptional spontaneous development of a chronic osteomyelitis mimicking a malignant tumor can be present without antibiotic therapy.

9 Acknowledgements

The histological sections were carried out by Peter Zimmermann in the laboratory for undecalcified histology run by the author's department for orthopedic surgery at the Kantonsspital Liestal and Stratec AG Oberdorf, Switzerland.

19.1 Implant removal—infected nonunion of the distal humerus

Jong-Keon Oh

1 Case description

A 39-year-old man injured his right arm while throwing a baseball 5 months prior to visiting the author's clinic. Injury films showed a low-energy spiral fracture of the distal humerus (AO/OTA Classification 12-A1) (**Fig 19.1-1**). Closed reduction and intramedullary nailing was attempted the day after injury. Immediate postoperative x-rays showed an unsuccessful attempt at nailing. Multiple-wedge fractures were iatrogenically created during the nailing and cerclage wires were used to fix the wedge fragments (**Fig 19.1-2**). A second procedure was done by the same surgeon 7 days after index nailing, probably because it was suspected that the initial nailing was unstable. This time the nail was removed and posterior plating was performed to achieve greater stability. The postoperative x-rays show posterior plating with a Y-plate (**Fig 19.1-3**). According to the medical records, swelling and redness developed, followed by discharge from the surgical wound 2 weeks after plating (no photographic documentation was available). The organisms identified by the tissue culture at the time of debridement were methicillin-resistant *Staphylococcus aureus* (MRSA) and *Enterobacter cloacae*. Vancomycin was administered intravenously on and off during the course of postoperative infection management at the previous hospital. Detailed information about the exact period of antibiotic treatment from the summarized transfer note was not available. The primary surgeon performed surgical debridement twice with implant retention. The patient was transferred to the author's institution 4 months later.

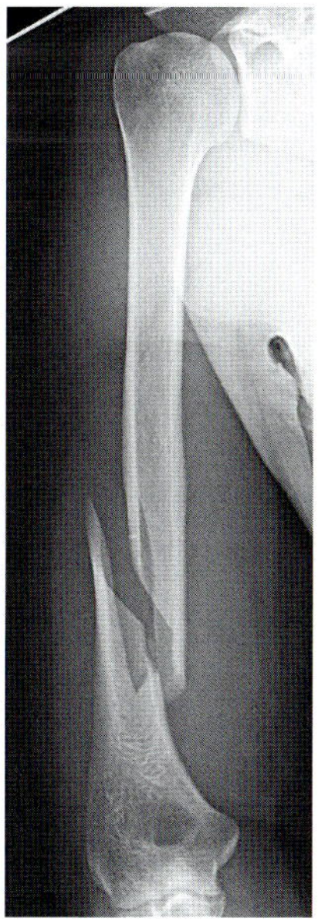

Fig 19.1-1 Initial injury x-ray shows low-energy spiral fracture of the distal humerus.

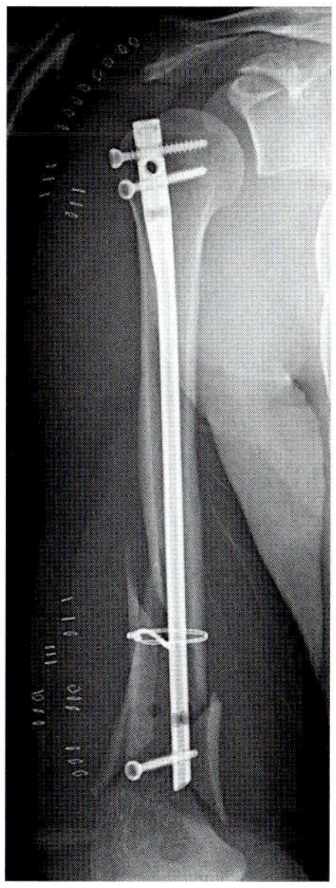

Fig 19.1-2 Postoperative x-ray shows an unsuccessful attempt at nailing. Multiple-wedge fractures were iatrogenically created by nailing and cerclage wiring was used resulting in soft-tissue stripping.

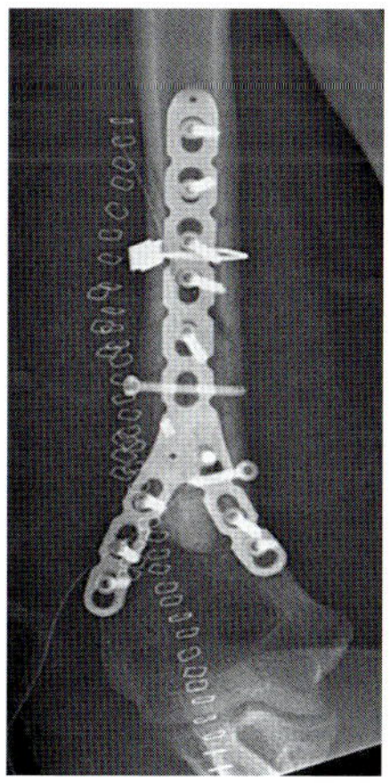

Fig 19.1-3 Postoperative x-ray after revision surgery performed 7 days after index nailing showed posterior plating with a Y-plate. Lag screws were used to fix the wedge fractures and cerclage wiring is also seen at the proximal part of the fracture site. Given the direction of lag screws and the wiring, a circumferential stripping of periosteum seems likely. The length of the plate is too short with only two bicortical screws placed into the proximal shaft.

Clinical examination showed a midline scar along the posterior arm with good soft-tissue coverage. A small draining sinus with purulent discharge was noted on the lateral side of the distal arm. The elbow was stiff with the range of motion from 10°, lacking full extension to 100° of flexion. Wrist drop was noted due to complete radial nerve palsy after the second surgery (nail removal and plating) by the primary surgeon (**Fig 19.1-4**). X-rays show resorption of bone around the fracture margins around the cerclage wiring and screw loosening. No signs of fracture healing were visible (**Fig 19.1-5**). Blood tests were conducted for screening and erythrocyte sedimentation rate (ESR) was elevated to 50 mm/h (normal range: 0–10 mm/h). C-reactive protein (CRP) level was slightly elevated to 5.8 mg/L (normal range: 0–5 mg/L). All other laboratory tests results were within the normal range.

2 Indications

Based on the history, the diagnosis of an infected nonunion of the distal humeral fracture with radial nerve palsy and stiff elbow joint was made. Initial management after postoperative infection was dictated by the well-known orthopedic principle, the so-called union-first strategy. The union-first strategy includes operative debridement, antibiotic suppression, and retention of hardware until fracture union occurs. Even after two attempts of surgical debridement and antibiotic suppression, pus drainage was persistent. Mostly it did not appear that the fracture was healing based on two main radiological findings:

1. The fixation construct did not afford enough stability from the beginning, as the plate length was too short and only two bicortical screws were placed at the proximal shaft. The fixation construct at this point (4 months postoperatively) with additional screw loosening is considered an unstable construct.
2. There were no radiographic signs of fracture healing. This represents a failure of the union-first strategy and surgical intervention including plate removal is mandatory.

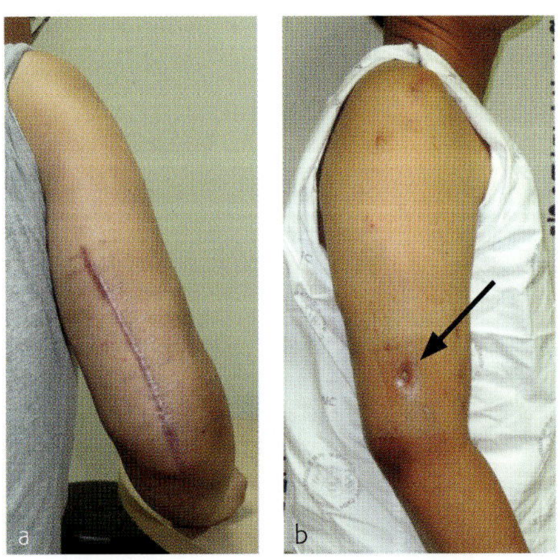
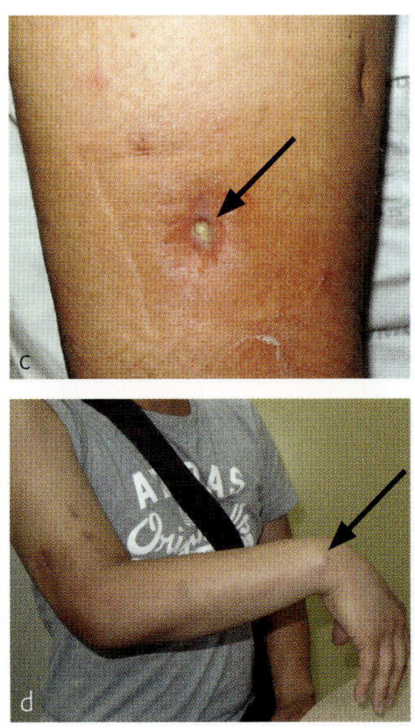

Fig 19.1-4a–d Clinical photographs.
a The midline scar along the posterior surface of the distal arm with good soft-tissue coverage.
b–c Small draining sinus with pus discharge was noted on the lateral side of the distal arm (arrows).
d The patient's elbow was stiff with the range of motion from 170° to 80° of flexion. Wrist drop was noted due to complete radial nerve palsy (arrow).

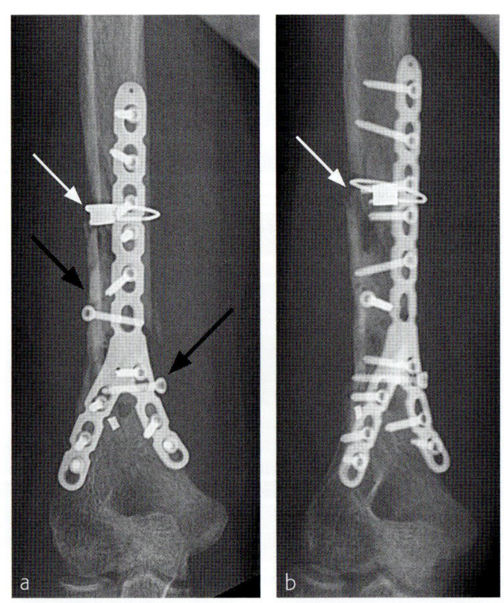

Fig 19.1-5a–b X-rays show resorption of bone around the fracture margins, especially near the cerclage wiring (white arrows) and screw loosening (black arrows). No signs of fracture healing were visible.
a AP view.
b Oblique view.

3 Preoperative planning

The problem was defined as an infected nonunion of the distal humeral fracture with radial nerve palsy. The author planned a staged reconstruction. Local soft-tissue condition was good enough for staged multiple reconstruction procedures. The patient was healthy and young—a type A host.

Stage 1: plate removal and radical debridement of infected and dead tissue. The author planned to fill the bone defect with antibiotic-loaded polymethylmethacrylate (PMMA) cement spacer, as significant bone defect after debridement was expected. Four grams of vancomycin hydrochloride were mixed with 40 g of PMMA bone cement. Exploration of the radial nerve and neurolysis, if possible, was planned. The planned extent of bone debridement was based on the analysis of previous procedures and radiological findings. The author thought that wedge fractures created by nail insertion were most likely devitalized by wiring and lag-screw placement in different directions ending up as sequestrum. Loosening of screws and bone resorption around the wires were the clues for this analysis. It was expected that resection of the bone from the level of the cerclage wire down to the most distal lag screw on the medial side would be performed (**Fig 19.1-5**). A temporary bridging external fixator across the elbow was planned to give stability. The procedure was performed in lateral position to use the previous posterior approach. Draping was done from fingers to shoulder and a sterilized pneumatic tourniquet was planned.

Stage 2: repeated debridement and definitive fixation with posterior plating. Exchange the PMMA cement spacer. The surgeon mixed 40 g bone cement with 4 g vancomycin hydrochloride based on the previous culture results. The patient was treated with 13.5 g piperacillin/tazobactam and 3 g vancomycin per day. The second-stage operation was planned 2–3 weeks after the stage 1 procedure as it was desirable to mobilize the elbow as early as possible.

Stage 3: polymethylmethacrylate cement spacer removal and autogenous bone graft. This final stage procedure was planned for 3–4 months after the second-stage procedure. Meanwhile aggressive rehabilitation to restore the elbow-joint motion and monthly follow-up with clinical examination were planned to ensure that the ESR/CRP levels had normalized before the bone graft and without clinical signs of recurrent infection. Systemic antibiotics therapy: 13.5 g piperacillin/tazobactam and 3 g vancomycin per day were introduced for 6 weeks after surgery.

4 Surgical approach

Surgical approaches were straightforward in this case as there was a prior long posterior incision (**Fig 19.1-4a**). It was planned to split the triceps muscle all the way up to the spiral groove to locate the radial nerve.

5 Surgical debridement and implant removal

A longitudinal skin incision was made over the previous operative scar. The plate was exposed by the triceps-splitting approach. All necrotic triceps muscles in contact with the plate were meticulously debrided. The plate was covered with infected granulation tissues and pus (**Fig 19.1-6a**). The plate was exposed more clearly by removing infected granulation tissues (**Fig 19.1-6b**). The plate was taken out without difficulty. Screw loosening was noted as expected based on the radiological findings. Plate removal exposed the posterior surface of the distal humerus (**Fig 19.1-6c**). Those previous wedge fragments that were expected to be devitalized and infected were removed and further resection margins from the proximal and distal fragments were chosen by the capacity to bleed at the resection margins (Paprika sign). Removal of wedge fragments was confirmed with image intensification (**Fig 19.1-7**). An intraoperative clinical photo shows the plate and dead bone fragments that were removed (**Fig 19.1-8**).

The radial nerve was identified at the spiral groove and intact continuity was verified (**Fig 19.1-9**). Neurolysis was performed by removing scar tissue around the nerve.

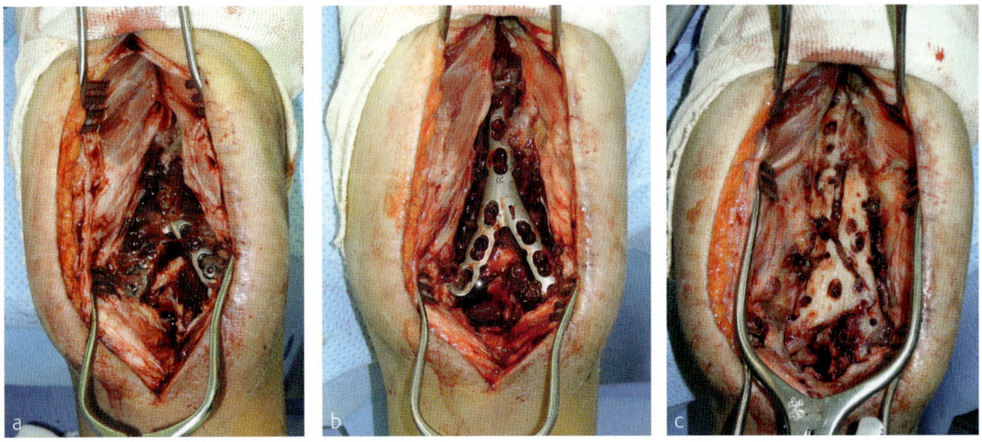

Fig 19.1-6a–c Intraoperative photographs.
- **a** Infected granulation tissue and pus covering the plate after a triceps-split approach.
- **b** The plate is more clearly exposed after debridement of surrounding infected tissues.
- **c** Plate removal exposed dead cortical bone surface with multiple screw holes, some of which are enlarged due to resorption around the loosened screws. Note also clearly visible nonunion gaps. Screw holes and nonunion gaps contained infected granulation tissues.

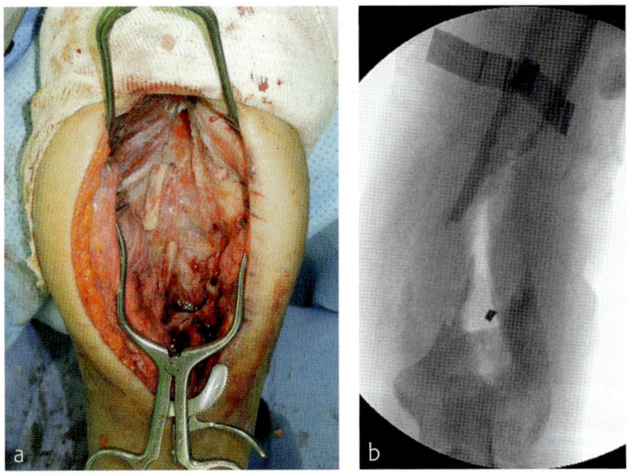

Fig 19.1-7a–b Intraoperative images.
- **a** Image taken after dead bone resection.
- **b** C-arm image shows the size of the bone defect after debridement.

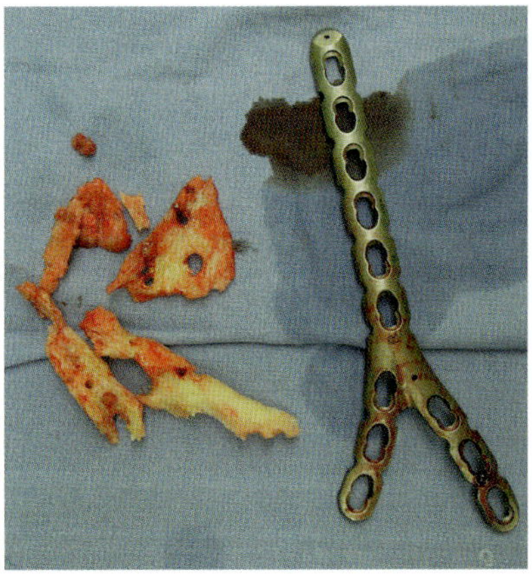

Fig 19.1-8 Removed dead bone fragments and the plate.

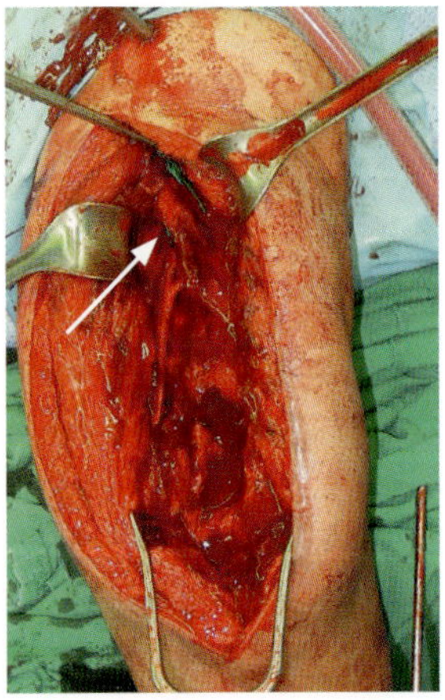

Fig 19.1-9 Intraoperative photograph shows the radial nerve identified at the radial groove (arrow).

6 Temporary fixation

The bone defect was then temporarily filled with an antibiotic-loaded (4 g of vancomycin in 40 g of PMMA powder) PMMA cement spacer (**Fig 19.1-10**). A flexible nail was introduced into the medullary canal to help stabilize the cement spacer within the defect. An induced membrane will form around the cement spacer and in turn the grafted bone will be contained by the induced membrane at the third-stage procedure. The spacer was shaped similar to the normal bone morphology at that level.

Temporary stabilization was necessary to maintain stability. A bridging external fixator was applied across the elbow joint. The positions of proximal Schanz screws were chosen not to hinder the definitive plate fixation at the second-stage procedure (**Fig 19.1-11**).

7 Postoperative management

Postoperatively the arm was kept in a comfortable position, passive wrist and finger extension and active flexion exercises were performed with functional bracing to rehabilitate the radial nerve palsy. Vancomycin was infused intravenously for 3 weeks after debridement. Intraoperative tissue culture revealed MRSA as the current infecting organism which confirmed the previous culture.

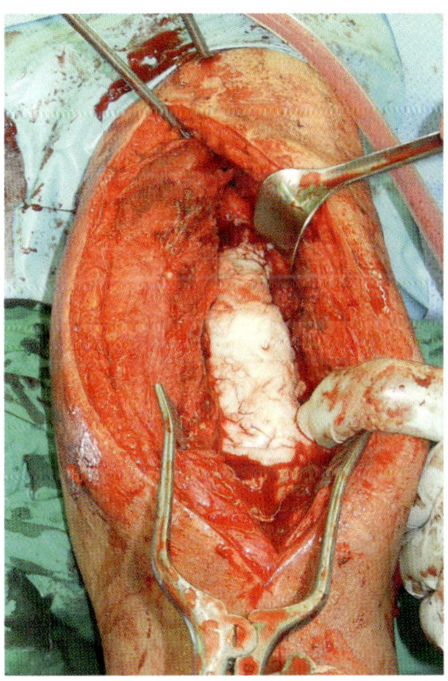

Fig 19.1-10 After bone resection the defect was filled with vancomycin-loaded polymethylmethacrylate cement spacer.

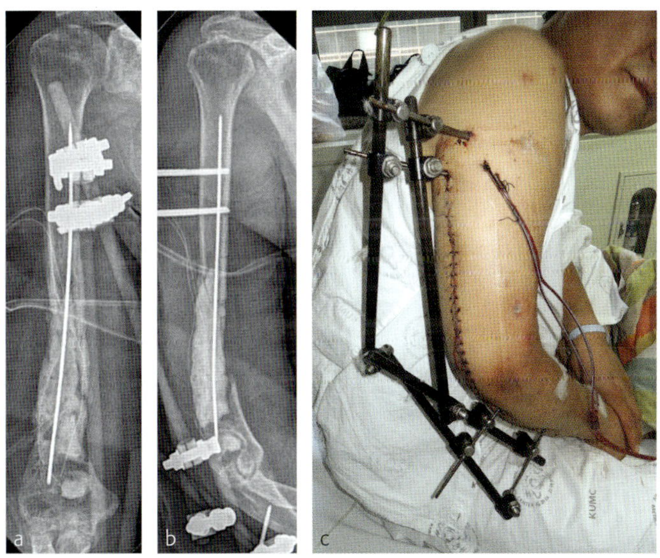

Fig 19.1-11a–c Postoperative images.
a–b X-rays show the size of the bone defect that is filled with polymethylmethacrylate cement spacer. Note the bridging external fixator. A flexible nail was used to help stabilize the cement spacer.
c The longitudinal surgical wound and bridging external fixator.

8 Reimplantation

8.1 Second-stage procedure

Three weeks after the first-stage debridement and temporary external fixation, the surgical wound was clinically clean and purulent drainage through the sinus tract had stopped following the initial debridement. The second-stage procedure was performed as planned. The external fixator was kept to maintain the length. The PMMA cement spacer was exposed by splitting the triceps again. Previous bone resection margins were carefully examined again and further resection was performed due to lack of bleeding at the cortical margin of the proximal fragment (**Fig 19.1-12**). Margins of surrounding soft tissues were meticulously trimmed off again. Trimmed tissues were prepared for another tissue culture. Then definitive fixation was carried out using an extraarticular locking compression plate distal humerus (LCP-DH). Additional plating was done along the medial side of the humerus across the bone defect. Then the bone defect was filled with an antibiotic-loaded PMMA cement spacer. Once the fixation was complete, the full range of elbow joint motion could be confirmed (**Fig 19.1-13**). The wound was closed over a suction drainage. Intravenous vancomycin was prescribed for 2 weeks. Suction drainage was removed 3 days after plating, followed by aggressive range-of-motion exercises.

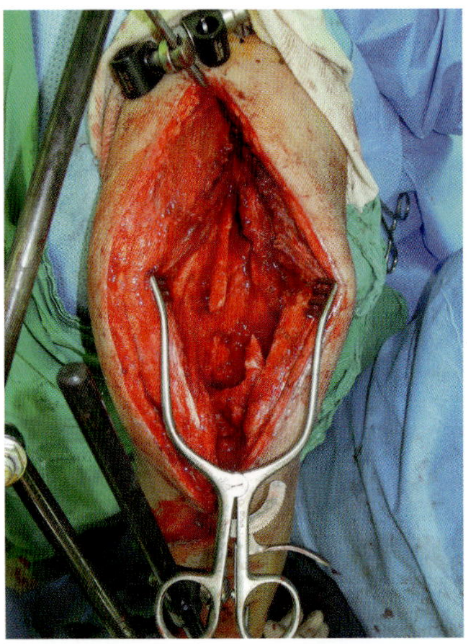

Fig 19.1-12 Intraoperative image shows the bone defect after cement removal.

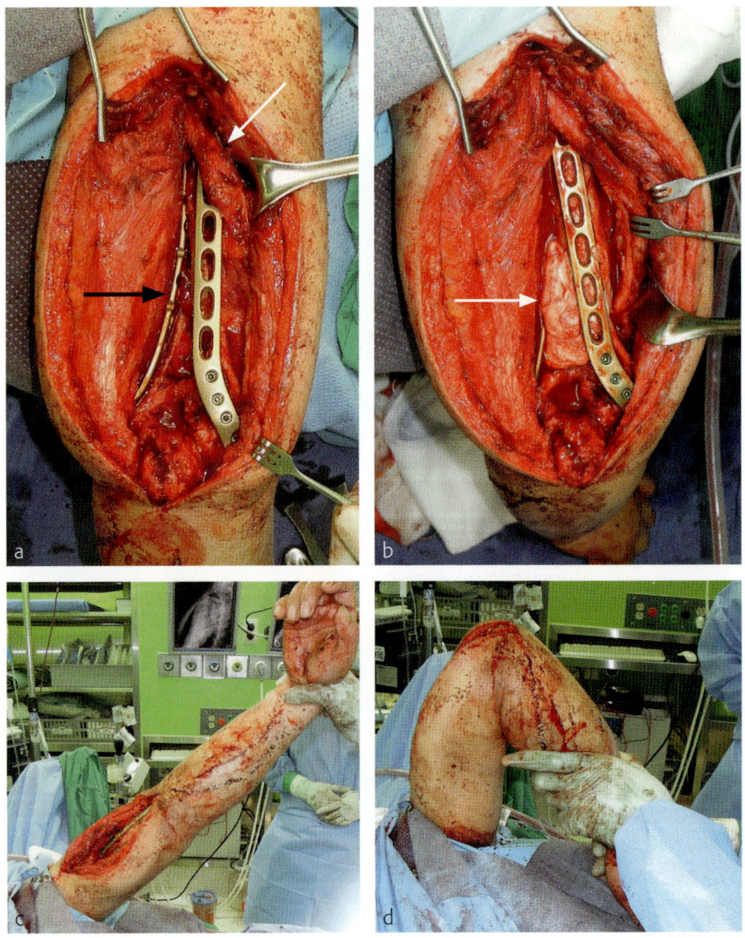

Fig 19.1-13a–d Intraoperative images.

a Posterior plating along the lateral column. The white arrow indicates the radial nerve under which the plate was slid. Additional plating (black arrow) at right angles to the posterior plate was performed along the medial side of the distal humerus.

b Bone defect was filled with a polymethylmethacrylate cement spacer (white arrow).

c–d Intraoperative elbow joint motion after fixation and cement spacer insertion.

Postoperative x-rays show a dual plating construct which was stable enough to commence vigorous rehabilitation 4 days postoperatively when the drain was removed (**Fig 19.1-14**).

The author followed up the patient with monthly laboratory tests and x-rays for 4 months postoperatively to ensure that the ESR/CRP levels normalized 4 weeks after the second-stage definitive fixation and stayed at the normal level for another 3 months. The patient was treated intravenously with piperacillin/tazobactam 3 x 4.5 g and vancomycin 3 x1 g per day for 6 weeks after surgery. No additional oral antibiotics were given because the serological marker was normalized after treatment with intravenous antibiotics. There were no signs of recurrence of infection during this period. The ESR and CRP levels were normalized. The patient regained elbow joint motion with 15° of flexion contracture and 95° of flexion by this time (**Fig 19.1-15**). Radial nerve palsy also fully recovered spontaneously.

8.2 Third-stage procedure

The same posterior approach was used to expose the cement spacer. A small amount of serous fluid collection was noted around the cement. Other than that tissues were clean and no gross evidence of infection was found. The cement spacer was removed with the use of a cement-removing chisel. Whitish-induced membrane was well formed around the cement spacer (**Fig 19.1-16**).

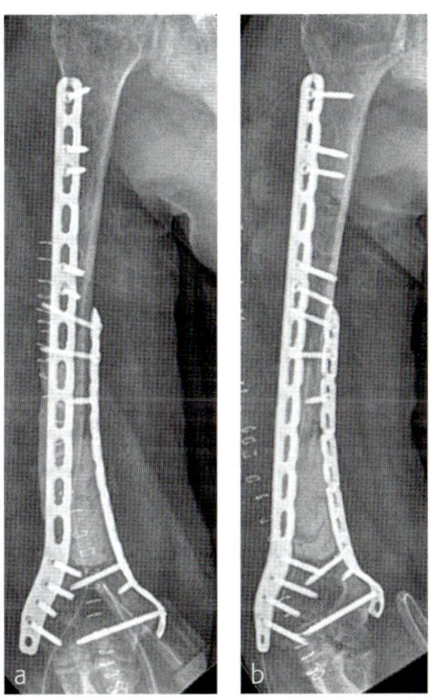

Fig 19.1-14a–b Postoperative x-rays show a dual plating construct.
a AP view.
b Lateral view.

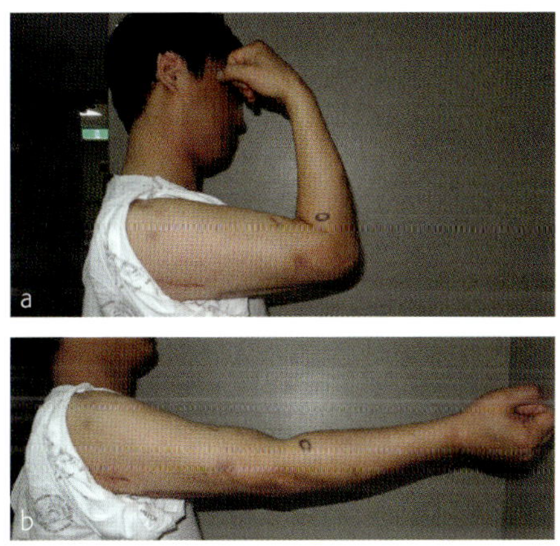

Fig 19.1-15a–b Four months after second-stage plating there is restoration of elbow joint motion without signs of infection.
a Flexion.
b Extension.

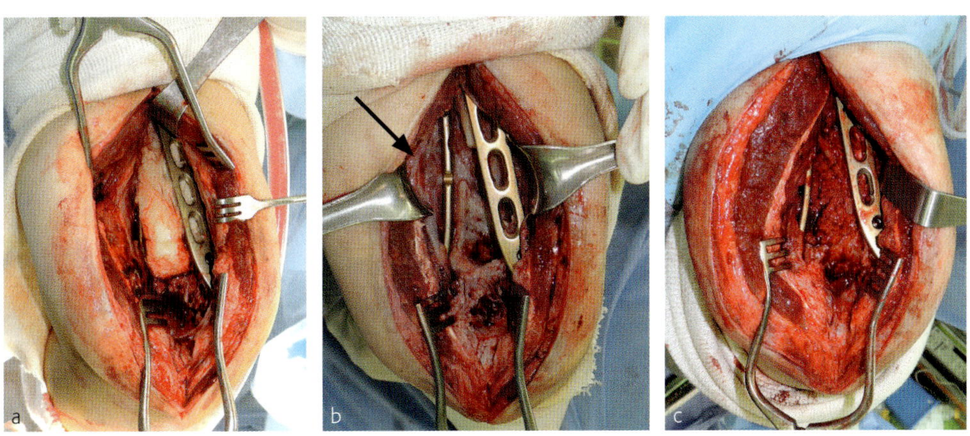

Fig 19.1-16a–c Intraoperative photographs.
a The cement spacer with clean surrounding soft tissues.
b Whitish-induced membrane (arrow) is visible after cement spacer removal.
c Cancellous bone graft filling the defect.

The bone defect was filled with autogenous cancellous bone graft taken from the ipsilateral iliac crest (**Fig 19.1-17a**).

The surgical wound was closed over a suction drain. Postoperative x-rays taken immediately after bone graft show grafted bone shadow along the medial column (**Fig 19.1-17**).

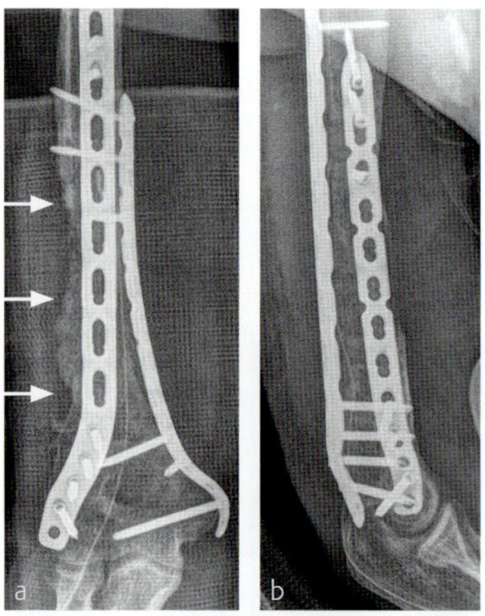

Fig 19.1-17a–b Postoperative x-rays show grafted bone that replaced the cement spacer (arrows).
a AP view.
b Lateral view.

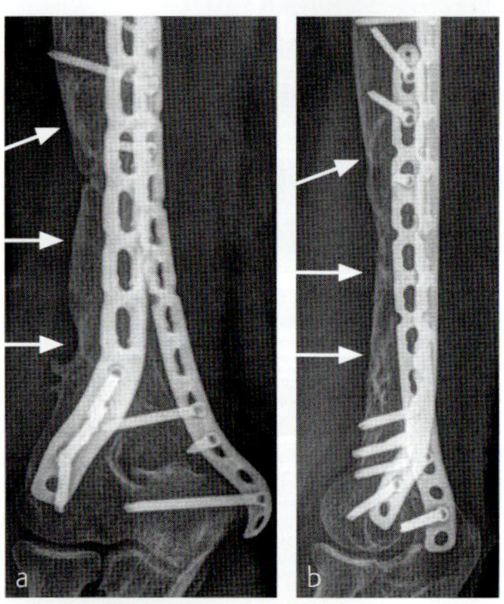

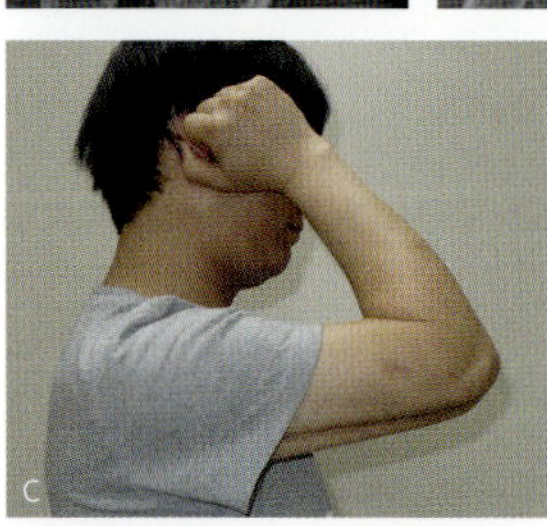

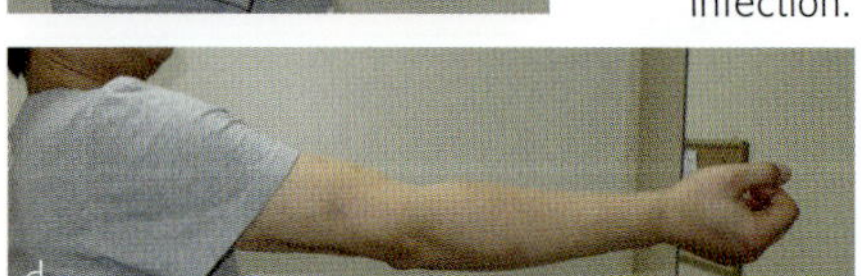

Fig 19.1-18a–d Follow-up images 6 months after bone graft.
a–b X-rays show consolidation of grafted bone (arrows).
c–d Range of motion of the right elbow without any signs of infection.

9 Outcome

On postoperative day 4, the drain was removed. Active range of motion was encouraged after this point. X-rays taken 6 months after bone grafting demonstrate consolidation and corticalization of the grafted bone. The patient recovered nearly full range of his elbow joint motion (**Fig 19.1-18**).

10 Pitfalls

- The union-first strategy for the management of acute postoperative infection after fracture fixation includes operative debridement, antibiotic suppression, and retention of hardware until fracture union occurs. This strategy works only when there is reasonable evidence for fracture healing while infection is being suppressed. It is not likely to succeed in the presence of a multidrug-resistant organism like MRSA.
- If there are no radiological signs of progressive fracture healing or the stability is not sufficient, remove the hardware and perform staged fracture fixation and bone reconstruction after radical debridement.

11 Pearls

- It is critical to have a plan for the whole staged reconstruction before commencing treatment. It is also important to inform the patient and his or her family about the treatment plan and possible complications and problems that may alter the surgeon's plans.
- Regarding the fixation construct, it is vital to consider a postoperative rehabilitation plan. In this case the patient presented with infected nonunion and a stiff elbow.
- An aggressive rehabilitation after definitive fixation at the second-stage procedure was planned. It took longer than expected for union after bone grafting, therefore, a dual plating construct was chosen that was the strongest fixation option available.

19.2 Implant removal—infected nonunion of the tibia

Jong-Keon Oh

1 Case description

A 66-year-old man injured his right leg in a traffic accident 17 months prior to visiting the author's clinic. Injury films demonstrated a high-energy open diaphyseal fracture of the distal tibia (AO/OTA Classification 42-C) (**Fig 19.2-1**). Photographic documentation of the initial wound was not available. Open reduction and intramedullary nailing was done primarily after debridement (**Fig 19.2-2**). The open wound was closed primarily and information about the exact soft-tissue condition before and after debridement was not available. Follow-up x-rays taken 7 months after the index operation show the removal of a proximal interlocking screw due to loosening and no callus formation at either the proximal or distal fracture sites (**Fig 19.2-3**). According to the medical records, at this time there was deep infection at the distal fracture site with purulent discharge. The causative organism was *Escherichia coli* by tissue culture. A second operation was performed by the primary surgeon to control the infection. There was segmental resection around the distal fracture site and reconstruction of the defect by bone transport technique with the use of an Ilizarov

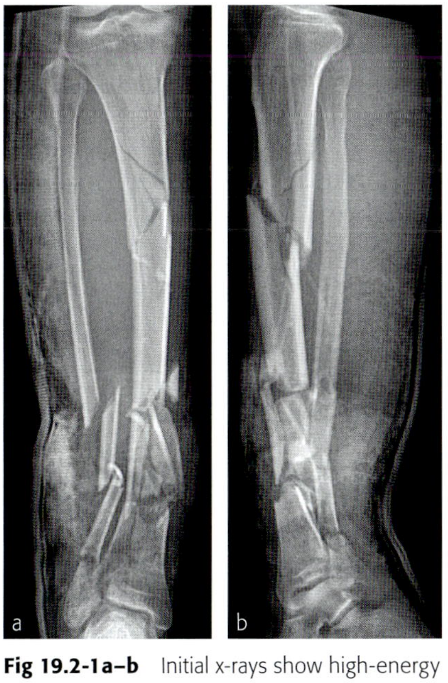

Fig 19.2-1a–b Initial x-rays show high-energy diaphyseal fracture of the right tibia.
a AP view.
b Lateral view.

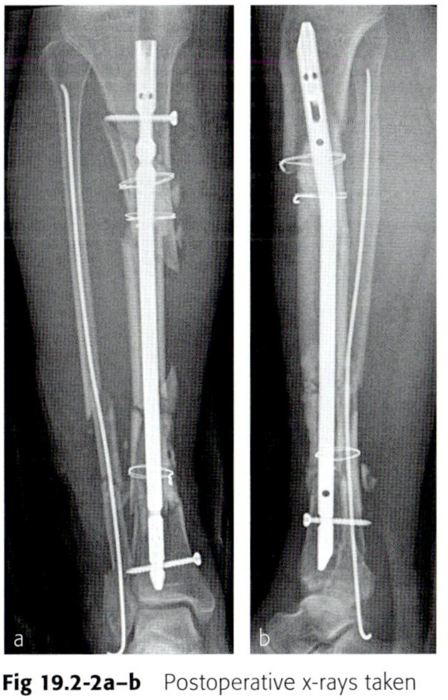

Fig 19.2-2a–b Postoperative x-rays taken immediately after the index operation show open reduction and cerclage wiring around both the proximal and distal fracture sites and nailing. This construct does not appear stable especially at the proximal fracture site as only one interlocking screw was used to stabilize the proximal fragment.
a AP view.
b Lateral view.

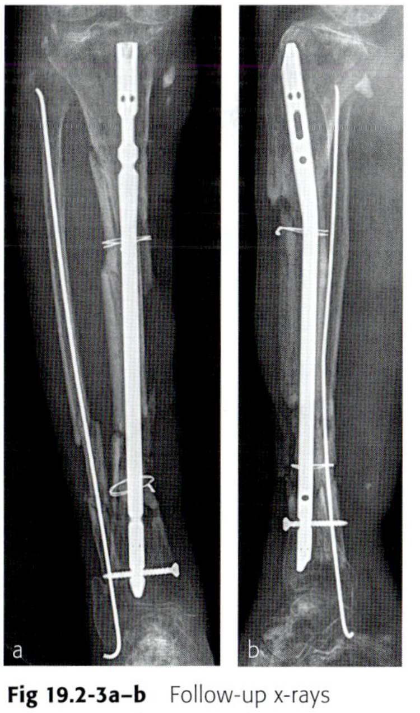

Fig 19.2-3a–b Follow-up x-rays taken 7 months after index operation demonstrate removal of the proximal interlocking screw due to loosening and no callus formation at either the proximal or distal fracture sites.
a AP view.
b Lateral view.

ring frame (**Fig 19.2-4**). The Ilizarov frame was removed 9 months after osteotomy. The patient was transferred to the author's clinic 1 month after frame removal. X-rays (17 months after injury) show double-level malalignment (10° valgus at the proximal regenerate bone column and 15° varus at the site of the distal docking site) with 17 mm shortening. Bridging callus formation along the medial cortex was not visible at the distal docking site with a visible fracture gap (**Fig 19.2-5**). There was tenderness over the distal nonunion site. The wound was covered well and there were no clinical symptoms and signs of infection for the past 9 months. The ankle was stiff with minimal motion present (**Fig 19.2-6**). Blood tests showed the erythrocyte sedimentation rate (ESR) was elevated to 35 mm/h (normal range: 0–10 mm/h). Other than that every laboratory test was within normal range including the C-reactive protein (CRP) level at 1.20 mg/L (normal range: 0–5 mg/L).

2 Indications

The patient had double-level malalignment (10° of valgus at the proximal regenerate bone column and 15° of varus at the distal docking site) with 17 mm shortening. Distal docking-site union was incomplete, so an additional surgical procedure was required to correct the deformity and to achieve solid union.

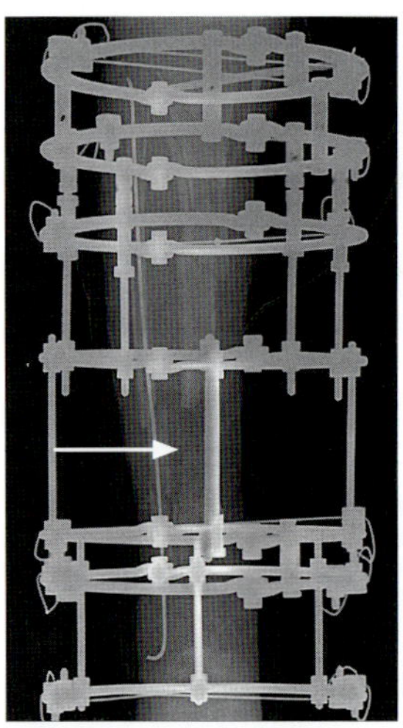

Fig 19.2-4 Segmental resection around the distal fracture site and bone transport with an Ilizarov frame was performed 9 months after injury.

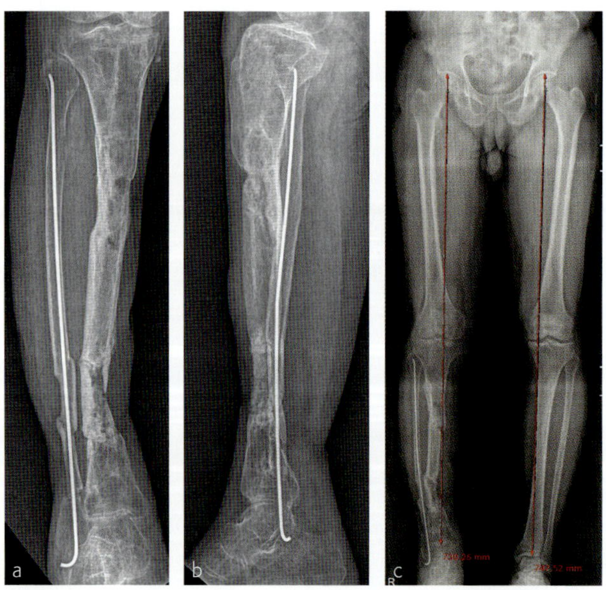

Fig 19.2-5a–c X-rays taken 1 month after frame removal show double-level malalignment (10° valgus at the proximal regenerate bone column and 15° varus malalignment present at the distal docking site) with 17 mm of shortening. Bridging callus formation along the medial cortex was not visible at the distal docking site with a visible fracture gap present.

- **a** AP view.
- **b** Lateral view.
- **c** Orthoradiogram view for comparative alignment.

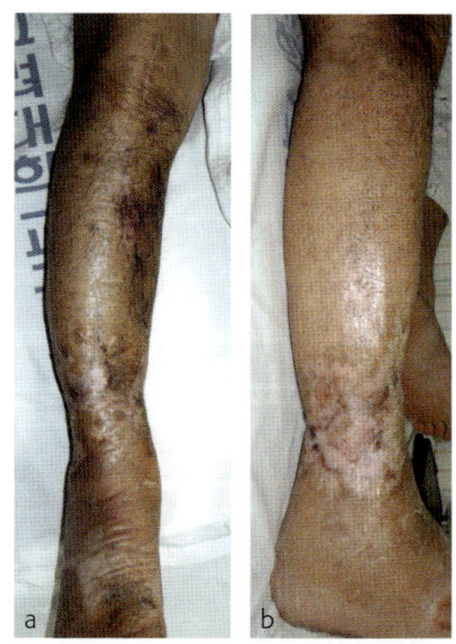

Fig 19.2-6a–b Clinical photographs just before correction and nailing. The wound was covered well and there were no clinical symptoms and signs of infection for the past 9 months.

3 Preoperative planning

Considering the patient's age, stiff ankle, and some expected length restoration after realignment, lengthening was not incorporated into the surgical planning. Acute correction with double-level osteotomy and nailing plus autogenous bone graft at the osteotomy sites was planned (**Fig 19.2-7**).

Although the ESR level was elevated, the author did not specifically plan for management of indolent infection as the patient had not shown any clinical signs of infection for the past 9 months. Intraoperative neutrophil count was planned to be used as a guide for possible but less likely staged operations, meaning debridement and temporary external fixation and polymethylmethacrylate (PMMA) cement spacer followed by second-stage reconstruction. The patient was positioned supine with the use of pneumatic tourniquet. It was believed that the femoral distractor may not be helpful as the bone quality was poor due to disuse osteoporosis resulting from the prolonged period of non-weight bearing. Instead it was planned to navigate a hand reamer through the central axes of the three main fragments after double-level osteotomy (Sofield osteotomy). A fibular osteotomy was planned only if the amount of deforming forces were big enough to hinder correction of tibial deformities.

4 Surgical approach

Surgical approaches were straightforward in this case as there were double-level deformities and the skin condition was acceptable to make longitudinal incisions directly over the anterior surface of the tibial crest (**Fig 19.2-8**).

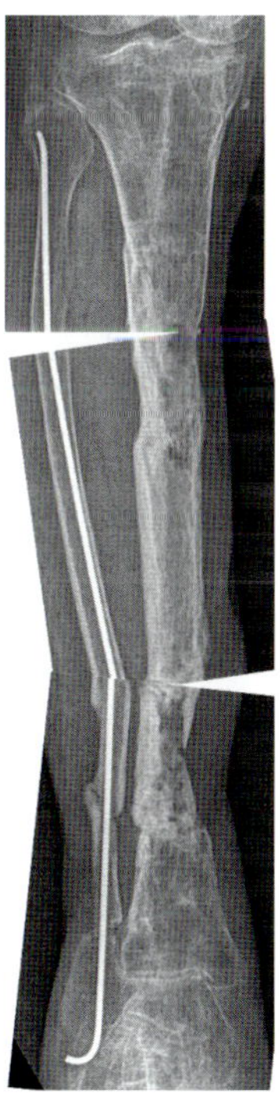

Fig 19.2-7 Double-level osteotomies centered over the center of rotation axes 1 and 2 were planned.

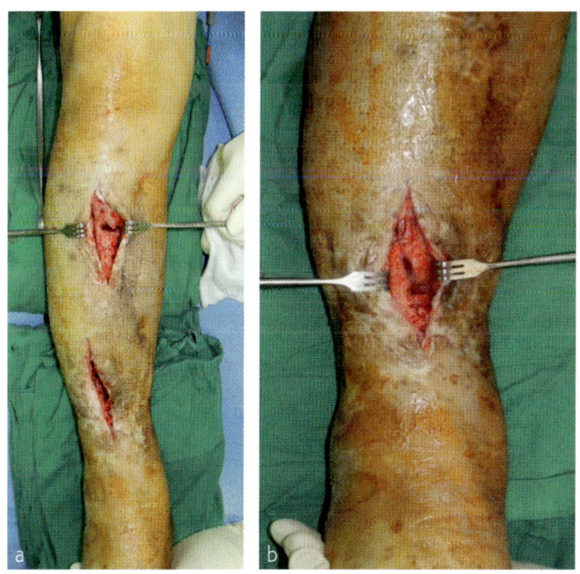

Fig 19.2-8a–b Direct longitudinal skin incisions were made over the osteotomy sites.

5 Surgical debridement

Upon opening the proximal malunion and distal nonunion sites, there were no clinical signs of infection. Intraoperative polymorphonucleocyte counts from both sites showed less than 1 per high-power field. Debridement was performed to remove the sclerotic bones around the osteotomy sites until healthy bone was exposed. Intraoperative photos were taken after debridement and nailing and show the size of the defects at both levels (**Fig 19.2-9**). These defects were filled with autogenous cancellous bone from the iliac crest.

6 Postoperative management

Postoperatively the leg was elevated with temporary immobilization in a long leg splint. Intravenous infusion of first-generation cephalosporin was prescribed according to the routine protocol for an elective clean surgery.

7 Outcome

Postoperative x-rays show correction of alignment and statically locked nailing (**Fig 19.2-10**).

On postoperative day 3, the drain was removed as the amount of drainage diminished to 7 mL/day. On postoperative day 4, the tissue culture from the proximal osteotomy site grew *E coli*. On postoperative day 5, the patient developed a spiking fever of 38.5° C and the drain tip culture revealed *E coli*. In response to this situation, antibiotics were started with β-lactamase inhibitor based on the culture results. The fever was not controlled even after antibiotic change but the surgical debridement was delayed mainly due to the surgeon's reluctance to face the reality of infection after successful reconstructive procedure including autogenous bone graft. Finally, a decision for surgical debridement was made on postoperative day 9 when purulent discharge through the proximal surgical wound was noted (**Fig 19.2-11**).

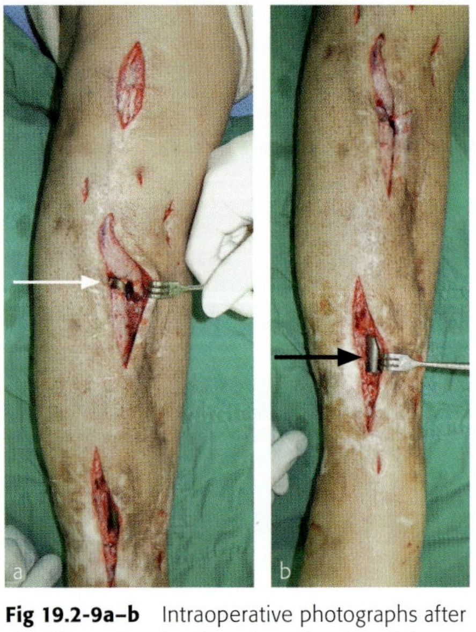

Fig 19.2-9a–b Intraoperative photographs after debridement and nailing show the size of the defects at both levels
(proximal: white arrow, distal: black arrow).

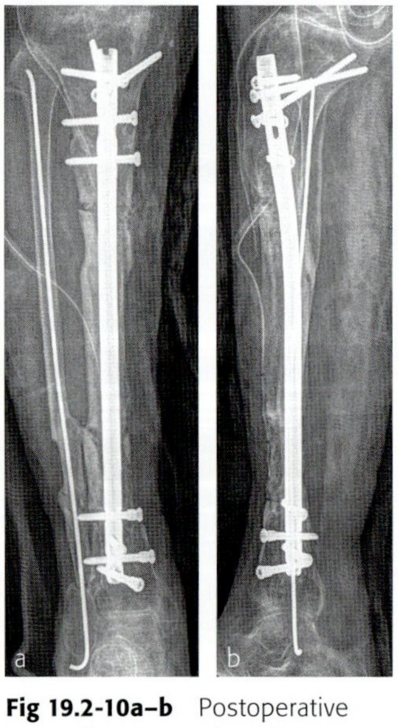

Fig 19.2-10a–b Postoperative x-rays show correction of alignment and statically locked nailing.

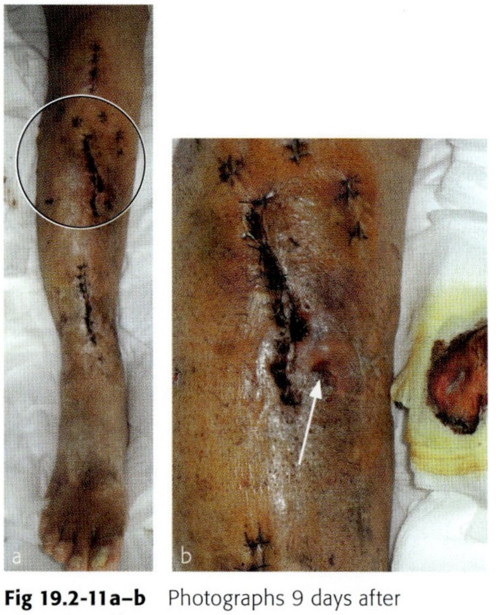

Fig 19.2-11a–b Photographs 9 days after reconstruction.

- **a** Note swelling and redness around the proximal osteotomy site (circle).
- **b** A close-up view shows purulent discharge from the focal sinus tract just medial to the main surgical wound (arrow).

8 Preoperative planning

Both the intraoperative tissue culture and the drain tip culture identically revealed *E coli* that was the infecting organism; this was identical to the infection after initial injury. The diagnosis is reactivation of an indolent infection. It also carries all features of acute deep postoperative infection. It is critical to have a roadmap for the whole treatment process that often includes multiple planned procedures. This patient now had serious postoperative deep infection with double-level nonunion with significant bone defect. All these problems cannot be solved by a single surgical procedure. A comprehensive treatment roadmap is needed to ensure the success of treatment.

First stage: urgent surgical debridement

1. Surgical debridement including all the bone graft.
2. External fixation along the medial side to maintain alignment. Schanz screw placement must not hinder repeated nailing at the second stage.
3. Nail removal, reaming of the medullary canal.
4. Insertion of antibiotic-loaded PMMA bead chain within the medullary canal, additional PMMA cement spacer at the defect.
5. Primary wound closure over a drain or temporary wound coverage with negative-pressure wound therapy (NPWT) closure.

Second stage: second debridement and definitive fixation

1. Performed 2–3 weeks after first-stage procedure.
2. Repeated debridement.
3. Repeated nailing and cement spacer at the bone defect over the two osteotomy sites.

Third stage: bone graft (Masquelet or induced-membrane technique)

1. After 3–4 months clinical observation for any signs of recurrence of infection.
2. Serial monthly laboratory testing for ESR/CRP levels.
3. When there are no clinical signs of infection and a normalized ESR/CRP level, remove cement spacer from the defect and autogenous bone graft.

9 Surgical approach

Previous incisions were used to perform debridement and implant removal.

10 Surgical debridement

Upon opening the proximal osteotomy site, pus was found and significant necrosis of the medial gastrocnemius and soleus muscles origins around the proximal osteotomy site (**Fig 19.2-12**). Based on this finding the author decided to remove the nail for a thorough and radical debridement. There was bloody pus around the proximal and distal interlocking screw holes. All the bone graft at both osteotomy sites was completely removed and the interlocking screw holes were curetted. The medullary canal was reamed to debride the infected granulation tissue from the medullary canal. Reaming the proximal metaphysis is not as efficient as reaming the diaphyseal area because the medullary canal is wide. Additional curettage was performed to further debride the proximal medullary canal.

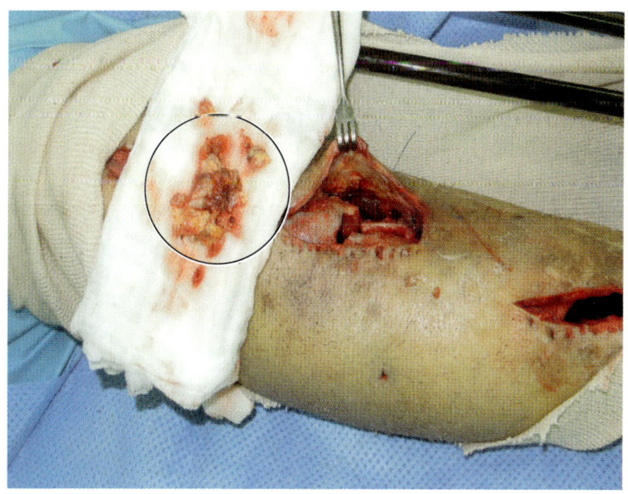

Fig 19.2-12 Intraoperative photograph shows the necrotic tissues removed around the proximal osteotomy site (circle).

Upon completion of the debridement the medullary canal was filled with an antibiotic-loaded PMMA cement bead chain and a cement spacer was placed to fill the bony defect and soft-tissue defect at the proximal wound (**Fig 19.2-13**) Both the incision for nail entry and the distal osteotomy sites (white arrows) were closed primarily without tension. The wound at the proximal osteotomy site (black arrow) was left open with NPWT due to tension upon trial closure. The negative pressure was kept at the lowest level of 25 mm Hg in an intermittent mode to try to maintain the local concentration of antibiotic release as high as possible.

11 Implant removal

Alignment was maintained with an external fixator along the medial side. And as revision nailing was planned at the second-stage operation in the roadmap, the Schanz screws were placed away from the nailing path (**Fig 19.2-14**). The original nail was removed through the previous incision once the external fixator was in place.

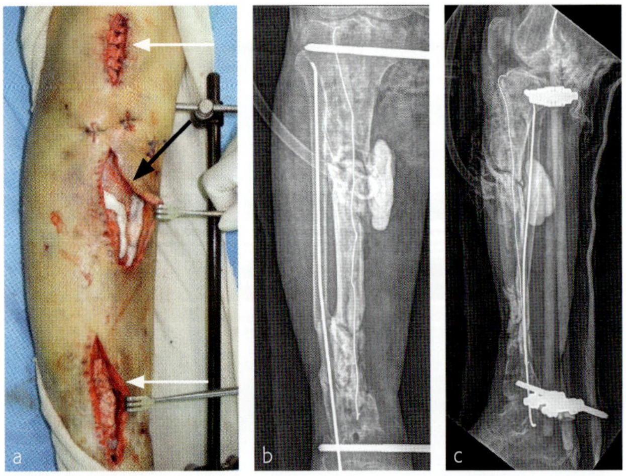

Fig 19.2-13a–c Intraoperative images.
- **a** The status of the soft tissues before wounds closure. Through the middle wound (black arrow) polymethylmethacrylate cement spacers are visible which were placed into the bone defect and dead space around the medial origin of the gastrocnemius and soleus muscles group.
- **b** AP x-ray view.
- **c** Lateral x-ray view.

12 Temporary fixation

Alignment was maintained with temporary external fixation along the medial side before the nail was removed (**Fig 19.2-13**). One Schanz screw was used in each fragment as the healed fibula acted as a strut on the other side.

13 Postoperative management

Postoperatively, a long leg split was used to add stability to the defect sites. The NPWT dressing was changed every 3 days in the operating room with the patient under local anesthesia.

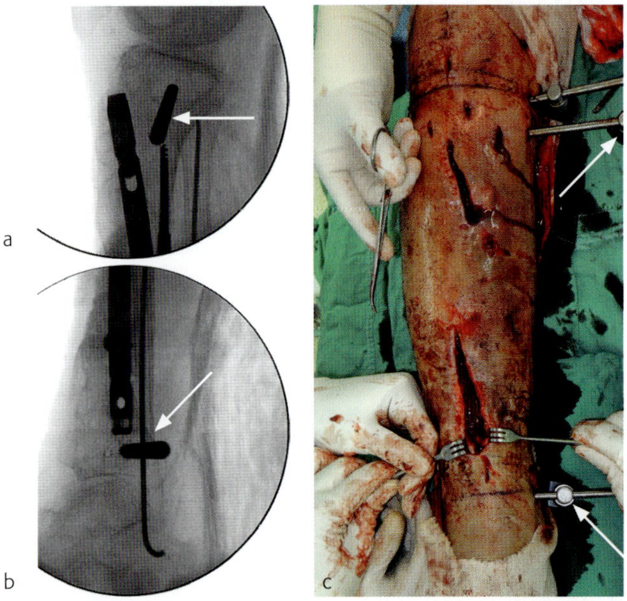

Fig 19.2-14a–c Intraoperative C-arm images (**a-b**) and photograph (**c**) taken after Schanz screw placement. Note the position of the Schanz screws (arrows) which will not interfere with nailing that was planned as a second-stage procedure after control of the infection.

14 Reimplantation

Fig 19.2-15 was taken 3 days after the first-stage debridement and shows the soft-tissue defect around the proximal osteotomy site. At this point the author decided to add a free flap as part of the second-stage operation.

The second-stage operation was performed 2 weeks after the first-stage debridement. The PMMA bead chain and spacers were removed and all surgical sites were debrided again. Devitalized gastrocnemius muscle tissue was further debrided (**Fig 19.2-16**). Surgeons then changed surgical gowns and draping before proceeding to revision nailing. Nailing was done and defects were again filled with PMMA spacers (**Fig 19.2-17**). After revision nailing, the patient was allowed to partially bear weight as tolerated once the anterolateral thigh perforator flap was stabilized. Postoperative x-rays show acceptable coronal plane alignment with 2.5 cm shortening. An apex anterior angulation at the proximal osteotomy site was noted (**Fig 19.2-18**).

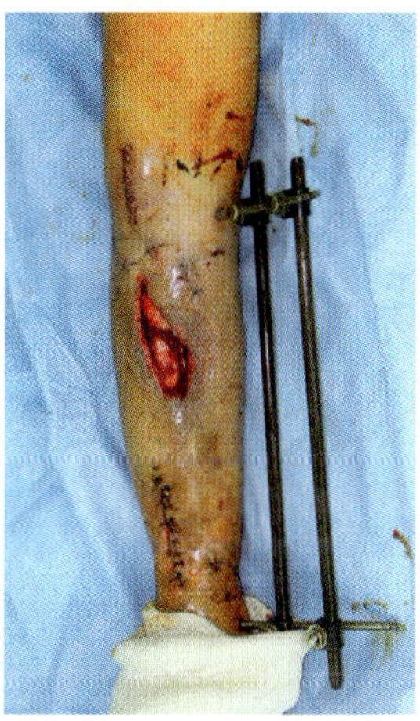

Fig 19.2-15 Clinical photograph 3 days after the first-stage operation shows a soft-tissue defect around the proximal osteotomy site.

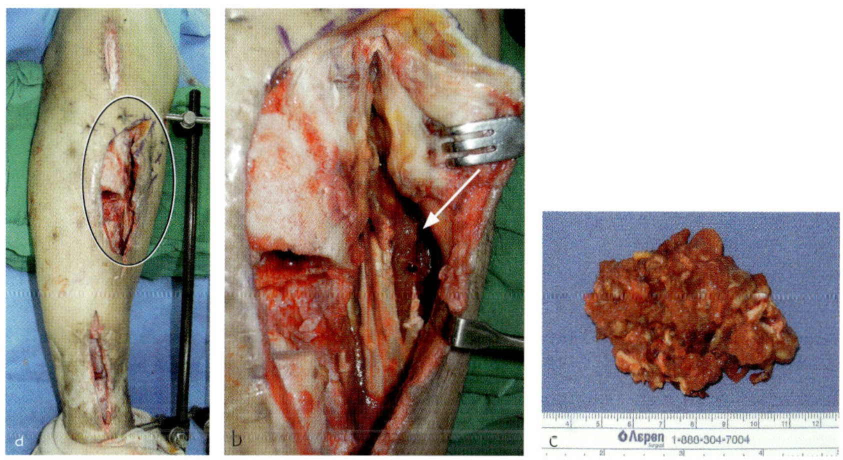

Fig 19.2-16a–c Intraoperative second-stage photographs.
a–b Discolored medial origin of gastrocnemius muscle (circle and arrow).
c All necrotic muscle tissue was debrided.

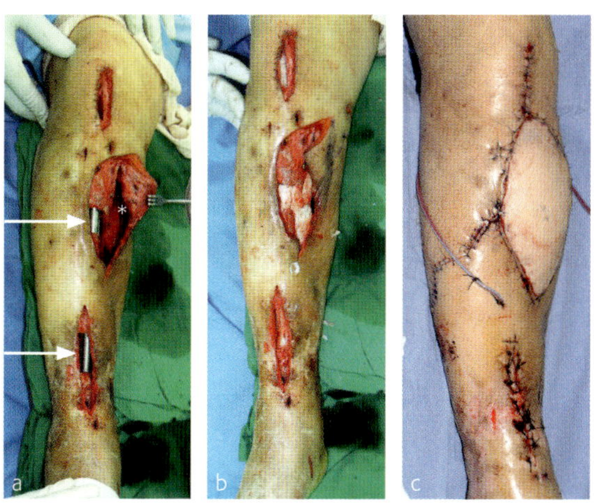

Fig 19.2-17a–c Intraoperative (**a–b**) and postoperative (**c**) photographs.
a The exposed nail due to bone defects on both osteotomy sites (white arrows). The asterisk indicates the dead space left after debridement of necrotic muscle.
b Bone defects and the dead space were filled with polymethylmethacrylate cement spacers.
c The skin defect was reconstructed with an anterolateral thigh perforator flap by a plastic surgeon.

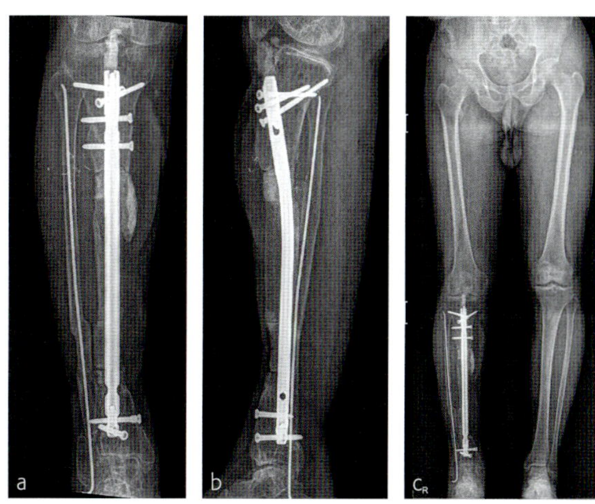

Fig 19.2-18a–c Postoperative x-rays show acceptable coronal plane alignment with 2.5 cm shortening. Apex anterior angulation at the proximal osteotomy site is noted.
a AP view.
b Lateral view.
c Full leg-length view.

The third-stage operation was performed 18 weeks after the second-stage operation.

During monthly follow-up, there was no sign of infection recurrence and the CRP level was normalized. The ESR was moderately elevated in contrast to the clinical findings and CRP level at this point. As there was no detectable reason for this moderately elevated ESR level, the author decided to perform a bone graft. The cement spacers were removed from the bone defects and the defects were filled with autogenous cancellous bone graft from the iliac crest. For the proximal osteotomy site, augmentation plating was done with a variable angle locking plate 2.7 (**Fig 19.2-19**). Postoperative x-rays show the grafted bone column (**Fig 19.2-20**).

The patient was given intravenous antibiotics sensitive to *E coli* for 2 weeks. Although it was believed the infection was completely controlled, intravenous antibiotics were prescribed to prevent recurrence of infection.

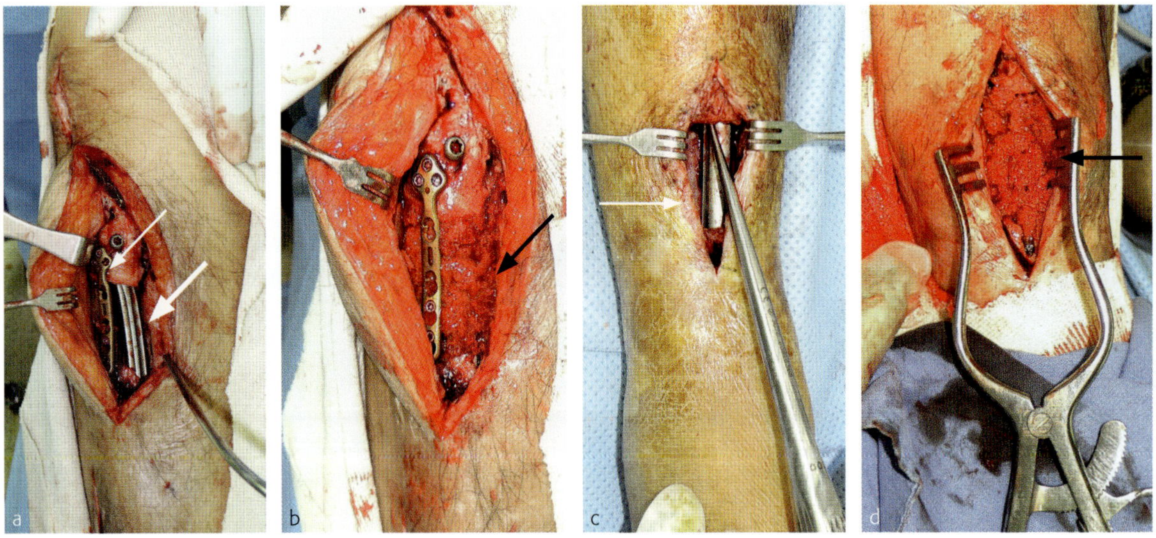

Fig 19.2-19a–d Intraoperative photographs.
a–b The extent of the proximal bone defect (thick white arrow) after polymethylmethacrylate cement spacer removal. Also note the locking plate 2.7 for augmentation (thin white arrow). This defect was filled with autogenous cancellous bone graft (black arrow).
c–d The white arrow indicates the distal bone defect around the nail and the black arrow indicates the grafted bone that fills the defect.

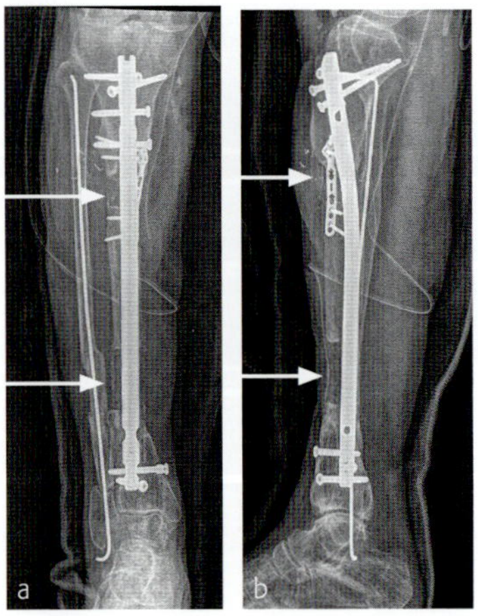

Fig 19.2-20a–b Postoperative x-rays show the grafted bone column (arrows).
a AP view.
b Lateral view.

15 Outcome

X-rays taken 6 months after bone graft demonstrate good fracture healing with circumferential remodeling of the grafted bone columns at both levels (**Fig 19.2-21**). There were no signs of recurrence of infection at this point. The patient was able to walk without support. He had some limping due to 2 cm shortening and stiffness of the ankle joint.

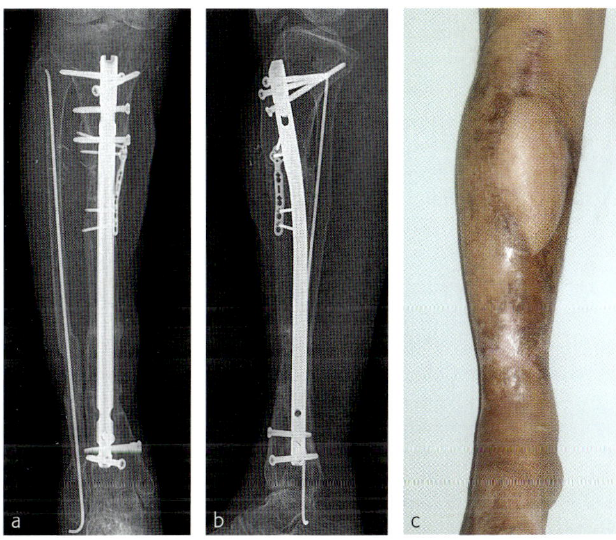

Fig 19.2-21a–c Six months after the third-stage operation (bone graft).
a–b AP (**a**) and lateral (**b**) x-rays show complete fracture healing and remodeling of grafted bone columns.
c Clinical photograph shows the status of the soft tissue at this time.

16 Pitfalls

- In this case the initial diagnosis was indolent infection with malalignment. An initial high-energy open fracture with a history of infection after poor initial management, prolonged period of external fixation, and elevated ESR. All these findings suggested the possibility of an indolent infection even in the absence of clinical signs of infection.
- Intraoperative polymorphonuclear counts cannot be used as a reliable indicator of the presence of infection.
- Acute postoperative infection (reactivation of indolent infection in this case) requires an urgent surgical debridement. In this case, on postoperative day 4, when the intraoperative tissue culture revealed *E coli* and fever, the surgeon should have performed an urgent surgical debridement. Initial decision making was to change antibiotic therapy. The surgical debridement was delayed significantly until postoperative day 9 when there was a purulent discharge from the surgical wound. This delay critically worsened the situation by giving the bacteria an opportunity to destroy bone and soft tissues. As a result of delay in debridement, the extent of debridement was significantly increased so that the free flap was necessary to cover the soft-tissue defect after debridement.

17 Pearls

- Consider indolent infection if:
  - The high-energy injury is initially not managed according to accepted principles.
  - There is history of multiple surgical procedures and infection.
  - There is elevated ESR/CRP levels.
- The first reaction to the postoperative infection is not empiric therapy with antibiotics but an urgent surgical debridement.
- The entire treatment roadmap has to be set up including all the staged definitive fixations and, if necessary, third-stage bone graft at the time of first-stage surgical debridement.

19.3 Implant removal—chronically infected total hip arthroplasty

Olivier Borens

1 Case description

A 63-year-old man underwent total hip arthroplasty (THA) for symptomatic arthritis of the right hip 2 years prior to presentation at the author's hospital (**Fig 19.3-1**).

Two weeks after the original operation, the patient dislocated his THA and was treated with closed reduction (**Fig 19.3-2**). A second dislocation occurred 1 month later. The treating surgeon decided to implant a double mobility cup to prevent further dislocations. Delayed healing of the wound and prolonged oozing was noted in the postoperative period. During this time, a culture swab was taken from the wound drainage, which demonstrated multisensitive *Staphylococcus aureus*. The surgeon chose nonoperative treatment using antibiotics with an oral cephalosporin. The clinical course revealed that the wound did not heal, and the surgeon decided to perform a two-stage exchange with prefabricated spacer (**Fig 19.3-3**).

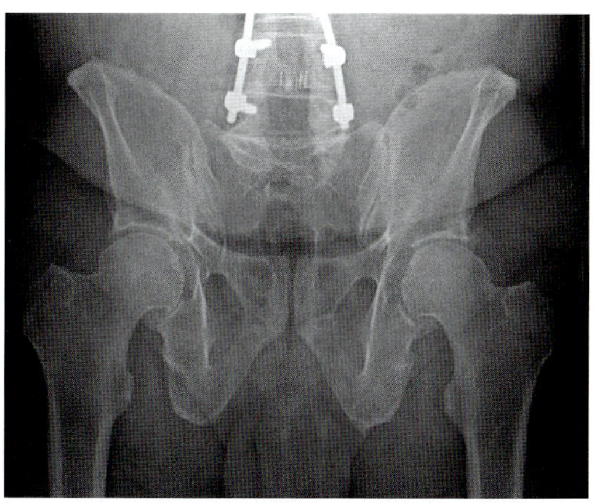

Fig 19.3-1 The patient underwent total hip arthroplasty for symptomatic arthritis of the right hip 2 years prior to presentation at the author's hospital.

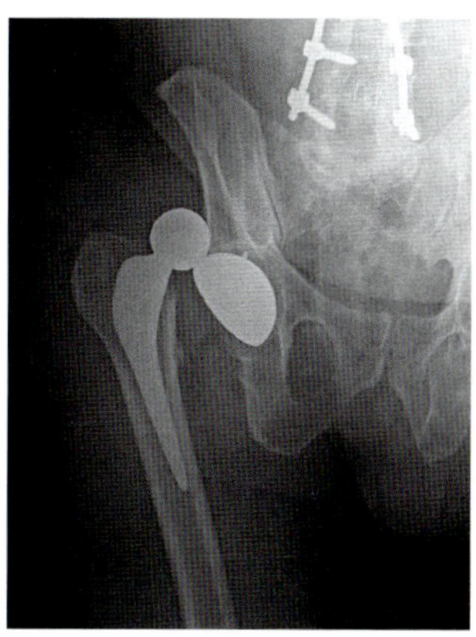

Fig 19.3-2 Two weeks after the original operation the patient dislocated his total hip arthroplasty.

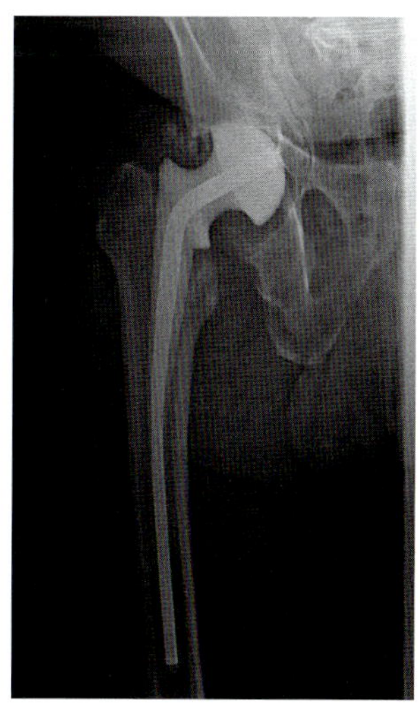

Fig 19.3-3 The clinical course revealed that the wound did not heal, so a two-stage exchange with prefabricated spacer was performed.

After a 3-month interval and with normalized inflammatory parameters (C-reactive protein [CRP], leukocyte count, and erythrocyte sedimentation rate) a revision stem with double mobility cup was implanted. The patient was treated for another 6 weeks with antibiotics with uneventful initial follow-up over 6 months. At that point, increasing pain was noted while walking and was not attenuated by antiinflammatory medication. The x-rays demonstrated loosening around the stem (**Fig 19.3-4**). Three months later (12 months after the last revision), the CRP level was 18 mg/L and erythrocyte sedimentation rate was elevated at 30 mm/h.

The patient was sent for specialist care, further investigation, and treatment.

2 Indications

Upon arrival at the author's outpatient clinic the patient walked bearing full weight with a right-sided limp due to pain from the right leg. The scar appeared calm, without redness or warmth. No pain was noted on palpation or when moving the hip joint.

3 Preoperative planning

The x-rays showed signs of loosening in Gruen zones 1 and 7 (**Fig 19.3-4**). The CRP level was 34 mg/L.

With these findings, it appeared likely that the patient had a persistent or recurrent infection of his THA. The author chose to proceed directly with a two-step exchange with a short interval instead of a one-step exchange due to multiple previous failed surgeries. As the prior antibiotic treatment was not well adapted and may have induced resistance, it was not clear whether an antibiofilm treatment was possible if a one-step exchange was used.

4 Surgical approach

A two-step exchange was performed with osteotomy of the proximal femur (Wagner osteotomy) and three cerclage wires were used for fixation of the proximal femur (**Fig 19.3-5**) after implantation of a handmade cement spacer (**Video 19.3-1**, **Video 10-1**, **Video 10-2**). Systemic antibiotics (amoxicillin-clavulanic acid 3 x 2.2 g/day) were given until the definitive microbiological results.

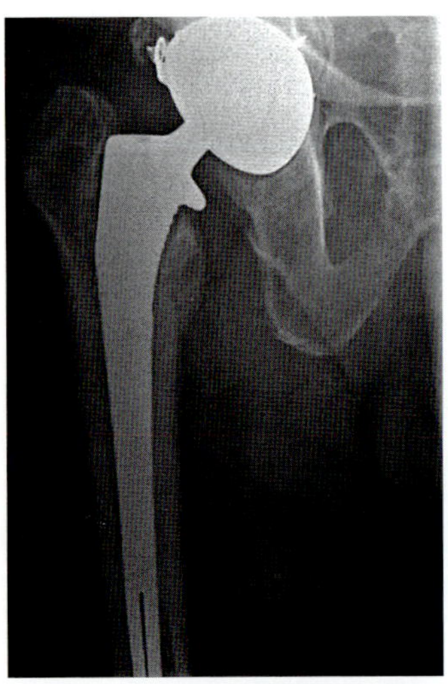

Fig 19.3-4 Loosening around the stem in Gruen zones 1 and 7.

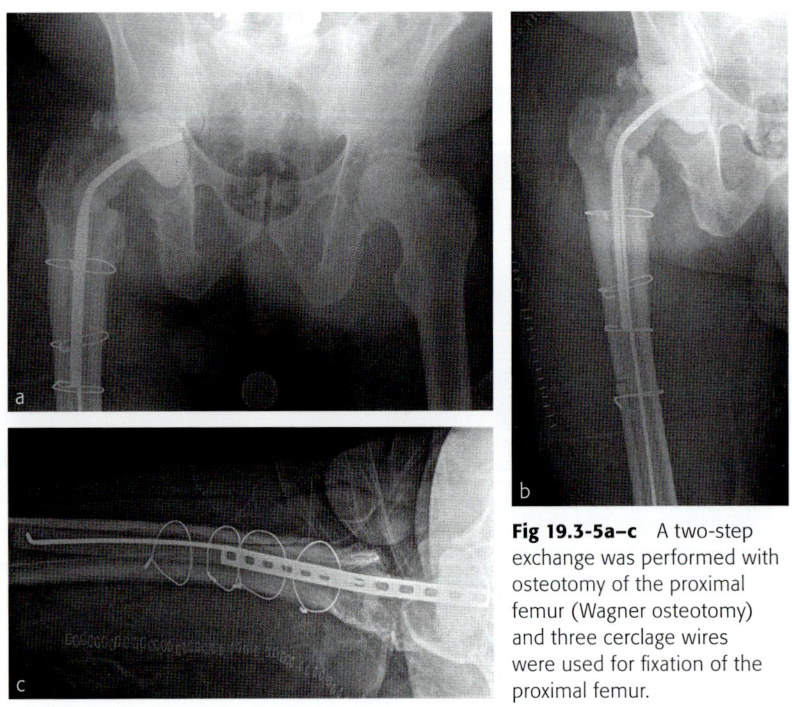

Fig 19.3-5a–c A two-step exchange was performed with osteotomy of the proximal femur (Wagner osteotomy) and three cerclage wires were used for fixation of the proximal femur.

Next the modular polyethylene liner is removed and an attempt is made to sublux the patella laterally: this author prefers subluxation to eversion; however, eversion can also be attempted at this time. If neither maneuver is successful, the next step is to peel off soft tissue from the lateral aspect of the patella; if this does not provide adequate exposure a formal lateral retinacular release can be performed. If exposure is still not adequate at this time, a quadriceps snip can be performed (**Fig 19.4-2**). The quadriceps snip is an apical extension of the arthrotomy across the quadriceps tendon (not in the quadriceps muscle) into the fibers of the vastus lateralis. A quadriceps snip is easy to perform and repair, heals reliably, and does not require a modification of the postoperative regimen. Tibial tubercle osteotomies (**Fig 19.4-4**) are used rarely in this author's practice, typically reserved for cases where there is a well-fixed, fully cemented tibial stem that requires removal (**Fig 19.4-5**).

The implants are removed with narrow osteotomes or a thin saw blade disrupting the cement mantle circumferentially. The femoral component is typically removed first, followed by the tibia and the patella last which is generally easily removed with an oscillating saw to cut off the body of the patella from the pegs which are removed with a high-speed burr.

Next, the proximal tibia is cut again to debride the surface using either an intramedullary or extramedullary cutting guide followed by a complete posterior synovectomy. In general there are large amounts of scar posteriorly and this tissue is removed until fat or muscle is seen in the posterior aspect of the knee. This not only further debrides infected synovium but also enhances exposure by releasing the tibia from the femur. The bony surfaces are all now carefully examined and all remaining cement or any residual bone that appears infected is removed followed by opening up the femoral and tibial canals with a drill or long cement removal tool so that they can be debrided as well and to allow for placement of the spacer. The entire wound is irrigated with sterile saline using pulsatile lavage. The knee is examined again to ensure all retained cement is removed along with any soft tissue or bone that appears infected, followed by spacer placement.

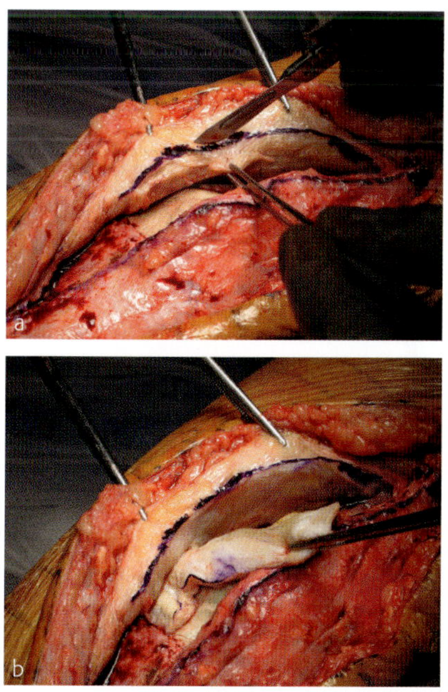

Fig 19.4-3a–b The border between the medial capsule and synovium has been marked out (**a**) to allow for sharp excision of the synovium (**b**).

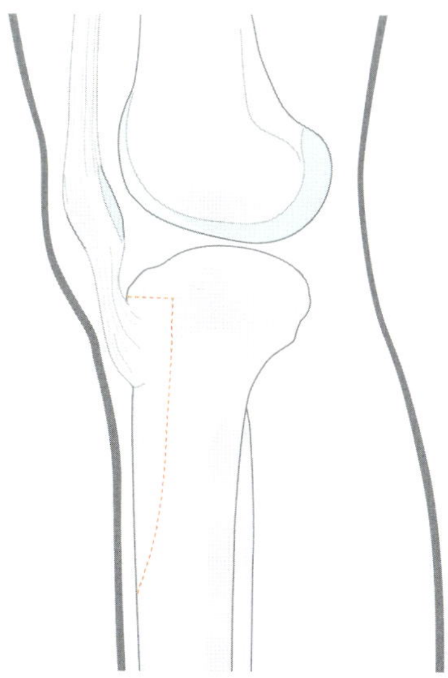

Fig 19.4-4 Tibial tubercle osteotomy as seen from the lateral view is made 5–8 cm in length tapering from proximally to distally and hinged open from medial to lateral leaving the lateral soft-tissue sleeve intact.

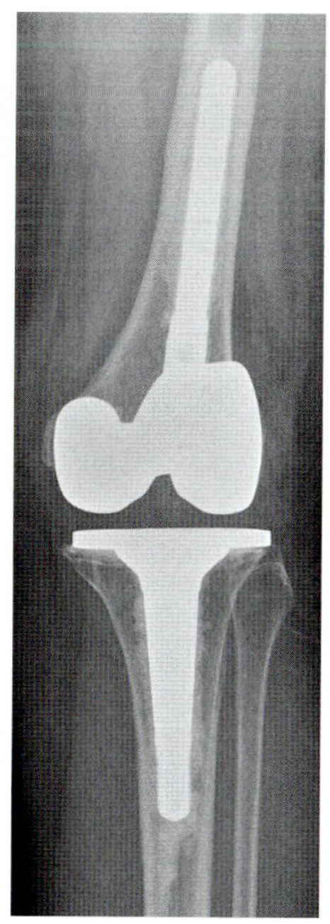

Fig 19.4-5 AP x-ray showing a fully cemented tibial stem that may require a tibial tubercle osteotomy to remove.

5 Temporary fixation with an antibiotic-loaded cement spacer

Antibiotic-loaded cement spacers are used routinely in contemporary practice to provide local antibiotic delivery and maintain soft-tissue tension, which facilitates the second-stage reconstruction. While the precise amount of antibiotics to be mixed into the cement is controversial, the author's preference is to use a high-viscosity cement mixed with approximately 4–6 g of antibiotics per 40 g package of cement. In general, high-viscosity cements elute the antibiotics better and a combination of antibiotics further promotes elution. The author's preference is typically a combination of vancomycin and tobramycin.

The choice between a static (**Fig 19.4-6**) and articulating spacer is again controversial; however, the author's preference usually is an articulating spacer (**Fig 19.4-7**). Articulating spacers may allow for greater postoperative range of motion (as was a concern in this case) and may facilitate the second-stage reconstruction as exposure is easier if the knee can be flexed and the soft tissues are generally more pliable. Although they can be made by hand (**Video 10-3**), the author prefers commercially available molds (**Fig 19.4-8**) that allow for more precise sizing along with the ability to adjust the thickness of the tibial spacer to optimize range of motion and stability. Static spacers are utilized if the soft-tissue envelope is compromised, if the remaining bone stock will not support an articulating spacer, or if the extensor mechanism is disrupted given the high risk of dislocation of an articulating spacer in this scenario.

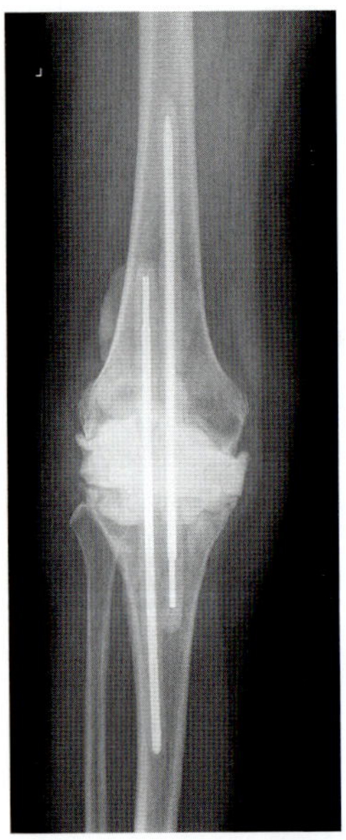

Fig 19.4-6 Static antibiotic spacer created with two threaded Steinmann pins that are coated with cement. One is placed up the femoral canal and one down the tibial canal and then they are allowed to overlap with additional cement placed into the knee joint to create a temporary knee fusion. A thin layer of cement is also placed between the extensor mechanism and the distal femur to facilitate exposure at the second stage.

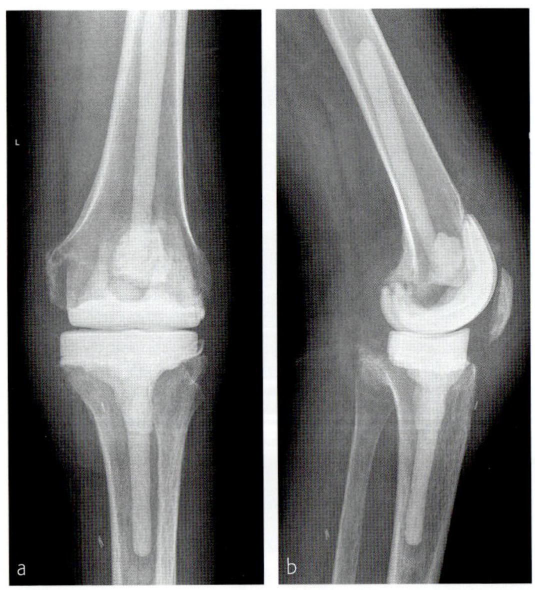

Fig 19.4-7a–b Views of the articulating spacer used for this case. Note the dowels of cement that have been placed into the canals. The tibial dowel of cement also stabilizes the tibial spacer, acting like a stem extension.

a AP view.
b Lateral view.

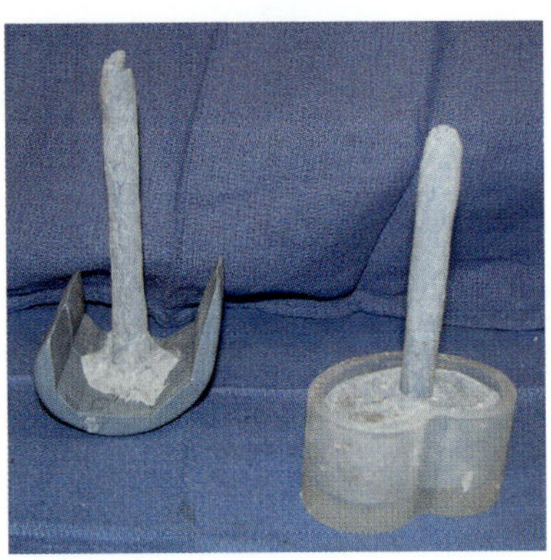

Fig 19.4-8 The articulating spacer has been made with commercially available molds. Stem extensions are added on to allow for local antibiotic delivery to the canals and to stabilize the tibial spacer. The tibial spacer mold allows the surgeon to adjust the thickness of the spacer to balance the flexion and extension gaps maximizing stability and range of motion. The intramedullary dowels are made first (approximately 10 mm in diameter and 10 cm in length) and allowed to fully dry and then inserted into the cement for the tibial spacer while it is hardening.

To make the spacer, the first step is to mix one 40 g batch of cement with the powdered antibiotics. The author has found that a stainless-steel baking sifter helps to mix the antibiotics and the powder portion of the cement (**Fig 19.4-9**). The first batch of cement is mixed early in the case, and dowels for the intramedullary canals are constructed by rolling the cement by hand into dowels that are approximately 10 mm in diameter by 10 cm in length which are allowed to completely harden. Once the femoral component has been removed, the femoral size is selected and one to two more batches of cement are mixed with antibiotics and placed into the mold, which is similarly allowed to harden completely. Finally, after the tibial component is removed, the flexion and extension spacers are checked with a spacer block to determine the optimal thickness of the tibial spacer (**Fig 19.4-10**); the author usually aims for a tibial spacer that is 2 mm thinner than the optimal tibial spacer block to ensure that the knee will not be too tight once the spacer is inserted. Once the tibial spacer size and thickness have been selected, another batch of cement is utilized to construct the tibial spacer and one of the previously made dowels is inserted into it to act like a stem extension; this will both deliver antibiotics into the tibial canal and stabilize the tibial spacer (**Fig 19.4-8**).

Once the tibial spacer has hardened, the tourniquet is released and hemostasis obtained; a bloody field at the time of final spacer insertion is desired to encourage a suboptimal cement mantle to facilitate spacer removal at the reimplantation. A final batch of cement is mixed with antibiotics and the tibial and femoral spacers are loosely cemented into place when the cement is in the later stages of hardening to intentionally obtain a poor cement mantle without interdigitation of cement into the remaining bone to facilitate removal at the second stage (**Fig 19.4-11**). Once the final batch of cement has hardened, the surgeon should assess overall stability of the construct and what range of motion is safe and will be allowed postoperatively. The arthrotomy is closed over a drain and the subcutaneous tissues and skin are closed with absorbable, nonbraided suture.

6 Postoperative management

A multidisciplinary approach to postoperative management is important to optimize outcomes. As previously outlined, collaboration with internal medicine and an infectious diseases specialist is critical to optimize any comorbidities that may be present and to monitor the response to antibiotic treatment. Patients may also require nutritional optimization.

Antibiotics are administered based on the sensitivities obtained from the intraoperative or preoperative cultures for 6 weeks with weekly measurements of the ESR and CRP levels. The antibiotics are then discontinued and 2 weeks later, the ESR and CRP levels are checked again, the knee is aspirated and the fluid sent for a synovial fluid WBC count, differential, and culture. In general, the author has found that while the ESR and CRP levels should decrease, they will not always return to normal prior to the proposed reimplantation at approximately 9 weeks after the first-stage procedure. Hence, there is no specific "cut-off" for determining infection resolution but the trend of these laboratory results should be downward and this trend should continue after antibiotic cessation. If the ESR and CRP levels increase

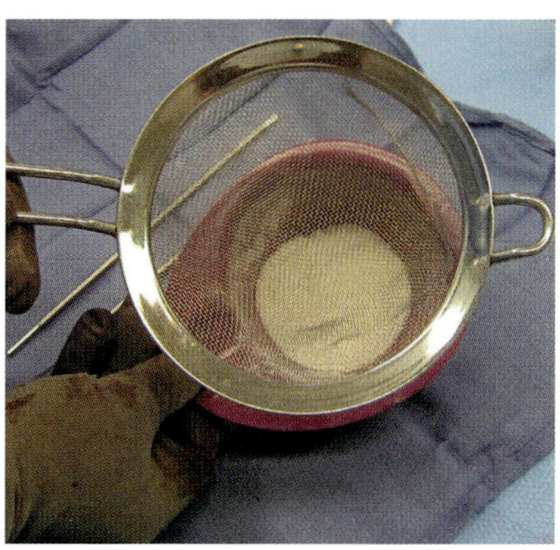

Fig 19.4-9 A stainless steel sifter assists with mixing the antibiotic and cement powder.

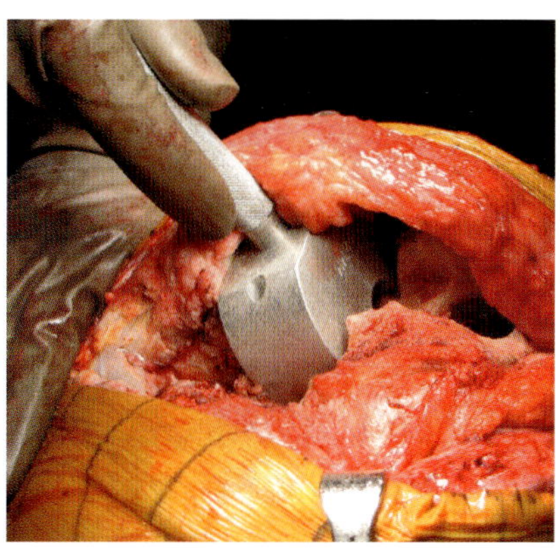

Fig 19.4-10 A spacer block is used to determine the thickness of the tibial spacer to be constructed.

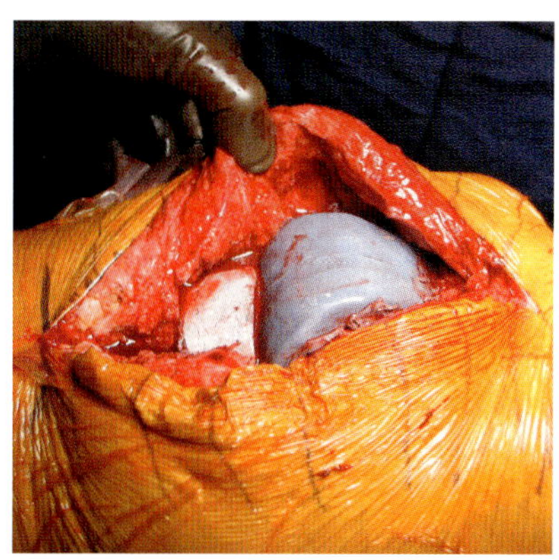

Fig 19.4-11 The final spacer is in place and stability and range of motion are assessed.

following discontinuation of antibiotic therapy, this is particularly concerning for persistence of infection. A synovial fluid WBC count over 3,000 cells/μL and a differential of > 80% are likewise concerning for persistent infection, as is a positive synovial fluid culture.

Following antibiotic spacer placement, patients are initially placed in a knee immobilizer, which is converted to a hinged knee brace on the first or second postoperative day. If there is any concern regarding the soft-tissue envelope, the knee should be immobilized for longer. The hinged knee brace is set to allow range of motion as was determined to be safe intraoperatively; in general the authors allow patients 0–90° range of motion and if the knee was stable intraoperatively, they are allowed to bear weight as tolerated while wearing the hinged knee brace. If there is any concern regarding knee stability or fixation of the spacer, more limited weight bearing is recommended.

7 Reimplantation

At 9 weeks postoperatively the patient is returned to the operating room where either a reimplantation procedure is performed or the spacer is exchanged; the second-stage procedure is only delayed if medical comorbidities or nutritional status requires optimization. This is a second chance to debride the knee joint and remove any devitalized or infected-appearing bone or soft-tissue. Multiple tissue and bone cultures (typically five or more) are obtained and an intraoperative frozen section can be used as a final check to confirm or deny persistent infection. The surgeon should be aware, however, that intraoperative frozen section interpretation can be challenging even for an experienced pathologist. Further, frozen sections are subject to sampling error (eg, if the wrong tissue samples are sent to the pathologist, they can be falsely negative). Gram stains have little value in the diagnosis of periprosthetic joint infection and their use is discouraged, as they are not sensitive enough and can also be falsely positive which only confuses management.

The spacer should be easily removed and the bony surfaces are cut again with a saw to both debride them once again and to prepare them for cementation of the revision components. After the bone surfaces are debrided the wound is again copiously irrigated with sterile saline using pulsatile lavage. The knee is prepared to accept the revision components which are inserted using a "hybrid" cementing technique where commercially available antibiotic-loaded cement (typically 0.5 g of gentamicin per 40 g package of cement) is placed near the articular portions of the implant; however, the stem extensions are not cemented but tightly press fit into the respective diaphysis of the tibia and femur (**Fig 19.4-12**). Additional or alternative antibiotics can be added to the cement, particularly if the infecting organism is not sensitive to gentamicin; however, usually, most surgeons prefer to not exceed 1 g of antibiotics per 40 g of cement when used for fixation of the revision implants as more than this may compromise the strength of the cement.

Prophylactic antibiotics are administered prior to the skin incision, and usually include a first-generation cephalosporin (such as cefazolin) and vancomycin; this may be altered, however, if the original infecting organism is not adequately covered by the above combination. Antibiotics are continued until final operative cultures are negative or continued if there is any concern regarding infection persistence. The decision to continue or discontinue antibiotics is usually made in conjunction with the infectious disease specialist.

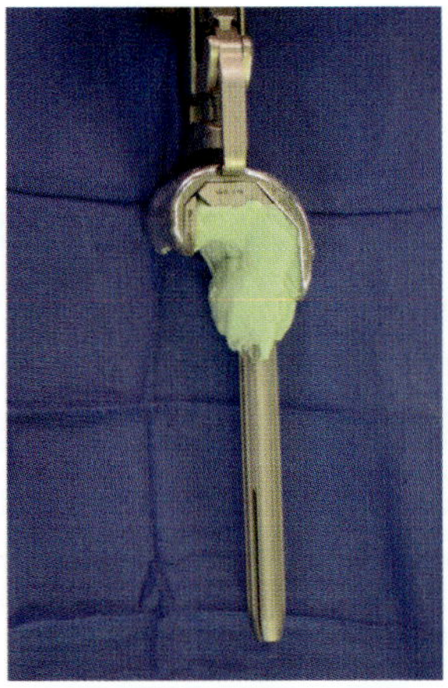

Fig 19.4-12 The revision components are inserted using a "hybrid" cementing technique where antibiotic-loaded bone cement is placed near the articular surfaces, and a cementless stem is tightly press fit into the diaphysis.

8 Outcome

The patient underwent removal of the infected TKA and placement of an articulating spacer (**Fig 19.4-7**); a plastic surgeon assisted with the exposure given the prior flap procedure. The patient received 6 weeks of intravenous antibiotics and his ESR and CRP levels showed progressive decreases; his wound healed uneventfully. His antibiotics were stopped and 2 weeks later, at 8 weeks postoperatively, the ESR level had decreased to 5 mm/h (normal range: 0–23 mm/h) and the CRP level was < 5 mg/L (normal range: less than 5 mg/L). The knee was aspirated and it showed 1,057 WBC/µL with a differential of 61% polymorphonuclear cells; cultures showed no growth.

At the time of reimplantation (9 weeks following removal of the infected arthroplasty) a plastic surgeon assisted with elevation of the prior flap and wound closure. The intraoperative frozen section was negative as was the final histopathology and all five tissue cultures. The revision implants were inserted with a "hybrid" cementing technique where the epiphyseal portion is cemented and the stem extensions are tightly press fit into the diaphysis (**Fig 19.4-12**, **Fig 19.4-13**). Antibiotics were discontinued 72 hours postoperatively. The patient, however, struggled to regain his range of motion, and 6 weeks after the reimplantation he had range of motion from a 5° flexion contracture to 75° of further flexion. He underwent a manipulation under anesthesia and 2 years postoperatively has range of motion from full extension to 100° of flexion.

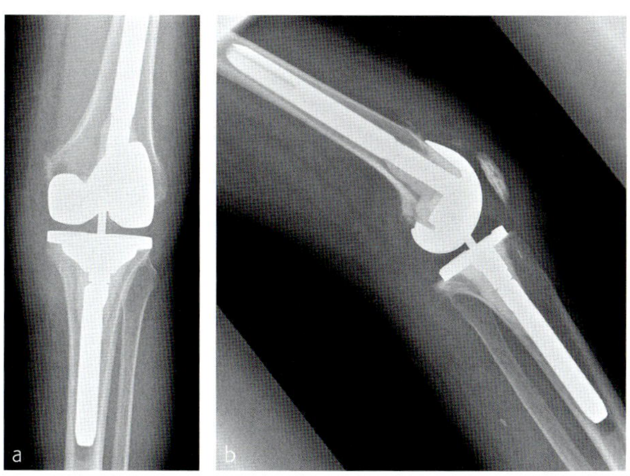

Fig 19.4-13a–b Views of the revision construct inserted with a "hybrid" cementing technique with cement in the epiphysis and stem extensions that are tightly press fit into the diaphysis.
a AP view.
b Lateral view.

9 Pitfalls

- Decision making: debridement alone is associated with a high rate of failure when treating a patient with chronically infected TKA.
- The surgical approach should be generous to allow for a complete synovectomy and the safe removal of implants and associated cement.
- Implant removal should commence at the interfaces between the implant and the cement mantle, and not between the cement mantle and the host bone as this can lead to excessive bone removal.
- Great care should be taken to remove any associated cement and infected-appearing bone and soft tissue; retained cement is probably the most common reason for recurrence of infection after spacer placement.
- The surgeon should strive for a "poor" cement mantle when inserting the temporary spacer by having a bloody field at the time of cementation.
- Medical and nutritional optimization between stages is important to optimize outcomes.
- It can be difficult to determine when the infection has been eradicated; the author typically relies on observation of the trend of the ESR and CRP; they should show steady decreases following removal of the implant but in many cases do not completely normalize prior to reimplantation at 9 weeks; if the ESR and CRP levels increase after cessation of antibiotic therapy, during the antibiotic "holiday", this is concerning for persistent infection.
- The surgeon should view the reimplantation procedure as a "second chance" to debride the wound, which should be done thoroughly to avoid the retention of any associated cement or nonviable infected-appearing bone or soft tissue.

10 Pearls

- Diagnosis: a patient with a painful, stiff, or otherwise symptomatic TKA should be evaluated for infection with a serum ESR and CRP followed by an aspiration of the joint if the serum tests are elevated or if the clinical suspicion for infection is high.
- Diagnosis: an aspiration of the knee joint is probably the most valuable single test, yielding a synovial fluid WBC count (optimal cut-off value for diagnosing infection approximately 3,000 cells/µL), differential (optimal cut-off value approximately 80%) and culture.
- Working closely with an infectious diseases specialist is helpful for optimizing antibiotic management.
- If surgical exposure is inadequate despite a thorough synovectomy, reestablishment of the space between the patellar tendon and tibia and a lateral retinacular release, the surgeon should have a low threshold to perform a quadriceps snip.
- Knowledge of the implants in place can facilitate their removal.
- If a static spacer is selected (as opposed to a mobile spacer), a thin layer of cement placed in the suprapatellar pouch will facilitate exposure at the second-stage procedure.
- The author strives to reconstruct the patella at the time of reimplantation, as Glynn et al suggest the outcomes are better if the patella is resurfaced as opposed to left unresurfaced at the second-stage reimplanation. If left unresurfaced, the patella tends to track laterally causing pain and instability. If bone loss of the patella is severe, impaction bone grafting is an easy and reliable solution for reconstruction yielding a convex structure that is easily captured in the femoral trochlea.
- Close collaboration with an infectious diseases specialist helps in the selection of antibiotics for inclusion in the cement spacer as well as following the first-stage procedure.
- Interestingly, failures of therapy seem oftentimes to be new infections, with new organisms identified at the time of reinfection in approximately two of three cases.

11 Further reading

Della Valle C, Parvizi J, Bauer TW, et al. Diagnosis of periprosthetic joint infections of the hip and knee. *J Am Acad Orthop Surg.* 2010 Dec;18(12):760–770.

Della Valle CJ, Berger RA, Rosenberg AG. Surgical exposures in revision total knee arthroplasty. *Clin Orthop Relat Res.* 2006 May;446:59–68.

Della Valle CJ, Sporer SM, Jacobs JJ, et al. Preoperative testing for sepsis before revision total knee arthroplasty. *J Arthroplasty.* 2007 Sep;22(6 Suppl 2):90–93.

Glynn A, Huang R, Mortazavi J, et al. The impact of patellar resurfacing in two-stage revision of the infected total knee arthroplasty. *J Arthroplasty.* 2014 Jul;29(7):1439–42.

Jacofsky DJ, Della Valle CJ, Meneghini RM, et al. Revision total knee arthroplasty: what the practicing orthopaedic surgeon needs to know. *J Bone Joint Surg Am.* 2010 May;92(5):1282–1292.

Kusuma SK, Ward J, Jacofsky M, et al. What is the role of serological testing between stages of two-stage reconstruction of the infected prosthetic knee? *Clin Orthop Relat Res.* 2011 April;469(4):1002–1008.

Parvizi J, Zmistowski B, Berbari EF, et al. New definition for periprosthetic joint infection: from the Workgroup of the Musculoskeletal Infection Society. *Clin Orthop Relat Res.* 2011 Nov;469(11):2992–2994.

Sah AP, Shukla S, Della Valle CJ, et al. Modified hybrid stem fixation in revision TKA is durable at 2–10 years. *Clin Orthop Relat Res.* 2011 Mar;469(3):839–846.

Sherrell JC, Fehring TK, Odum S, et al. The Chitranjan Ranawat Award: Fate of two-stage reimplantation after failed irrigation and débridement for periprosthetic knee infection. *Clin Orthop Relat Res.* 2011 Jan;469(1):18–25.

Tetreault MW, Wetters NG, Aggarwal V, et al. The Chitranjan Ranawat Award: Should prophylactic antibiotics be withheld prior to revision surgery to obtain appropriate cultures? *Clin Orthop Relat Res.* 2014 Jan;472(1):52–56.

Van Thiel GS, Berend KR, Klein GR, et al. Intraoperative molds to create an articulating spacer for the infected knee arthroplasty. *Clin Orthop Relat Res.* 2011 Apr;469(4):994–1001.

Yi PH, Frank RM, Vann E, et al. Is potential malnutrition associated with septic failure and acute infection after revision total joint arthroplasty? *Clin Orthop Relat Res.* 2015 Jan;473(1):175–182.

Zmistowski B, Tetreault MW, Alijanipour P, et al. Recurrent periprosthetic joint infection: persistent or new infection? *J Arthroplasty.* 2013 Oct;28(9):1486–1489.

19.5 Implant removal—infected total knee replacement

Stephen L Kates, Christopher J Drinkwater

1 Case description

A 43-year-old woman with severe diffuse pigmented villonodular synovitis (PVNS) had previously undergone extensive subtotal synovectomy as well as direct popliteal fossa exposure for open resection of extraarticular PVNS, followed by radiation therapy. She had not had recurrence of PVNS but went on to develop progressively worsening arthritic changes with subchondral cysts and recurring swelling. She underwent total knee replacement (TKR).

Six months after TKR she developed swelling and knee pain. The knee was aspirated and cultures were positive for methicillin-sensitive *Staphylococcus aureus*. The C-reactive protein (CRP) level was 235 mg/L. She then underwent irrigation, debridement, and polyethylene exchange in the hope of preserving her implants. She was treated with intravenous vancomycin. X-rays 2 months later demonstrated radiolucent lines at the bone-cement interface suggesting that the prosthesis was being undermined by the infectious process, representing infectious loosening of the implants (**Fig 19.5-1**).

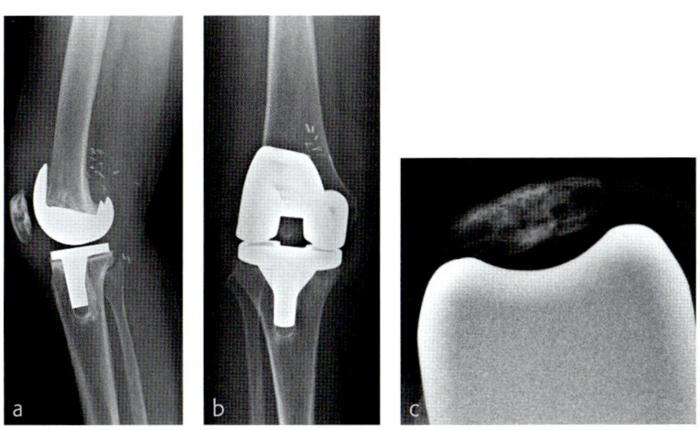

Fig 19.5-1a–c Radiolucent lines at the bone-cement interface and implant migration suggest that the prosthesis is being undermined by the infection. These x-rays were made 8 months after the initial total knee replacement procedure. Initial postoperative x-rays did not demonstrate any radiolucent lines or varus alignment.

2 Indications

The patient had persistent severe pain in the infected total knee joint which is refractory to irrigation and debridement and is also causing debilitating loss of function and disruption to a satisfactory lifestyle. While she is not systemically ill, the patient requested the infected TKR be explanted in an attempt to reduce pain and cure the infection as a two-stage surgery. In the presence of radiographic changes, debridement, irrigation, and polyethylene exchange are contraindicated.

3 Preoperative planning

When preparing for implant removal, an entire set of cement osteotomes and removal tools is preferred (**Fig 19.5-2**). In the event that these are unavailable, the standard set of osteotomes and a large bone tamp are the minimum required instruments. A small oscillating saw, typically pneumatically operated, is extremely useful to saw through the cement of the femoral and tibial implants. This allows for a cleaner removal of the implants and preservation of bone stock. The authors do not recommend the use of the Gigli saw as it seems to sacrifice more bone than is necessary.

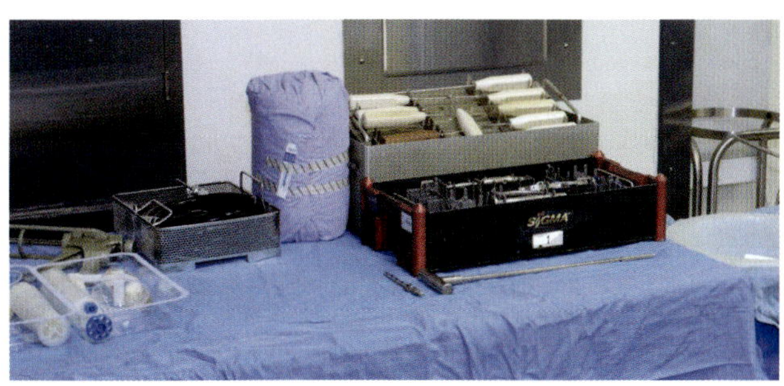

Fig 19.5-2 A set of cement osteotomes and prosthesis-specific removal tools.

4 Surgical approach

A medial parapatellar arthrotomy (which was the prior surgical approach) is used for TKR. Typically, the pneumatic tourniquet is used to reduce bleeding and improve visualization of the operative field. The thickened joint capsule and tendon tissue are encountered and must be carefully dissected and retracted to provide complete exposure of the infected prosthesis (**Fig 19.5-3**). It may be necessary to extend the original exposure proximally and distally. To obtain this exposure, it is necessary to have a full set of knee joint retractors available. In some cases, the patellar clamp used to implant the patellar button may be used to gently evert the patella.

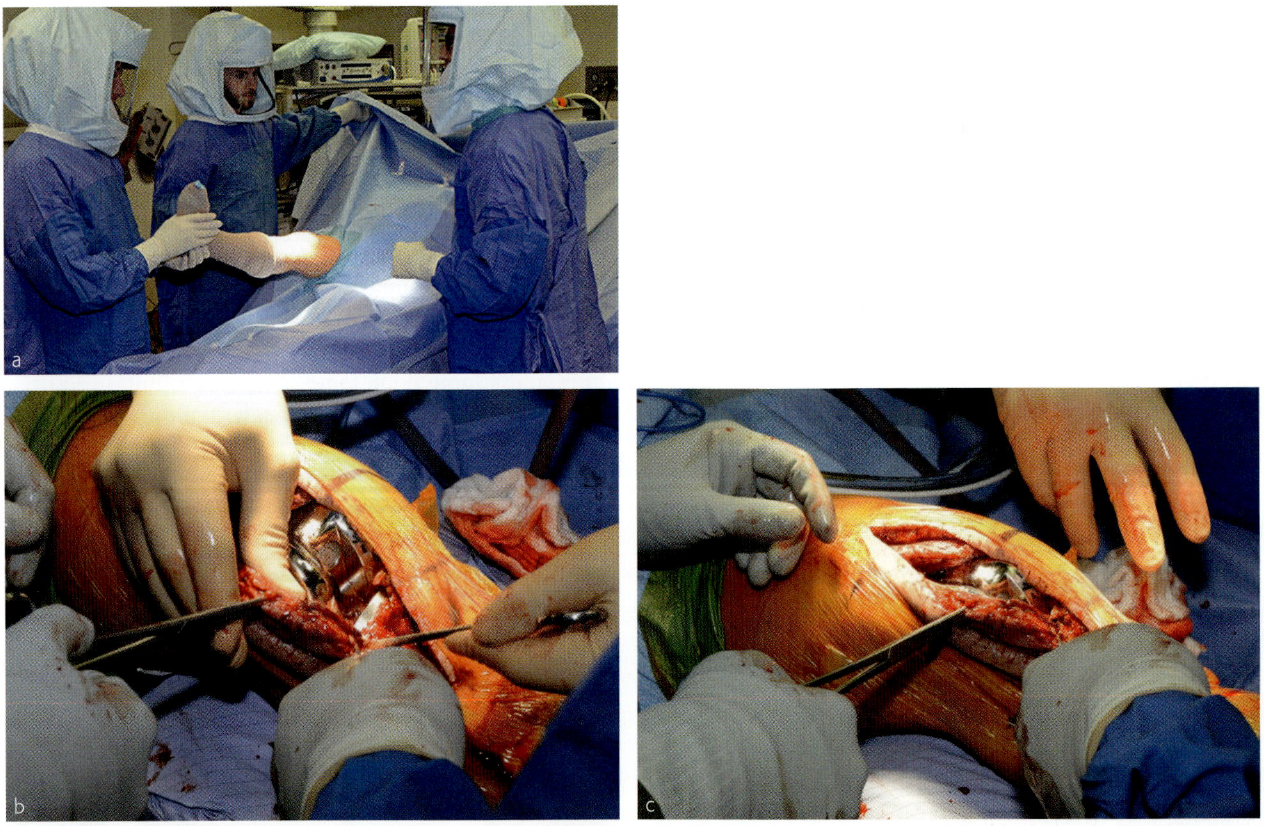

Fig 19.5-3a–c Surgical approach.
a Draping the extremity free enables good exposure. Sterile technique is used throughout the procedure.
b Careful exposure of the prosthesis is achieved by gently exposing the femoral and tibial implants.
c The patellar implant is now exposed enabling proper explantation.

5 Surgical debridement

Surgical debridement is conducted methodically and during the course of the procedure (**Fig 19.5-4**, **Fig 19.5-5**, **Fig 19.5-6**). This involves drainage of any purulent liquid, removal of infected synovial tissue, removal of all remaining bone cement, removal of all implants, and brushing or reaming the intramedullary canal of the femur and tibia. Special attention must be paid to the recess behind the femur to be certain that all infected tissue, cement, and debris are removed. Irrigation with a jet-pulsed saline lavage tool is useful to better visualize the remaining devitalized tissue and cement.

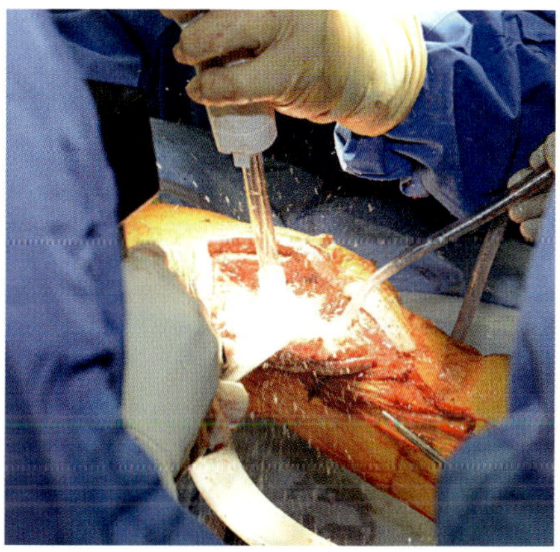

Fig 19.5-4 Jet lavage used during debridement.

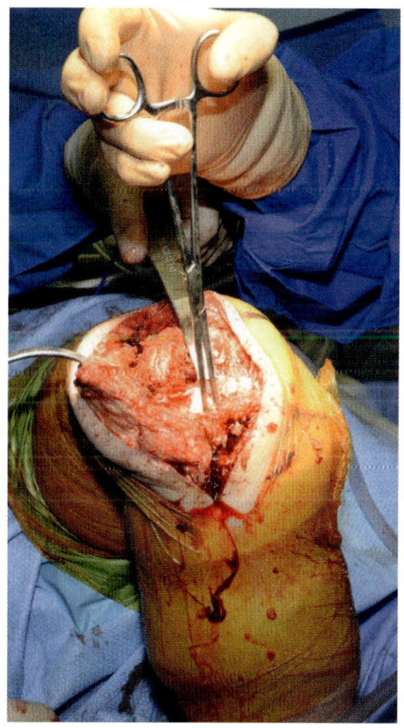

Fig 19.5-5 Removal of cement from the tibial canal often requires use of a longer clamp to extract cement fragments.

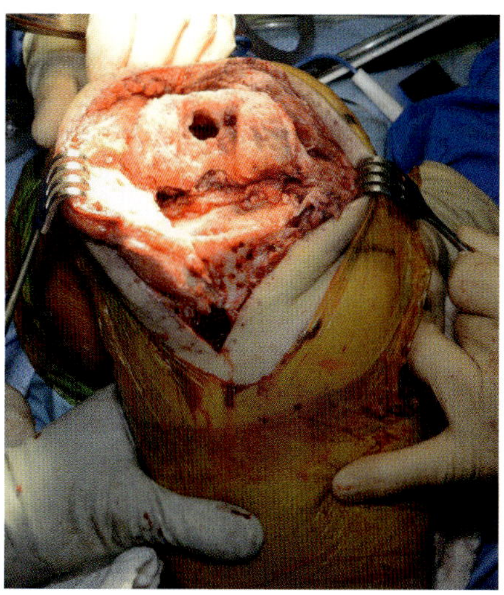

Fig 19.5-6 Debridement has been successfully completed and the joint is ready for antibiotic spacer placement.

6 Implant removal

It is easier to remove the femoral implant initially in a methodical manner as shown in **Fig 19.5-7**, **Fig 19.5-8**, **Fig 19.5-9**. Once the femoral implant has been loosened, it can be driven off the distal femur and in a distal direction with a V-shaped tamp.

Next, the tibial implant is removed. The cement-bone interface is freed with a small oscillating saw (a 1 cm wide blade is best) and cement chisels. A dogleg-shaped chisel works well in the posterior aspect of the tibial implant where a normal chisel cannot easily reach. When the implant has been slightly loosened, it can be driven upward with the V-shaped tamp.

The patella implant is best removed with the small oscillating saw with 1 cm blade. If any cement remains in the lug holes of the patellar implant, a high-speed round or football-shaped burr can be used to carefully remove the cement.

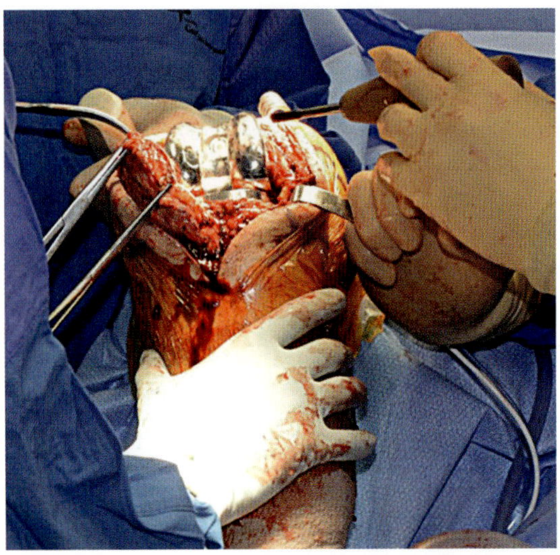

Fig 19.5-7 A cement chisel is used to free the bone-cement interface at the femoral implant.

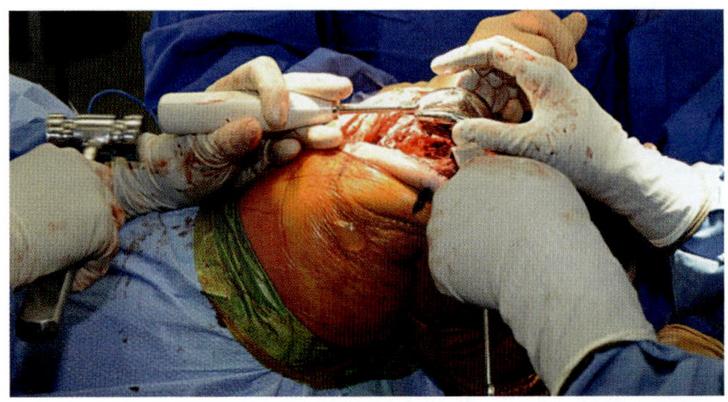

Fig 19.5-8 The femoral implant is removed with a V-shaped tamp.

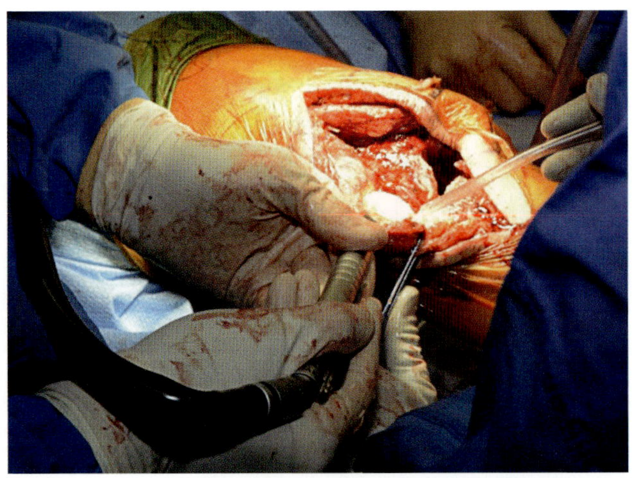

Fig 19.5-9 The bone-cement interface is freed with a small oscillating saw.

7 Temporary fixation

A temporary articulating antibiotic spacer (**Video 10-3**) is now created using factory molds (**Fig 19.5-10**, **Fig 19.5-11**). The cement is loaded with gentamicin and vancomycin, which will elute over the first week after implantation. Although these are anatomically shaped implants, they do not function as well as a TKR. They maintain the space for the next effort at replacement.

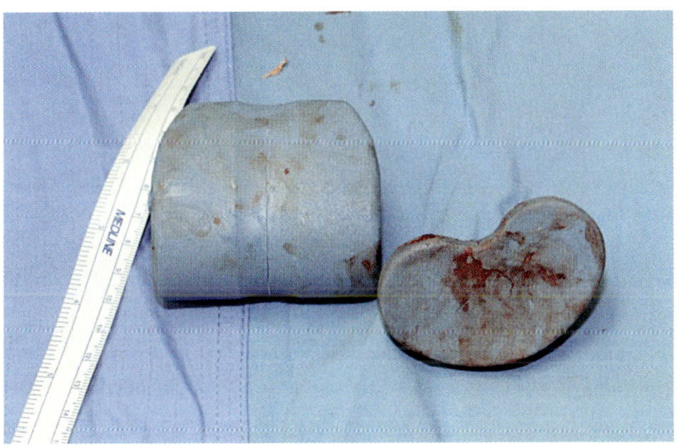

Fig 19.5-10 A molded temporary antibiotic spacer.

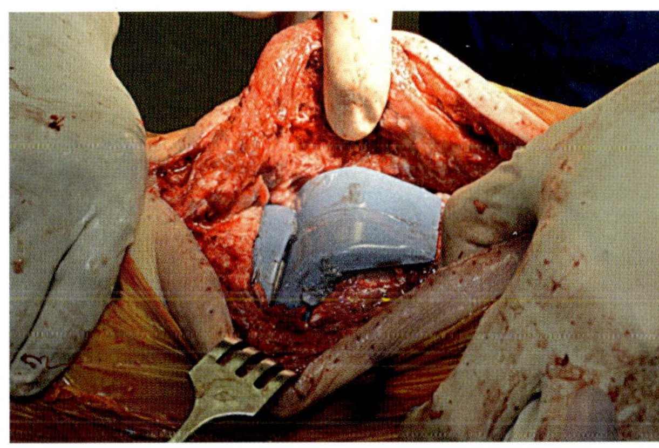

Fig 19.5-11 Molded antibiotic spacer installed in the joint space.

8 Postoperative management

Postoperatively, the patient is managed in a removable hinged knee brace (**Fig 19.5-12**). Weight bearing as tolerated is permitted. The infection itself is managed using a central venous line with intravenous antibiotics. The antibiotic cefazolin was administered intravenously and a 6-week period of antibiotic therapy was prescribed with the help of the infectious diseases physician. Monthly CRP levels and erythrocyte sedimentation rates (ESR) were checked. When the CRP reached a low level (typically 1 mg/L or less), reimplantation was scheduled.

9 Reimplantation

At 6 weeks after explantation of the infected TKR, the patient was ready for reimplantation. The ESR and CRP levels were reduced nicely from preoperative values. The patient completed a 6-week course of cefazolin. The incision healed well without drainage (**Fig 19.5-13**).

After appropriate discussion with the patient, TKR was planned. Standard surgical preparation was performed and positioning was typical for revision TKR (**Fig 19.5-14**).

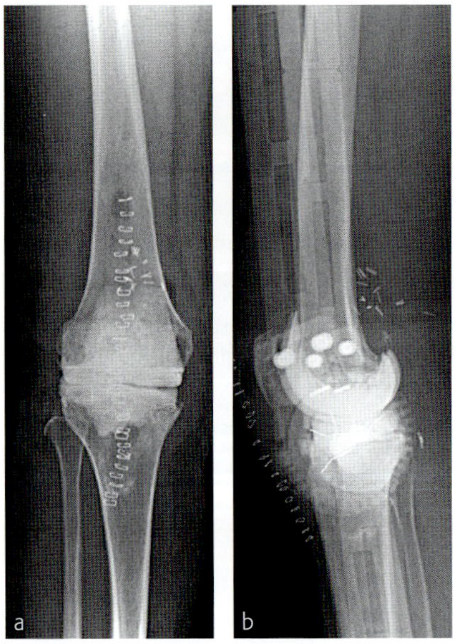

Fig 19.5-12a–b Postoperative x-rays following the explantation of total knee replacement demonstrate acceptable positioning of the cement spacers. These x-rays were taken with a hinged knee brace in place.

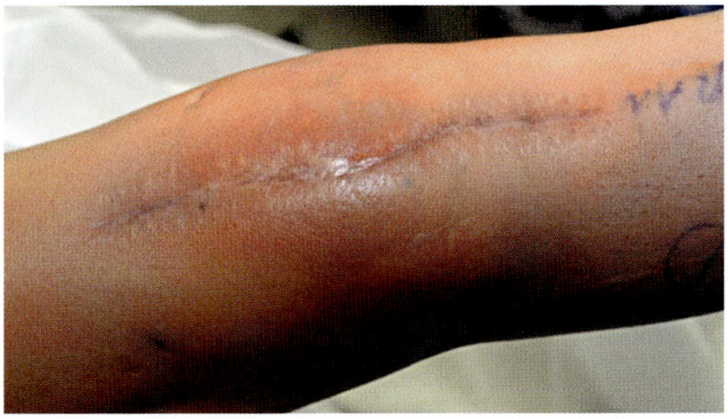

Fig 19.5-13 The incision healed well 6 weeks after explantation.

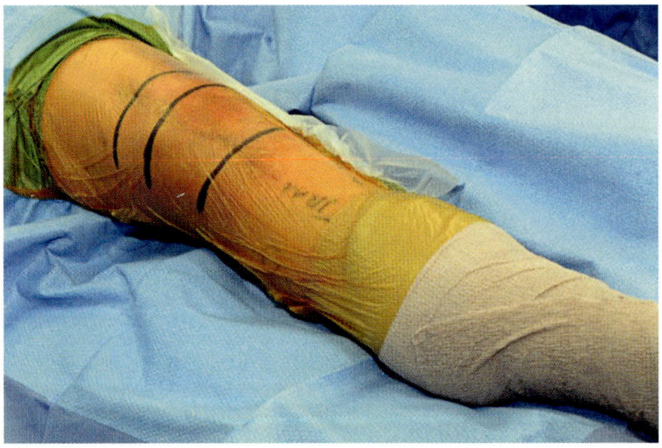

Fig 19.5-14 Standard surgical preparation and positioning for revision total knee replacement.

Surgical exposure in this situation can be tedious. Careful surgical dissection is essential to find appropriate tissue planes. The quadriceps mechanism is exposed and the medial arthrotomy is performed (**Fig 19.5-15**).

Once the spacer is exposed, it is usually necessary to remove it in pieces (**Fig 19.5-16**). Osteotomes and a mallet are used to remove the spacer.

After the spacer is removed, methodical debridement is performed and the bones are prepared for reinsertion of TKR. The degree of bone deficit will determine the need for primary or revision implants. In this case, minimal bone loss was present and primary implants were used for revision. The completed exposure is shown in **Fig 19.5-17**. Intraoperative Gram stain, aerobic and anaerobic cultures, and frozen section were sent for analysis during surgery. The frozen section showed one nucleated cell per high-power field and no evidence of acute inflammation. At this time, 2 g of intravenous cefazolin were administered for surgical prophylaxis.

At this point, standard TKR technique is used to finish the procedure. Cefazolin was continued for 24 hours after the revision surgery and then discontinued. The intraoperative cultures were negative for bacterial growth.

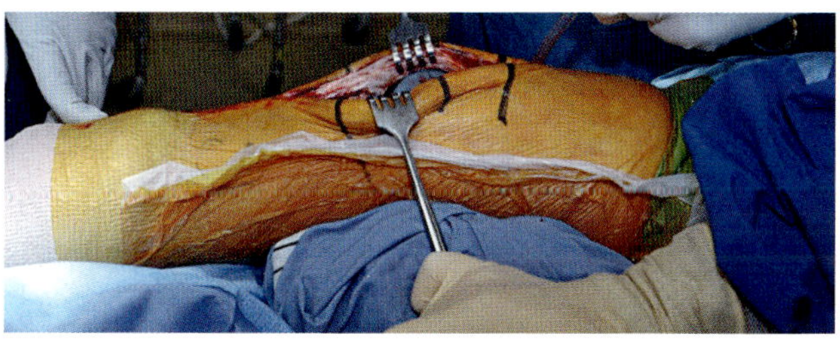

Fig 19.5-15 Careful surgical exposure and dissection is essential to perform medial arthrotomy.

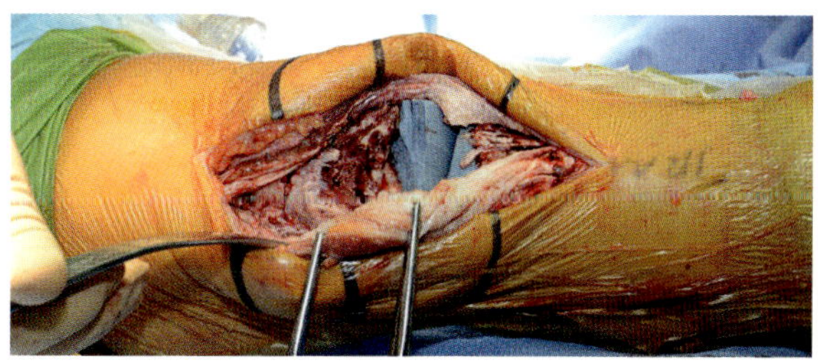

Fig 19.5-16 After exposure it is usually necessary to remove the spacer with osteotomes and a mallet.

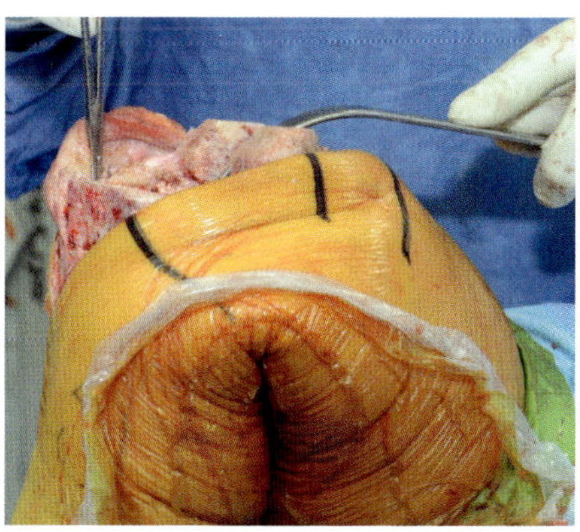

Fig 19.5-17 Completed exposure in preparation for total knee replacement.

10 Outcome

The x-rays in **Fig 19.5-18** demonstrate a satisfactory TKR. Primary knee implants were used in this case for revision. Oftentimes, it will be necessary to use constrained or hinged prostheses that should be available at the time of the second-stage surgery.

In this case, the incision was properly healed at 2 weeks and staples were removed. The patient started physical therapy on postoperative day 1. She regained range of motion of 0–105° by 4 months and was satisfied with the outcome. Her CRP and ESR levels returned to the normal range. There was no evidence of recurrence of infection. **Fig 19.5-19** shows x-rays taken at 9 months.

11 Pitfalls

- Diagnosis and decision making: it is essential to have a correct microbiological diagnosis prior to the debridement and explantation surgery. This can avoid use of an incorrect antibiotic regimen and incorrect antibiotics in the spacer. A common error seen in practice is the use of repeated irrigation, debridement, and spacer exchange. Typically, an irrigation and debridement procedure should be done no more than once prior to a definitive debridement and explantation. Surgical judgment should include a careful assessment of the viability of soft tissues in and around the knee joint. The presence of necrotic tissue should bias the surgeon toward an early second-look debridement after explantation. In some cases, an early arthrodesis may be required. The presence of gangrene or gas-forming organisms may necessitate amputation as a definitive early procedure. Although uncommon, this is sometimes necessary in such cases.

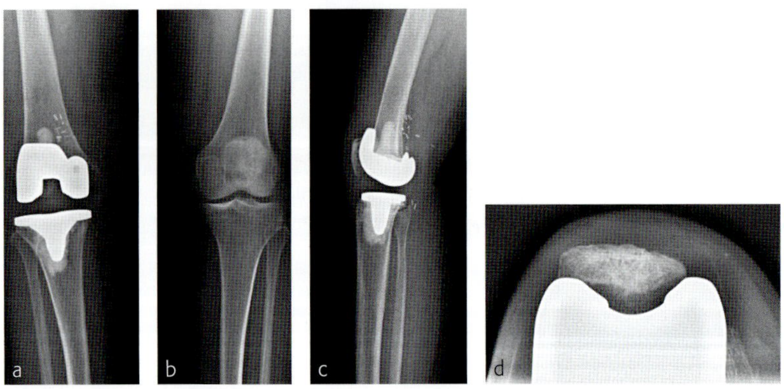

Fig 19.5-18a–d Postoperative x-rays demonstrate that satisfactory total knee replacement has been accomplished on AP (**a**–**b**), lateral (**c**), and patellar (**d**) views.

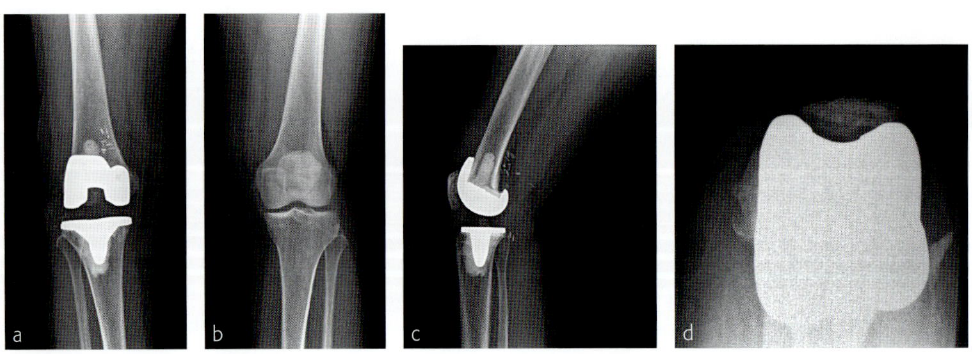

Fig 19.5-19a–d X-rays demonstrate satisfactory total knee replacement appearance at 9 months after revision of total knee replacement.

- Surgical approach: typically, the prior surgical incision and arthrotomy are reused. It may be necessary to extend the incisions proximally and distally to achieve better exposure. In some cases, partial release of the patellar tendon attachment may be required to achieve exposure. Excellent exposure is essential to successfully perform a good debridement and implant removal. This can be particularly challenging when patients have undergone multiple prior surgeries with scarred tissues. Obesity also considerably complicates the situation.
- Implant removal: preparation for implant removal dramatically expedites the process. This includes having the correct cement chisels, a small oscillating saw, antibiotic cement, and molds, as needed. Depending on the particular situation, it can be challenging to remove the implants. This is particularly the case with long-stem revision knee replacements that are solidly fixed but actively infected. In such cases, it is essential to have a full set of cement removal chisels, reamers, and a good strategy to successfully remove the revision implants.
- Temporary fixation: in most cases, the use of internal polymethylmethacrylate (PMMA) spacers represents the best strategy. These are typically made of antibiotic-laden PMMA cement. Bracing the extremity in a hinged knee brace is usually necessary to provide enough stability for the patient to be mobilized after surgery.
- Rehabilitation: in most cases, the patient will be able to bear weight on well-made PMMA spacers with a hinged knee brace. Therapy is directed at mobilization and ambulation. Work on range of motion is usually not possible until definitive revision is performed.
- Reimplantation: the primary pitfall with reimplantation is reinfection. This is best avoided by careful preoperative assessment for infection before reimplantation surgery. The preoperative assessment consists of diagnostic workup, clinical assessment, radiographic assessment, and needle aspiration of the joint space with microbiological analysis. Prior to implanting the new TKR, a frozen section of the synovial tissue is useful to rule out acute inflammation. During reimplantation, always obtain new tissue specimens for microbiological analysis. If the intraoperative cultures are positive after reimplantation, long-term antibiotic management will likely be required.
- Failure of therapy: in some cases, the first stage of explantation will fail to clear the infection or control it. At this time, it will be necessary to have a team discussion about treatment goals. Options for treatment include repeated debridement and antibiotic spacer replacement, conversion to an arthrodesis, or in severe cases amputation may be required. There exists a small percentage of patients who decline to have any additional treatment after explantation is performed. For these patients, long-term bracing and suppressive antibiotic therapy may be needed.

12 Pearls

- Decision making: when performing explantation of a TKR, the keys to success are correct diagnosis, meticulous preoperative planning, and working as a team with an infectious diseases physician. Surgery should be scheduled when adequate help is available to safely perform the procedure.
- Surgical approach: meticulous attention to detail, obtaining wide exposure, and having adequate personnel to help are essential.
- Implant removal: careful attention to breaking down the bone-cement interface with the oscillating saw followed by use of cement-removal chisels greatly simplifies the process of implant removal.
- Temporary fixation: cement-spacer molding and fabrication should permit early mobilization of the patient. Carefully making these with factory molds or hand molding are essential. Some limited fixation with cement to host bone is desirable to prevent dislocation.
- Definitive revision—second stage: careful exposure dramatically simplifies reimplantation. Having primary implants, a constrained knee system, and a hinged system available offers many options and improves the chances for success.
- Antibiotic management: use only specific antibiotics to which the organism is sensitive. Ask an infectious diseases physician for advice on dosage and duration of therapy.

19.6 Implant removal—infected total shoulder arthroplasty

Arthur Grzesiak, Alain Farron

1 Case description

A 59-year-old male baker with type 2 diabetes mellitus and arterial hypertension underwent left total shoulder arthroplasty for symptomatic osteoarthritis treated conservatively for many years (**Fig 19.6-1**, **Fig 19.6-2**).

The recovery process was good and the patient returned to part-time work 3 months after surgery. Five months postoperatively he fell down the stairs and developed a significant left shoulder and pectoral hematoma. The x-rays taken at that time showed no fracture or displacement of the prosthesis.

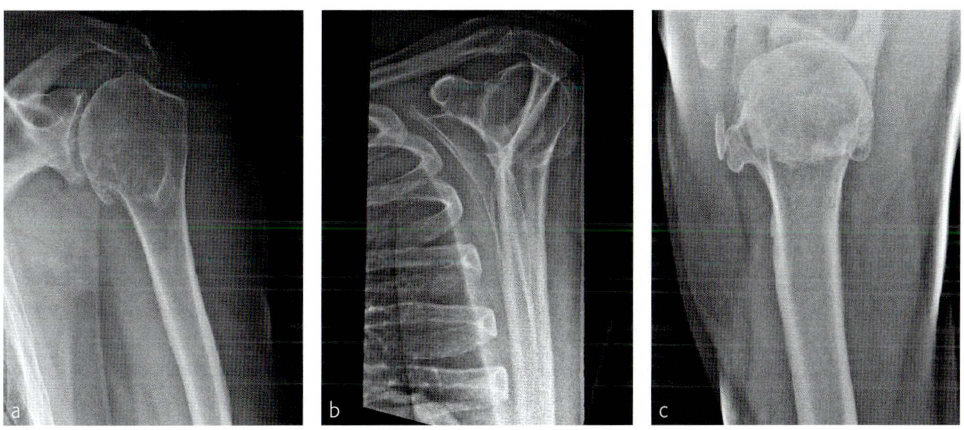

Fig 19.6-1a–c Preoperative situation of the left shoulder with a pronounced arthritis.
a AP view.
b Lateral Neer view.
c Axial view.

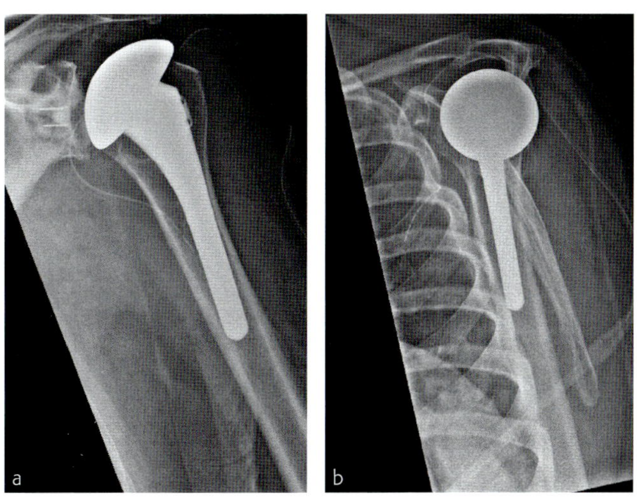

Fig 19.6-2a–b Postoperative images of the left total shoulder prosthesis.
a AP view.
b Lateral Neer view.

Eight months postoperatively the patient complained of pain at rest and during the night that increased with activities of daily living. He presented with a left prepectoral tumefaction and erythema (**Fig 19.6-3**). A computed tomographic scan showed no signs of osteolysis or prosthetic loosening but demonstrated a pectoralis major muscle hematoma with several small collections of gas (**Fig 19.6-4**). A joint aspiration was performed; the fluid aspirated remained sterile.

The clinical examination showed a relatively good left shoulder range of motion (ROM) with 110° active flexion and abduction, 30° external rotation, and internal rotation to L5. The strength was conserved but movement provoked pain in the rotator cuff. The x-rays were normal (**Fig 19.6-5**). The C-reactive protein (CRP) level was increased at 72 mg/L and the patient had no fever.

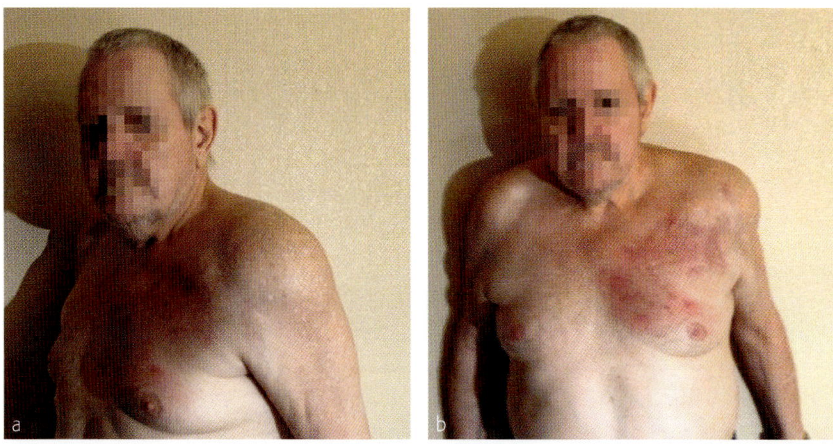

Fig 19.6-3a–b Erythema and pectoral swelling at the 10-month follow-up.

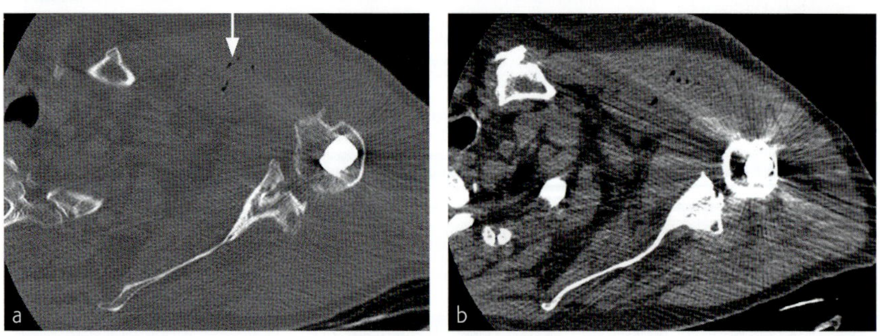

Fig 19.6-4a–b Computed tomographic scans of the left shoulder show voluminous hematoma under the pectoralis major muscle. The arrow (**a**) shows gas pockets that are highly suspicious of infection.

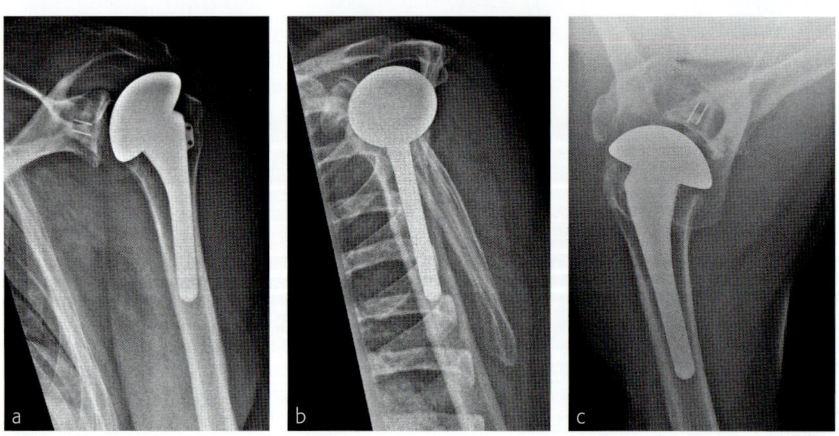

Fig 19.6-5a–c X-rays show left shoulder replacement at the 10-month follow-up.
a AP view.
b Lateral Neer view.
c Axial view.

2 Indications

At 10 months after the left total shoulder arthroplasty, the patient noted his shoulder was more painful and presented with clinical signs highly suspicious for a low-grade infection:

- Pain at rest, worse with movement
- Posttraumatic hematoma left pectoralis major with gas in the soft tissue
- Erythema around the surgical site and the hematoma
- Rising CRP level

Low-grade infections caused by less virulent organisms often present with few impressive clinical findings. Typical signs like implant loosening, osteolysis, or fistula can be absent or develop late, sometimes after years. A detailed history and high index of suspicion are mandatory, even ahead of negative joint aspiration (which can be false negative in up to 20% of cases).

The goals of the proposed treatment are:

- Identification of the responsible causative organism and establish its sensitivities
- Definitive control and hopefully eradication of infection
- Pain free and satisfactory shoulder function to allow the patient to continue his profession and resume activities of daily living

3 Preoperative planning

The responsible organisms are unidentified and the symptoms have lasted for more than 3 weeks. Additionally, the skin conditions are not calm. The authors decided to perform a two-stage exchange of the prosthesis with a temporary spacer. The interval between the two operations permits identification of the organism, planning the antibiotic therapy, and improving the skin conditions. The decision about the length of the interval is determined after obtaining the antibiogram and according to the local soft-tissue situation.

The procedure is performed with the patient under general anesthesia in beach chair position. Antibiotics, if given before, should be stopped more than 2 weeks before the operation to increase the chances of identifying the responsible organism.

The surgeon should be prepared to deal with intraoperative humeral shaft fracture and have fixation hardware ready, such as plates or cables. Sometimes prosthetic components are so well fixed that a bone window or even an osteotomy is necessary to explant them. Surgeons performing prosthetic explantation should be familiar with those techniques.

Surgical debridement is performed with scalpel or electrocautery. Slotted-teeth curettes of different sizes are advantageous, especially for bone debridement.

If prefabricated spacers are used, the surgeon should obtain different sizes to best match the patient's anatomy. If the surgeon plans to custom-make the spacer, it is essential to use heat-resistant antibiotic powder, as the polymethylmethacrylate cement reaches a high temperature during polymerization.

4 Surgical approach

The intervention is performed through the deltopectoral approach which offers several advantages:

- Excellent visibility of rotator cuff, humeral head, proximal shaft, glenoid
- Distally extensible if necessary
- It is the standard approach for total shoulder arthroplasty

A subscapularis tenotomy allows good intraarticular exposure and permits easy displacement of the humeral head and diaphysis anteriorly.

5 Surgical debridement

All necrotic tissues, bone fragments, and the synovial membranes are debrided. The surgeon must carefully remove all remaining sutures from previous surgeries as they are foreign bodies that could harbor bacteria. The humeral diaphysis is cleaned with slotted-teeth curettes to remove the fibrous tissues of the interface between bone and implant. After debridement the wound is irrigated with 9 L of saline solution using a pulsatile lavage device.

In this case the subscapularis and supraspinatus tendon were not found intraoperatively.

6 Implant removal

The arthroplasty implant can be removed with standard explant systems. Some manufacturers allow detachment of the prosthetic head first. In that way a special or universal extractor with a sliding hammer device can be connected to the stem. If the surgeon is not familiar with the components in place, he or she should refer to the manufacturer for advice and special explant instruments. The removal of the prosthetic head offers the advantage of allowing direct access to the bone-stem interface. If the stem is not retractable by simple hammering with the extractor, the surgeon must free the bone-implant interface by use of flexible osteotomes, or chisels between them. Excessive force can create humeral shaft fractures, so consider a controlled shaft osteotomy if the stem remains solidly affixed to the shaft.

The cemented glenoid component can be removed with standard osteotomes and chisels. In this case the glenoid polyethylene was loosened and removed by hand. The surgeon should remove all the polymethylmethacrylate cement as it represents a foreign body, which is typically covered by bacterial biofilm.

The same principle applies to cement around prosthetic stems. In this case the humeral stem was not cemented.

All the prosthetic components were sent for sonication. A minimum of three tissue samples were harvested and underwent microbiological cultures. Then empiric antibiotic therapy was started intravenously—in this case with 2.2 g of coamoxicillin.

7 Temporary fixation

A custom-made spacer is formed with 40 g of PMMA cement charged with supplementary antibiotics (2 g of vancomycin and 4 g of gentamicin). It is armed with a one-third tubular plate to enhance its stability (**Fig 19.6-6**). The implanted spacer helps to eradicate the infection by providing local antibiotics in a much higher concentration than could by achieved with oral or intravenous antibiotics. Mechanically, it protects the soft tissues from retraction, which could make a secondary arthroplasty difficult and allows early mobilization of the limb which helps to diminish muscle atrophy and articular stiffness.

The shoulder was reduced with the spacer and the mobility and stability tested to ensure that postoperative mobilization was possible. The subscapularis tendon was sutured and the wound closed layer by layer with nonresorbable simple stiches.

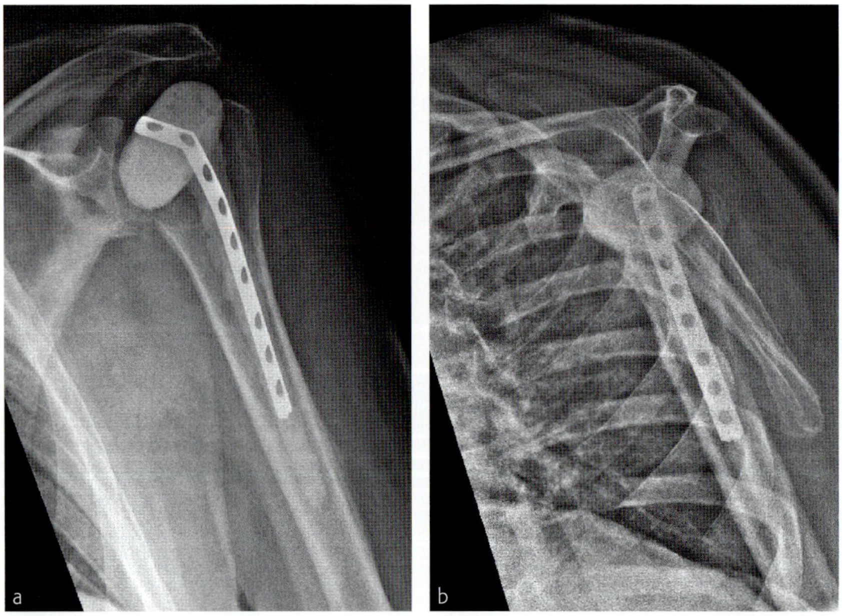

Fig 19.6-6a–b Postoperative views of the cemented spacer.
a AP view.
b Lateral Neer view.

8 Postoperative management

The postoperative management consists of a 4-week period of immobilization in a sling and swath-like commercial shoulder immobilizer. Postoperative x-rays (AP and lateral Neer views) are taken to verify the spacer position and exclude iatrogenic fractures (**Fig 19.6-6**).

Hand, wrist, and elbow are mobilized immediately. Shoulder mobilization is started when pain control is satisfactory, avoiding abduction and flexion below 30° for 4 weeks, then free ROM is allowed as tolerated.

In this case, the sonication and tissue samples cultured positive for *Staphylococcus epidermidis*. According to the antibiogram (**Table 19.6-1**), coamoxicillin was replaced by flucloxacillin 2 g every 6 hours intravenously for 2 weeks, followed by cotrimoxazole 3 times per day orally until the implantation of the new prosthesis.

The scar and surrounding soft tissues rapidly demonstrated a good resolution of infection. The CRP dropped to normal levels within 2 weeks.

The clinical parameters and the organism's sensitivity to rifampin permit a shoulder arthroplasty reimplantation after a short interval of 2 weeks. In cases of rotator-cuff absence, the surgeon can implant a reverse total shoulder prosthesis to achieve better mobility. If this option is not possible, an exchange of the spacer for a hemiarthroplasty is advantageous. Spacers can produce excessive glenoid wear over time because of its nonpolished surface. Hemiarthroplasty will not achieve a better function compared a spacer but can significantly reduce wear and the risk of secondary glenoid destruction.

Because of quick pain relief and satisfactory function of his shoulder, the patient initially refused a second intervention. The antibiotic therapy was conducted for a total of 3 months and then stopped. The shoulder remained asymptomatic.

At the 8-month follow-up the patient was satisfied with his left shoulder with only occasional pain. The ROM was limited with 90° flexion and abduction, 10° external rotation, and internal rotation to L5. The x-rays show a well-positioned spacer without glenoid wear (**Fig 19.6-7**). At that time, the patient agreed to undergo a second-stage procedure.

Staphylococcus epidermidis **(8 x 10E2 germs/mL)**	
Antibiogram	I
Penicillin G	R
Oxacillin	S
Flucloxacillin	S
Amoxicillin	R
Amoxicillin/clavulanic acid	S
Gentamicin	S
Tetracyclin	S
Doxycyclin	S
Erythromycin	S
Clarithromycin	S
Clindamycin	S
Cotrimoxazole	S
Ciprofloxacin	S
Levofloxacin	S
Rifampin	S
Vancomycin	S
Teicoplanin	S
Fusidic acid	R
1. *Staphylococcus epidermidis*	

Table 19.6-1 The antibiogram obtained after cultures of sonication fluid. Note the organism's sensitivity to rifampin. This is a good prognostic factor.
Abbreviations: I, intermediate; N, not defined; R, resistant; S, sensitive.

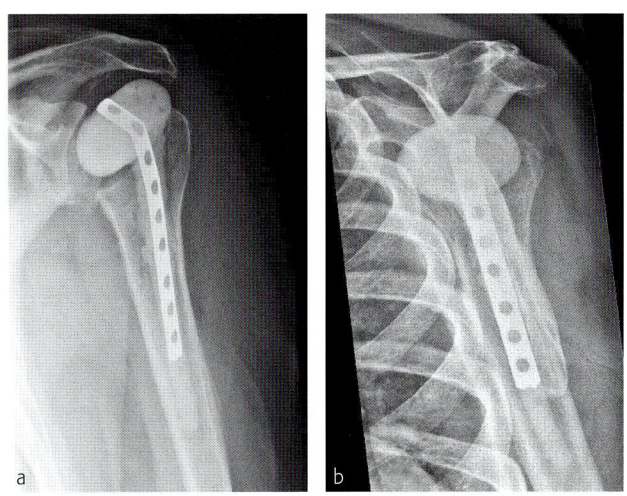

Fig 19.6-7a–b The situation remains stable 10 months after spacer implantation with no additional glenoid wear.

9 Reimplantation

The second stage was performed 10 months after the first stage. It consisted of spacer removal and placement of a hemiarthroplasty.

Normally, the second stage includes a major debridement but in this case the infection was considered to be resolved for more than 10 months and the soft tissues were calm.

The authors used standard antibiotic prophylaxis as for primary arthroplasty with 1.5 g intravenous cefuroxime 20 minutes before the skin incision which was continued until final microbiological culture results.

The positioning of the patient was identical to the first stage: beach chair position under general anaesthesia. The same deltopectoral approach was used.

In this case the spacer was removed by hand without any special instruments and was sent for sonication.

The glenoid did not demonstrate excessive wear. The hemiarthroplasty was performed following the standard surgical technique of the manufacturer. An anatomical, noncemented stem was used.

Wound closure was performed in the usual way over an intraarticular suction drain, which is normally removed on the second day.

Postoperative x-rays (AP and lateral Neer views) to verify the prosthesis' position showed an iatrogenic displaced periprosthetic fracture (**Fig 19.6-8**). The authors decided to treat it conservatively.

The postoperative management consisted 6 weeks of immobilization in a sling and swathe-like commercial shoulder immobilizer. Normally, hand, wrist, and elbow are mobilized immediately and shoulder mobilization is started when pain control is satisfactory, with active flexion and abduction of maximum 90° without external rotation. Free motion in all directions is allowed after 6 weeks.

In this case shoulder mobilization was delayed until the 6-week follow-up visit, when x-rays confirmed no additional displacement of the fracture.

The sonication fluid cultures remained sterile and cefuroxime was stopped on postoperative day 5.

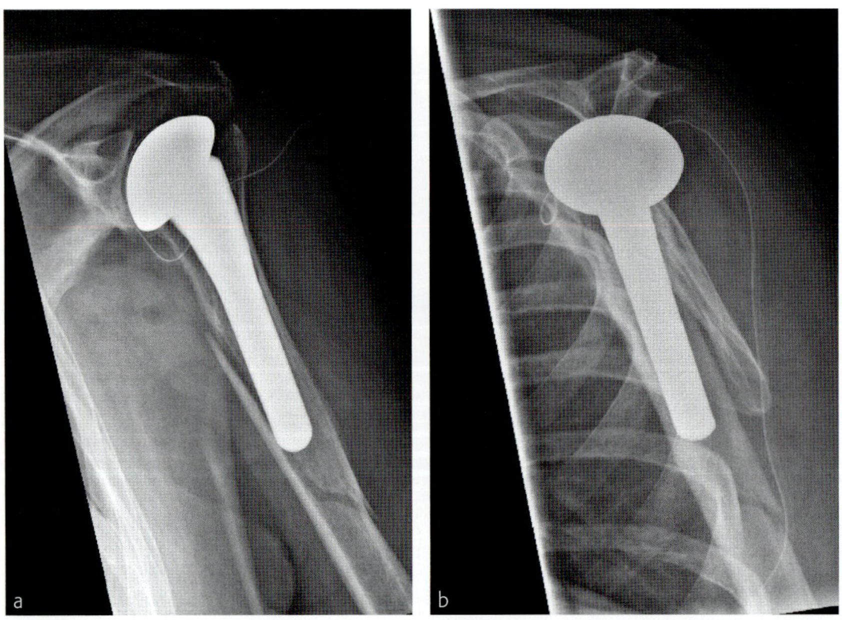

Fig 19.6-8a–b X-rays taken on postoperative day 1. Minimally displaced periprosthetic shaft fracture.
a AP view.
b Lateral Neer view.

10 Outcome

At 3-month follow-up, the patient was asymptomatic. The left shoulder ROM was satisfactory with 90° flexion, 80° abduction, 20° external rotation, and internal rotation to L5. In the strength examination, the left shoulder strength was slightly diminished in abduction and internal rotation. These findings reflected the absent supraspinatus and subscapularis tendons.

Radiologically, the fracture is healing nondisplaced with good callus formation (**Fig 19.6-9**).

11 Pitfalls

- Normal skin flora like *Propionibacterium acnes* or *S epidermidis* provoke low-grade infections and a positive culture can be misinterpreted as a contamination: correlate the results with the clinical history and presentation.
- Plan surgical approach according to the "worst-case scenario". It should be usable or extensile should something go wrong, eg, in case of an intraoperative fracture or need for an osteotomy.

12 Pearls

- If possible delay antibiotic prophylaxis until tissue samples for microbiology are harvested—you diminish false-negative results.
- Make your hand-made spacer with a bent K-wire distally—in case of spacer fracture or intentional fragmentation remove the distal blocked parts without osteotomy.

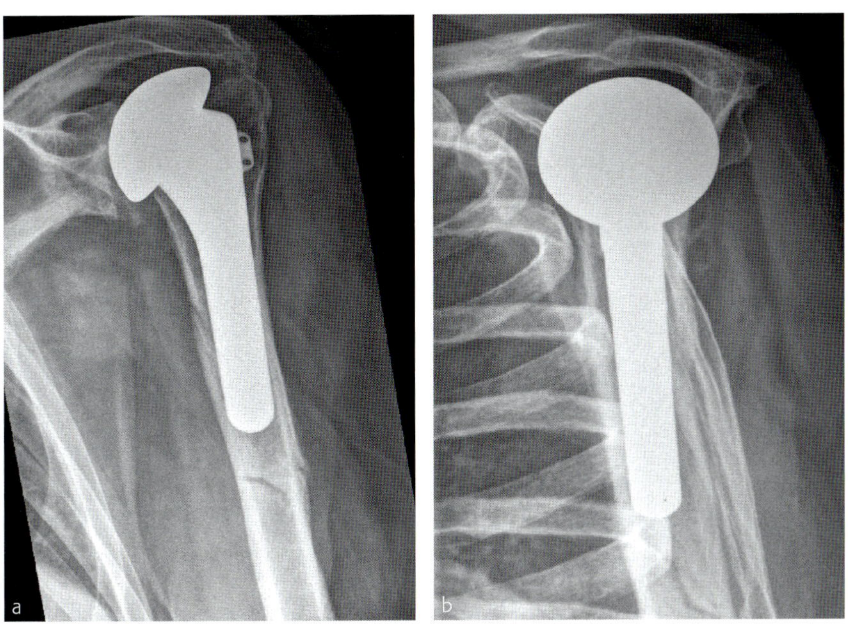

Fig 19.6-9a–b Three months after hemiarthroplasty. The periprosthetic fracture shows callus formation and no secondary displacement.
a AP view.
b Lateral Neer view.

19.7 Implant removal—acutely infected total ankle arthroplasty

Lisca Drittenbass, Xavier Crevoisier, Mathieu Assal

1 Case description

A 71-year-old woman presented with a 2-week history of increasing pain, redness, and swelling of her left ankle with fever and chills for the past 36 hours. She had undergone total ankle arthroplasty 6 years before. Her only other pertinent medical history included recurrent depression. Physical examination revealed increased warmth, erythema, induration, and tenderness about the distal leg and ankle. Skin was intact without drainage or abscess formation. Distal pulses were present, and sensation was intact in both lower limbs. Laboratory results demonstrated white blood cell count of 13,300 cells/µL, hemoglobin level 11.4 g/dL, and C-reactive protein (CRP) level of 210 mg/L. X-rays of the left ankle showed radiolucency around the tibial component with cyst formation (**Fig 19.7-1**). A tentative diagnosis was made of acute late periprosthetic joint infection of the left ankle arthroplasty.

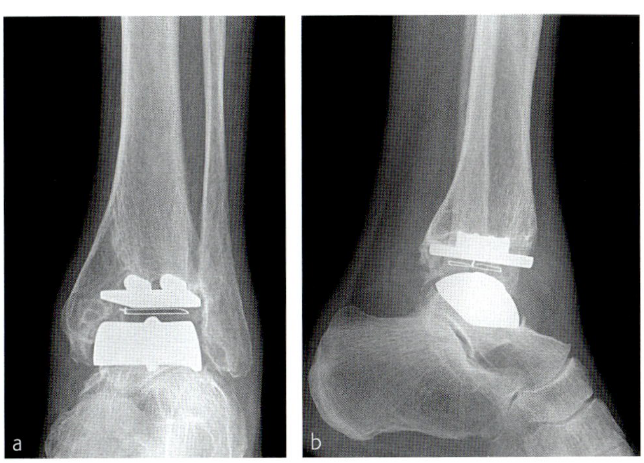

Fig 19.7-1a–b Preoperative x-rays of the left ankle show some areas of radiolucency around the tibial component with cyst formation.
a AP view.
b Lateral view.

2 Indications

Because of the presumed diagnosis, emergency surgical treatment was indicated without prior aspiration of the joint due to the critical clinical situation of an acutely ill, febrile patient with unstable blood pressure. Since preoperative x-rays showed periprosthetic bone resorption and bone cysts, retention of the components was not recommended. The surgical plan was for a two-stage procedure with urgent debridement, removal of all components, placement of a gentamicin-loaded cement spacer, and temporary external fixation as a first step. A one stage procedure consisting of irrigation, debridement, polyethylene exchange, and retention of the implants was not an option due to x-ray evidence of implant loosening.

Eight weeks after the initial procedure final reconstruction included removal of the spacer and external fixator with an ankle arthrodesis by means of an interposition iliac crest corticocancellous bone graft and fixation with screws and anterior plate. The indication for an arthrodesis was based on a patient with a sedentary lifestyle and low functional demands who was seeking a permanent solution and not opposed to sacrificing joint mobility. Revision arthroplasty was considered to carry a higher risk of needing further surgery in the future and was therefore not proposed.

The literature to our knowledge does not currently provide a standardized algorithm for treatment of prosthetic joint infection of the total ankle. Furthermore, it is not clear whether algorithms allowing short intervals for two-stage procedures for infected arthroplasty of the knee and the hip can be safely applied to the ankle. The long interval of 8 weeks between stages was allowed for 6 weeks of curative antibiotic treatment followed by an antibiotic-free interval of 2 weeks prior to the final reconstruction.

3 Preoperative planning

Removal of the implant required the necessary instrumentation, including specially shaped chisels. The patient was positioned supine with a pad under the ipsilateral buttock to position the forefoot pointing to the ceiling (**Fig 19.7-2**). No tourniquet was used. Intravenous antibiotics were administered intraoperatively after all microbiological samples were obtained. The patient was placed under general anesthesia in the setting of acute infection affecting the limb.

For the second-stage intervention the same protocol was applied except for the use of a thigh tourniquet.

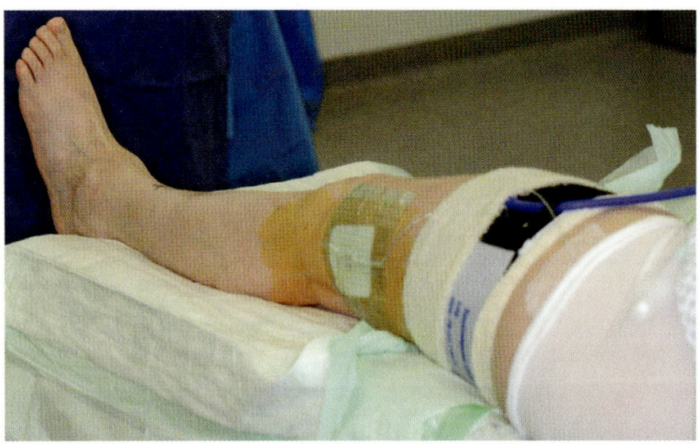

Fig 19.7-2 The patient was positioned supine with a pad under the ipsilateral buttock to position the forefoot pointing to the ceiling. A tourniquet was applied but not inflated.

4 Surgical approach and debridement

An anterior approach to the ankle was made through the existing anterior midline incision, extending from 8–10 cm proximal of the joint line down to the lateral aspect of the talonavicular joint (**Fig 19.7-3**). Following the skin incision, substantial purulent liquid was noted. The extensor retinaculum was exposed while carefully protecting the medial branch of the superficial peroneal nerve in the distal portion of the incision during subcutaneous dissection. Splitting off the retinaculum was performed and the joint capsule was accessed through the interval between the tibialis anterior tendon medially and the extensor hallucis longus laterally. Intraoperative status revealed pus in the ankle joint space with stable implants. The neurovascular bundle consisting of the anterior tibial artery and the deep peroneal nerve was identified in the proximal portion of the interval and retracted laterally. The fat tissue on the joint capsule was incised using ligatures for the transverse vessels crossing this area.

After thorough irrigation and debridement, all necrotic and fibrotic soft tissue was meticulously removed. All devitalized and septic tissues were removed by use of a Luer rongeur. The anterior rim of the tibia was sparingly removed to fully expose the implant (**Fig 19.7-4**). Cysts above the tibial implants were revealed. Purulent fluid and six tissue samples were retrieved for microbiological and histological testing. Empiric intravenous antibiotic treatment was initiated with coamoxicillin after obtaining all samples.

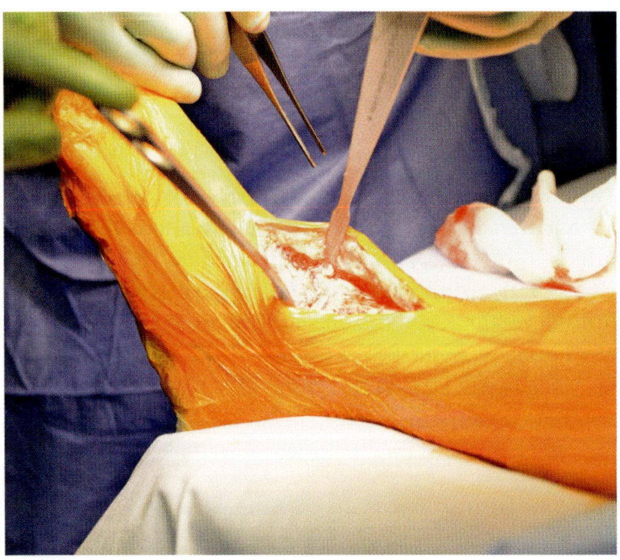

Fig 19.7-3 Anterior approach to the ankle.

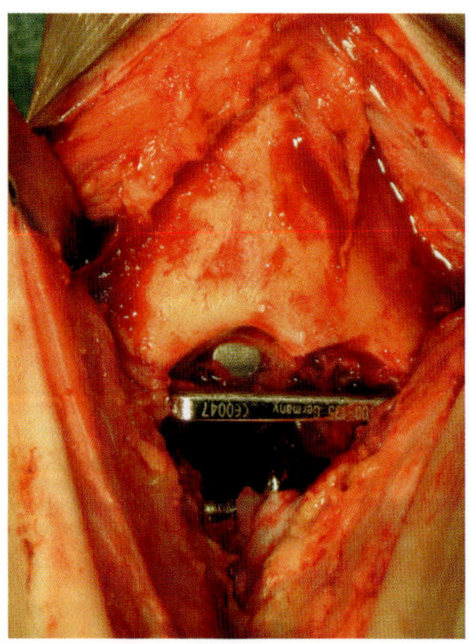

Fig 19.7-4 Cysts above the tibial implant.

5 Implant removal

The polyethylene component was removed with Kocher forceps. Different size chisels were used around the tibial and talar implants to facilitate their removal (**Fig 19.7-5**). Fibrotic tissue underneath the remaining bone surface was removed thoroughly and abundant rinsing with an antiseptic polyhexanide solution was performed using a pulsatile jet-lavage irrigation system.

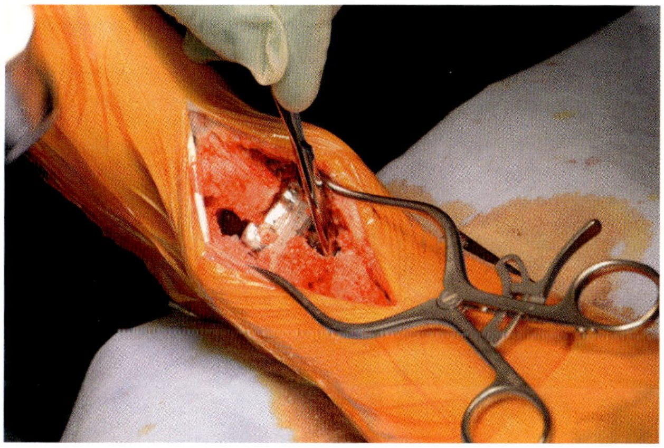

Fig 19.7-5 Implant removal using different size chisels around the tibial and talar implants.

6 Temporary fixation

A high-viscosity gentamicin-loaded polymethylmethacrylate (PMMA) spacer was molded to fill the cavity. The wound was closed primarily over two drains. A medial tibiocalcaneonavicular external fixator was applied to achieve temporary stabilization of the ankle without compromising access to the wound for frequent dressing changes (**Fig 19.7-6**).

7 Postoperative management (1)

Postoperative x-rays are shown in **Fig 19.7-7**. The drains were removed within 48 hours postoperatively, and the dressings were changed daily until the wound was dry. The external fixator was left in place for 8 weeks until the second intervention was performed. The patient was mobilized with partial weight bearing of 15 kg for the entire period. Microbiological samples revealed infection with methicillin-sensitive *Staphylococcus aureus*, and treatment was continued with flucloxacillin 4 x 2 g intravenously daily for 14 days. Rifampin 2 x 450 mg intravenously daily was added after the wound had become completely dry. After 2 weeks the patient was discharged and antibiotic treatment was continued with ciprofloxacin 2 x 750 mg per day orally and rifampin 2 x 450 mg per day orally for 4 weeks. All antibiotics were discontinued 2 weeks before the second surgery.

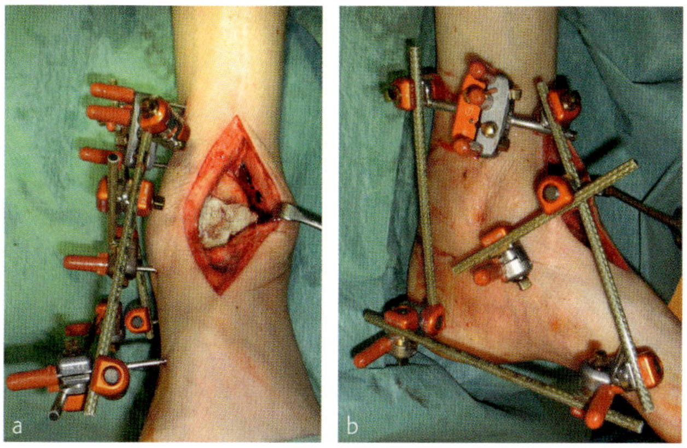

Fig 19.7-6a–b A medial tibiocalcaneonavicular external fixator was applied to achieve temporary stabilization of the ankle.

a AP view.

b Lateral view.

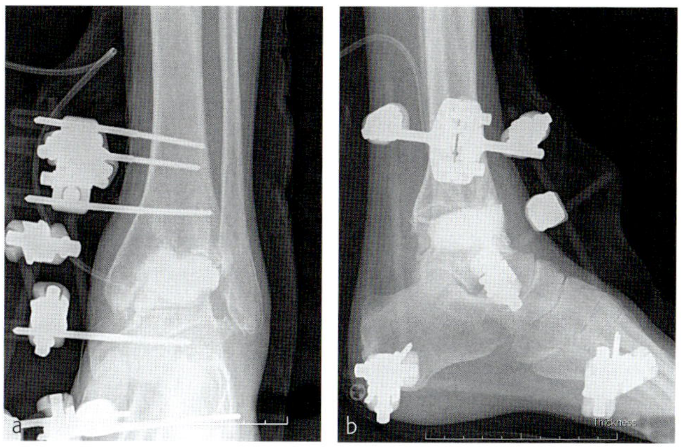

Fig 19.7-7a–b Postoperative x-rays after implant removal show the cavity filled with a cement spacer and stabilization with an external fixator.

a AP view.

b Lateral view.

8 Ankle arthrodesis

Eight weeks after the removal of the infected implant the final reconstruction was performed. This consisted of removal of the external fixator and PMMA spacer, followed by tibiotalar arthrodesis. Preoperative laboratory results had revealed regression of the CRP level to 5 mg/L and white blood cell count to 7,300 cells/µL.

The operation started with removal of the external fixator. The previous anterior approach to the ankle joint was used and the PMMA spacer was removed revealing a clean ankle cavity. Six tissue samples were obtained for microbiological examination following which a general prophylactic antibiotic (cefuroxime 1.5 g) was administered intravenously. Thorough debridement and irrigation were performed, and a 1 mm layer of bone was removed to obtain a clean bone surface.

Three large corticocancellous struts were harvested from the ipsilateral anterior iliac crest. Next an oblique fibular osteotomy was performed through a direct lateral approach 7 cm proximal to the tip of the lateral malleolus. A 7 mm slice was removed and the remaining edges were made smooth. The medial third of the fibula was removed with an oscillating saw. The bone graft struts were placed in a manner to span the cavity between the tibia and the talus and fixed with two cannulated 4.0 mm screws. One screw was placed from posterolateral aiming from proximal to distal and one from lateral beginning in the lateral process of the talus aiming proximally. The ankle was maintained in neutral position. The remaining fibula was fixed to the tibia with one 3.5 mm cortical screw. To augment stability a contoured reconstruction plate was applied anteriorly and fixed with five screws. The wound was closed over a drain layer by layer with nonabsorbable sutures for the skin.

9 Postoperative management (2)

Postoperative x-rays are shown in **Fig 19.7-8**. Intravenous antibiotics were continued until final histology and bacteriology revealed no infection. No further antibiotics were administered. A lower-leg split combicast was used for postoperative immobilization. The patient remained nonweight bearing for 6 weeks and then began partial weight bearing with increasing weight for an additional 4 weeks with a lower-leg combicast boot for a further 8 weeks.

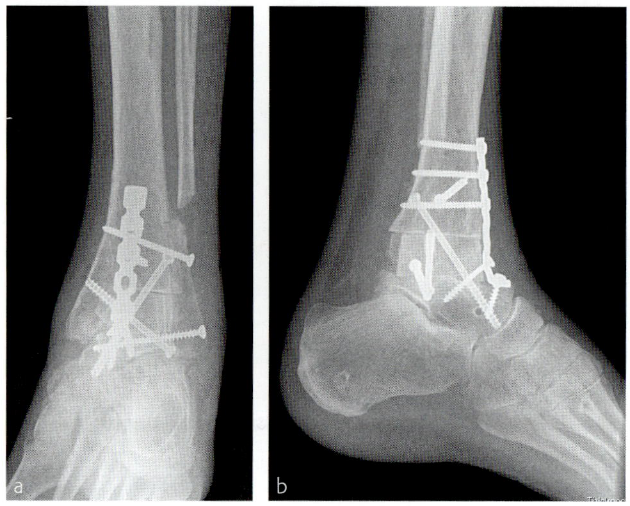

Fig 19.7-8a–b Postoperative x-rays after ankle arthrodesis.
a AP view.
b Lateral view.

10 Outcome

All wounds healed uneventfully. At 6 months the patient presented with a fluid gait and only occasional pain. Clinically, the ankle remained in a well-aligned neutral position. X-rays at 6 months demonstrated solid union with no signs of graft resorption or infection, and at 2 years they remained unchanged (**Fig 19.7-9**). The patient was highly satisfied with the outcome with no pain or limitation in her daily activities.

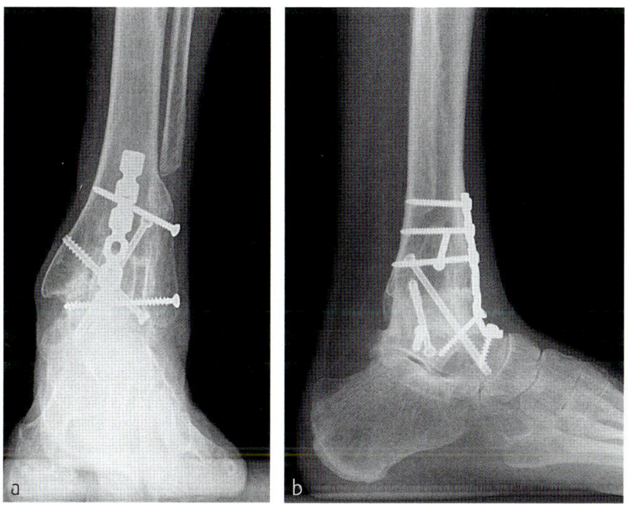

Fig 19.7-9a–b X-rays at 2 years demonstrated solid union with no signs of graft resorption or infection.
a AP view.
b Lateral view.

11 Pitfalls

- Delayed or missed diagnosis of infection
- Wrong strategy for removal of implants
- Removing too much bone stock
- Failing in adequate debridement of contaminated bone and soft tissues
- Surgical wound breakdown

12 Pearls

- Any prosthetic joint that becomes painful with an elevated CRP level should raise suspicion of infection; appropriate steps should be taken to confirm or rule out infection.
- Appropriate preoperative planning is mandatory and includes:
  - Identification of implants
  - Approach
  - Instruments for implant removal and bone debridement
  - Perfect knowledge of implant revision or tibiotalar fusion techniques

  This will minimize bone loss and improve the postoperative functional result.
- Surgical wound complications can be minimized with good surgical technique (minimizing dissection and gentle soft-tissue handling) and appropriate postoperative immobilization with stable external fixation.
- Treatment of prosthetic joint infection requires a team approach specialized in this field. This will substantially improve healing rates and outcomes.

19.8 Implant removal—chronically infected total elbow arthroplasty

Anjan P Kaushik, John C Elfar

1 Case description

A 72-year-old left-handed woman underwent semiconstrained cemented right total elbow arthroplasty (TEA) at another institution 15 years prior to presentation. She developed a deep infection 13 years after the original surgery and underwent implant removal and debridement that included radial head resection, and single-stage immediate reimplantation of a semiconstrained TEA with antibiotic-impregnated cement. Microbiology reports of cultures from the second procedure demonstrated growth of methicillin-resistant *Staphylococcus aureus* (MRSA). **Fig 19.8-1a–c** display the elbow x-rays 2 years after one-stage revision and presentation to the authors' institution. Lytic areas adjacent to the cement interface prompted a computed tomographic scan, which demonstrated further lucencies around the implant (**Fig 19.8-1d–e**).

The patient continued to have symptoms, which included limited range of motion (ROM), persistent edema, erythema of the elbow joint, and pain with use of the right elbow. The previous incision was well healed, without any sinus tracts or drainage. Laboratory studies revealed an elevated erythrocyte sedimentation rate (ESR) of 65 mm/h and C-reactive protein (CRP) level of 18 mg/L. Repeated elbow aspiration demonstrated the presence of MRSA infection on culture. The patient also had a history of bilateral total knee and bilateral total hip arthroplasties. Her left hip arthroplasty had been revised for aseptic loosening 7 years before.

Treatment options for this patient with chronically infected TEA were discussed with her, including resection arthroplasty, two-stage component removal and later reimplantation, and long-term antibiotic suppression. After discussion with her primary physician and an infectious diseases specialist for preoperative medical optimization, considering her extensive medical history, she elected to undergo extensive debridement and resection arthroplasty.

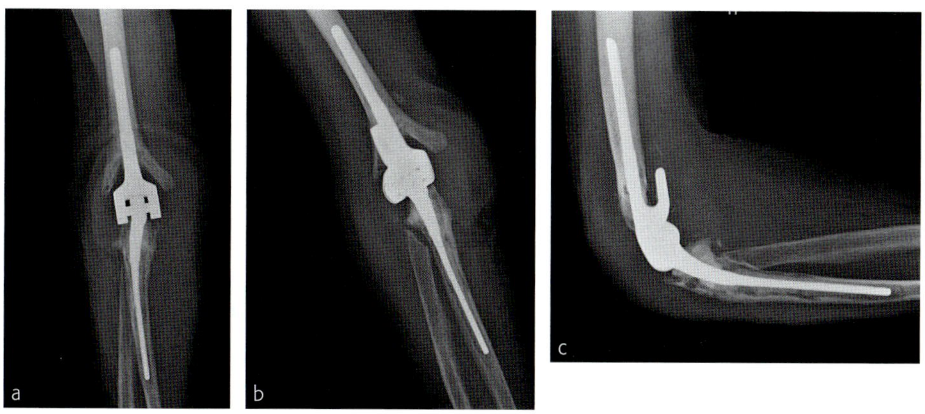

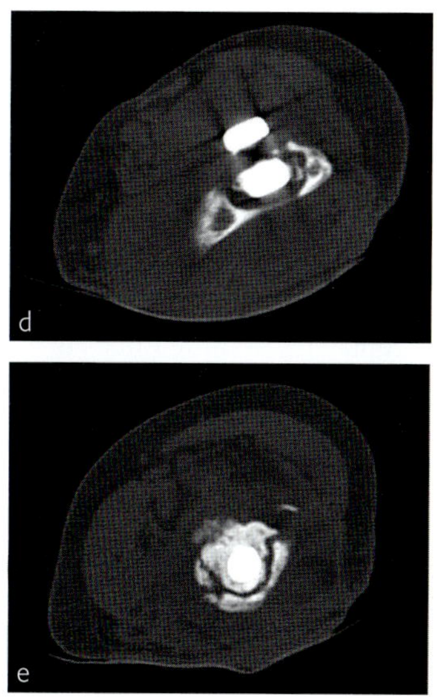

Fig 19.8-1a–e Preoperative images of the right elbow.
a AP view.
b Oblique view.
c Lateral view.
d–e Computed tomographic scans (axial cuts).

2 Background: etiologies and risk factors

Management of TEA complicated by infection can be challenging, and failure to eradicate the causative pathogens may necessitate resection arthroplasty. Infection rates after primary TEA have been reported to be in the range of 3–8% [1–6], but one series demonstrated rates up to 12% [7]. Improvements in surgical technique and implants, particularly the routine use of antibiotic-impregnated cement and avoidance of postoperative hematomas, have reduced the incidence of periprosthetic infections [3, 8].

Contributing factors to infection include the thin soft-tissue envelope around the elbow, previous procedures to the elbow, prior infections, inflammatory arthritides (rheumatoid arthritis: adult and juvenile forms), and immunocompromised host, which often results from treatment with disease-modifying antirheumatic drugs (DMARDs) or steroids [5, 9–11]. Rheumatoid patients given extensive drug regimens consisting of nonsteroidal antiinflammatory drugs (NSAIDs), steroids and DMARDs are at risk for immunosuppression, which can adversely affect surgical outcome [12]. A recent systematic review [8] has indicated concern over the recent rise in infections secondary to DMARD use. Delayed wound healing and prolonged postoperative wound drainage, as well as reoperation are also significant risk factors for infection [8–10, 13].

Revision or complex elbow surgery is also associated with higher infection rates. In one series [14], 3 (23%) of 13 patients who underwent conversion of a spontaneously fused or ankylosed elbow to TEA had infections. Infection rates for TEA performed for posttraumatic causes such as distal humeral fractures have been variable, ranging from 1–2% [15, 16] up to 5–6% [1, 17, 18]. Selected indications for TEA in the setting of trauma show a much higher incidence of infection-related failure, as is the case with gunshot wounds resulting in comminuted fractures around the elbow, which have a failure rate of 28% due to deep infection [19].

Patients with hemophilia undergoing TEA may also be at risk for periprosthetic infection, although only a small series [20] has been reported to date, in which 1 (14%) of 7 arthroplasties became infected. Total elbow arthroplasties in patients younger than 40 years were not found to increase the rate of infection significantly: 2 (4%) of 55 cases had deep infection in one series [21]. Obese patients (body mass index > 30) have a higher TEA revision rate than nonobese patients, however, the implant survival rate for deep infection was similar between these groups [22].

3 Indications: elbow resection arthroplasty

Principles for surgical treatment acquired from prosthetic joint infections in total hip and total knee arthroplasties may be applicable to the elbow [8, 23, 24]. In the treatment algorithm proposed by Bernard Morrey's group [25] at the Mayo Clinic, the most significant factors affecting outcome for revision arthroplasty for infection include duration of symptoms, patient health status, bacteriology, component fixation, bone stock, and careful surgical technique.

In the case presented, the indication for resection arthroplasty included chronic infection with a highly virulent organism (MRSA), which had failed prior one-stage revision with antibiotic-impregnated cement. Moreover, the long-term presence of the infection was a factor. Most patients with a long-term infection in a total joint arthroplasty are treated with two-stage revision. This patient with a long-term infection with a resistant organism is not always a candidate for reimplantation. Such patients should be informed that reimplantation is not always possible. This patient's fragile medical status also favored an attempt to perform a single procedure instead of multiple surgeries. Furthermore, the presence of presumably uninfected hip and knee arthroplasties raises the possibility that a chronic infection in one part of the body may eventually seed those uninvolved sites. For this reason, long-term suppressive antibiotics were not favored.

The most common treatment option for chronic TEA infections is resection arthroplasty but if the patient cannot tolerate surgery, chronic suppressive antibiotics can be administered indefinitely [9, 10]. Resection arthroplasty may be the best salvage treatment in patients who have low functional demands or who cannot medically undergo multiple extensive surgeries. The goals of surgery are to offer pain relief and to maintain adequate ROM with stability. Resection arthroplasty need not be a final solution, as the decision to proceed to a second-stage revision procedure can be made at a later date. Consultation with the infectious diseases specialist is recommended. The treatment regimen of the infection included 6 months of antibiotic treatment. After this period, eradication of the infection is confirmed with a bone biopsy from the operative site prior to the consideration of reimplantation.

4 Preoperative planning and workup

Preoperative imaging with AP, lateral, and oblique elbow x-rays should be completed to evaluate if the component fixation is stable or loose, and to examine the extent of cement penetration. Computed tomography may also assist in determining stability. Examination should focus on the patient's neurological status, elbow stability, ROM, and active muscle function, particularly active triceps motor function. A complete blood count, ESR, and CRP should also be obtained, with the CRP level serving as a baseline with which to trend the resolution of infection postoperatively [9, 25, 26]. An attempt to obtain preoperative cultures from the elbow joint should be completed with needle aspiration.

Diagnostic indications of an infected elbow arthroplasty include presence of a sinus tract and wound drainage, persistent joint inflammation or pain symptoms more than 30 days, radiographic evidence of loosening, abnormal laboratory values, and a culture positive for an organism on aspiration [26].

The surgeon should obtain operative reports from the primary TEA and other subsequent procedures, and should have details of the implants and cement technique used. Specific attention should be given to the disposition of the ulnar nerve and to the cement technique used, which present critical elements of the operative plan. Previous culture results are also helpful. In the operating room, the availability of a high-speed burr, osteotomes, curettes, implant-specific extraction instrumentation, pulsatile lavage, and antibiotic cement should be confirmed.

Intraoperative medication management in rheumatoid patients taking DMARDs and other antiinflammatories may follow the guidelines detailed by Howe and colleagues [12]. As far as duration of surgery, in the authors' experience, 2 hours are typically allowed for revision of a loose prosthesis and up to 2 additional hours allowed for each component that is believed to be well fixed. This means that this example case was booked for 4 hours for resection arthroplasty.

5 Surgical approach

A posterior triceps-sparing approach, as detailed by Bryan and Morrey [27], is commonly used. The use of a sterile tourniquet is appropriate but exsanguination with a compressive Esmarch bandage is discouraged to avoid the possibility of dissemination of infectious material from the joint. Tourniquet use is confined to 2 hours, with the first 90 minutes allowed during the beginning of the case and the final 30 minutes reserved for any new cement implantation and closure over a drain. For the standard approach, a midline incision is made through the scar of the previous surgery, and meticulous soft-tissue handling is emphasized, with the elevation of thick medial and lateral flaps and avoidance of skin pinching with forceps. Sinus tracts should be excised. Extension of the prior incision is often necessary in both the proximal and distal directions to gain additional exposure. The ulnar nerve is freed and retracted medially, and the posteromedial triceps is reflected subperiosteally, maintaining continuity with the forearm fascia [9, 25, 27]. All efforts to preserve or reattach the triceps insertion should be made. Further soft-tissue releases are completed until the previously placed implants are fully visualized. Any fluid remaining in the joint and loose connective tissue or pseudomembranes intimately associated with the implant should be sent for microscopic examination and cultures with antibiotic sensitivity testing.

6 Surgical debridement and implant removal: intraoperative steps

A thorough surgical debridement of the soft tissues should be completed, and specimens should be sent for cultures as well as frozen-section pathology. In equivocal cases, such as those with no growth on preoperative aspiration cultures, examination by the pathologist can be helpful for surgical decision making [28].

Removal of loose implants is generally straightforward, with implant-specific instruments for extraction. The bushing and pin connecting the humeral component to the ulnar component should be removed, followed by the ulnar component if it is loose. The humeral component can then be extracted with the appropriate clamp if it is loose. The components, cement fragments, and pseudomembranes associated with the implants should all be removed with the use of osteotomes, curettes, rongeurs, a motorized router, and a high-speed burr if this is possible [9, 26]. Creating a small window in the posterior cortex of the distal humerus can streamline the removal process; however, maintaining the structural integrity of the humeral shaft and distal humeral condyles is important for stability in a resection arthroplasty [9]. A nylon brush can be inserted into the medullary cavities by hand or as an attachment to the pulsatile lavage [26]. Intraoperative image intensification can be used to localize cement fragments deeper in the canal that need to be retrieved. All attempts should be made to preserve bone stock during the cement extraction and joint debridement. This is because the integrity of the shaft of the humerus and the proximal ulna are integral to the function of the forearm. Sacrifice of the humeral shaft in particular is discouraged.

Well-fixed implants, on the other hand, pose a significant technical challenge in revision arthroplasty, and osteotomies of the humerus or ulna are occasionally necessary. In the case presented, the ulnar component was loose and was easily removed. The humeral component, however, was well fixed; therefore, a 4 cm long x 1 cm wide posterior humeral trapezoidal osteotomy was completed with osteotomy of the lateral epicondyle, as depicted in **Fig 19.8-2**.

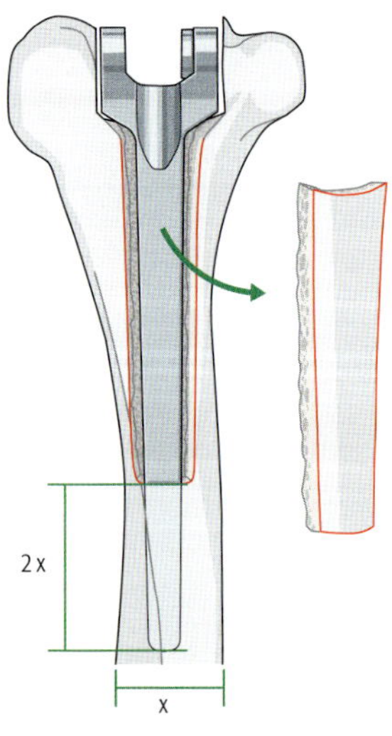

Fig 19.8-2 Osteotomy of the posterior humeral cortex for improved exposure during explantation of the humeral component.
Adapted from Cheung et al [9].

Planning the length of a humeral osteotomy is important, so if reimplantation is chosen in future, a revision humeral stem will bypass the osteotomized window by two cortical diameters proximally [9, 25]. On the ulnar side, a longitudinal osteotomy on the proximal medial part of the ulna can offer exposure to slide flexible osteotomes distally to extract the implant. A pencil-tipped burr can then be passed into the ulnar medullary cavity to remove cement fragments [9]. In both the humeral and ulnar osteotomies, the cortical windows should be preserved for bone stock to be later repaired to the humerus or ulna with suture or cerclage fixation [25]. Resorbable sutures for repair are preferred over cerclage wires. Particularly during osteotomy steps, the radial nerve should be protected along the humerus and the ulnar nerve along the ulna.

After extensive debridement of the bone, soft tissue, and cement, pulsatile irrigation is then completed with normal saline. An antibiotic-impregnated cement spacer or cement beads can be placed. These are placed as far into the medullary canals of the humerus and ulna as possible. Antibiotics commonly used include vancomycin and tobramycin. Beads can be linked by absorbable suture or by stainless steel wire and allow more surface area for elution of the antibiotics [9, 26]. In patients for whom a resection arthroplasty is considered a possible end point, bead- or cement-based elution of antibiotics can be problematic. The triceps muscle, fascia, and skin flaps should be handled meticulously and closed with monofilament sutures to reduce the chances of reinfection. Closed circuit drain suction is commonly used to reduce the incidence of hematoma formation.

For resection arthroplasty, ulnohumeral stability is mainly achieved by preserving, if possible, the medial and lateral humeral condyles, with which the residual olecranon articulates [25]. These condyles can be deepened and contoured to accommodate the proximal ulna as an articulation [9]. In some instances, one or both condyles must be removed to remove the implant, as in the present case. In such a situation, the condyle(s) can be reimplanted if the bone is viable. However, in some instances bone destruction in the setting of infection can result in nonviable bone in the condyles and may become a source of persistent infection. In this case, the lateral condyle was removed as part of the osteotomy to remove the well-fixed humeral stem. It was partially reimplanted to bolster the medial condyle and to act as a buttress against medial subluxation of the forearm in the postoperative period. The medial column was left intact.

7 Postoperative management

Postoperatively, the elbow is immobilized in extension and the drain can be removed within 1–2 days, after output diminishes to less than 20 mL every 8 hours. Cultures are followed for speciation, and an infectious diseases consultation is made for appropriate antibiotic selection according to sensitivities. An in-hospital nutritionist consultation can also be helpful for wound healing.

Intravenous antibiotics are maintained for at least 6 weeks, and serial complete blood count, ESR, and CRP serological levels are drawn to monitor for resolution of infection and inflammation [9, 25]. In cases where infection does not resolve via clinical symptoms, serological markers, or reaspiration, a repeated irrigation and debridement may be performed [26]. If the patient cannot medically tolerate additional procedures, long-term suppressive antibiotics may be the only remaining option.

8 Outcome

This particular case was selected because of the long-term history of an infection that was difficult to treat. The patient underwent resection arthroplasty without complication. Postoperative x-rays are shown in **Fig 19.8-3**. The idea of possible reimplantation in future was left open. Most patients with an infected TEA seek a plan toward reimplantation as soon as possible. Every effort should be undertaken to understand, in consultation with the infectious diseases specialist, the duration of postresection antibiotics that will be necessary to eradicate the infection. Even after this period, which in this case was predicted to be 6 months, further diagnostic testing is necessary to prove that the infection was indeed fully treated. It is only based on the results of additional testing with open or guided biopsy that the possibility of reimplantation can be visited. As a result of these considerations, in the authors' practice, the majority of patients with a complex long-term history of infection with MRSA are treated with resection arthroplasty as an end point. Little data can predict a patient's appropriateness for future reimplantation, and this must be communicated in such cases.

As noted above in this case the ulnar stem was loose and the humeral stem was well fixed, so a posterior humeral cortex osteotomy was completed to help with exposure of the proximal portion of the humeral stem for removal. This cortical window was repaired with resorbable suture after debridement. Cement removal, extensive debridement, and

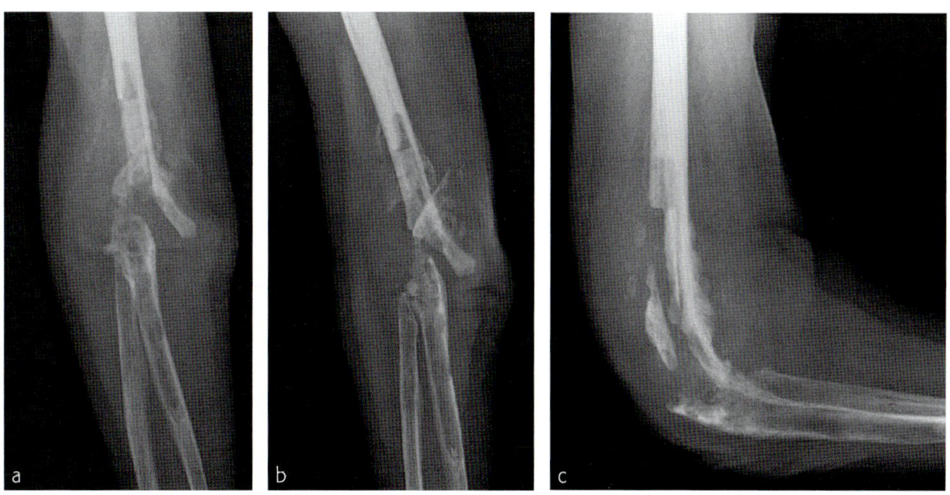

Fig 19.8-3a–c Postoperative x-rays of the right elbow.
a AP view.
b Oblique view.
c Lateral view.

irrigation were completed, and the medial condyle and shaft were contoured to encircle the remaining olecranon. Wound closure was completed and the triceps insertion was maintained. A drain was placed and a splint applied after dressing the incision.

Postoperatively, the infectious diseases specialist recommended intravenous vancomycin through a peripherally inserted central catheter line for 8 weeks and continued oral supplementation for 6 months. Intraoperative cultures again found MRSA growth that was susceptible to vancomycin. The patient was kept in a removable elbow brace locked at 60° short of full extension for 2 weeks and later fitted with a contoured thermoplast posterior long-arm splint. Physical therapy was started for passive and active-assisted ROM after 2 weeks. Weekly blood samples demonstrated improvements in the CRP and ESR levels, and the patient clinically improved with decreased elbow edema and an incision that healed uneventfully. Elbow ROM improved to an arc of 20° at full extension, to 120° of flexion.

9 Pitfalls

- The most commonly chosen treatment option for chronic TEA infections is resection arthroplasty but if the patient cannot tolerate surgery, long-term suppressive antibiotics can be administered indefinitely.
- The use of a sterile tourniquet is appropriate but exsanguination with a compressive Esmarch bandage is discouraged to avoid the possibility of dissemination of infectious material from the joint.
- Meticulous soft-tissue handling is emphasized to avoid devastating skin breakdown or triceps insufficiency. Elevation of thick medial and lateral flaps and avoidance of skin pinching with forceps is recommended.
- All attempts should be made to preserve bone stock and the integrity of the humeral condyles during the cement extraction and joint debridement.
- Well-fixed implants pose a significant technical challenge in revision arthroplasty, and osteotomies of the humerus or ulna are occasionally necessary. Planning the length of a humeral or ulnar osteotomy is important, so that if reimplantation is chosen in future, a revision stem will bypass the osteotomized window by two cortical diameters.
- In cases where infection does not resolve postoperatively, a repeated irrigation and debridement may be performed. If the patient cannot medically tolerate additional procedures, long-term suppressive antibiotics may be the only remaining option.

10 Pearls

- Resection arthroplasty may be the best salvage treatment in patients who have low functional demands or who cannot medically undergo multiple extensive surgeries.
- A thorough surgical debridement of the soft tissues should be completed, and specimens should be sent for cultures as well as frozen-section pathology.
- The implants, cement fragments, and pseudomembranes associated with the implants should all be removed with the use of osteotomes, curettes, rongeurs, and a high-speed burr. Creating a small window in the posterior cortex of the distal humerus can streamline the removal process.
- Intraoperative image intensification can be used to localize cement fragments deeper in the humeral and ulnar canals that need to be retrieved.
- In resection arthroplasty requiring osteotomies, suture fixation of osteotomy cortical windows with resorbable sutures is preferred over cerclage wires or other metallic fixation.
- For resection arthroplasty, ulnohumeral stability is mainly achieved by preserving, if possible, the medial and lateral humeral condyles with which the residual olecranon articulates.
- An antibiotic-impregnated cement spacer or cement beads can be placed.
- A suction drain should be used, and the elbow is immobilized in extension.
- Consultation with an infectious diseases specialist is highly recommended for antibiotic management and monitoring of infection resolution.

11 Other surgical alternatives and outcomes

Various options to treat an infected TEA include open or arthroscopic irrigation and debridement with retention of components, single-stage immediate exchange arthroplasty, two-stage revision arthroplasty, cemented arthrodesis, a distal humeral or total humeral tumor prosthesis, and long-term antibiotic suppression.

Debridement with retention of components is generally only reserved for cases where the symptom duration is less than 30 days, components are well fixed, the patient is in good health with a good soft-tissue envelope, and bacteriology on aspiration reveals *S aureus* and not *Staphylococcus epidermidis* [4, 25]. Open debridement typically involves a posterior approach, disarticulation of the components, removal of the bushings, extensive debridement, irrigation, and addition of antibiotic-impregnated cement beads or powder, insertion of new bushings, and closure. This procedure has a success rate of 70% eradication if *S aureus* is the offending organism, but is associated with a high complication rate [4]. Complications include wound breakdown, triceps avulsion or insufficiency, and peripheral nerve injury [4, 29]. Arthroscopic irrigation and debridement with synovectomy has also been reported, with successful eradication of methicillin-sensitive *S aureus* in one case [30], but this is not a recommended treatment alternative.

Single-stage immediate revision arthroplasty, which has been studied more in the lower extremity, is an option in patients who have had a prior infected elbow arthroplasty or prior septic native elbow. In one case series of *S aureus* infections, five of six elbows that underwent immediate exchange TEA had resolution of infection, and the other required resection arthroplasty [31]. The indications for single-stage revision TEA are limited [25, 32]; however, and in the present case, prior single-stage reimplantation was not successful at eradicating infection. It is probably true that special consideration should be given to the consequences of failure to eradicate the infection in patients who are candidates for single-stage revision. This consideration should naturally include the presence of arthroplasties in other joints that are at risk for seeding. If a single-stage revision has a higher likelihood of failure than a two-stage revision, then two-stage revision should be strongly considered in such patients who have other joints susceptible to seeding.

Staged exchange arthroplasty has been shown in some series to be somewhat successful for eradication of infection and preservation of implant and elbow function [4, 9, 26]. Indications for surgical treatment include favorable health of the patient to tolerate a revision procedure, sufficient bone stock in the humerus and ulna for reconstruction, evidence of loose components, and symptom duration of more than 30 days [25]. Persistent wound drainage or wound dehiscence also warrants early operative intervention [13].

During second-stage revision elbow arthroplasty (reimplantation), the same posterior incision is used and adhesions are released to expose the ulnohumeral joint. The cement spacer and/or beads are removed, and at least three tissue and fluid samples are again sent to pathology for frozen-section microscopic examination to confirm the absence of organisms and inflammation. If histology reveals no acute inflammation, the surgeon can proceed with preparing the medullary canals of the humerus and ulna for the new implants [9, 26]. The bone surfaces are irrigated well and dried prior to introducing the antibiotic cement. A cement restrictor may be used to limit extension proximally in the humerus. If humeral or ulnar osteotomies were performed in the first stage, the cortical windows are replaced and stabilized with cerclage cables after the appropriately sized long-stemmed implants are inserted. Allograft struts can be used as an augment option [9, 25]. The incision is again carefully closed over a drain, and a long-arm splint in extension is maintained for 48 hours to limit hematoma formation and tension on the closure. No further antibiotics are needed, and patients are allowed to work with physical and occupational therapy for elbow ROM. Lifetime restrictions limiting lifting to < 4.5 kg and repetitive lifting < 1 kg are similar to those after primary TEA [9].

A unique salvage treatment option is the use of a tumor endoprosthesis such as a total humeral replacement or distal humeral replacement. This may be used in patients who have failed multiple elbow and/or shoulder revision arthroplasties; however, the literature [33] is limited to case reports, and this method has not been extensively studied.

Cemented arthrodesis for periprosthetic infection is another possible solution, however, this has been associated with an unacceptably high complication rate and revision rate secondary to reinfection, hardware failure, or fibrous nonunion [34].

12 References

1. **Baksi DP, Pal AK, Baksi D.** Prosthetic replacement of elbow for intercondylar fractures (recent or ununited) of humerus in the elderly. *Int Orthop.* 2011 Aug;35(8):1171–1177.
2. **Schneeberger AG, Meyer DC, Yian EH.** Coonrad-Morrey total elbow replacement for primary and revision surgery: a 2- to 7.5-year follow-up study. *J Shoulder Elbow Surg.* 2007 May-Jun;16(3 Suppl):S47–54.
3. **Morrey BF, Adams RA.** Semiconstrained arthroplasty for the treatment of rheumatoid arthritis of the elbow. *J Bone Joint Surg Am.* 1992 Apr;74(4):479–490.
4. **Yamaguchi K, Adams RA, Morrey BF.** Infection after total elbow arthroplasty. *J Bone Joint Surg Am.* 1998 Apr;80(4):481–491.
5. **Kim JM, Mudgal CS, Konopka JF, et al.** Complications of total elbow arthroplasty. *J Am Acad Orthop Surg.* 2011 Jun;19(6):328–339.
6. **Krenek L, Farng E, Zingmond D, et al.** Complication and revision rates following total elbow arthroplasty. *J Hand Surg Am.* 2011 Jan;36(1):68–73.
7. **Kasten MD, Skinner HB.** Total elbow arthroplasty. An 18-year experience. *Clin Orthop Relat Res.* 1993 May;(290):177–188.
8. **Voloshin I, Schippert DW, Kakar S, et al.** Complications of total elbow replacement: a systematic review. *J Shoulder Elbow Surg.* 2011 Jan;20(1):158–168.
9. **Cheung EV, Adams RA, Morrey BF.** Reimplantation of a total elbow prosthesis following resection arthroplasty for infection. *J Bone Joint Surg Am.* 2008 Mar;90(3):589–594.
10. **Spormann C, Achermann Y, Simmen BR, et al.** Treatment strategies for periprosthetic infections after primary elbow arthroplasty. *J Shoulder Elbow Surg.* 2012 Aug;21(8):992–1000.
11. **Tachihara A, Nakamura H, Yoshioka T, et al.** Postoperative results and complications of total elbow arthroplasty in patients with rheumatoid arthritis: three types of nonconstrained arthroplasty. *Modern Rheumatol.* 2008 Oct;18(5):465–471.
12. **Howe CR, Gardner GC, Kadel NJ.** Perioperative medication management for the patient with rheumatoid arthritis. *J Am Acad Orthop Surg.* 2006 Sep;14(9):544–551.
13. **Jeon IH, Morrey BF, Anakwenze OA, et al.** Incidence and implications of early postoperative wound complications after total elbow arthroplasty. *J Shoulder Elbow Surg.* 2011 Sep;20(6):857–865.
14. **Peden JP, Morrey BF.** Total elbow replacement for the management of the ankylosed or fused elbow. *J Bone Joint Surg Br.* 2008 Sep;90(9):1198–1204.
15. **Mansat P, Nouaille Degorce H, Bonnevialle N, et al.** Total elbow arthroplasty for acute distal humeral fractures in patients over 65 years old - results of a multicenter study in 87 patients. *Orthop Traumatol Surg Res.* 2013 Nov;99(7):779–784.
16. **Chalidis B, Dimitriou C, Papadopoulos P, et al.** Total elbow arthroplasty for the treatment of insufficient distal humeral fractures. A retrospective clinical study and review of the literature. *Injury.* 2009 Jun;40(6):582–590.
17. **Throckmorton T, Zarkadas P, Sanchez-Sotelo J, et al.** Failure patterns after linked semiconstrained total elbow arthroplasty for posttraumatic arthritis. *J Bone Joint Surg Am.* 2010 Jun;92(6):1432–1441.
18. **Prasad N, Dent C.** Outcome of total elbow replacement for distal humeral fractures in the elderly: a comparison of primary surgery and surgery after failed internal fixation or conservative treatment. *J Bone Joint Surg Br.* 2008 Mar;90(3):343–348.
19. **Demiralp B, Komurcu M, Ozturk C, et al.** Total elbow arthroplasty in patients who have elbow fractures caused by gunshot injuries: 8- to 12-year follow-up study. *Arch Orthop Trauma Surg.* 2008 Jan;128(1):17–24.
20. **Marshall Brooks M, Tobase P, Karp S, et al.** Outcomes in total elbow arthroplasty in patients with haemophilia at the University of California, San Francisco: a retrospective review. *Haemophilia.* 2011 Jan;17(1):118–123.
21. **Celli A, Morrey BF.** Total elbow arthroplasty in patients forty years of age or less. *J Bone Joint Surg Am.* 2009 Jun;91(6):1414–1418.
22. **Baghdadi YM, Veillette CJ, Malone AA, et al.** Total elbow arthroplasty in obese patients. *J Bone Joint Surg Am.* 2014 May 7;96(9):e70.
23. **Achermann Y, Vogt M, Spormann C, et al.** Characteristics and outcome of 27 elbow periprosthetic joint infections: results from a 14-year cohort study of 358 elbow prostheses. *Clin Microbiol Infect.* 2011 Mar;17(3):432–438.
24. **Rand JA, Morrey BF, Bryan RS.** Management of the infected total joint arthroplasty. *Orthop Clin North Am.* 1984 Jul;15(3):491–504.
25. **Cheung EV, Yamaguchi K, Morrey BF.** Treatment of the infected total elbow arthroplasty. In: Morrey BF, Sanchez-Sotelo J, eds. *The Elbow and Its Disorders.* 4th ed. Philadelphia, Pa: Saunders Elsevier; 2009:862–874.
26. **Peach CA, Nicoletti S, Lawrence TM, et al.** Two-stage revision for the treatment of the infected total elbow arthroplasty. *Bone Joint J.* 2013 Dec;95-B(12):1681–1686.
27. **Bryan RS, Morrey BF.** Extensive posterior exposure of the elbow. A triceps-sparing approach. *Clin Orthop Relat Res.* 1982 Jun;166:188–192.
28. **Ahmadi S, Lawrence TM, Morrey BF, et al.** The value of intraoperative histology in predicting infection in patients undergoing revision elbow arthroplasty. *J Bone Joint Surg Am.* 2013 Nov;95(21):1976–1979.
29. **Duquin TR, Jacobson JA, Schleck CD, et al.** Triceps insufficiency after the treatment of deep infection following total elbow replacement. *Bone Joint J.* 2014 Jan;96-B(1):82–87.
30. **Mastrokalos DS, Zahos KA, Korres D, et al.** Arthroscopic debridement and irrigation of periprosthetic total elbow infection. *Arthroscopy.* 2006 Oct;22(10):1140.e1–3.
31. **Gille J, Ince A, Gonzalez O, et al.** Single-stage revision of peri-prosthetic infection following total elbow replacement. *J Bone Joint Surg Br.* 2006 Oct;88(10):1341–1346.
32. **Yamaguchi K, Adams RA, Morrey BF.** Semiconstrained total elbow arthroplasty in the context of treated previous infection. *J Shoulder Elbow Surg.* 1999 Sep-Oct;8(5):461–465.
33. **Wang ML, Ballard BL, Kulidjian AA, et al.** Upper extremity reconstruction with a humeral tumor endoprosthesis: a novel salvage procedure after multiple revisions of total shoulder and elbow replacements. *J Shoulder Elbow Surg.* 2011 Jan;20(1):e1–8.
34. **Otto RJ, Mulieri PJ, Cottrell BJ, et al.** Arthrodesis for failed total elbow arthroplasty with deep infection. *J Shoulder Elbow Surg.* 2014 Mar;23(3):302–307.

20 Pediatric osteomyelitis

Theddy Slongo

1 Introduction

In contrast to adults, who generally develop osteomyelitis due to an open bone injury or as a complication after a surgical procedure (osteosynthesis, joint replacement), pediatric osteomyelitis is usually acquired via a hematogenous route [1, 2], often without an obvious cause. Therefore, the diagnosis is often made late after other causes of fever or illness are considered. Especially in young children, a delayed diagnosis and late initiation of therapy often leads to severe and permanent damage [3].

The age of the child is crucial. In younger children, osteomyelitis is often coupled with purulent arthritis leading to joint destruction if the diagnosis is missed or delayed [4]. Early diagnosis and an early start to therapy are therefore paramount. As a rule we can say that the younger the child the more important it is to treat early to prevent long-term sequelae.

1.1 Occurrence and socioeconomic background of osteomyelitis

Children get osteomyelitis in the 21st century depending on their socioeconomic background. While the hematogenous osteomyelitis occurs in developed countries, in less developed countries or regions with poor medical care, local osteomyelitis caused by open wounds or fractures and poor hygienic care, and lack of antibiotics is more commonly seen [5–7].

1.2 Age of onset

Almost 80% of all cases of hematogenous osteomyelitis occur in childhood, with 80–90% occurring in the first 2 years of life. The pathophysiology shown below explains why in this age group osteomyelitis is almost always accompanied by septic arthritis. Osteomyelitis in childhood is a metaphysitis which usually involves the joint.

After puberty, with the closure of the growth plate, pediatric osteomyelitis demonstrates an identical pathology pattern to that seen in adults [8].

1.3 Morphology and anatomy

The emergence of hematogenous osteomyelitis and osteoarthritis according to age is directly related to the morphological structure of the epiphysis and metaphysis in children (**Fig 20-1**).

With septic inflammation comes an increase in pressure in the metaphyseal and diaphyseal area of the bone with reduction of blood supply, which interferes with the immune system response to the infection. Systemic antibiotics also have reduced access to the site of infection [4].

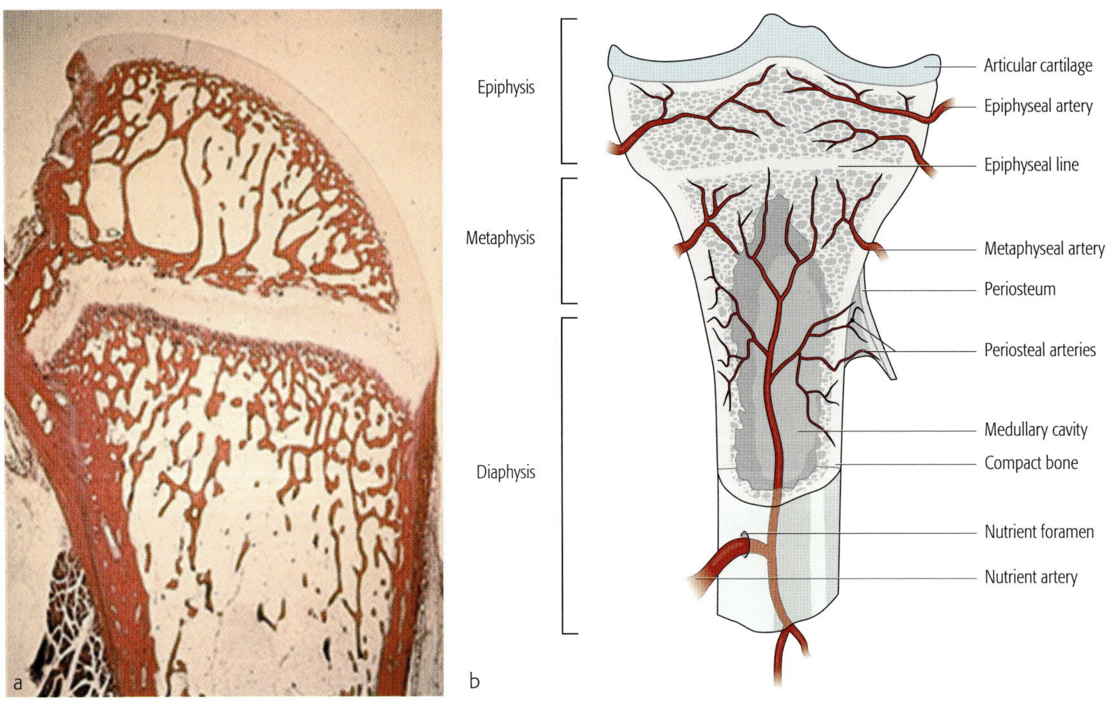

Fig 20-1a–b Vascularity of the epimetaphyseal region in the proximal tibia.
a Histological cross-section through the epimetaphyseal region with no vessels passing the growth plate.
b Cross-section with different vessels; note that all vessels for the epiphysis are not coming from the metaphysis.

1.4 Timing and pathophysiology

Time is one of the most important determinants for the outcome of osteomyelitis and septic arthritis. The younger the child, the less time may elapse before treatment. The critical time limit should not exceed 24–48 hours. Systemic antibiotics may limit the inflammatory process, but will not improve the outcome. **Table 20-1** shows this relationship as a function of the type of inflammation and age [8].

The pathophysiology differs between osteomyelitis and septic arthritis. Awareness of these differences is important for an early diagnosis and an important factor for the outcome. **Table 20-2** gives a helpful overview of the pathophysiological differences.

Days	Change	Method			
		MRI	BS	S	X-ray
0–3	Pain Inflammation/hyperemia	+	+		
3–5	Soft-tissue swelling Marrow edema/thrombosis	+	+ -	+	
7(10)–14	Osteoporosis/osteolysis Coalescence/bone perforation	+	+	 +	+
10–14	Reaction of the periosteum Reparation				+
	Sclerosis				+

Table 20-1 The significance of clinical and paraclinical signs from the first symptoms to chronic infection.
Abbreviations: MRI, magnetic resonance imaging; BS, bone scan; S, sonography.

Osteomyelitis	Purulent arthritis
→ Hematogenic infection of the medullary zone particularly the metaphyseal segment	→ Hematogenic or direct osteogenic infection of the synovia
→ Inflammatory increase of interosseous pressure within the first 24–48 hours	→ Hyperemia/enrichment of the synovia with granulocytes, these secrete proteolytic enzymes (collagenase)
→ Capillary leak, limitation of the blood circulation within the following 3–7 days; hyperemia of the periphery	→ Destruction of joint cartilage within 2–6 days
→ Breakthrough of the infection through the cortex to the subperiosteal space and to the epiphysis	→ Effusion formation with increasing intraarticular pressure leads to circulatory disorder and necrosis
→ Destroying bone matrix followed by osteolysis	→ Destruction of the capsule → joint dislocation
→ Involvement of the soft tissue and perforation (fistula) through the skin	→ Formation of fibrin also leads to malnutrition of the cartilage
→ Additional hematogenic seed with new infection is possible	→ Destruction of the cartilage leads to ankyloses of the joint
	→ A long-lasting hyperemia in the hip leads to coxa magna

Table 20-2 The pathogenic and pathophysiological steps during a bone or joint infection in childhood.

1.5 Etiology

A summary of the medical literature and personal experience is described for the development of acute osteomyelitis:

- Acute osteomyelitis usually occurs in children.
- It is usually a hematogenous infection from remote focus.
- The most common organisms responsible include:
  - *Staphylococcus aureus*
  - *Streptococcus pyogenes*
  - *Hemophilus influenzae*
  - Gram-negative organisms
- *Salmonella* infections are often seen in children with sickle-cell anemia.
- The site of infection is usually the metaphysis of long bones.

1.6 Location of pediatric infections

Table 20-3 shows the frequency of body sites of osteomyelitis and septic arthritis. It summarizes the author's own clinical data and literature survey.

For an early diagnosis of septic arthritis and osteomyelitis it is important to combine different aspects, such as patient history, clinical findings, and visual findings. The analysis and synthesis of this combination of factors determines early treatment. In addition, the subsequent diagnostic workup results give us the definitive diagnosis (**Table 20-4**).

Osteomyelitis	**%**
• Femur	26
• Tibia	25
• Humerus	12
• Fibula/radius/phalanges/calcaneus	5

Septic arthritis	
• Knee joint	40
• Hip joint	23
• Elbow joint	14
• Ankle joint	13

Table 20-3 Frequency of osteomyelitis and septic arthritis in specific body sites.

Patient history	**Clinical findings**	**Laboratory tests**
• Relieving posture • Fever • Malaise, fatigue • Pain • Previous infection	• Local tenderness • Fever • Swelling/warmth • Poor function/pseudoparalysis	• WBC/ESR/CRP • Rheumatoid factor/titer • Positive blood cultures • Kidney function BUN/creatinine
Visual diagnostics	**Surgical**	
• Plain x-ray in two planes • Sonography • Bone scan (if localization is unclear) • MRI postprimary if situation is unclear • CT scan (2-D reconstruction)	• Even if limited suspicion of infectious arthritis, always aspirate the joint with patient under anesthesia, independently of the duration of symptoms • Gram stain, culture and sensitivity, cell count, and differential • If results are positive (purulent fluid) proceed to arthrotomy and drainage • If subperiosteal liquid is present, surgical approach recommended if history longer than 48 hours	

Table 20-4 Summary of different diagnostics and their implications for further treatment.
Abbreviations: MRI, magnetic resonance imaging; WBC, white blood cell; ESR, erythrocyte sedimentation rate; CRP, C-reactive protein; BUN, blood, urea, nitrogen; MRI, magnetic resonance imaging; CT, computed tomographic.

To avoid unnecessary antibiotic therapy or surgery it is important to understand the differences in diagnostic workup between a septic and a reactive arthritis as shown in **Table 20-5.**

1.7 Therapeutic algorithm

The following author's clinical list (inpatient care) (**Table 20-6**) offers a safe algorithm for adequate treatment; this treatment must be adapted to the bacteriological results (resistance) as soon as possible. This treatment algorithm is adapted from the treatment modalities of Nade [9].

Examination	Normal	Noninfectious effusion	Septic effusion
Quantity of effusion	< 3.5 mL	Often > 3.5 mL	Often > 3.5 mL
Transparency	Transparent	Transparent	Cloudy
Color	Clear	Yellowish	Yellow-greenish
Viscosity	High	High	Different, often low
White blood cells, cells/µL	< 200	200–2,000	> 100,000
Polymorphic leukocytes	< 25%	< 25%	> 75%
Bacteriology	Negative	Negative	Frequently positive
Glucose, mmol/L	Similar to serum	Similar to serum	50% of serum value

Table 20-5 The laboratory examination results of joint fluid comparing septic and reactive arthritis in childhood.

Intravenous antibiotics	Joints	Osteomyelitis
• According to the most frequent pathogens: – *Staphylococcus aureus* – *Streptococcus* – Gram-negative bacteria • Adaptation of the antibiotics upon receipt of possible resistances – Immobilization • Hip joint – Skin traction • Other joints – Plaster-cast splints • Suspicion of osteomyelitis – Plaster-cast splint of the corresponding extremity	• If suspicious – Always aspirate and/or lavage • Particularly for hip joint – Effusions > 8 mm must always be aspirated	• Even if sonography shows no subperiosteal liquid to be visible, but bone scan is positive, start with antibiotics • Regularly repeat sonography • Consider obtaining MRI scan of body site • Plain x-rays should be obtained after 10–12 days; at this time radiological changes become visible • If there is appearance of fluid collection or bony lesions are noted, surgery is indicated to drain the fluid and debride the site

Table 20-6 Algorithm for safe treatment, to be adapted to bacteriological results.
Abbreviation: MRI, magnetic resonance imaging.

1.8 Prognosis of pediatric infections

A good prognosis if there is:

- Early diagnosis (patient history not longer than 48 hours prior to the start of therapy)
- Pathogen-specific antibiotics used rather than empiric treatment
- Rapid clinical improvement noted (improvement of the symptoms within 24–48 hours)
- No visible radiological or sonographic findings

A bad prognosis if there is:

- A time interval between symptoms to start of therapy > 5 days
- Persistence of symptoms
- An appearance of subluxation or dislocation on plain x-rays
- An appearance of joint or bone abnormality on plain x-rays
- Inadequate antibiotic therapy
- Too short a course of antibiotic therapy (4–6 weeks orally)

The best prognosis occurs if there is:

- A time interval between diagnosis to therapy < 3 days
- Radiological bone alterations or lesions visible early and consequently a combined approach to treatment
- Combined antibiotic therapy and surgery

2 Summary

- Untreated or late recognition or diagnosis of osteomyelitis and septic arthritis has serious implications for the child.
- Early diagnosis is essential, including aspiration of a joint or fluid collection.
- The antibiotic therapy must be started immediately.
- If the symptoms do not disappear within 48 hours or bony lesions or articular changes are noted, surgical intervention should be undertaken immediately.
- Failure to recognize the need for a change in therapy can have devastating consequences for the child.

3 References

1. **Carmody O, Cawely D, Dodds M, et al.** Acute haematogenous osteomyelitis in children. *Ir Med J.* 2014 Oct;107(9):269–270.
2. **Street M, Puna R, Huang M, et al.** Pediatric acute hematogenous osteomyelitis. *J Pediatr Orthop.* 2015 Sep;35(6)634–639.
3. **Faden H, Grossi M.** Acute osteomyelitis in children. Reassessment of etiologic agents and their clinical characteristics. *Am J Dis Child.* 1991 Jan;145(1):65–69.
4. **Yagupsky P, Bar-Ziv Y, Howard CB, et al.** Epidemiology, etiology, and clinical features of septic arthritis in children younger than 24 months. *Arch Pediatr Adolesc Med.* 1995 May;149(5):537–540.
5. **Christiansen P, Frederiksen B, Glazowski J, et al.** Epidemiologic, bacteriologic, and long-term follow-up data of children with acute hematogenous osteomyelitis and septic arthritis: a ten-year review. *J Pediatr Orthop B.* 1999 Oct;8(4):302–305.
6. **Bickler SW, Rode H.** Surgical services for children in developing countries. *Bull World Health Organ.* 2002;80(10):829–835.
7. **Lauschke FH, Frey CT.** Hematogenous osteomyelitis in infants and children in the northwestern region of Namibia. Management and two-year results. *J Bone Joint Surg Am.* 1994 Apr;76(4):502–510.
8. **Bonhoeffer J, Haeberle B, Schaad UB, et al.** Diagnosis of acute haematogenous osteomyelitis and septic arthritis: 20 years experience at the University Children's Hospital Basel. *Swiss Med Wkly.* 2001 Oct 6;131(39-40):575–581.
9. **Nade S.** Choice of antibiotics in management of acute osteomyelitis and acute septic arthritis in children. *Arch Dis Child.* 1977 Sept;52(9):679–682.

20.1 Osteomyelitis of the distal tibia

Theddy Slongo

1 Case description

A 3-year-old boy presents with a 5-day history of increasing pain in the left lower leg. After 2 days of fever (38.5° C), his mother notices swelling in the left distal lower leg. The child is not able to walk on the affected extremity.

The family physician's primary diagnosis was pharyngitis and probably a trauma of the lower leg. Blood examination shows a mild leukocytosis. Therapy was to medicate the fever and bed rest.

Two days later, an increasing fever (up to 40° C) developed with increasing pain and swelling of the left lower leg. The child was taken back to the family physician who administered antibiotics (amoxicillin/clavulanic acid). Advice to the mother was to call again the following day if he was not better. There was no improvement the next day, so the child was sent to the children's hospital.

1.1 Clinical examination

- 3-year-old boy with weakened condition, fever 39.5° C
- Unable to walk
- Local left lower leg examination demonstrated swelling, warmth, redness, and tenderness in the distal third of the leg
- Inguinal lymph nodes swollen and painful

1.2 Additional examination

Laboratory workup:

- White blood cell count > 30,000 cells/µL
- Erythrocyte sedimentation rate > 40 mm/h
- C-reactive protein > 300 mg/L

X-ray: lower leg AP and lateral; normal lateral view of the bone; some swelling of the soft tissue is noted (**Fig 20.1-1**).

Because of the obvious localized symptoms, the next examination for this age group is sonography (**Fig 20.1-2**, **Fig 20.1-3**).

Both the distal tibia and the joint are examined with ultrasound. A clinical picture of the examination technique is shown in **Fig 20.1-3a**.

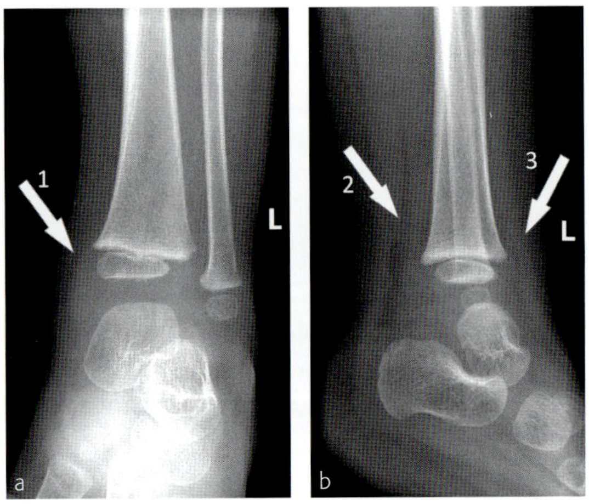

Fig 20.1-1a–b X-rays of the lower leg.

a AP view. Medial arrow 1 shows an effusion of the ankle joint.

b Lateral view. Arrow 2 shows the posterior swelling between the fascial layers. Arrow 3 shows the pus penetrating the fascia creating a subcutaneous abscess.

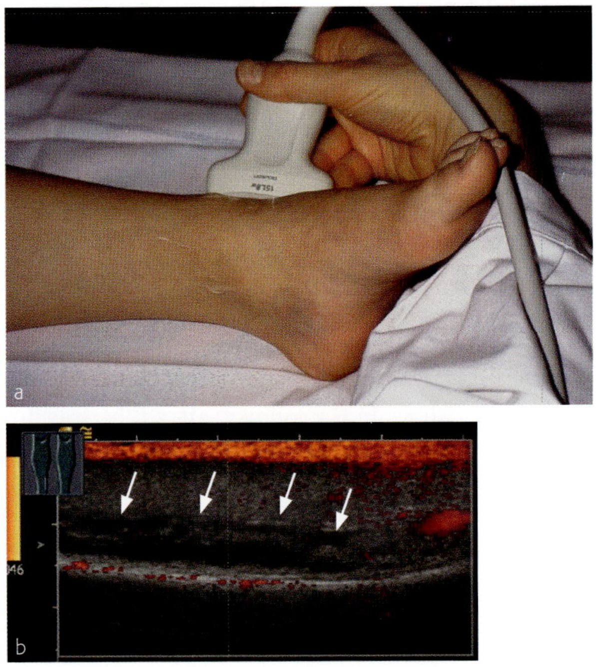

Fig 20.1-3a–b Ultrasound examination of the distal tibia.

a Photograph of ultrasound examination technique.

b Ultrasound image showing the abscess over the cortex surface (arrows).

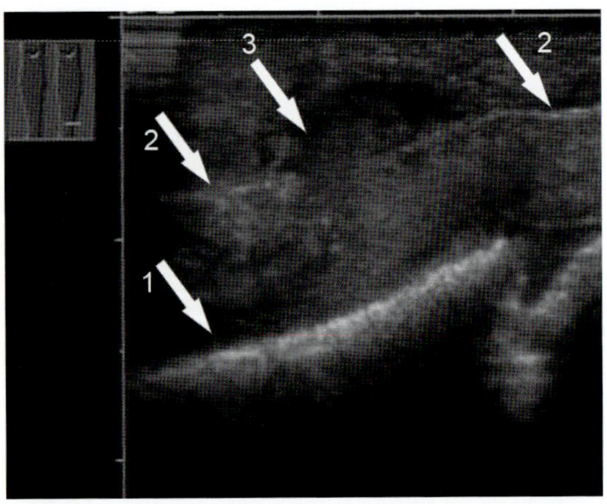

Fig 20.1-2 Sonographic image. Arrow 1 shows the ankle joint effusion; arrow 2, the fascial layer swelling; and arrow 3, the pus penetrating the fascia creating a subcutaneous abscess.

2 Indication

The clinical and patient history and results of the blood examination and sonography are clear indications for surgical intervention. Delay will increase the risk for a systemic sepsis and additional damage of the distal tibial physis.

3 Preoperative planning

Sonographic localization of the process was concordant with x-ray findings and helped with planning of an anterolateral approach; if needed, from the same incision, the posterior tibia can also be explored. In **Fig 20.1-1** the medial arrow 1 shows an effusion of the ankle joint. On the lateral view arrow 2 shows the posterior swelling between the fascial layers.

4 Patient positioning

The child is positioned supine. The leg is draped sterilely over the knee joint so that the knee can be bent and the lower leg moved freely (**Fig 20.1-4**).

The author prefers to have the knee bent and positioned on a mobile, sterile leg holder (**Fig 20.1-5**).

A nonsterile tourniquet is used on the thigh (300 mm Hg).

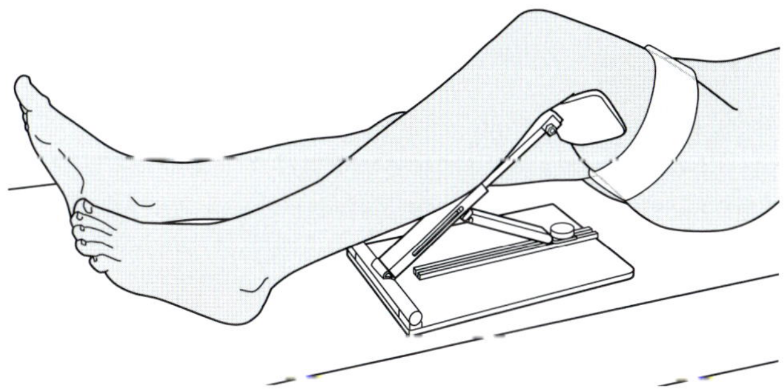

Fig 20.1-4 The child is positioned supine. The leg is draped sterilely over the knee joint so that the knee can be bent and the lower leg moved freely.

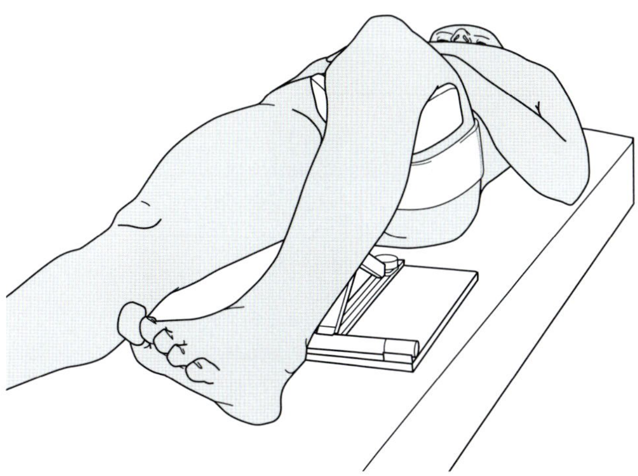

Fig 20.1-5 The knee is bent and positioned on a mobile, sterile leg holder.

5 Surgical approach

A 12–15 cm long skin incision is performed as shown in **Fig 20.1-6**. After the incision of the fascia, exposure of the tendons and muscles is achieved by blunt dissection.

As was evident on the sonography, the pus has perforated the periosteum and the deep fascia so the pus drained under pressure.

6 Surgical debridement

After irrigation of the different areas around the muscles and subperiosteal space, the ankle joint must also be opened.

The capsule is opened, irrigated, and drained.

Because the origin of the infection is in the bone, the cortex must be opened widely by chisel or burr (**Fig 20.1-7**).

The bone is drained for 3–4 days.

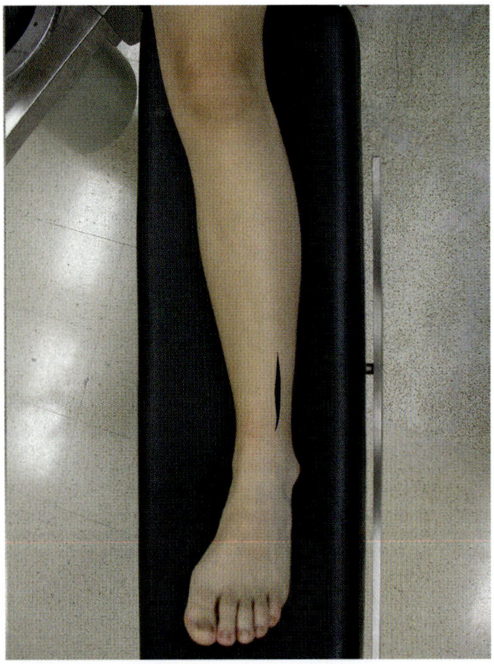

Fig 20.1-6 A 12–15 cm long skin incision is made.

7 Temporary fixation

For pain management and care, it is recommended to apply a dorsal lower leg plaster cast, or better, a fiberglass cast split or a prefabricated splint. The author prefers a precontoured U-cork splint (**Fig 20.1-8**) which is easy to change for wound control and nursing, and is also washable.

In more critical cases and in older children, application of a small external fixator for immobilization and elevation of the leg is recommended.

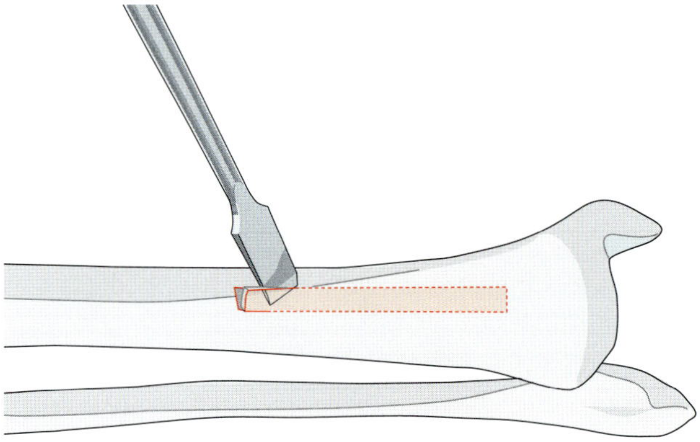

Fig 20.1-7 The origin of the infection is in the bone so the cortex must be opened widely by chisel or burr.

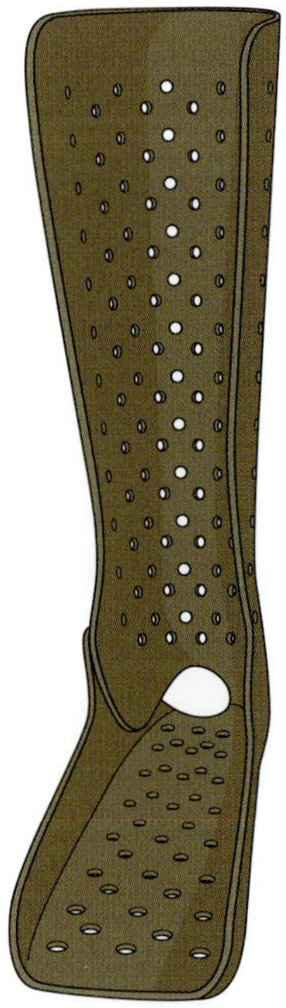

Fig 20.1-8 A precontoured U-cork splint.

8 Postoperative management

The child should receive intravenous antibiotics for at least 7–14 days depending on the blood test results; it is recommended to initiate a longer-term intravenous approach. The author recommends a central venous catheter. This is more comfortable for the child and prevents multiple new painful venopunctures.

The drains remain in place for at least 2–3 days.

After wound healing, a lower leg soft cast is applied for at least 4–6 weeks until there is evidence of good bone consolidation of the bone window.

Long-term oral antibiotics are continued until the C-reactive protein level has normalized, typically at least 4–6 weeks.

9 Outcome

In this case the healing occurred without complication as expected. In the long-term follow-up no axial deviation and no growth arrest was seen. Function of the ankle joint returned to normal after 8 weeks.

10 Pitfalls

Regarding the child's age, the symptoms, and the local situation, the diagnosis should not have been missed or the symptoms should not have been misinterpreted for such a long time. In this case the algorithm shown in **Table 20-3** would lead to the correct diagnosis earlier, permitting more timely treatment.

11 Pearls

The correct interpretation of symptoms leads to early diagnosis and treatment with intravenous antibiotics. In most cases antibiotic therapy within the first 24 hours can prevent surgery. A high index of suspicion for the diagnosis of infection is essential.

20.2 Osteomyelitis of the proximal humerus

Theddy Slongo

1 Case description

A 14-year-old boy presented with recurrent fever for 3 weeks and increasing pain in the left shoulder. The boy had a history of falling onto the left shoulder during gymnastics.

The first consultation with his general practitioner was approximately 10 days after the onset of symptoms.

The diagnosis of this consultation was painful swelling of the left shoulder and proximal humerus compatible with trauma. X-rays showed no fracture (**Fig 20.2-1**). The recommendation of the general practitioner was pain medication, arm sling, and to return for assessment if the symptoms did not resolve after a few days.

In a second consultation 5 days later the boy had the same symptoms, increasing pain, and more swelling. He had normal body temperature. Blood tests showed C-reactive protein (CRP) level between 80–90 mg/L and white blood cell count of 12,000 cells/μL. Therapy at this time was use of a sling, to continue with pain medication, and prescription steroids.

On the follow-up examination the patient had increasing swelling and pain. The general practitioner sent the boy to the local hospital for further investigation.

New blood tests showed CRP level > 250 mg/L and white blood cell count > 20,000 cells/μL.

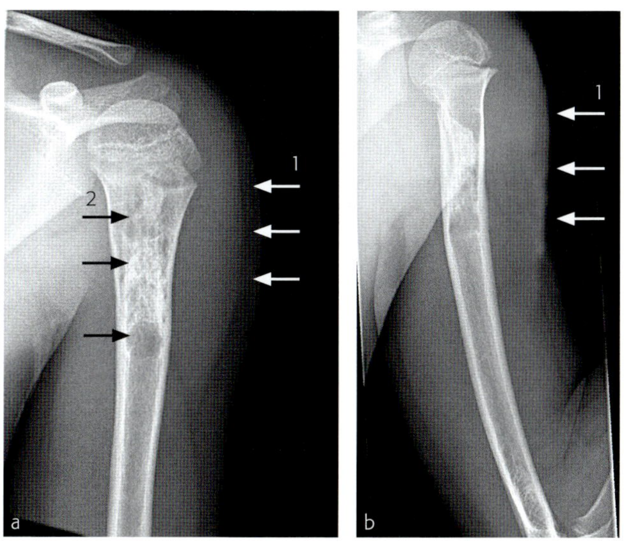

Fig 20.2-1a–b Initial x-rays made by the general practitioner 3 weeks before admission to the author's hospital. These x-rays were completely misinterpreted as "normal". On the AP (**a**) and lateral (**b**) views we see the following pathological signs:

1 Important swelling of the region of the deltoid muscle.
2 Pathological changes of the metaphyseal proximal part of the humerus with sclerotic and osteolytic zones.

These signs are highly suspicious for an active process in the bone and soft-tissue infection or an aggressive tumor.

Sonography was obtained showing a subcutaneous cystic mass 14.7 cm long and 3.8 cm thick (**Fig 20.2-2**). In addition, a computed tomographic (CT) scan was performed (**Fig 20.2-3a–c**).

For the treating pediatrician and the radiologist the situation was unclear and they decided to perform a needle aspiration of the cystic lesion which yielded a lot of pus.

Diagnosis at transfer was subcutaneous abscess. The child was transferred with this diagnosis to the author's clinic.

1.1 Clinical examination

At admission to the author's clinic emergency department the boy presents with these symptoms:

- Hyperemic shoulder and humeral region
- Doughy swelling
- Painful and pseudoparalytic shoulder

1.2 Additional examination

In this case no additional examinations were carried out. The prior sonography pictures, CT scan with 2-D reconstruction, and blood tests were obtained.

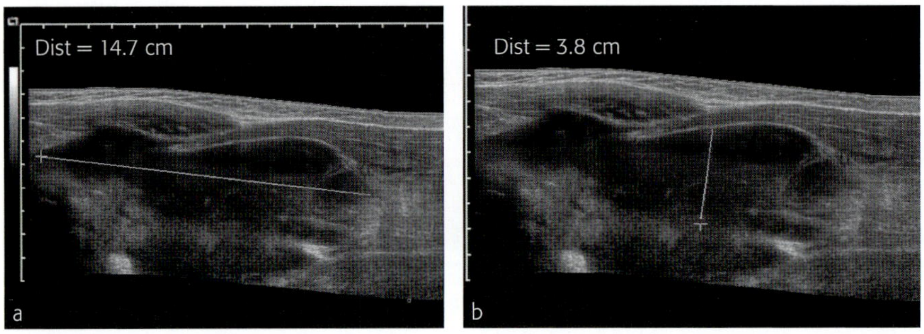

Fig 20.2-2a–b The ultrasound images show a large abscess in the proximal humerus 14.7 cm long and 3.8 cm thick. The defect in the cortical bone is also shown. This is a sign that the infection or process comes from the bone.

2 Indication

According to the history, blood examination values, and radiological investigation, the diagnosis of an advanced osteomyelitis with bone fistula was established (**Fig 20.2-3d–f**).

3 Preoperative planning

Since there was no doubt about the active osteomyelitis, intravenous antibiotics were started (ie, clindamycin). Even though the boy was 14-years-old at the time of admission, the proximal physis was still open. The parents were informed about potential complications of growth arrest or malalignment.

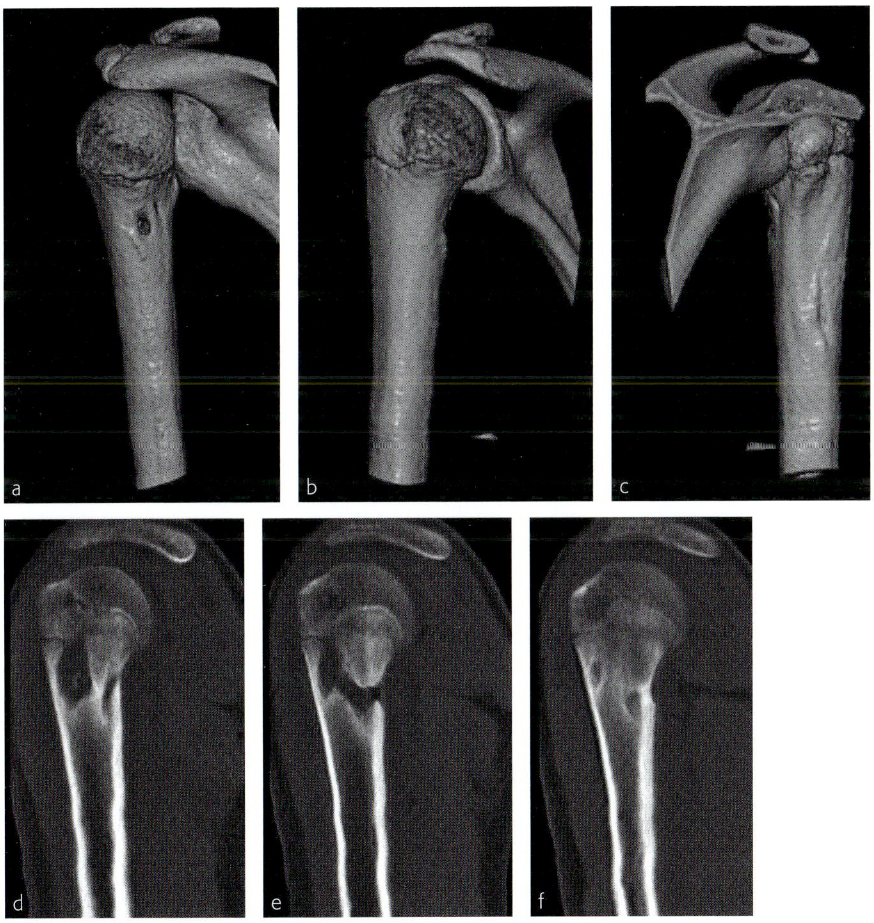

Fig 20.2-3a–f 3-D CT scans (**a–c**) and 2-D (**d–f**) x-rays.

a–c In the 3-D reconstructions of these computed tomographic scans only the perforation on the anteromedial side is shown. These images demonstrate that 3-D reconstructions are less helpful for diagnosis than the more informative 2-D x-rays.

d–f 2-D x-rays clearly show the large lytic zone in the metaphysis and the perforation of the cortex which is responsible for the abscess in the proximal humerus. However, the physis is still not involved.

4 Surgical approach

Because the abscess extended in a circular fashion through the intermuscular and subcutaneous tissues, it was important to discuss which approach was the least traumatic and best for curettage of the proximal humerus.

The incision was made at the anterior sulcus along the anterior border of the deltoid muscle—the deltopectoral approach (**Fig 20.2-4**), making a blunt dissection of the muscle (**Fig 20.2-5**). The exposure was easy because of the large intermuscular abscess, so the dissection was mostly accomplished by the process.

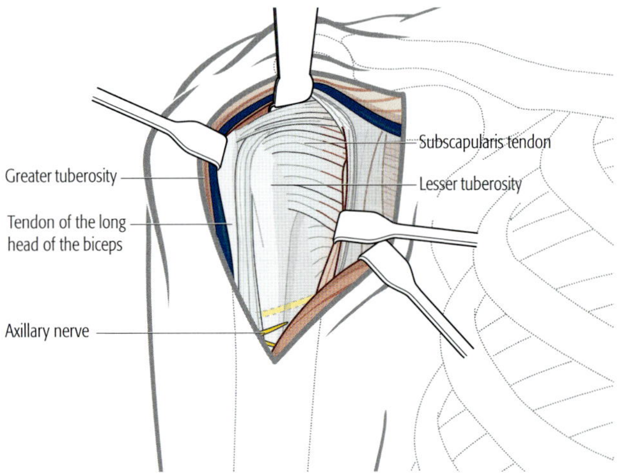

Fig 20.2-4 The approach to the proximal-medial humerus was made by a deltopectoral approach, along the anterior border of the deltoid muscle.

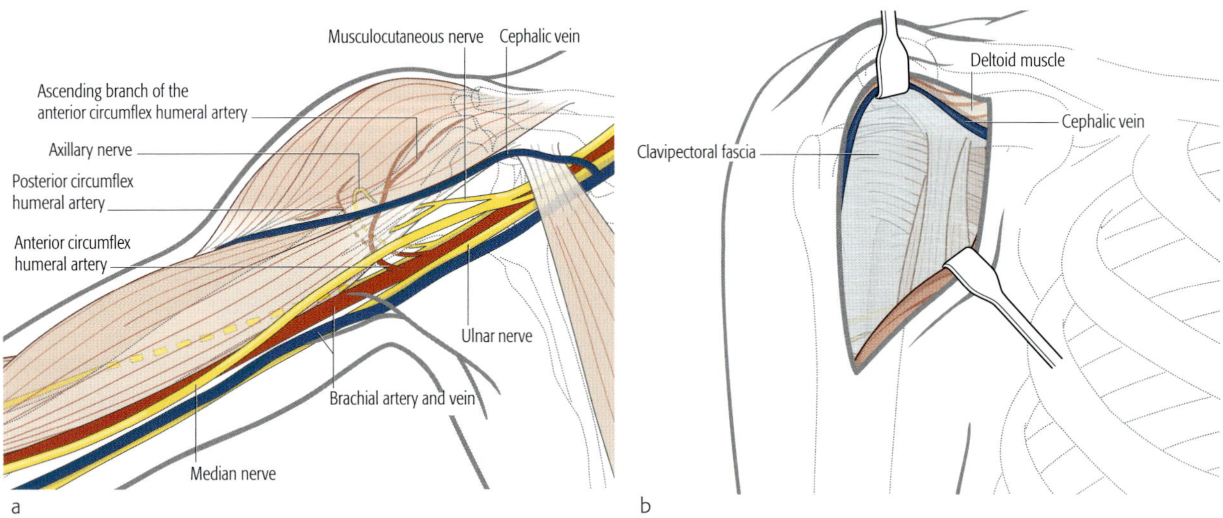

Fig 20.2-5a–b Nerve and vascular damage can be prevented with the preparation along the anterior border of the deltoid muscle; careful attention must be paid to the cephalic vein so rounded smooth retractors are recommended. In this case the dissection was nearly completely performed by the abscess.

5 Surgical debridement

Once all the muscles were dissected at least 2/3 of the circumference of the proximal humerus was exposed well.

The bony fistula at the anterior aspect of the humerus was visible.

Before opening the cortex of the proximal humerus and performing curettage, the different abscesses between the muscles were debrided and washed out.

Two drains were inserted, one more proximally and posterior, the other more distally and anterior.

The bone was then opened using a long cortical window more from the medial side (as shown on the postoperative x-rays) (**Fig 20.2-6**). The reason for that approach was the thin cortex on the medial side which could easily be perforated by finger pressure.

Then, the infected and destroyed cancellous metaphyseal bone was removed leaving a big hole in the proximal metaphysis.

The fistula was also debrided using a curette.

As the pus was mostly located in the soft tissue and intermuscular area and less in the metaphysis, no drain was placed in the bone cavity. A gentamicin-impregnated sponge was placed in the large metaphyseal hole. The wound was then closed with a few deep stiches.

6 Temporary fixation

In this case, the bone was still stable with a medial cortical defect so no fixation was needed. It was believed that the weakness created by presence of the medial defect was unlikely to fracture.

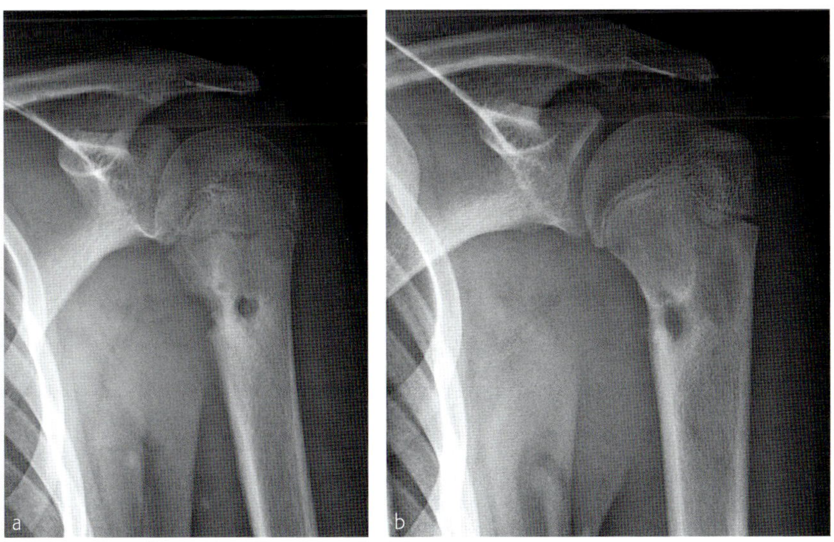

Fig 20.2-6a–b The postoperative x-rays show the medial defect where the large window was made. In this region the cortex was thin. In addition, we can see the bigger hole of the fistula after curettage.

a AP view.
b Lateral view.

7 Postoperative management

While the subcutaneous drain was in place for 3 days the arm was immobilized in the bed within a sling (**Fig 20.2-7**).

According to the bacteriology results, *Staphylococcus aureus*, sensitive to nearly all antibiotics, grew in the culture. Clindamycin was continued intravenously for 10 days according to the hospital guidelines. After 10 days, the antibiotic therapy was continued orally for 1 week after CRP level had normalized.

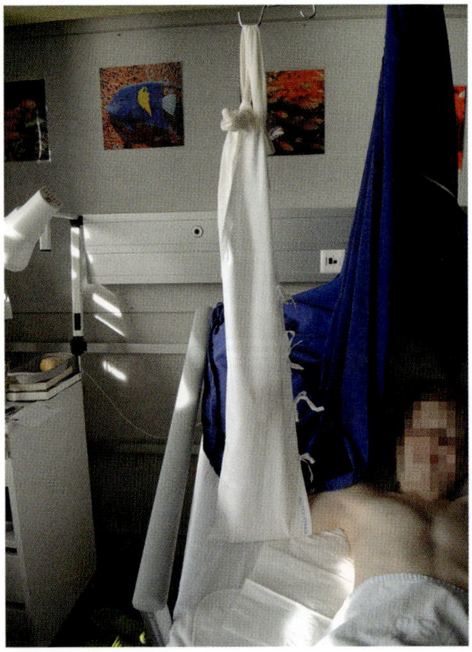

Fig 20.2-7 Immobilization of the arm using a sling.

8 Outcome

The further clinical evolution and follow-up was not problematic. X-rays after 1 month showed the bone defect appeared larger and there was concern about healing (**Fig 20.2-8**). X-rays 2 months later demonstrated that the defect began to fill up (**Fig 20.2-9**). After 1 year, the bone defect was completely healed and the bone appeared to be normal (**Fig 20.2-10**). Functionally the shoulder was also normal and the patient was pain free.

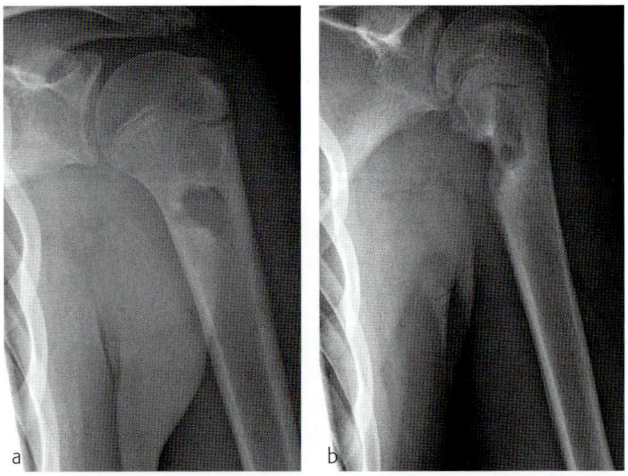

Fig 20.2-8a–b The first follow-up x-rays show that the bone defect is larger than visualized immediately postoperatively. This could indicate an ongoing active infection, but the clinical situation (ie, no swelling, no pain) and the blood laboratory tests (ie, C-reactive protein level nearly normal) show that there is no active process and that this resorption is the normal reaction of the bone.

a AP view.
b Lateral view.

9 Pitfalls

Even when all symptoms suggested an osteomyelitis (ie, pain, swelling, fever, and abscess), those symptoms were misinterpreted and the diagnosis was delayed for a long time; the clearly abnormal x-rays were interpreted as normal (see **Fig 20.2-1**). In such cases, there are undesirable long-term results, growth problems or malunion [1–3].

10 Pearl

In these neglected cases the result can be complications, such as septicemia and long-term growth problems. However, extensive exploration and debridement of the bony abscess resulted in these problems being avoided and there was a functional and anatomically normal outcome (**Fig 20.2-10**). The shoulder mobility was symmetrical, and the head of the humerus as well as the joint appeared normal.

11 References

1. **Ilharreborde B.** Sequelae of pediatric osteoarticular infection. *Orthop Traumatol Surg Res.* 2015 Feb;101(1 Suppl):S129–137.
2. **Nduaguba AM, Flynn JM, Sankar WN.** Septic arthritis of the elbow in children: clinical presentation and microbiological profile. *J Pediatr Orthop.* 2016 Jan;36(1):75–79.
3. **Carmody O, Cawley D, Dodds M, et al.** Acute haematogenous osteomyelitis in children. *Ir Med J.* 2014 Oct;107(9):269–270.

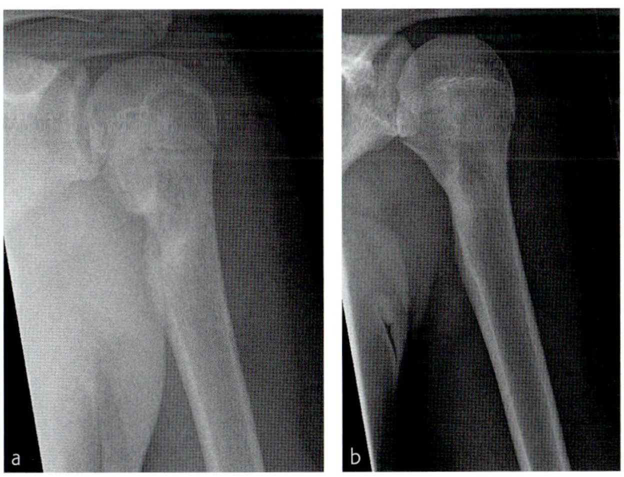

Fig 20.2-9a–b The second follow-up x-rays after 3 months show progressive healing with normal bone formation and decreasing defect.
a AP view.
b Lateral view.

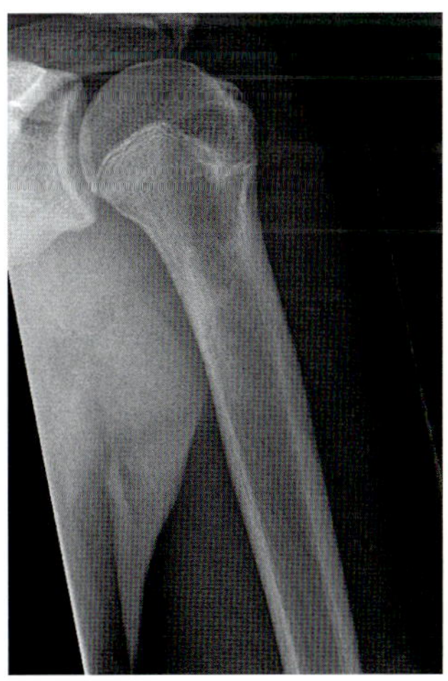

Fig 20.2-10 The follow-up x-ray after 1 year shows full recovery with normal bone structure.

20.3 Postoperative osteomyelitis of the tibia

Theddy Slongo

1 Case description

A 14.5-year-old girl sustained a ski injury (ie, torsion of the leg when the right ski was fixed). This injury resulted in a closed, long spiral isolated tibial fracture with a long butterfly fragment (AO Pediatric Classification 42t–D/5.2). No other injuries were present (**Fig 20.3-1**).

The child was transferred to a local hospital for treatment. The surgeon performed "old-fashioned" open reduction and external fixation (ie, wide exploration and a screw in every hole) and plating of the tibia (**Fig 20.3-2**).

After 5 days the patient went home. At this time, according to the girl's mother, there was marked swelling and the whole lower leg was still painful. Over the next 2 weeks, the child was always in pain with a low temperature and the anterior part over the suture had an increasing hyperemia. After 16 days she returned to the surgeon for a postoperative visit.

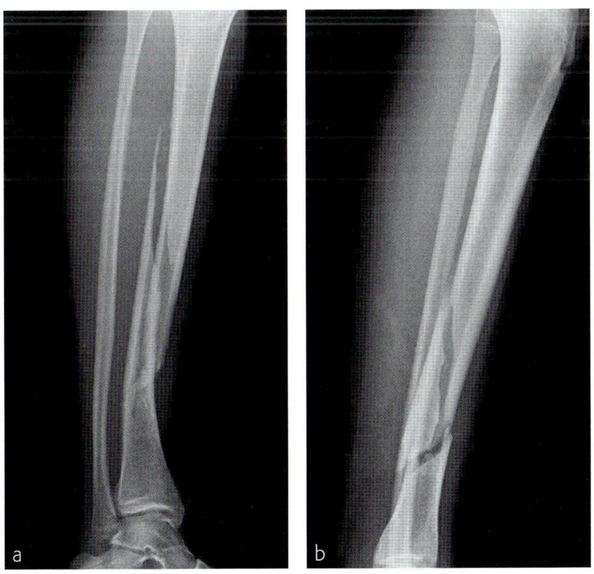

Fig 20.3-1a–b Initial x-rays show a minimally displaced and not severely angulated comminuted isolated tibial shaft fracture. Since the fibula is intact, a too rigid fixation can cause healing problems even in children. Therefore, nonoperative treatment can also be discussed.
a AP view.
b Lateral view.

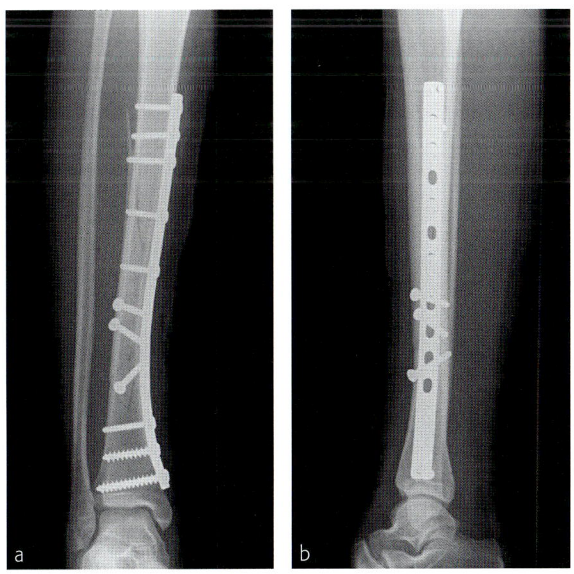

Fig 20.3-2a–b Postoperative x-rays show a dynamic compression plate osteosynthesis in a rigid fashion; in addition there are three lag screws for the butterfly fragment. To make such an anatomical osteosynthesis with absolute stability, a wide approach is necessary.
a AP view.
b Lateral view.

1.1 Clinical examination 16 days postoperatively

The patient had a weakened condition with elevated temperature (~38° C), severely swollen lower leg, severe local hyperemia, and secretion from the distal wound. Blood testing demonstrated a white blood cell count > 15,000 cells/µL. A new x-ray was taken which added no new information (**Fig 20.3-3**). The decision was made to start oral antibiotics and revisit the case in 3–5 days.

Over the next 3 weeks the situation did not markedly change. After starting antibiotics, the swelling and local hyperemia decreased. After 10 days of antibiotic therapy, all the symptoms were slowly returning. So 5 weeks after the operation the attending surgeon ordered a computed tomographic scan (**Fig 20.3-4**). The decision was made to continue antibiotics because there were no obvious signs of osteomyelitis or bone sequestrum.

After 7 weeks, two blisters had formed in the distal third of the wound (**Fig 20.3-5**). In addition, a new x-ray was taken showing some callus formation in the proximal fracture region, with no healing reaction in the distal part (**Fig 20.3-6**). At this time, the child was sent to the author's clinic.

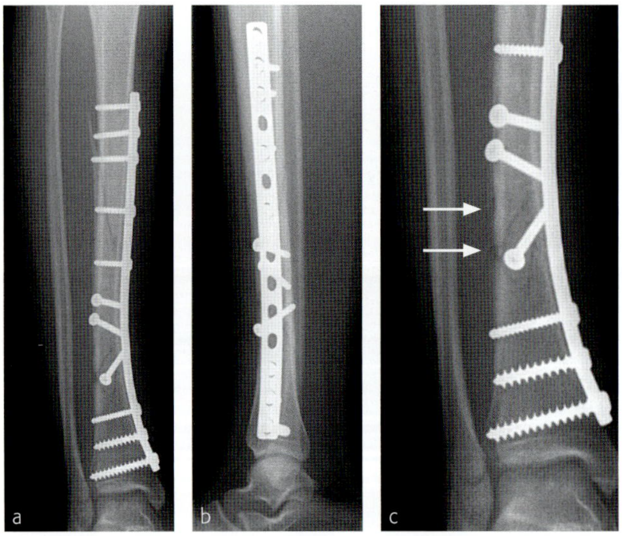

Fig 20.3-3a–c
a–b After 16 days new x-rays were taken because the patient returned with swelling and pain. The radiologist and the surgeon interpreted these new pictures as unobtrusive. But some resorption and irregularity on the lateral cortex is visible.
c The detailed view clearly shows this resorption (arrows).

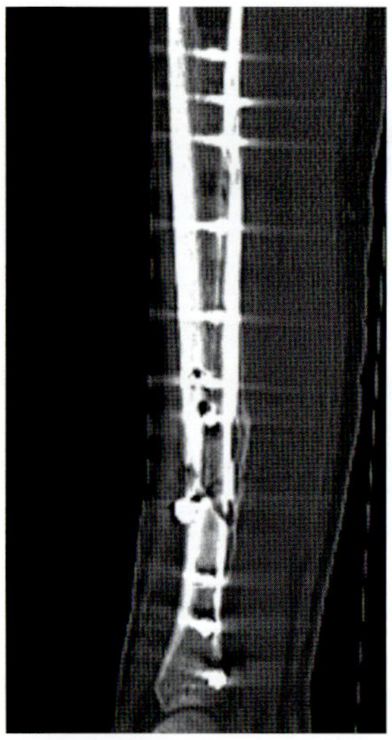

Fig 20.3-4 In this 2-D computed tomographic scan cut the resorption zone is much clearer; this was initially misinterpreted.

1.2 Clinical examination on presentation at the author's clinic

The 14.5-year-old girl was 7 weeks postoperative with no fever. The local situation showed slight swelling, slight hyperemia, the proximal wound had healed, and the distal wound had two fistulas with cloudy liquid draining (**Fig 20.3-5**).

1.3 Additional examination

When the child was sent to the author's clinic, the prior examinations and radiological investigations were obtained. Together with the information on the clinical situation (**Fig 20.3-5**) there was no need for further examinations.

A bone scan could have been discussed, but in children a necrotic or avital bone is rare and during the planned revision it can be checked clinically.

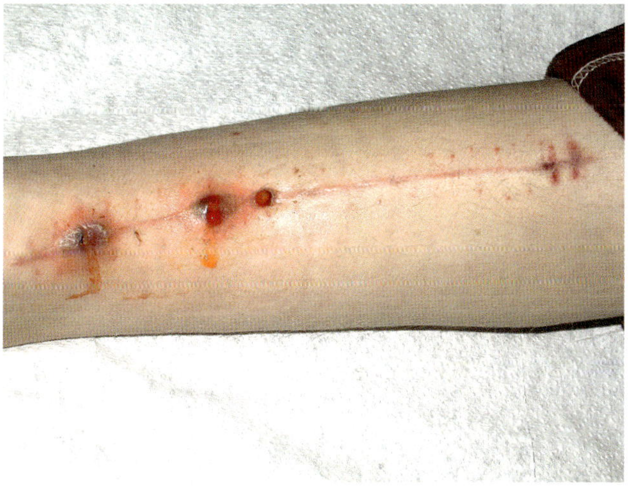

Fig 20.3-5 The first clinical picture of the local situation showing the blisters and swollen distal lower third of the leg.

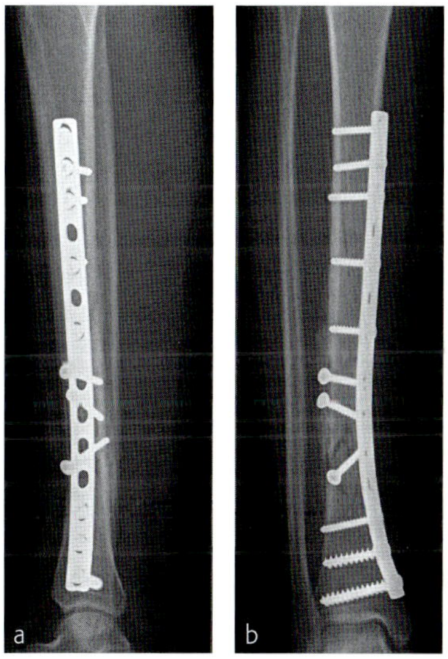

Fig 20.3-6a–b Because of a swollen, painful leg and blisters in the distal third a new x-ray was taken after 7 weeks: in the upper part there is some healing but in the distal part progressive resorption is a sign of infection.
a AP view.
b Lateral view.

2 Indication

This was an infected plate osteosynthesis with insufficient management of the situation. In addition, there were two fistulas with purulent drainage. Therefore, there was a clear indication for immediate revision surgery.

3 Preoperative planning

1. Removal of the plate followed by local debridement and removal of all potential dead bone.
2. Fixation with a ring fixator and cleaning of the wound with negative-pressure wound therapy (NPWT) closure dressing.

The goal is to treat the infection and close the wound as a secondary healing without additional surgery, and to fix the nonunion with the ring fixator up to complete bone healing, with no change to fixation.

4 Surgical approach

1. The patient is in supine position with no tourniquet with preparation and draping of the right leg above the knee.
2. Reopening of the wound along the first incision and excision of the fistulae.
3. Removal of the plate because the screws were still well fixed in the proximal part, however, almost all distal screws were loosened.

5 Surgical debridement

Once the plate was removed, it was clear that the first surgeon had stripped nearly all the periosteum from the tibia. Surrounding 50% of the length of the plate was a large cavity of infection with pus, and only in the proximal half had the soft tissue adhered to the plate.

Three small, free sequestrae were removed which were not seen on the x-ray or the computed tomographic scan. The large butterfly spiral wedge was not in contact with the periosteum and was white.

Since the main proximal and distal fragments had good blood supply, they were left in situ. In children this is permitted because of the increased ability for rapid healing and revascularization.

6 Temporary and definitive fixation

1. Placement of a ring fixator for good stabilization allows for full weight bearing on the one hand and biological distraction/compression on the other hand.
2. Application of an NPWT dressing for wound closure. To apply such a dressing in combination with an external fixator a special liquid rubber was used around the pins to achieve an airtight closure (**Fig 20.3-7**, **Fig 20.3-8**, **Fig 20.3-9**).

Due to the patient's age there was high healing potential so the goal was to have a stable and dynamic fixation that could be used to assist healing. **Fig 20.3-10** shows the postoperative x-ray with the ring fixator in situ; the small bone defect is visible from where the small sequestra was removed, most clearly visible on the lateral view **Fig 20.3-10a**.

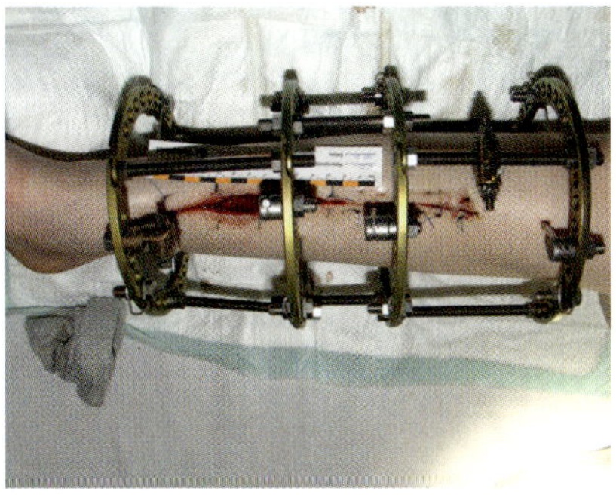

Fig 20.3-7 Clinical situation after debridement and wound cleaning and before application of negative-pressure wound therapy closure. In the region where the fistulas and blisters were resected the wound was left open. This was a good approach for the negative pressure wound therapy closure.

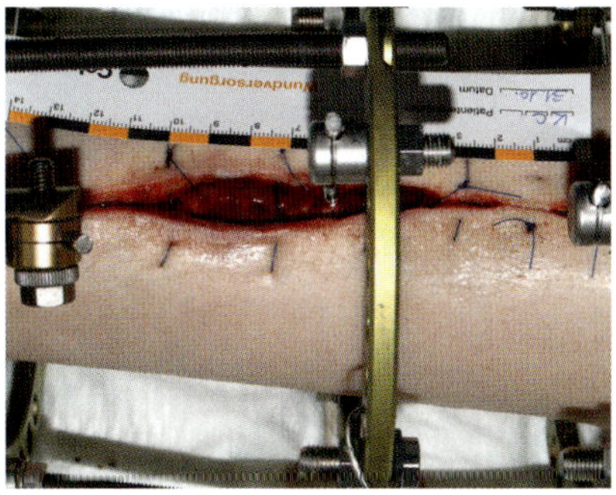

Fig 20.3-8 Bleeding bone after removal of the three small sequestrae. One half-pin was inserted directly into the large butterfly segment to hold it in place.

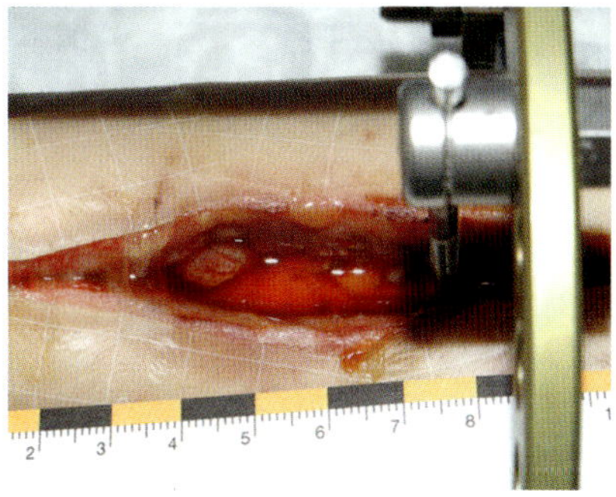

Fig 20.3-9 Situation during the first negative-pressure wound therapy closure exchange.

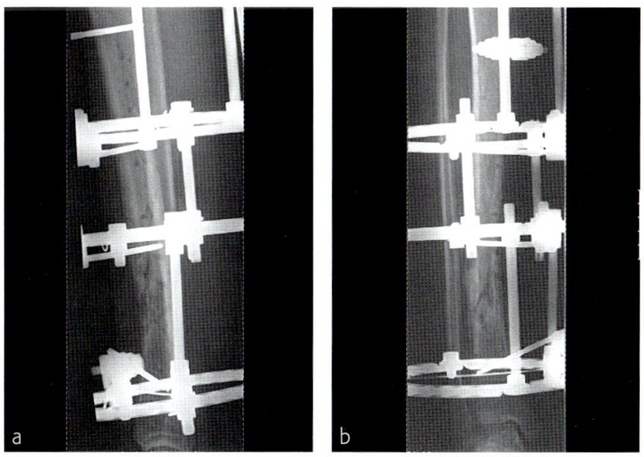

Fig 20.3-10a–b Some days after plate removal and debridement: the ring fixator is fixing the fracture.

a On this lateral view the bone defect on the anterior aspect is clearly visible.

b The AP view shows a good alignment of the fracture and fragments.

7 Postoperative management

The first NPWT dressing was left in place for 3 days before it was changed. During this short time there was a clear improvement; the base of the wound and the bone appeared red and healthy, which was evidence for revascularization (**Fig 20.3-11**).

The child was positioned in the bed or wheelchair with the leg in an elevated position. Because of the duration of symptoms and the length of time for which the child had taken antibiotics, the pediatric infection specialist advised stopping the oral antibiotics [1–3]. The focus was on the local treatment. The circulation could be stimulated and accelerated with wound care. This is sufficient management in a healthy child.

Over the next 3 weeks, the NPWT treatment was continued and there was rapid healing and closure of the wound. At this time the child was allowed to walk with partial weight bearing as tolerated (**Fig 20.3-12**, **Fig 20.3-13**).

After 4 weeks the child was discharged from the clinic in a good general condition. Further follow-up care was provided by the homecare nurse. The child was followed up in the clinic every 2 weeks.

Six weeks after beginning treatment in the author's clinic, there was good healing and integration of the free butterfly fragment. In addition, good callus formation was also visible (**Fig 20.3-14**).

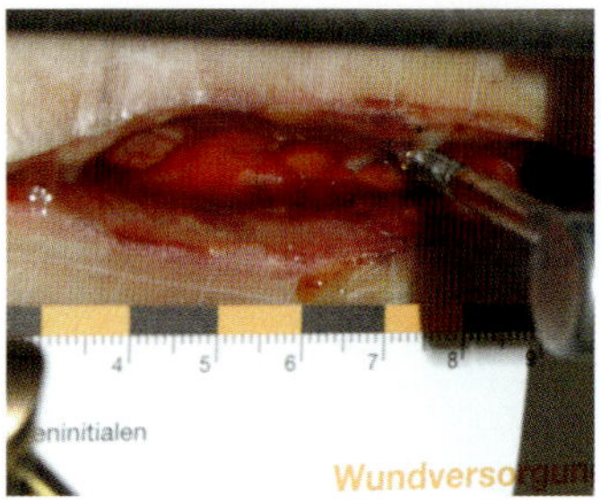

Fig 20.3-11 Detailed view of when the negative-pressure wound therapy closure was exchanged the second time. To check the healing progress, a scale was always used for photographic documentation. The skin protection for the negative-pressure wound therapy closure dressing is also visible.

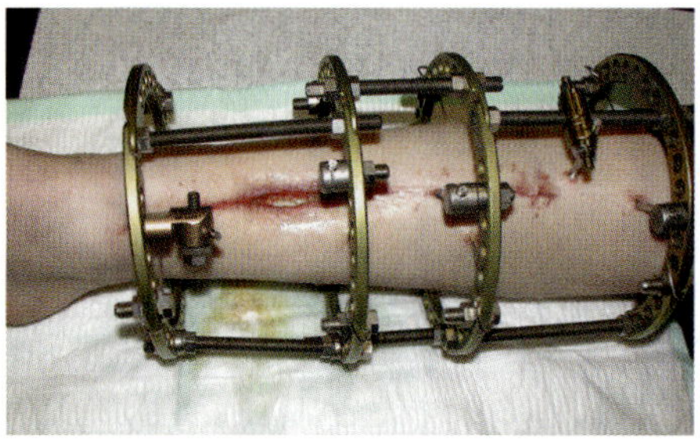

Fig 20.3-12 Clinical situation after 3 weeks of negative-pressure wound therapy closure. At this point the therapy was stopped. Now the patient was allowed and stimulated to walk bearing full weight.

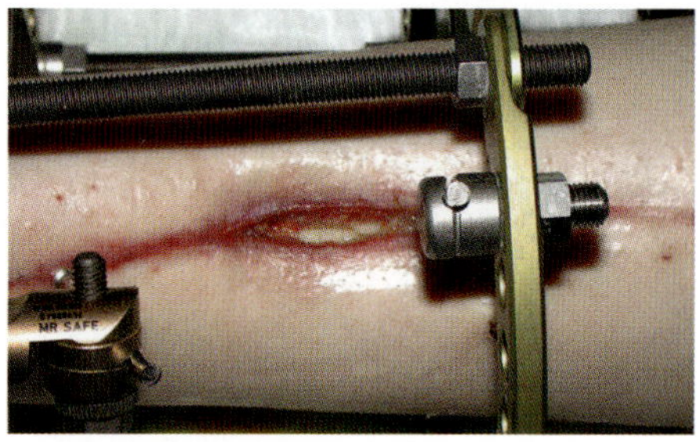

Fig 20.3-13 One week after the negative-pressure wound therapy closure was stopped, on the one hand the wound has reduced in size, but on the other hand, there is some secretion. The bacteriological examination (sterile secretion) showed no infection.

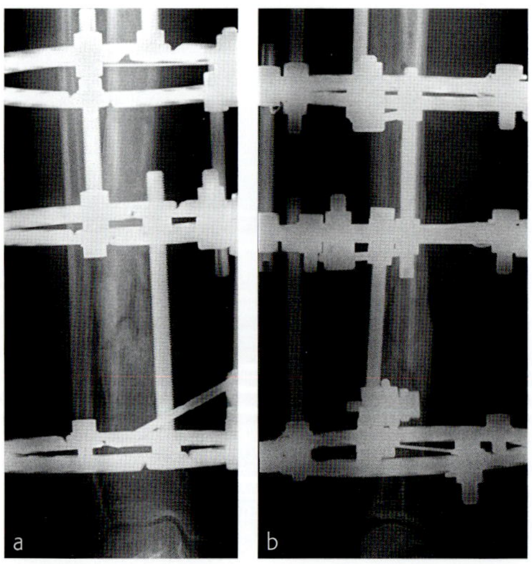

Fig 20.3-14a–b These new x-rays taken 6–7 weeks after the author's treatment show a progressive consolidation and integration of the fragment, and no new resorption. The fracture line between the main distal fragment and the long butterfly fragment is still present.
a AP view.
b Lateral view.

8 Outcome

The x-rays after 10 weeks (**Fig 20.3-15**, **Fig 20.3-16**) showed sufficient healing and the skin condition was also good, which meant a completely healed wound, no swelling, and no sign of infection.

The ring fixator was removed with sedation and a functional, removable fiberglass splint was applied.

Two weeks later, a new x-ray was performed to check for fracture or signs of instability (**Fig 20.3-17**).

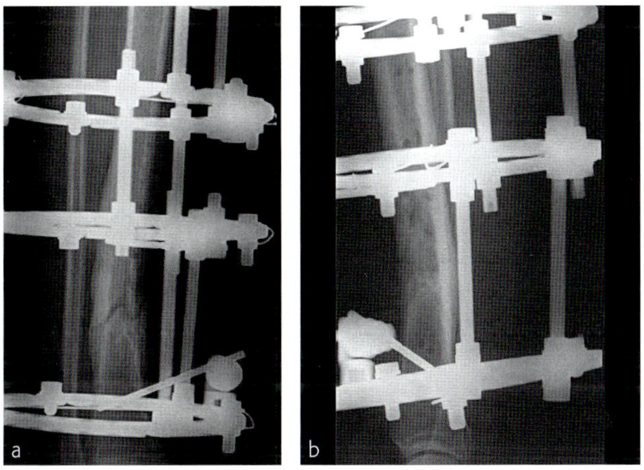

Fig 20.3-15a–b Ten weeks after application of the ring fixator there remains a line in the distal part of the fracture. But now more bridging callus is visible, especially on the lateral side. The ring fixator was removed and replaced by a custom-made fiberglass splint.
a AP view.
b Lateral view.

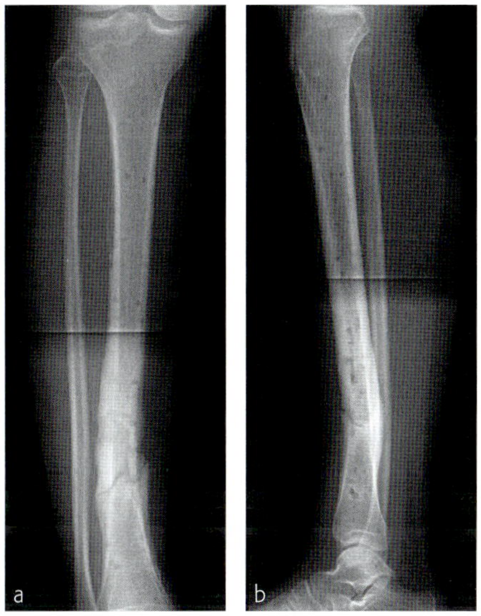

Fig 20.3-16a–b Three days after the fixator was removed the patient experienced some pain, so a new x-ray was taken. However, there was no difference to the x-ray with the fixator in place. The posterior consolidation was better than the anterior consolidation.
a AP view.
b Lateral view.

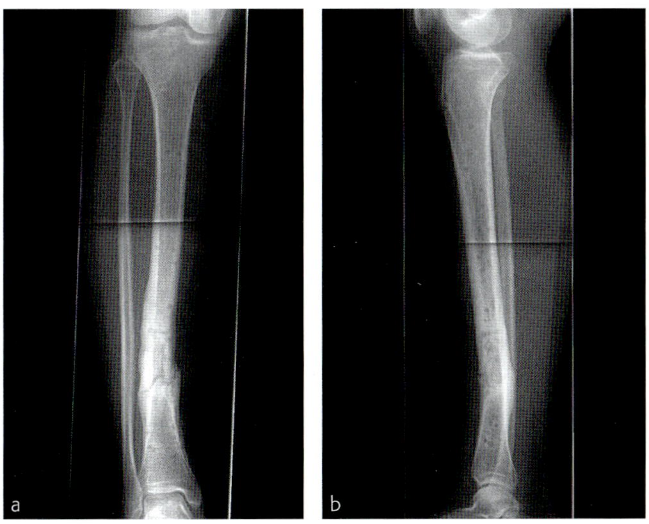

Fig 20.3-17a–b Two weeks later, a new x-ray was performed to check for fracture or signs of instability. There was no negative evolution and healing was occurring.
a AP view.
b Lateral view.

The child was walking without any problems with the removable splint. There was no pain and no other pathological signs. The x-ray 6 months after initial revision shows a slow but continuous consolidation and remodeling. Only a small fissure on the anterior cortex was visible. Visually and radiologically there is a slight recurvatum (**Fig 20.3-18**). At this time, sports activities were allowed.

The further follow-up visits were all uneventful (**Fig 20.3-19**, **Fig 20.3-20**). The child returned to normal function and activity. There was no leg-length discrepancy visible. Cosmetically, the patient and the parents were also happy. Follow-up visits ceased after 2 years.

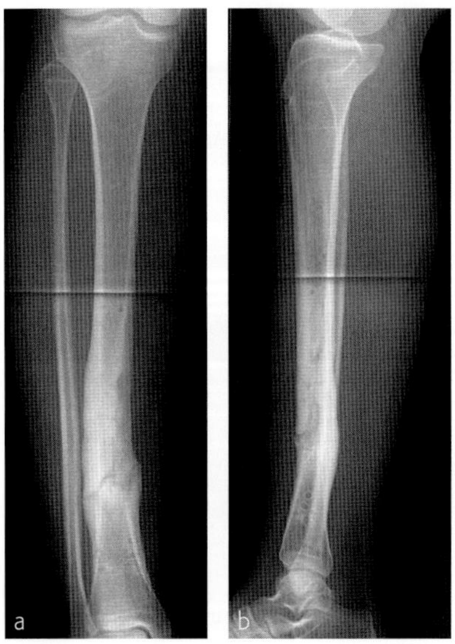

Fig 20.3-18a–b Healing was progressing well 2.5 months later; there was no local pain and the wound was completely closed. The patient was allowed to do low-impact sports activities like jogging, swimming, and bicycling.
a AP view.
b Lateral view.

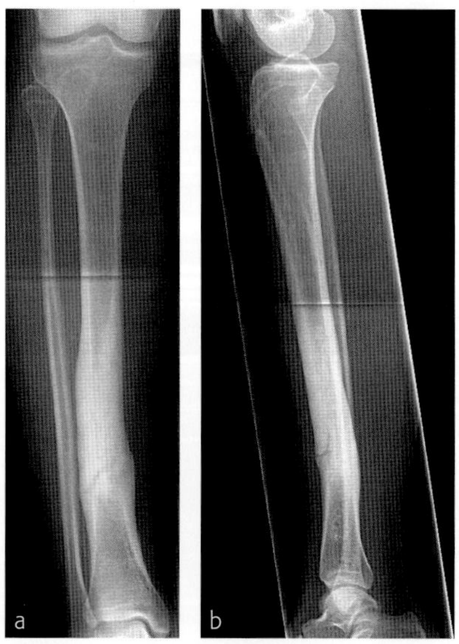

Fig 20.3-19a–b The next x-rays and clinical controls were made 5 months later. The patient had no problems. There is now full consolidation even though a fine fracture line is visible
a AP view.
b Lateral view.

9 Pitfalls

- The initial osteosynthesis was inappropriate for this fracture and given the age of the child; this fracture could also have been treated with a normal, well-molded long-leg plaster cast, healing within 6 weeks.
- The technique of the plate osteosynthesis does not correspond to today's biological specifications. For a child, this type of fixation is too rigid.
- The signs of the infection were misinterpreted and recognized too late.
- Inadequate therapy for the infection was provided.

10 Pearls

- Because of the good health of the child, the infection could be solved within a short time.
- The acceptance of the ring fixator by the child and her parents led to a good outcome.
- There was early solid consolidation and healing without functional restriction.

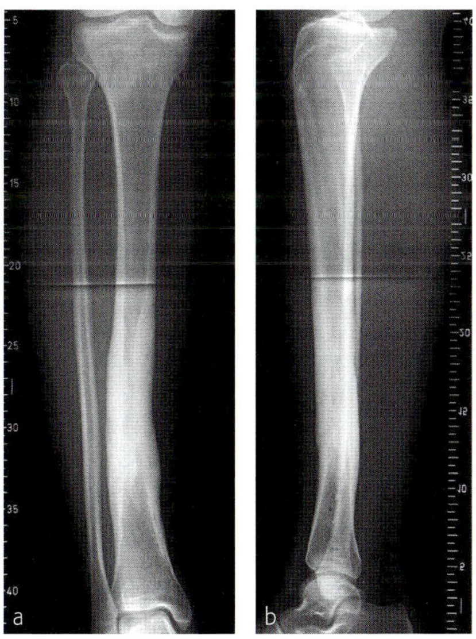

Fig 20.3-20a–b The last follow-up x-ray after 2 years shows full remodeling and the start of tibial recanalization. Radiologically there is slight varus in the AP view (**a**) and recurvation in the lateral view (**b**). Clinically this was not a problem and the patient and her parents were happy.

11 References

1. **[No authors listed].** Will oral antibiotics suffice in osteomyelitis? *Arch Dis Child.* 2015 Mar;100(3):278.
2. **Keren R, Shah SS, Srivastava R, et al.** Comparative effectiveness of intravenous vs oral antibiotics for postdischarge treatment of acute osteomyelitis in children. *JAMA Pediatr.* 2015 Feb;169(2):120–128.
3. **Schroeder AR, Ralston SL.** Intravenous antibiotic durations for common bacterial infections in children: when is enough enough? *J Hosp Med.* 2014 Sep;9(9):604–649.

20.4 Osteomyelitis/septic arthritis of the proximal femur in a toddler

Theddy Slongo

1 Case description

After 10 days of subfebrile temperature, a mother noticed that her 16-month-old boy no longer wanted to bear weight on the right leg. She waited another day and when the situation did not improve, the mother took the toddler to a pediatrician. In the meantime, his condition had worsened with a temperature over 38° C.

The pediatrician diagnosed pharyngitis and swollen lymph nodes. The mother reported later that the pediatrician did not examine the legs or hip of her child. He prescribed medication to reduce the fever and an antibiotic.

Over the next 2 days the condition remained unchanged. The mother reported to the pediatrician that the boy exhibited severe pain with movement of the right leg. After a new consultation, the pediatrician sent the toddler for a pelvic x-ray. The diagnosis was normal x-ray, no pathology noted (**Fig 20.4-1**).

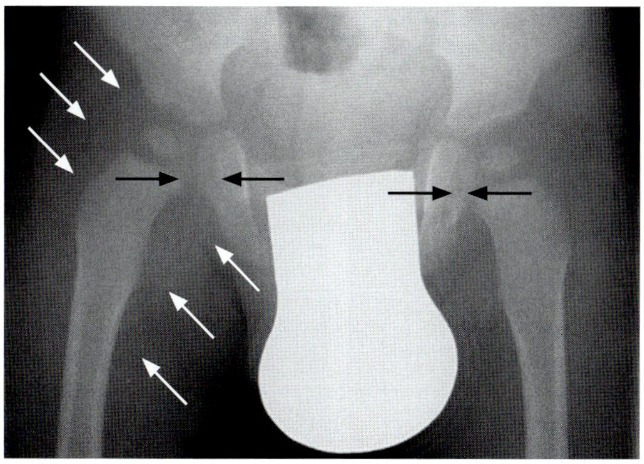

Fig 20.4-1 The initial x-ray taken by a private radiologist. The diagnosis was a normal hip. But there are different pathological signs in the right proximal femoral region and in the hip. Wider joint space (black arrows), lower transparency of the soft tissue in the proximal femur (white arrows), and irregular bone structure.

The pediatrician referred him to the pediatric clinic of the author's children's hospital because of this unclear situation. Age, symptoms, and pseudoparalysis in the absence of neurological signs (ie, meningitis) strongly suggest that the toddler has osteomyelitis or osteoarthritis [1].

1.1 Clinical examination 17 days after the first symptoms

The boy was seen first by a pediatrician at the clinic:

- 16-month-old toddler in severely reduced condition, not moving his right leg, passive movement painful, swollen right thigh and inguinal region
- Fever 39° C
- Boy shows a septic condition; an immediate intravenous antibiotic therapy (cefuroxime) was started [2–4]

1.2 Additional examination

Blood testing: white blood cell count more than 40,000/ µL and C-reactive protein level nearly 200 mg/L. A blood culture was performed.

X-rays of the right hip and femur (**Fig 20.4-2**) revealed a severe, progressive destruction of the upper femur and an extended joint space.

A consultation together with the pediatric surgeon was arranged: the surgeon decided to explore the proximal femur and hip joint. For him no additional investigations were indicated; his diagnosis was neglected osteomyelitis/septic arthritis.

The pediatrician requested a sonography (**Fig 20.4-3**). The interpretation of the sonography was not absolutely clear; the radiologist reported an infection with pus. Therefore, a bone scan was also performed showing a hyperperfusion in the whole proximal femoral part and in the hip joint (**Fig 20.4-4**).

The toddler was sent to pediatric surgery [5].

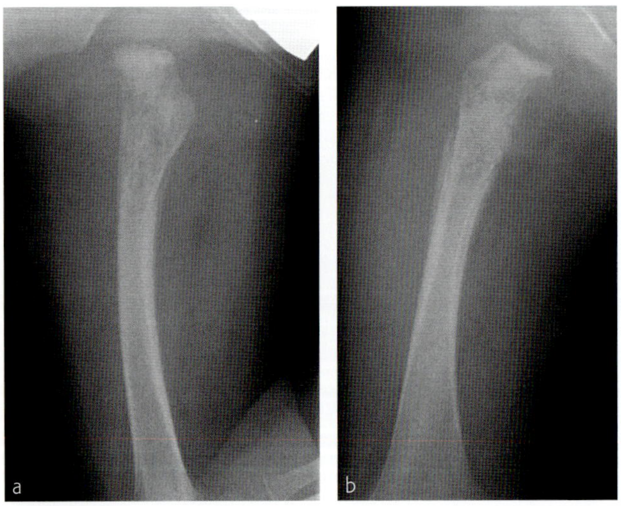

Fig 20.4-2a–b These x-rays were taken 17 days after onset of symptoms. There is a progressive destruction of the upper femur and an extended joint space.

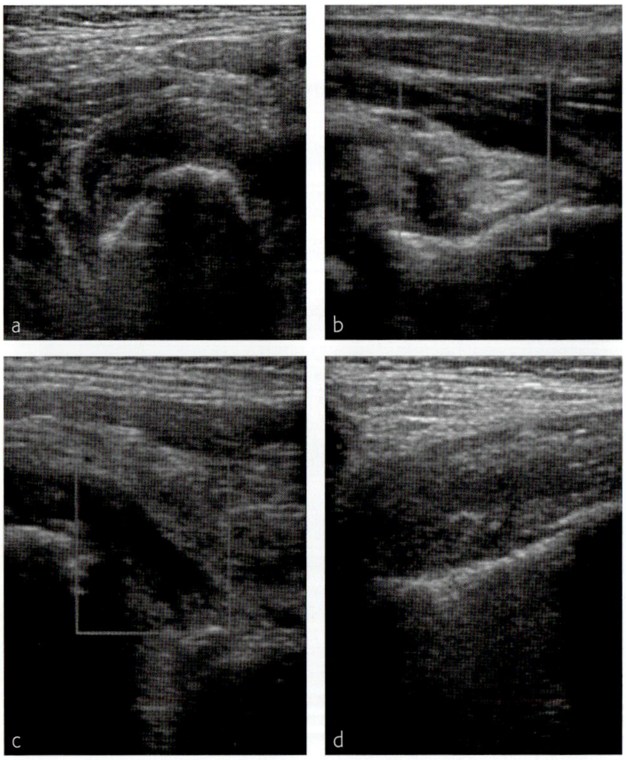

Fig 20.4-3a–d The interpretation of this sonography was difficult because the majority of the capsule was destroyed so the clear structure of the joint and the capsule was misinterpreted. An obvious effusion in the hip joint was not seen.

2 Indication

From a surgical point of view, the indication for an intervention was absolutely necessary [2]; only an exploration, evacuation of pus, and irrigation and drainage of the joint can prevent a total disaster, such as avascular necrosis (AVN) of the hip and the proximal femur. However, there was a high risk that AVN could not be prevented after such a long time. Risks were discussed in detail preoperatively with the parents.

3 Preoperative planning

The most difficult step in the preoperative planning was planning the correct approach. In addition, it was important to discuss with the parents the whole postoperative procedure: long-term intravenous antibiotic therapy, the possibility of further operations, and functional deficit.

4 Surgical approach

To minimize additional surgical damage the author decided to perform two separate approaches: a classic lateral approach for the femur, and an inguinal incision and blunt dissection in the medial window for the hip [6].

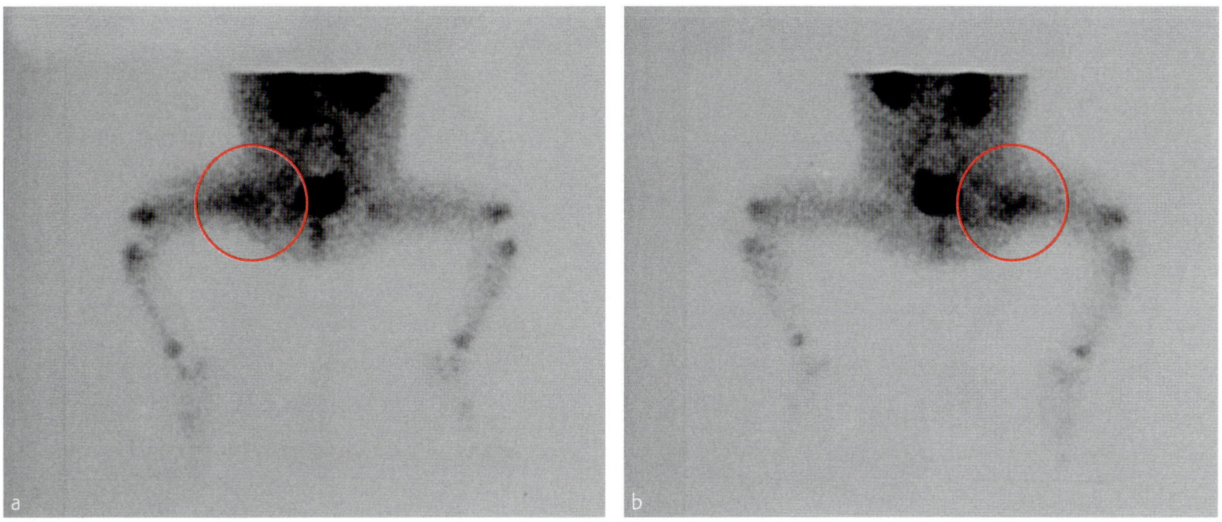

Fig 20.4-4a–b On these unnecessary bone scans the same information is shown as seen on the x-ray.
a Anterior view.
b Posterior view.

5 Surgical debridement

Step 1: Lateral approach

A lateral incision was made from the tip of the greater trochanter up to the middle of the thigh, then a classic opening of the fascia and subvastus lateralis approach to the femur.

After opening the fascia, a lot of pus was evacuated offering a spontaneous view of the lateral femur. The dissection of the muscle was done by the abscess. The periosteum was also destroyed.

Then the femur was opened using a lateral bony window of 1 x 5 cm. Thorough irrigation was performed. Two drains were placed: one in the medullary canal, one subfascially. Then the skin was closed loosely.

Step 2: Inguinal approach (**Fig 20.4-5**)

Using an inguinal incision, ie, distal along the inguinal ligament, the fascia was prepared. After opening the fascia, exposure was achieved between the vessels on the medial side and the psoas muscle with the nerve on the lateral side following the path of the abscess. The capsule of the hip joint was completely destroyed. Intensive irrigation of the hip joint was performed (using 1 L of fluid) which was subluxed by a gentle traction on the leg. Once the femoral head was cleared and clean, the cartilage was visible and appeared light gray in color, indicating a nutrition problem. The femoral head was then perforated with a sharp needle and no bleeding was visible. An irrigation drain was then installed in the hip joint for 48 hours.

6 Temporary and definitive fixation

After the operation the child was positioned and fixed in an abduction brace (Lörracher splint) that is normally used to treat hip dysplasia (**Fig 20.4-6**). This fixation was applied both to reduce pain and to stabilize the hip in a centered position.

7 Postoperative management

Over the next 48 hours the hip joint was irrigated over the drain; the lateral two drains provided evacuation of the pus.

Antibiotics were administered for 14 days through a central vein catheter (**Table 20.4-1**) [4]. Then for 4 more weeks oral antibiotics were given until all blood parameters were normalized.

The Lörracher splint was removed after 4 weeks and the toddler started to walk. The x-ray (**Fig 20.4-7**) after 5 weeks shows a defect on the proximal femur and some asymmetry in the hip joint.

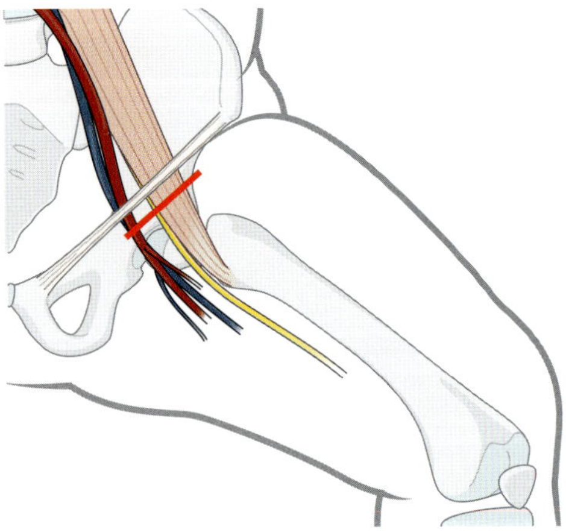

Fig 20.4-5 Clinical intraoperative view of a toddler's left inguinal region. The 4–5 cm incision is made along the inguinal skin line. Then the medial window is used in a modified way: the two vessels are medial, the femoral nerve together with the psoas muscle are lateral.

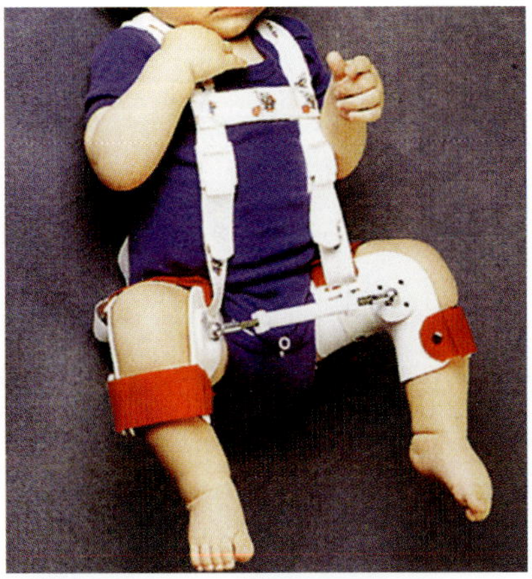

Fig 20.4-6 Postoperatively the patient was immobilized in a mobile abduction brace, a Lörracher splint, which allows concentric stable movement of the hip joint.

Diagnosis	Pathogen	First choice therapy (single shot and interval)	Duration, days	Maximum dosage	Alternatives/remarks
Osteomyelitis acute	*S aureus* *S pyogenes* *H influenzae* *K kingae*	Age < 5 years Cefuroxime 50 mg/kg every 8 h IV → Cefuroxime axetil 30 mg/kg every 8 h orally	IV > 7–10 IV + orally 28	4.5 g	Amoxicillin clavulanate 50 mg/kg every 8 h IV
		Age > 5 years Clindamycin 15 mg/kg every 6 h IV → Clindamycin 15 mg/kg every 8 h orally	IV > 7–10 IV + orally 28	1.8 g	Amoxicillin clavulanate 30 mg/kg every 8 h orally
Osteomyelitis chronic	*Staphylococcus* *Enterobacteriaceae*	Always interdisciplinary consultation between surgeon and infectious diseases specialist Therapy started after biopsy and culture			
Arthritis acute	*S aureus* *S pyogenes* *Neisseriaceae* *K kingae*	Age < 5 years Cefuroxime 50 mg/kg every 8 h IV → Cefuroxime axetil 50 mg/kg every 8 h orally (sic!)	IV > 7 IV + orally 21	4.5 g	Amoxicillin clavulanate 50 mg/kg every 8 h IV
		Age > 5 years Clindamycin 15 mg/kg every 6 h IV → Clindamycin 15 mg/kg every 8 h orally Gonorrhea ceftriaxone 2 g every 24 h IV x 7 days	IV > 7 IV + orally 21	1.8 g	Amoxicillin clavulanate 30 mg/kg every 8 h orally
Lyme arthritis (mostly gonarthritis)	*Borrelia burgdorferi*	Ceftriaxone 80 mg/kg every 24 h IV	14	2 g	Amoxicillin 20 mg/kg every 8 h orally × 28 days Age > 8 years Doxycycline 1–2 mg/kg every 12 h orally x 28 days

Table 20.4-1 Antibiotic therapy of skeletal infection according to age, diagnosis, and pathogen.
Data translated into English by the author and with permission from Schöni M, Simonetti G, Aebi C, eds. *Berner Datenbuch Pädiatrie.* Verlag Hans Huber Hogrefe AG Bern; 2015:355.

Abbreviations: *S aureus*, *Staphylococcus aureus*; *S pyogenes*, *Staphylococcus pyogenes*; *H influenzae*, *Haemophilus influenzae*; *K kingae*, *Kingella kingae*; IV, intravenous.

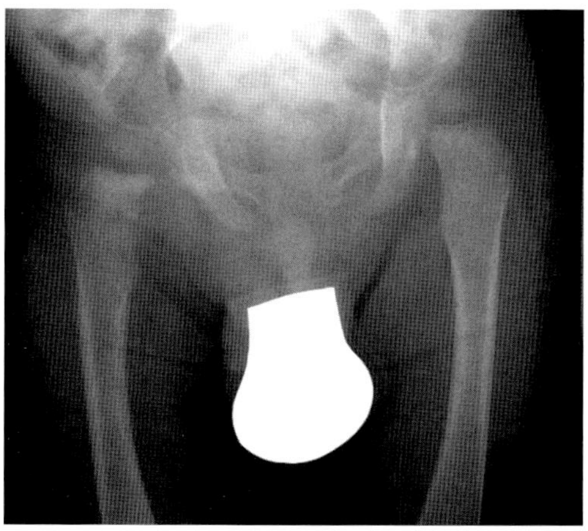

Fig 20.4-7 The 5-week postoperative x-ray demonstrates the initial as well as the operative bone defect but no new destruction.

8 Outcome

Over the next few months the child developed normally and was walking without a limp. The first real follow-up x-ray was taken 6 months after surgery. At this time, there was no sign of AVN and there was good healing of the proximal femur. A typical phenomenon—the head within the head—was seen as a good sign as new bone was forming around the original ossification center of the head, but also the beginning of a coxa magna (**Fig 20.4-8**).

In principle it was pleasing to see this positive evolution of the hip. Further follow-up examinations are absolutely necessary.

In x-rays **Fig 20.4-9**, **Fig 20.4-10**, and **Fig 20.4-11** both the positive and negative developments over the next 9 years can be seen.

These changes were observed: increased shortening of the femoral neck, development of a flat and wide femoral head (but still well contained), overgrowth of the greater trochanter, and some reaction on the acetabular side. The joint space at this time was still normal.

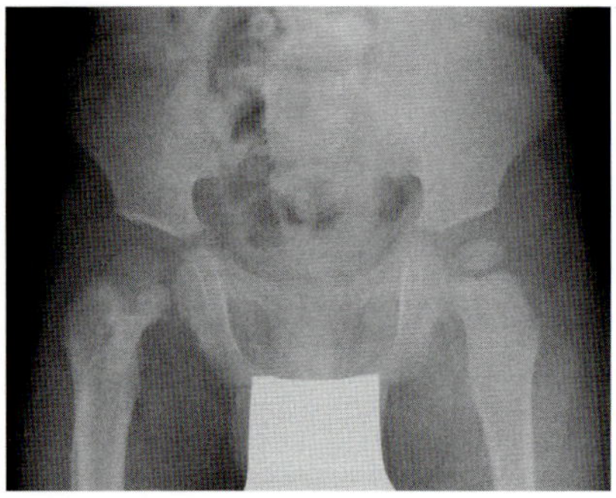

Fig 20.4-8 The 6-month postoperative x-ray shows a special phenomenon: the head within the head sign around the old head. This means that at the time of the infection around the head new bone formation is visible as a circle. Femoral healing is also visible.

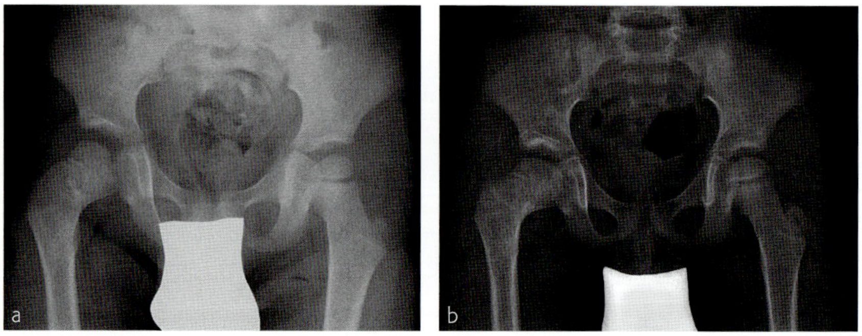

Fig 20.4-9a–b X-rays taken 4 years postoperatively.

a A good situation: no sign of avascular necrosis, integration of the head within the head sign, wide joint space, and good femoral bone consolidation.

b The beginning of some articular reaction is visible.

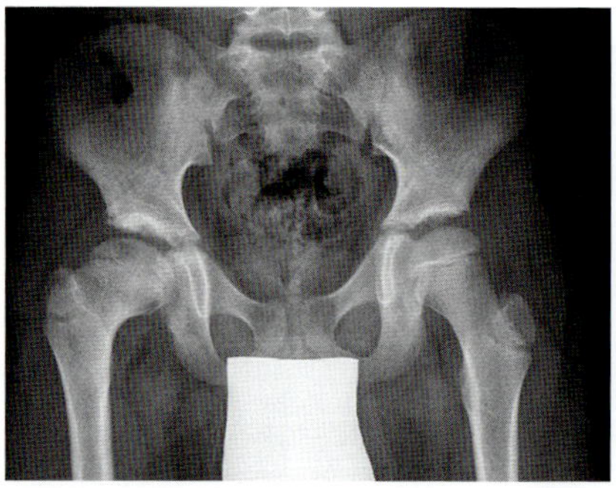

Fig 20.4-10 X-ray taken 6 years postoperatively shows a flat femoral head but spherical and congruent to the acetabulum is a slight sign of a transient avascular necrosis. The situation is similar to the evolution of a Perthes disease. The femur appears nearly normal.

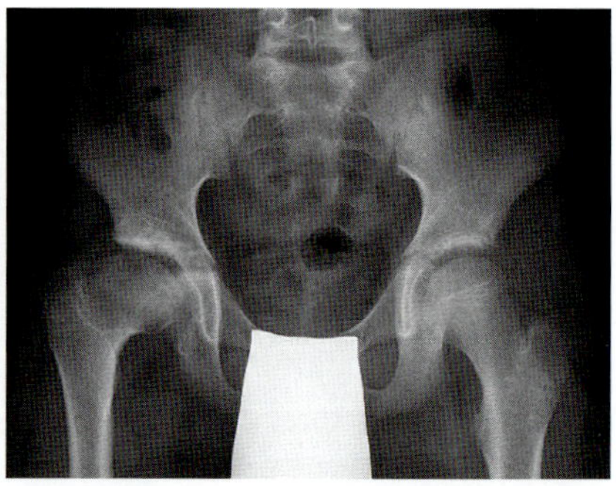

Fig 20.4-11 X-ray taken 8 years postoperatively demonstrates a premature closure of the femoral head physis but still a spherical containment; the greater trochanter overgrowth proximally simulates a coxa vara.

At 11 years, 9.5 years after the infection and surgery, the boy's situation worsened and he developed severe hip pain.

The function was poor and the child was limping, the right leg was 2 cm shorter than the left leg.

X-ray and clinical symptoms were typical for a mixed intraarticular and extraarticular impingement by compression of the minor gluteal muscle between high greater trochanter and acetabulum (**Fig 20.4-12, Fig 20.4-13**). On the other side a smaller joint space is visible, a lateralization of the femoral head, and in addition some reaction on the acetabular side.

At this time a surgical hip dislocation was performed for inspection of the hip joint and to perform a relative femoral neck lengthening [7, 8]. Intraoperative findings were severe damage of the labrum, damage of the articular cartilage in an area of 2 cm x 0.5 mm between 10 and 2 o'clock (**Fig 20.4-14**).

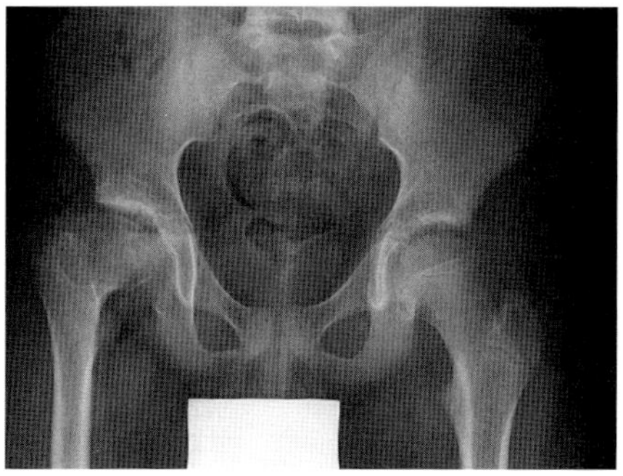

Fig 20.4-12 Between 8 and 9 years postoperatively the femoral head started to migrate laterally and proximally; the tip of the greater trochanter is now at the level of the lateral acetabular rim. At this time the child had rapidly increasing hip pain. The two reasons for this are damage to the lateral and anterior acetabular rim and labrum, and an impingement of the minor gluteal muscle between the greater trochanter and acetabulum.

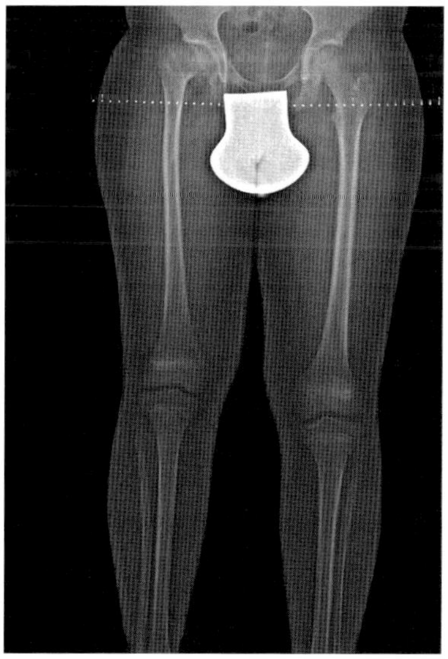

Fig 20.4-13 The full leg-length standing x-ray shows the resulting leg-length deficit of 3.5 cm; the leg axis is still correct.

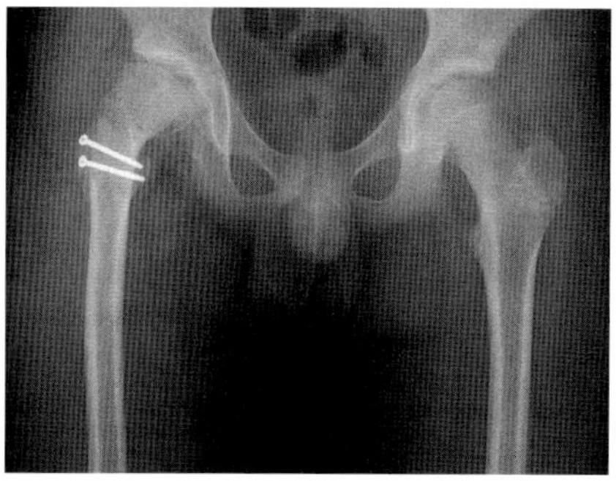

Fig 20.4-14 The situation was greatly improved 3 weeks after surgical hip dislocation and relative femoral neck lengthening. The range of motion was nearly symmetrical to the left side, and the child had no pain. This x-ray shows clearly the effect of the relative neck lengthening and that the neck-shaft angle was always normal.

Unfortunately, at this time, it was not determined that the hip was unstable and the postoperative x-ray documents this instability; therefore an abduction brace was applied for some time (**Fig 20.4-15**). However, after 6 weeks, due to the instability, a triple pelvic osteotomy was performed (**Fig 20.4-16**).

As is evident in the x-ray (**Fig 20.4-17**), the hip could be stabilized but the process of destruction was progressing rapidly. The hip joint nearly disappeared and in addition the hip function decreased but the child was pain free.

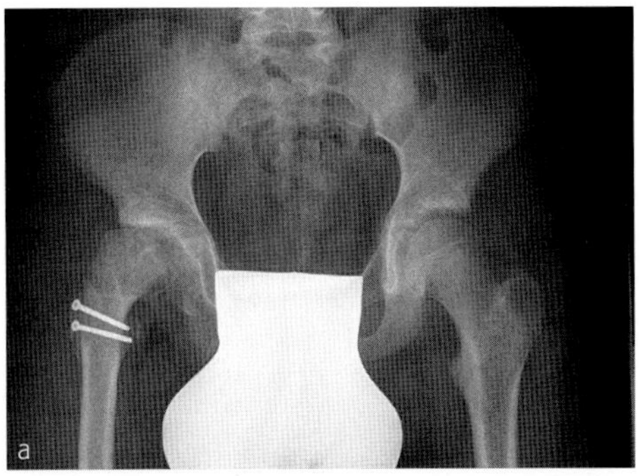
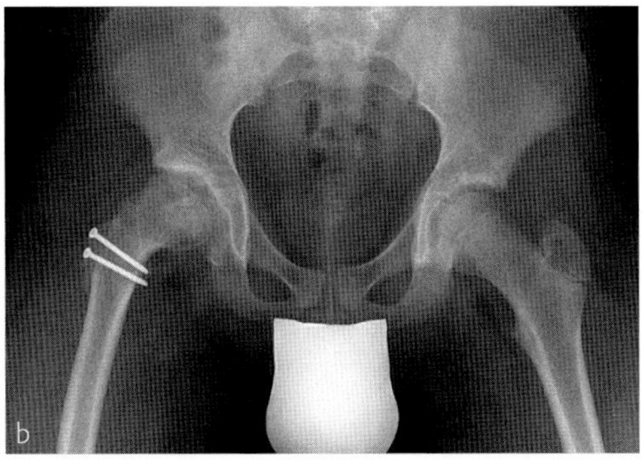

Fig 20.4-15a–b Three weeks after surgery an x-ray for healing assessment was performed.
a The hip is no longer stable.
b The adduction x-ray shows a recentering of the femoral head so an adduction brace was applied.

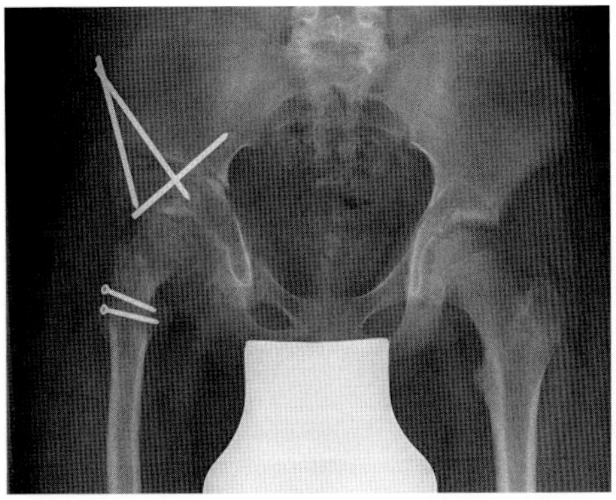

Fig 20.4-16 Five weeks after the triple osteotomy the hip is well covered but not optimally centered; there is still some lateralization. On the other hand, the joint space has become narrower.

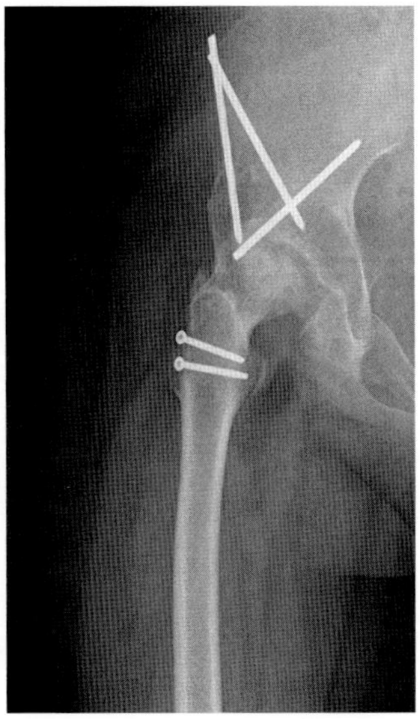

Fig 20.4-17 Eight months after the triple osteotomy, the child's hip is pain free. However, all planes of movement were reduced. In the sagittal plane the flexion was still relatively good up to 100°. Because of the leg-length discrepancy, in principle a bone lengthening should be performed. But in this particular situation it would be problematic because of the high pressure on the hip joint during and after lengthening.

9 Pitfalls

- Ignorance of the typical symptoms at the beginning and delay in the therapy can cause an initial AVN of the femoral head as well as necrosis of the proximal femur. In addition the child can develop septicemia with septic shock.
- Awareness of the unstable situation of the hip after the surgical hip dislocation and the relative femoral neck lengthening. The triple osteotomy should be performed at the same time.
- From clinical experience and the literature, once you have such a neglected infectious situation, initially one can treat the problem. The destructive process is ongoing but often remains inactive as long there is no new trauma. The new intervention with the triple osteotomy was such a trauma and reactivated the destructive process.

10 Pearls

- Initially and later, there was no AVN despite the delay in treatment.
- The child functioned well over a long period.

11 References

1. **Bergdahl S, Ekengren K, Eriksson M.** Neonatal hematogenous osteomyelitis: risk factors for long-term sequelae. *J Pediatr Orthop.* 1985 Sep-Oct;5(5):564–568.
2. **Keren R, Shah SS, Srivastava R, et al.** Comparative effectiveness of intravenous vs oral antibiotics for postdischarge treatment of acute osteomyelitis in children. Pediatric Research in Inpatient Settings Network. *JAMA Pediatr.* 2015 Feb;169(2):120–128.
3. **Schroeder AR, Ralston SL.** Intravenous antibiotic durations for common bacterial infections in children: when is enough enough? *J Hosp Med.* 2014 Sep;9(9):604–609.
4. **Slongo T.** Mikrobiologische Diagnostik häufiger Infektionskrankheiten [Microbiological diagnosis of common infectious diseases]. In: Schöni M, Simonetti G, Aebi C, eds. *Berner Datenbuch Pädiatrie.* Bern: Verlag Hans Huber Hogrefe AG; 2015:355.
5. **[No authors listed]** Will oral antibiotics suffice in osteomyelitis? *Arch Dis Child.* 2015 Mar;100(3):278.
6. **Dieckmann R, Hardes J, Ahrens H, et al.** [Treatment of acute and chronic osteomyelitis in children.] *Z Orthop Unfall.* 2008 May-Jun;146(3):375–380. German.
7. **Albers CE, Steppacher SD, Schwab JM, et al.** Relative femoral neck lengthening improves pain and hip function in proximal femoral deformities with a high-riding trochanter. *Clin Orthop Relat Res.* 2015 Apr; 473(4):1378–1387.
8. **Leunig M, Ganz R.** Relative neck lengthening and intracapital osteotomy for severe Perthes and Perthes-like deformities. *Bull NYU Hosp Jt Dis.* 2011;69 Suppl 1:S62–67.

21 Treatment of infection with limited resources

Zhao Xie

1 Introduction

Infection is a problem that does not discriminate between patients based on socioeconomic status, race, place of residence, or ethnicity. As such, infections happen all over the world after trauma and after surgery. Some patients will be unable to afford treatment and the cost of newer technologies. In some settings, the institution treating patients with infection may lack the ability to provide newer technologies or high-cost implants. Nonetheless, there are safe, basic methods of treatment available in such cases. This chapter focuses on the use of basic implants or no implants and proven surgical methods for treating bone infections.

2 Basics

Surgical debridement is a fundamental principle for management of deep-bone or soft-tissue infection. Basic principles include establishing the diagnosis which can often be done with careful physical examination, a thorough history, plain x-ray, and needle aspiration of the suspected area of infection. Some infections are easy to diagnose whereas others may require more effort to establish the correct diagnosis. For additional information about diagnosis of infection, see chapter 7 Diagnostics.

3 Etiology

A fundamental aspect of infection treatment is understanding the etiology of the infection. Much of this understanding can be gained by obtaining a careful history from the patient or his or her family (**Fig 21-1**). Was there a trauma? Was there a puncture? Has the patient been ill? How long have symptoms been present? Where are the symptoms located? Has a fever been noted? Is there local redness, swelling, or drainage from the area of concern? Has the patient been exposed to others with similar problems?

4 Wound types

Most cases of bone infection will have an associated wound. Detailed management of such wound problems is covered in chapter 13 Soft-tissue infections and chapter 14 Open wounds. For the purposes of this chapter, the author reviews basic methods for management of the infected extremity including preferred management strategies.

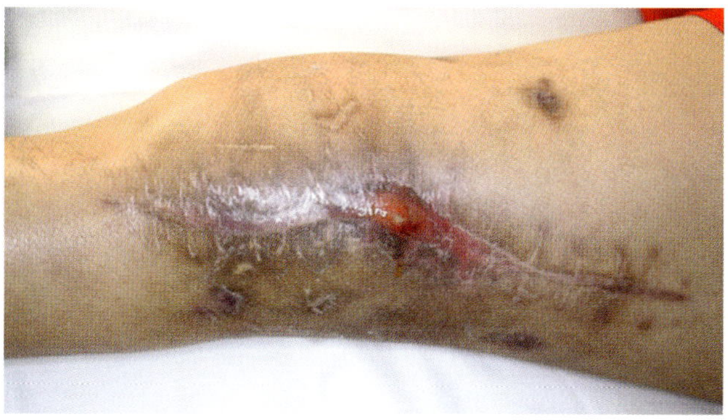

Fig 21-1 Patient was referred to the author's hospital 18 months after initial fracture of both lower limbs in a motor vehicle crash. He was diagnosed definitively with a methicillin-resistant *Staphylococcus aureus* infection involving the distal part of the left femur. He was previously treated with vancomycin intravenously prior to transfer to the author's center. On examination, he had healed surgical incisions of his left thigh with active drainage, and a functional ankylosis of his left knee joint.

5 Symptoms

Basic symptoms of infection have been covered thoroughly in the previous chapters in this book. The classic findings of redness, increased warmth, pain, swelling, and drainage are likely to be seen in most patients with bone infection. When treating patients with limited resources, patients will often present late to receive care(**Fig 21-2a**). This may be due to attempted treatment at another facility or for socioeconomic reasons. Beyond common symptoms, scars and skin discoloration can often be seen in patients with a delay in care (**Fig 21-2b**).

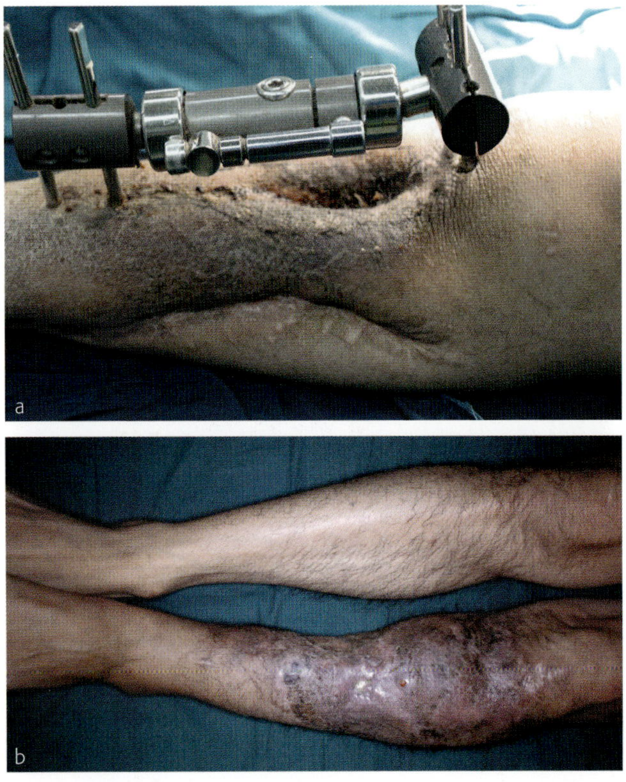

Fig 21-2a–b Results of delayed care.
a Unilateral commercial external fixator present on the left femur with open wound treatment.
b Scars and skin discoloration are noted as signs of a chronically indent.

6 Diagnostic workup

The fundamental diagnostic workup should be conducted in all cases. This includes a detailed history and physical examination. Plain x-rays are frequently useful to understand the underlying bone condition and the presence of implants, foreign material, and sequestered bone fragments. Needle aspiration of the suspected infection site is worthwhile in many cases.

6.1 Laboratory

A peripheral white blood cell (WBC) count should be available at most centers and the C-reactive protein (CRP) is another useful serum marker, if available. In cases with active drainage, WBC count and CRP can be normal, or merely above the line. This finding may also be noted in nondraining infection situations.

Procalcitonin is more sensitive but WBC count and CRP are cheaper and more appropriate ways to confirm the diagnosis of infection.

6.2 Microbiology

Gram stain and aerobic/anaerobic cultures are the basic microbiological studies that should be performed in most cases. Sequestra are the most valuable samples and deep-wound cultures are helpful to find the bacteria. The "antibiotic holiday" can be useful before surgery to improve the chance of an accurate diagnosis. Postoperative antibiotics should be adjusted when a definitive bacterial culture has been obtained.

6.3 Radiology

Plain x-rays are the most useful radiological study to order for the patient with a bone infection. They can be used to identify the location of sequestra, the fixation of the bone defect, and the anatomical type of osteomyelitis (**Fig 21-3**). Rarely, for a deep site of infection, such as deep in the pelvis, a computed tomographic scan would be beneficial. Ultrasound, if available, is another simple and inexpensive method to localize a fluid collection.

7 Basics of bone management

The basics of bone management will follow from an accurate diagnosis. The diagnosis should include the site of infection; suspected extent of infection; presence of a fracture, of surgical implants, of foreign material; or sequestered bone (**Fig 21-3**). All these diagnostic criteria are critical to make a precise surgical plan, including the choice of incision, extent of bony resection, management of the dead space, and fixation of the fracture [1].

7.1 Principles

A fundamental principle of bone infection management is debridement of all necrotic bone tissue. This can sometimes be difficult to determine. Bone that is bleeding is usually safe to retain. Sequestered fragments of bone or necrotic bone material behave like foreign bodies and should be removed in all cases. Mechanical debridement is the best method to remove the nidus of infection, and the extent of debridement affects prognosis [2]. Additionally, the presence of purulent fluid will require drainage in all cases. There is no substitution for good surgical bone debridement in cases involving the bone.

7.2 Specific methods

The author demonstrates with photographs several innovative yet simple and less costly methods of managing bone infection. **Fig 21-4** shows how to use internal fixation under infection circumstance. **Fig 21-5** demonstrates how to use bone cement to temporarily fix the bone.

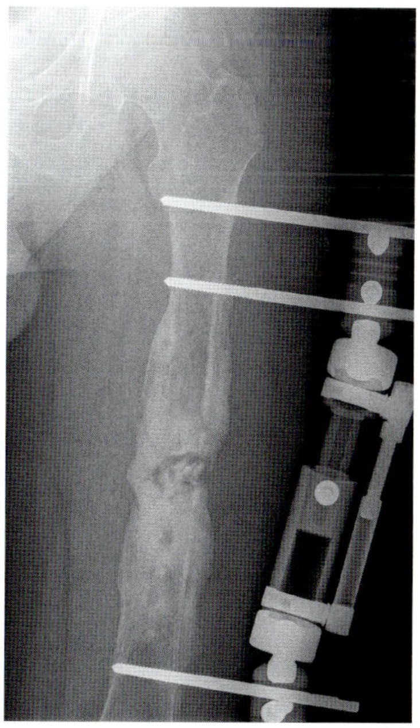

Fig 21-3 X-ray shows an external fixator in situ with an established nonunion, involucrum, and sequestrum of bone.

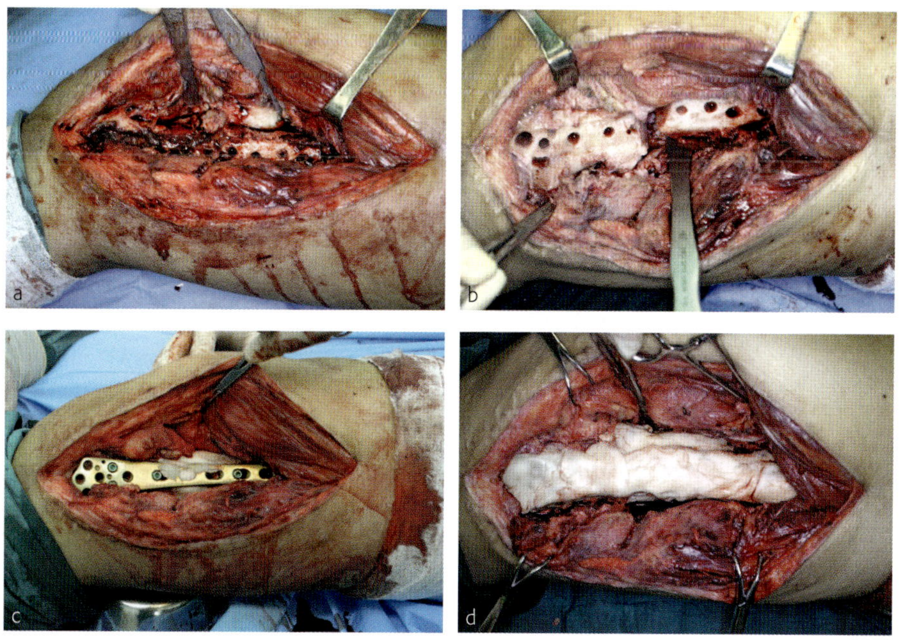

Fig 21-4a–d Internal fixation is not advised when the infection is diagnosed clinically or bacteriologically. These consecutive pictures show a locking plate that was placed and wrapped in antibiotic cement. The wrapped plate is a compromise when a bulky external fixator is contraindicated. The patient eventually had successful wound healing primarily and bone union ultimately.

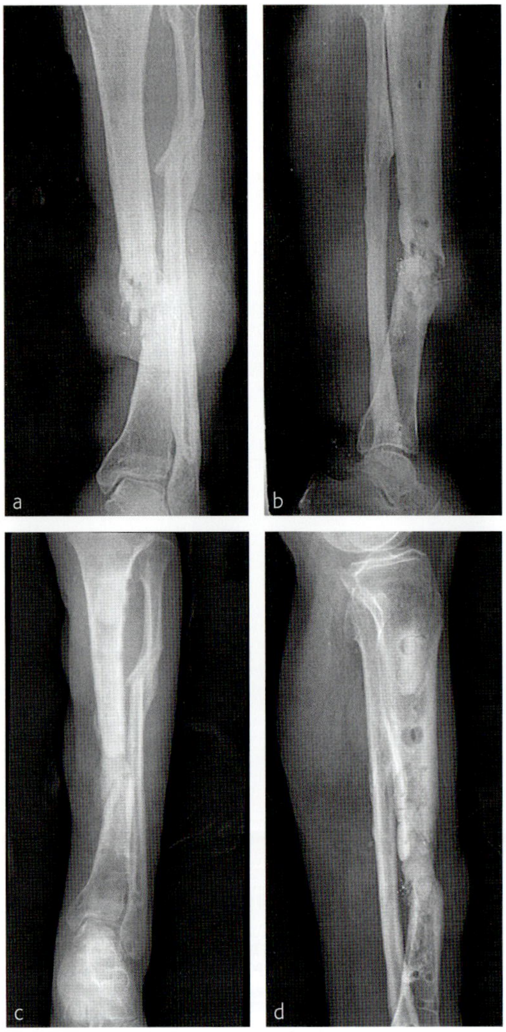

Fig 21-5a–d This patient suffered from trauma with an open fracture 8 years ago. The initial debridement was carried out and external fixation was placed. After the fourth day, the wound became infected. Redness and swelling was observed. The patient had another debridement and was discharged due to socioeconomic reasons.

a–b X-rays of the patient's left leg when he first was admitted to the author's hospital after the surgery. Bacterial culture was confirmed of methicillin-resistant *Staphylococcus aureus* infection.

c–d Antibiotic cement was placed after debridement without any internal or external fixation. The cement can still stabilize the bone if the patient cooperates in situations of limited resources.

7.3 Masquelet technique

The Masquelet technique has many forms. Among the simplest forms is meticulous bone debridement followed by placement of a polymethylmethacrylate block spacer containing antibiotic powder into the bone void left by debridement. This void can be managed successfully in many cases with the block spacer that imparts some stability to the extremity, directly treats the infection, and promotes a biological membrane to form around the spacer (**Fig 21-6**). After the infection has been controlled, the spacer can be carefully removed retaining the biologically induced membrane. The cavity left behind by the spacer can then be filled with autogenous bone graft which can be obtained from the patient's pelvic region (**Fig 21-7**). This patient acquired bone union 6 months after surgery (**Fig 21-8**) and the plate was removed at his final follow-up (**Fig 21-9**).

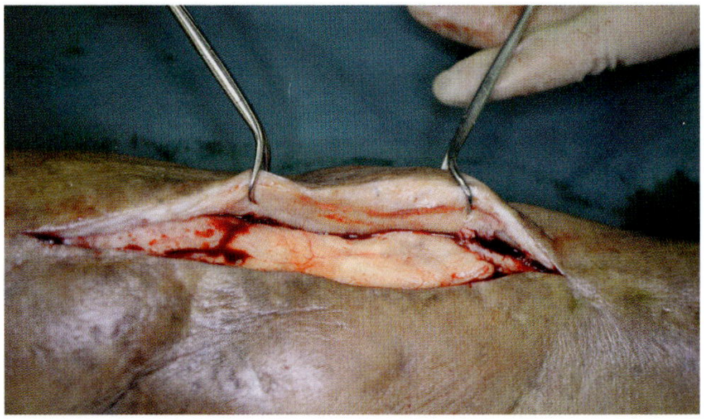

Fig 21-6 The same patient as in **Fig 21-5**. The white biological membrane was carefully examined above the surface of the bone cement.

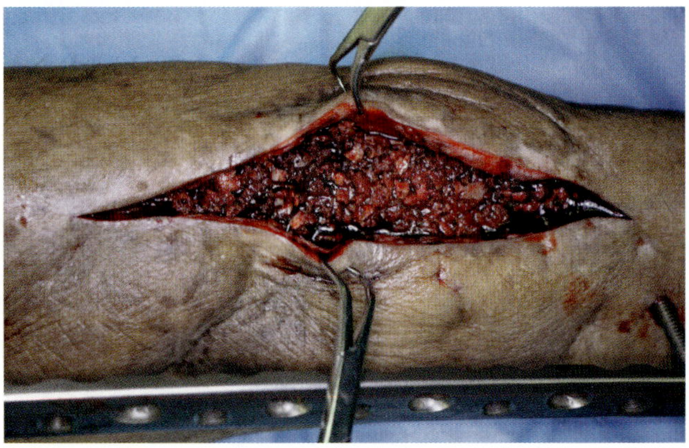

Fig 21-7 Autogenous cancellous bone was grafted from the iliac crest after the bone cement was removed.

7.4 Debridement and casting/splinting

In some cases bone debridement can be performed, such as drainage of an intramedullary abscess with removal of sequestered bone. Following wound management, the leg may be immobilized in plaster until healing has occurred.

7.5 External fixation methods

Although new commercial external fixation is typically costly, there are some less costly alternatives available (see **Fig 21-2a**).

For example, the locking compression plate (LCP) works like a unilateral external fixator. The characteristic angle-stable framework of the LCP allows for complete consolidation of the fracture and does not depend on the friction between plate and bone, but the holding force between the locking screw and the cortical bone [3]. Some experts report the successful use of an LCP as an external fixator. Unlike a bulky, traditional external fixation the LCP is concealed, and thus more aesthetic, better tolerated, and compatible with activities of daily living (**Fig 21-10**). Other advantages are further outlined by Kloen [4], including stability, ease of removal, and less radiographic silhouette.

7.6 Antibiotic management

Antibiotic management is a fundamental treatment method required to help the patient overcome his or her infection. This is covered in greater detail in chapter 5 Systemic antibiotics.

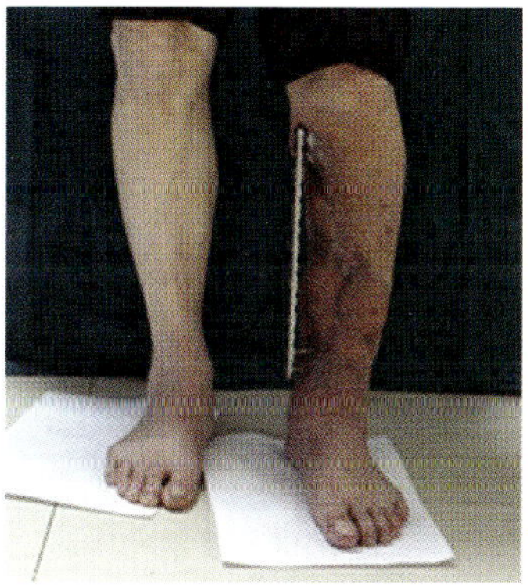

Fig 21-8 The patient can fully bear weight 6 months after surgery.

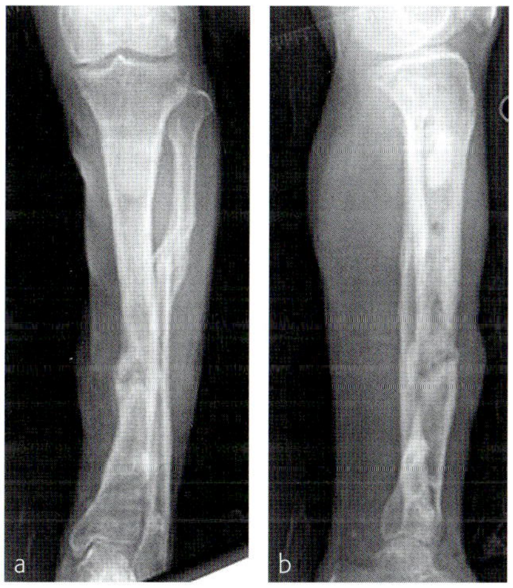

Fig 21-9a–b The plate was removed at his final follow-up 18 months after surgery.

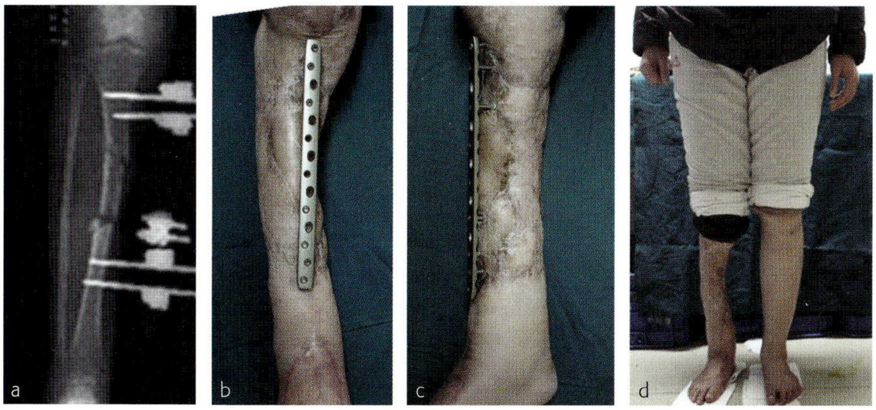

Fig 21-10a–d A female patient who suffered from posttraumatic osteomyelitis with segmental dead bone in the midtibia.
a An external fixator is present on the medial aspect of the right tibia.
b–c Dead bone was removed using meticulous debridement. A Masquelet technique with a locking compression plate acting as an external fixator was performed.
d The patient went on to bone union and her plate was removed in the surgical examination room as an outpatient.

8 Conclusion

Infection is a problem that affects patients from all regions of the world and people of all socioeconomic classes. Because some centers and some patients have limited means to treat these infections, it is important to be familiar with some basic methods for management of the infection. Some of these techniques are time-honored and have been used by surgeons for more than 100 years. Others are newer, more innovative methods developed more recently. The author has presented these methods in the hope that they will be useful to surgeons.

9 References

1. **Motsitsi NS.** Management of infected nonunion of long bones: the last decade (1996–2006). *Injury.* 2008 Feb;39(2):155–160.
2. **Simpson AH, Deakin M, Latham JM.** Chronic osteomyelitis. The effect of the extent of surgical resection on infection-free survival. *J Bone Joint Surg Br.* 2001 Apr;83(3):403–407.
3. **Miller DL, Goswami T.** A review of locking compression plate biomechanics and their advantages as internal fixators in fracture healing. *Clin Biomech (Bristol, Avon).* 2007 Dec;22(10):1049–1062.
4. **Kloen P.** Supercutaneous plating: use of a locking compression plate as an external fixator. *J Orthop Trauma.* 2009 Jan;21(1):72–75.

10 Acknowledgments

Jian Zhong Xu, MD, and Sheng Peng Yu, MD, contributed to this chapter.

Glossary

Antiseptic coverage
Coverage of a wound with a moist dressing that includes an antiseptic to be changed each day with the objective of preventing a superinfection until the wound has healed or the wound is closed by suture or plastic surgery.

Arthritis, septic, infectious
Staging as defined by Gächter. There are four stages based on the degree of severity.

Bacteria, difficult-to-treat
In terms of implant-associated infections, bacteria are considered difficult to treat if there are few or no antibiotics available that can reliably eliminate the bacteria including those bound within the biofilm. In other words, the likelihood of successful treatment is not high unless curative antibiotic therapy is administered following removal of the implant. Difficult-to-treat bacteria include:

- Rifampin-resistant staphylococci
- Enterococci
- Small-colony variants (SCV) primarily of staphylococci but also of *Salmonella spp.*, *Escherichia coli*, *Pseudomonas aeruginosa*
- Enterobacteria and *Pseudomonas aeruginosa* that are resistant to quinolones
- Fungi
- Methicillin-resistant *Staphylococcus aureus* (MRSA)
- Vancomycin-intermediate sensitivity *Staphylococcus aureus* (VISA)
- Vancomycin-resistant *Staphylococcus aureus* (VRSA)
- Vancomycin-resistant enterococci (VRE)

Infections with unknown pathogens that have been clearly detected in histological tests are also difficult to treat.

Biofilm
Microorganisms adhering to the surface of implants and which are embedded in a glycoprotein matrix. Bacteria and fungi in biofilm are metabolically inactive or have low metabolic activity and thus less susceptible to most antibiotics.

Brodie abscess
An intramedullary abscess form of primary chronic osteomyelitis. This is characterized by a central inflammatory focus that is differentiated from a broad, sclerotic bone margin and is usually localized in the metaphysis, frequently in the tibia. It mainly affects adolescents and young adults with an above-average immune status.

Coagulase reaction
Method for differentiating staphylococci: *Staphylococcus aureus*, which forms a clot when mixed with fibrinogen-containing plasma, is coagulase-positive. Nearly all other pathogenic staphylococci, eg, *Staphylococcus epidermidis*, are coagulase-negative.

Debridement
Debridement is used to reduce the bacterial count at the site of infection and optimize the conditions for antibiotic therapy. The critical steps include:

- Removal and replacement of the implants in cases of hematogenous infections lasting longer than 3 weeks or if an exogenous infection after surgery
- Removal of the tissue surrounding the implant and necrotic bone
- Excision of often extensive joint-capsule protrusions and fistulas containing detritus
- Adequate wound drainage to prevent postoperative hematoma
- Open synovectomy with joint infections (stages 3 and 4)
- Tissue samples must be collected from the periprosthetic area or "implant bed"

Gram staining
Christian Gram developed a staining technique in which bacteria surrounded by a thick cellular wall composed of peptidoglycans turn blue (gram-positive bacteria) and those with only a thin cellular wall with an additional outer lipid membrane turn red (gram-negative bacteria).

Healing in periprosthetic infections

Healing in periprosthetic infections is defined as meeting the following criteria:

- No history or clinical signs of infection symptoms
- Normalization of C-reactive protein (CRP) < 10 mg/L and/or erythrocyte sedimentation rate (ESR) < 20 mm/h
- No radiological signs of infection > 24 months after the first infected revision

Healing is considered likely to occur in relapse-free patients between 12 and 24 months. A persistent infection (or relapse) occurs with recrudescent infection with the same microorganisms and is not time-dependent. A new infection is defined as occurrence of an infection with different microorganisms.

Infection classification

Infection classification based on time of initial manifestation after surgery		
Osteosynthesis	Early infection	≤ 2 wk
	Delayed infection	3–10 wk
	Late infection	≥ 10 wk
Joint replacement	Early infection	≤ 3 mo
	Delayed infection	3–24 mo
	Late infection	≥ 24 mo
Infection classification based on pathogenesis		
Exogenous	Inoculation from outside (perioperative) usually manifesting within the first 2 years	
Hematogenous	Inoculation via the bloodstream at any time	

Inoculum effect

Bacterial density is higher in abscesses than in standardized resistance testing (> 10^6 CFU/mL vs 10^5 CFU/mL). The inoculum effect refers to the decreasing efficacy of certain antibiotics, eg, β-lactam antibiotics, with increasing microbial counts, which must be taken into account during therapy. This is the reason why with implant-associated infections the focus of infection must be eradicated using careful debridement prior to antibiotic treatment.

Low-grade infection

With implant-associated infections, low-virulent, otherwise nonpathogenic bacteria such as *Staphylococcus epidermidis* take advantage of the fact that the body's defences against infection are weakened due to a locally acquired granulocyte defect in the immediate vicinity of the implant. These bacteria can also establish themselves as a biofilm on the surface of the implant. This leads to an exogenous infection with delayed manifestation that is restricted to the immediate vicinity of the foreign body.

Minimum inhibitory concentration (MIC) and pharmacodynamics

The minimum inhibitory concentration (MIC) corresponds to the antibiotic level at which bacteria are inhibited. The relationship between the antibiotic level and the MIC can be used to estimate how long the antibiotic level will remain above the MIC between dosages. In the case of all β-lactams (penicillins and cephalosporins), it is beneficial to maintain the antibiotic level above the MIC at the focus of infection for as long as possible. For severe infections (eg, endocarditis or periprosthetic infection), it is therefore advisable to determine the MIC.

MRSA

Methicillin-resistant *Staphylococcus aureus*. Although it is no longer currently used in clinical applications, methicillin is an indicator of resistance to flucloxacillin, amoxicillin/clavulanic acid, and cephalosporins.

MRSE

Methicillin-resistant *Staphylococcus epidermidis* (see MRSA).

Open fracture

Gustilo-Anderson open fracture classification

Grade	Criteria
1	Clean wound, wound < 1 cm in length, simple fracture
2	Wound > 1 cm in length without extensive soft-tissue damage
3a	Open fracture with adequate periosteal coverage of the fractured bone despite an extended soft-tissue damage, caused by high-energy trauma
3b	Open fracture with extensive soft-tissue loss, periosteal stripping, and bone exposure
3c	Open fracture associated with an arterial injury requiring repair

Osteomyelitis

Infection of the bone and bone marrow. Osteomyelitis is classified as acute or chronic, depending on progression. An etiological distinction is drawn between exogenous and hematogenous osteomyelitis. Exogenous infections may spread from a wound, eg, a pressure ulcer, or penetrate the bone via an open fracture, a surgical access site, or a postoperative wound with impaired healing.

PCR

The polymerase chain reaction (PCR) is a method used to identify bacterial DNA. With PCR bacteria can be detected even if they have already been killed. This means that eubacterial PCR can occasionally identify bacteria that cannot be cultivated. It is considerably more difficult to interpret the PCR with polymicrobial findings. In addition, molecular biological analysis only enables the identification of isolated resistances (eg, MRSA or rifampin resistance). Presently the method is constantly undergoing further development.

Proof of infection

Meeting at least one of the following criteria satisfies proof of infection:

- Abscess with pus discharge, possibly following incision
- Presence of a fistula
- Microbiological identification of the same pathogen in at least two samples (tissue samples, sonication of foreign bodies)
- Histological testing of periprosthetic tissue/implant bed: total of more than 20–25 granulocytes in 10 fields of view at 400x magnification

Sensitivity

Likelihood of a test detecting a true positive value with a positive test result.

$$P(\text{positive result} \mid \text{true positive}) = \frac{\text{Number of true positives}}{\text{Number of true positives} + \text{number of false negatives}}$$

Sepsis

Acute systemic inflammatory response that forms an organism's reaction to an infection. Often life-threatening, high risk of hematogenous spread to endoprosthetic implants, especially with *S aureus*.

Sequestrum

Infected, necrotic bone fragment that no longer has a stable connection to vital bone.

Single-shot

Single antibiotic dosage administered as a prophylaxis prior to surgical procedures.

SIRS

Systemic inflammatory response syndrome. This is referred to as sepsis if it is caused by an infection. In addition to a detected or presumed focus of infection, at least two of the following criteria must be met to confirm a diagnosis of sepsis:

- Body temperature > 38°C or < 36°C
- Heart rate > 90 beats/min (tachycardia)
- Tachypnoea: breathing rate > 20 breaths/min or hyperventilation with pCO_2 < 32 mm Hg
- Leukocytosis (> 12,000 cells/µL) or leukopenia (< 4,000 cells/µL) or left shift (ie, > 10% immature leukocytes in the differential blood count)

Small-colony variants (SCV)

Bacterial populations (usually *Staphylococcus aureus*) that form small colonies due to their slow growth. These occur during prolonged exposure to antibiotics and cause chronic and recurrent infections. They are highly resistant to antibiotics not showing a reliable in vitro/in vivo correlation.

Sonication
Procedure for detecting bacterial colonies fixed in the biofilm on explants. The biofilm is removed from foreign bodies using ultrasound. The bacteria are released and can then be cultivated in the appropriate media.

Specificity
Likelihood of a test to detect a true negative value with a negative test result.

$$P\ (\text{negative result} \mid \text{true negative}) = \frac{\text{Number of true negatives}}{\text{Number of true negatives} + \text{number of false positives}}$$

Spondylitis
Bacterial or abacterial inflammation of one or more vertebrae.

Spondylodiscitis
Bacterial or abacterial inflammation of one or more intervertebral disc spaces and the adjacent vertebrae. It is virtually always attributable to spondylitis in adults.

Therapy with antibiotics
We differentiate between prophylactic (preventive) preemptive, empiric and targeted therapy.

Index

Page numbers in *italics* refer to figures and/or tables

E

F

G

H

M

N

O

P

R

S

T

U

V

W

X

Z